Physical Therapy Research

2ND EDITION

Physical Therapy Research

PRINCIPLES AND APPLICATIONS

Elizabeth Domholdt, PT, EdD

Professor and Dean, Krannert School of Physical Therapy
University of Indianapolis
Indianapolis, Indiana

W.B. SAUNDERS COMPANY
An Imprint of Elsevier Science
Philadelphia   London   New York   St. Louis   Sydney   Toronto

W.B. SAUNDERS COMPANY
An Imprint of Elsevier Science

The Curtis Center
Independence Square West
Philadelphia, Pennsylvania 19106

Library of Congress Cataloging-in-Publication Data

Domholdt, Elizabeth
   Physical therapy research : principles and applications / Elizabeth Domholdt.—2nd ed.

   p. ; cm.

   Includes bibliographical references and index.

   ISBN 0–7216–6963–8

   1. Physical therapy—Research.   I. Title.
   [DNLM: 1. Physical Therapy.   2. Research.   WB 25 D668p 2000]

   RM708 .D66 2000
   615.8'2'072—dc21   99–047086

Editor: Andrew Allen
Designer: Nicholas Rook
Production Manager: Frank Polizzano
Manuscript Editor: Tina Rebane
Illustration Coordinator: Lisa Lambert
Indexing Supervisor: Angela Holt
Cover Designer: Nicholas Rook

PHYSICAL THERAPY RESEARCH: PRINCIPLES AND APPLICATIONS   ISBN 0–7216–6963–8

Printed in the United States of America.

Last digit is the print number: 9   8   7   6   5   4   3

Foreword

Domholdt's *Physical Therapy Research,* 2nd edition, arrives as physical therapy faces the dawn of a new and challenging millennium. The landscape of research in physical therapy is changing radically as calls for "evidence-based practice in physical therapy" are heard all around us. Clinicians are under increasing pressure to keep up-to-date and to base their practice more firmly on "evidence." In the face of growing external threats, many clinicians are calling for research that will "prove" (tomorrow, if possible) that what we do "works"! Researchers, in response to increasing demands for evidence on the effectiveness of physical therapy services, are aggressively pursuing clinical outcomes research. Academic faculties are being asked to develop a cadre of future physical therapists who can draw on the growing body of scientific evidence to manage patients and to train tomorrow's researchers to conduct high-quality, clinically relevant research. Physical therapy research methods and skills need to match contemporary needs of the profession.

In Chapter 1, Domholdt posits that research is the creative process by which professionals systematically challenge their everyday practices. The challenge is to choose the right methods to match the research questions that need to be addressed. When I was first introduced to research in physical therapy as a student some 26 years ago, the message was clear: the road to valid research in physical therapy led through experimental research methods. Anything less was "soft science" or, at best, inadequate. Domholdt's second edition of *Physical Therapy Research* attests to how far the profession's thinking about research has evolved over the past 26 years. In addition to traditional research methods covered in her first edition, this second edition provides the reader with a vastly expanded discussion of nonexperimental research techniques essential to responding to the calls for relevant data on clinical outcomes and effectiveness of specific physical therapy services, the foundation for evidence-based practice. This second edition introduces the reader to the importance of methods for developing scientific case reports, qualitative research methods, epidemiologic principles and tools, outcomes and survey research methods, and the application of each to physical therapy practice. Expanded sections on data analysis provide the reader with an introduction to statistical tools appropriate to nonexperimental as well as experimental research designs. As such, this second edition provides the consumer and student researcher with an important foundation for the development and use of research to meet these demands for evidence-based practice in physical therapy.

Throughout my review of Domholdt's work, I was reminded of an equation set forth by Shaughnessey and colleagues (1994), which states that the usefulness of any source of information is equal to its relevance, multiplied by its validity, divided by the work required to extract the information. Readers of the second edition of *Physical Therapy Research* will find this work achieves high relevance, high validity, and low work required to extract the critical information needed by consumers and producers of research alike. It will become a highly valued resource for those who seek a thorough introduction to research methods needed for contemporary physical therapy research.

Alan M. Jette
Boston University

REFERENCE

Shaughnessy AF, Slawson DC, Bennett JH: Becoming an information master: a guidebook to the medical information jungle. *J Fam Pract.* 1994;39:489–499.

Preface

Physical therapists share a deeply held belief that the exercise of our professional expertise, in partnership with the patients or clients with whom we work, makes a difference in their lives. This deeply held belief is a positive force when it leads to the high levels of professionalism and commitment that are demonstrated by therapists around the globe on a daily basis. This belief, however, can also serve as a negative force when it leads practitioners to the uncritical acceptance of all of physical therapy practice.

The purpose of research, then, is not to justify what we do. Rather, research is needed to determine which of the many things we do as physical therapists can be justified. This is an important distinction. The former leads to a search for weak evidence that supports our current practices; the latter leads to a search for strong evidence that can help us change and improve our practices on the basis of the evidence.

Evidence-based practice in physical therapy can be realized only by a joint effort of the producers and consumers of research. This is a textbook that will serve most of the needs of research consumers and can serve many of the foundational needs of research producers. It does so by using straightforward language and relevant examples to capture the diversity and complexity of research that is of interest to physical therapists. In addition, consumers and producers of research who require more detail on a given topic will find that each chapter is well-referenced with a mix of contemporary and classic citations.

The text is divided into two parts: principles and applications. The first 24 chapters present the principles of research that both consumers and producers of research need to know. The final four chapters are designed to help consumers and producers of research apply these principles as they evaluate the literature and design and implement projects.

The first edition of this text provided a solid grounding in traditional research design and analysis, as well as an introduction to emerging research topics such as qualitative and single-system designs. This second edition maintains the solid grounding in traditional research topics and provides expanded coverage of a number of traditional and emerging topics of importance to physical therapy research: outcomes research, epidemiology, qualitative design, single-system design, case reports, and survey research. The data analysis components of the text have been upgraded accordingly to include the statistical tools used with these research approaches. Effect size, power analysis, sensitivity, specificity, receiver–operator curves, odds ratios, survival analysis, and logistic regression are some of the new topics that have been added throughout the text.

Successful completion of this edition required the assistance of many individuals. The Vice-President and Provost at the University of Indianapolis, Lynn Youngblood, EdD, has always supported my desire to remain an active scholar while fulfilling my administrative and teaching duties for the University. During the 1998–99 academic year he tolerated my benign neglect of some administrative duties in favor of completing this revision. The faculty and staff of the Krannert School of Physical Therapy carried on just fine despite the many days that I blocked out to work on "the book," and everybody kept their eye-rolling to a minimum when hearing of yet another milestone or roadblock on the way to the completion of this edition!

Carol Baker, PT, a colleague and friend, was instrumental in getting the revision done within the twentieth century. She worked on almost every chapter by identifying new references and providing substantive and editorial feedback to the revisions. She deserves special recognition for her assistance in reorganizing and updating the over 200 references on measurement tools in Chapter 19. Christine Guyonneau, MLS, reference librarian at the University of Indianapolis, once again provided valuable feedback to the chapter on locating the literature—an area that has undergone and is continuing to undergo rapid change. Ted Worrell, EdD, PT, SCS, FACSM, a University of Indianapolis colleague who recently joined the Duke University faculty, provided feedback to the epidemiology and outcomes chapters. Jan Gwyer, PhD, PT, a colleague from Duke University, provided input into new areas that should be included in this edition. Denise Wass, MS, PT, and Reneé Van Veld Khalid, MS, PT, former students and now colleagues, provided, respectively, proofreading and photocopying services, and input into the revision of the glossary.

Finally, I have to thank my husband of 16 years, Gary Shoemaker, for all he brings to my life. He's a steady guy with an understated sense of humor that grabs you when you least expect it. During the year of serious work on this revision, his ability to make me look up from the computer screen to laugh at his day, at the news, at the dogs, and even at myself, has been a life-saver!

Elizabeth Domholdt
Indianapolis, Indiana

Contents

SECTION 1 **Research Fundamentals**

1 **Research in Physical Therapy** **3**
Definitions of Research 4
Reasons for Developing Research in Physical Therapy 7
Barriers to Research in Physical Therapy 9
History of Research in Physical Therapy 11
Summary 13

2 **Theory in Physical Therapy Research** **15**
Definitions of Theory 15
Scope of Theory 19
Relationship Between Theory, Research, and Practice 25
Summary 26

3 **Research Ethics** **27**
Boundaries Between Practice and Research 28
Moral Principles of Action 29
Informed Consent 31
Research Codes of Ethics 32
Research Risks 35
Summary 36

SECTION 2 **Research Design**

4 **Research Problems, Questions, and Hypotheses** **41**
Developing Answerable Research Problems 41
Criteria for Evaluating Research Problems 46
Summary 48

5 **Research Paradigms** **49**
Quantitative Paradigm 50
Qualitative Paradigm 54

Single-System Paradigm 58
Relationships Among the Research Paradigms 59
Summary 60

6 Design Overview 62
Identification of Variables 63
Design Dimensions 67
Control 71
Summary 76

7 Research Validity 77
Internal Validity 78
Construct Validity 88
External Validity 91
Relationship Among Types of Validity 93
Summary 94

8 Selection and Assignment of Subjects 95
Significance of Sampling and Assignment 95
Populations and Samples 96
Probability Sampling 97
Nonprobability Sampling 103
Assignment To Groups 105
Sample Size 109
Summary 110

SECTION 3 Experimental Designs

9 Group Designs 115
Single-Factor Experimental Designs 115
Multiple-Factor Experimental Designs 118
Summary 123

10 Single-System Design 125
Problems With Group Designs 125
Characteristics of Single-System Designs 126
Single-System Designs 127
Limitations of Single-System Designs 132
Summary 132

SECTION 4   **Nonexperimental Designs**

11   **Overview of Nonexperimental Research**   **137**
Description   138
Analysis of Relationships   142
Analysis of Differences   144
Summary   146

12   **Clinical Case Reports**   **148**
Contributions of Case Reports to Theory and Practice   149
Purposes of Case Reports   150
Format of Case Reports   152
Summary   153

13   **Qualitative Research**   **154**
Assumptions of the Qualitative Paradigm   154
Qualitative Designs   155
Qualitative Methods   159
Summary   168

14   **Epidemiology**   **170**
Ratios, Proportions, and Rates   171
Screening and Diagnosis   180
Nonexperimental Epidemiological Designs   184
Summary   187

15   **Outcomes Research**   **189**
Purpose of Outcomes Research   190
Frameworks for Outcomes Research   191
Measurement Tools for Outcomes Research   193
Design Issues for Outcomes Research   196
Summary   201

16   **Survey Research**   **204**
Scope of Survey Research   204
Types of Information   206
Types of Items   206
Implementation Overview   207
Mailed Questionnaires   208
Interviews   215
Summary   217

SECTION 5   **Measurement**

17   Measurement Theory   221

Definitions of Measurement   222
Scales of Measurement   222
Types of Variables   225
Statistical Foundations of Measurement Theory   225
Measurement Frameworks   230
Measurement Reliability   231
Measurement Validity   235
Summary   237

18   Methodological Research   239

Reliability Designs   239
Validity Designs   244
Summary   247

19   Measurement Tools for Physical Therapy Research   248

Anthropometric Characteristics   249
Arousal, Mentation, and Cognition   251
Community and Work Integration, Self-Care, and
    Home Management   252
Gait, Locomotion, and Balance   254
Integumentary Integrity   257
Muscle Performance   257
Neuromotor Development and Sensory Integration   261
Pain   261
Range of Motion and Joint Integrity and Mobility   262
Sensory Integrity   265
Ventilation, Respiration, Circulation, Aerobic Capacity,
    and Endurance   265
Summary   267

SECTION 6   **Data Analysis**

20   Statistical Reasoning   277

Data Set   278
Frequency Distribution   278
Central Tendency   283
Variability   284
Normal Distribution   287
Sampling Distribution   289

Significant Difference   291
Errors   295
Power   297
Statistical Conclusion Validity   297
Summary   299

21   Statistical Analysis of Differences: The Basics   300
Distributions for Analysis of Differences   301
Assumptions of Tests of Differences   302
Steps in the Statistical Testing of Differences   304
Statistical Analysis of Differences   304
Summary   323

22   Statistical Analysis of Differences: Advanced and Special Techniques   325
Advanced ANOVA Techniques   326
Analysis of Single-System Designs   336
Survival Analysis   340
Hypothesis Testing with Confidence Intervals   341
Power Analysis and Effect Size   344
Summary   345

23   Statistical Analysis of Relationships: The Basics   347
Correlation   348
Linear Regression   356
Summary   358

24   Statistical Analysis of Relationships: Advanced and Special Techniques   360
Reliability Analysis   360
Multiple Regression   367
Logistic Regression   370
Factor Analysis   372
Summary   376

SECTION 7   Being a Consumer

25   Locating the Literature   379
Types of Information   380
Types of Professional Literature   380
Focused Literature Search   380
Ongoing Literature Search   389
Obtaining Literature Items   391
Summary   392

26   Evaluating the Literature   394
Elements of a Research Article   395
Guidelines for Writing About Published Research   395
Evaluation of Single Studies   395
Evaluation of Review Articles   403
Conducting a Conceptual Review of the Literature   405
Summary   408

SECTION 8   Implementing Research

27   Implementing a Research Project   413
Proposal Preparation   414
Human Participants' Protection   418
Funding   420
Obtaining Participants   426
Data Collection   428
Data Analysis   433
Summary   435

28   Publishing and Presenting Research   436
Publication of Research   436
Presentation of Research   441
Summary   444

APPENDIXES

A   Random Numbers Table   447

B   Table: Areas in One Tail of the Standard Normal Curve   453

C   Questions for Evaluating a Research Article   455

D   Guidelines for Preparing a Journal Article Manuscript   459

E   Sample Manuscript for Hypothetical Study   465

F   Sample Platform Presentation Script with Slides   491

GLOSSARY   501

INDEX   513

Research Fundamentals

Research in Physical Therapy

Definitions of Research
    Research Challenges the Status Quo
    Research Is Creative
    Research Is Systematic

Reasons for Developing Research in Physical Therapy
    Body of Knowledge
    Efficacy of Physical Therapy
    Improvements in Patient Care

Barriers to Research in Physical Therapy
    Lack of Familiarity with the Research Process

Lack of Statistical Support for Research
Lack of Funds for Research
Lack of Time
Ethical Concerns About Use of Human and Animal Subjects
Overcoming Barriers

History of Research in Physical Therapy

Research in physical therapy is the process by which we determine whether what we do as physical therapists makes a difference in the lives of the people we serve. In the rapidly changing and increasingly accountable world of health care it is no longer enough to say that we do good work; it is no longer enough to casually note that patients feel better after our treatments. Rather, physical therapists must be willing to both *search* for evidence about the effectiveness of our practices and then *modify* our practices in response to the evidence that is found. Physical therapists who accept this challenge of evidence-based practice also accept another challenge: that of learning about research in physical therapy. A working knowledge of research design and analysis is a prerequisite to evaluating existing evidence and producing new evidence.

This book provides physical therapists with a framework for understanding and applying the systematic processes of research. As with other fields of study, research is ever-changing and a text can only represent research thought at a particular point in time. This text does, however, present both traditional research methods as well as emerging approaches. Just as physical therapists involved with research must challenge their beliefs about physical therapy, researchers must be willing to challenge their ideas about research.

Learning about research in physical therapy can be challenging. First, it involves developing a diverse set of knowledge and skills in research design, statistical analysis, and writing. At the same time these new skills are being mastered, the status quo is being challenged by questioning the conventional wisdom of the profession. The combination of trying to learn new material while simultaneously challenging previously held beliefs can engender frustration with the new material and doubt about one's previous learning. Some physical therapists are unable to cope with such uncertainty and retreat to anecdotes and intuition as the basis for their work in physical therapy. Others delight in the intellectual challenge of research and commit themselves to developing an evidence-based practice. Such therapists balance the use of existing but unsubstantiated practices with critical evaluation of those same practices through regular review of the professional literature and thoughtful discussion with colleagues. In addition, these therapists may participate in clinical research that tests the assumptions under which they practice.

This introductory chapter defines research, examines reasons for and barriers to implementing physical therapy research, and puts physical therapy research into a historical context. Based on this foundation, the rest of the book presents the *principles* needed to understand research and suggests guidelines for the *application* of those principles for interpretation and implementation of research.

■ DEFINITIONS OF RESEARCH

Research has been defined by almost every person who has written about it. Charles Franklin Kettering, engineer and philanthropist, had this to say:

> "Research" is a high-hat word that scares a lot of people. It needn't; . . . it is nothing but a state of mind—a friendly, welcoming attitude toward change. . . . It is the problem-solving mind as contrasted with the let-well-enough-alone mind. It is the composer mind instead of the fiddler mind. It is the "tomorrow" mind instead of the "yesterday" mind.[1(p91)]

Otto Payton, a physical therapist who has written widely about physical therapy research, indicates that "research should begin with an intellectual itch that needs scratching." [2(p8)] Leslie Portney and Mary Watkins,[3] and Denise Polit and Bernadette Hungler,[4] who have written texts on research in physical therapy and nursing, all emphasize the organized, systematic nature of research. Three important characteristics about research emerge from these different views: first, research challenges the status quo; second, it is creative; and third, it is systematic.

Research Challenges the Status Quo

The first characteristic is that research challenges the status quo. Sometimes the results of research may support current clinical practices; other times the results point to areas of treatment that are not effective when put to a systematic test. But whether research does or does not lead to a revision of currently accepted principles, the guiding philosophy of research is one of challenge. Is this treatment effective? Is it more effective than another treatment? Would this person recover as quickly without physical therapy? Is physical therapy management superior to pharmacological or surgical management for a given condition? The status quo can be challenged in several ways; three examples follow.

One way of challenging the status quo is to identify gaps in our knowledge that represent common practices not substantiated by scientific evidence. Because much of our practice as physical therapists is based on the collective wisdom of past professionals, we forget that much of this practice has not been verified in a systematic way. This situation is not unique to physical therapy. In 1987 a shortened form of the report of the Quebec Task Force on Spinal Disorders was published in the journal *Spine* as a monograph for clinicians.[5] Among other things, this task force evaluated the clinical literature related to care of activity-related spinal disorders and identified which of a variety of treatments were supported by evidence within the literature. Figure 1–1 shows a modified version of a segment of one of the figures produced within the monograph. The unshaded areas of the figure represent treatments—including common practices of physical therapists and physicians—that lack scientific evidence for their effectiveness, in the judgment of the task force. The dark-shaded areas represent treatments that the task force judged to be contraindicated on the basis of scientific evidence. The remaining light-shaded boxes highlight those few treatments for which the task force found scientific evidence. Thus, very little scientific support was found for many common treatments for activity-related spinal disorders.

A second approach to challenging the status quo is to systematically test the effects of common practices. Delitto and colleagues[6] did this when they designed a randomized clinical trial to determine whether patients with a certain pattern of low back signs and symptoms benefited more from a treatment approach designed to match their signs and symptoms than they did from a general, unmatched treatment. The patients within their study all had signs and symptoms that would lead many therapists to adopt a treatment approach combining sacroiliac joint mobilization, extension exercises, and avoidance of flexed postures. Their challenge to the status quo could be restated as follows:

THERAPEUTIC MODALITY	Acute low back pain	Chronic low back pain
Bed rest for < 2 days to promote rest		
Orthosis to promote rest		
Systemic medication to diminish spasm		
Thermotherapy to reduce pain		
Cryotherapy to reduce inflammation		
Mobilization/manipulation to increase range of motion		
Massage to diminish spasm		
Electroanalgesia to diminish pain		
Strengthening exercises to increase strength		
Stretching exercises to increase range of motion		
Home exercises to increase endurance		
Postural information to increase function		
Functional training to increase function		
Surgery to alter joint tissue		
Chemonucleolysis to alter joint tissue		

FIGURE 1–1. Partial summary of evidence compiled by the Quebec Task Force on Spinal Disorders on the effectiveness of therapeutic modalities in the treatment of acute and chronic low back pain without radiating symptoms. The dark shading indicates that the treatment is contraindicated on the basis of scientific evidence; the light shading indicates that the usefulness of the treatment has been demonstrated by either randomized or nonrandomized controlled trials, and no shading indicates that there is no scientific evidence to support the treatment.
Modified from Quebec Task Force on Spinal Disorders. Scientific approach to the assessment and management of activity-related spinal disorders: treatment of activity-related spinal disorders. *Spine*. 1987;12(suppl):S22–S30.

Therapists classify patients with low back pain according to signs and symptoms and differentiate their treatments on the basis of these classifications. However, there is really no evidence to show that a specific match between classification and treatment leads to better results than offering nonspecific treatments. Therefore, let's see if patients who receive a treatment that is matched to their classification really have better outcomes than those who receive nonspecific treatment.

Patients with low back syndrome who fit an extension-mobilization category (their symptoms improved with extension movement tests, worsened with flexion movement tests, and they had signs of sacroiliac regional pain) were treated with either a matched mobilization and extension routine or with an unmatched program of flexion exercises. They found that the patients in the matched group improved faster than the unmatched group, as measured by scores on a standardized functional outcome test. Thus, this challenge to a common set of clinical procedures yielded support for those procedures.

A third way of challenging the status quo is to test novel or traditionally avoided treatments. A long-held and only recently challenged assumption of physical therapists is that traditional resistive muscle strengthening is inappropriate for individuals with central nervous system pathology. Damiano and colleagues[7] challenged this in their study of quadriceps femoris muscle strengthening in children with spastic diplegic cerebral palsy. They found that the children demonstrated increased quadriceps femoris muscle force, no concurrent increase in hamstring muscle force, and decreased knee flexion at heel-strike after a 6-week quadriceps femoris muscle strength training program. Thus, the results of their challenge to this commonly held belief suggest that therapists should reexamine these beliefs as well as the treatment implications that flow from these beliefs.

Thus, these three challenges to the status quo identified gaps in the knowledge of physical therapy practice, provided support for one set of clinical practices, and suggested a need for review of another set of clinical beliefs. Research is about these kinds of challenges, presumably with the hope that what we currently do will be supported, but with the willingness to add to our research base or change our practice when support for what we do as physical therapists is lacking.

Research Is Creative

The second characteristic of research is that it is creative. Rothstein believes that many physical therapists are quick to accept an authoritarian view of physical therapy: "Our teachers and our texts tell us how it should be, and we accept this in our eagerness to proceed with patient care."[8(p895)] Researchers are creative individuals who move past the authoritarian teachings of others and look at physical therapy in a different way.

For example, most physical therapists who work with patients who have had strokes or amputations strive for their patients to exhibit as symmetric a gait pattern as possible. Winter, a biomechanist, was creative enough to ask whether a symmetric gait is the most efficient gait for an individual with unilateral dysfunction:

> At the outset, the author would be cautious about gait retraining protocols which are aimed at improved symmetry based on nothing more than an idea that it would automatically be an improvement. It is safe to say that any human system with major structural asymmetries in the neuromuscular skeletal system cannot be optimal when the gait is symmetrical.[9(p362)]

Researchers thrive on the creative intellectual processes that lead to the development of new ways of conceptualizing their disciplines. Creative aspects of physical therapy research are emphasized in Chapter 2, which presents information about the use of theory in physical therapy, and Chapter 4, which provides a framework for the development of research problems.

Research Is Systematic

The third characteristic of research is that it is systematic. In contrast, much of our clinical knowledge is anecdotal, or is passed on through "ecclesiastical succession" [10(p3)] from prominent therapists who teach a particular treatment to eager colleagues or students. Anecdotal claims for the effectiveness of treatments are colored by the relationship between the physical therapist and patient and do not control for factors, other than the treatment, that may account for changes in the condition of the patient. The systematic nature of research attempts to isolate treatment effects from other influences that are not ordinarily controlled in the clinic setting. Much of this text is devoted to presenting the systematic principles that underlie research methods: Sections 2–4 (Chapters 4 through 16) cover research design, Section 5 (Chapters 17 to 19) discusses measurement in physical therapy, and Section 6 (Chapters 20 through 24) introduces data analysis.

■ REASONS FOR DEVELOPING RESEARCH IN PHYSICAL THERAPY

There are at least three reasons for doing physical therapy research: (1) to establish a body of knowledge for physical therapy, (2) to determine the efficacy of physical therapy treatments, and (3) to improve patient care in physical therapy. Each of these reasons is examined in the sections that follow.

Body of Knowledge

The body of knowledge rationale for physical therapy research is related to the concept of a profession. The characteristics of a profession have been described by many authors, but include several common elements. Houle divided the characteristics of a profession into three broad groups: conceptual, performance, and collective identity characteristics (Table 1–1).[11] One of the critical performance characteristics is mastery of the theoretical knowledge that forms the basis for the profession.

Physical therapists have been accused of being beggars and borrowers of information from anatomy, physiology, kinesiology, psychology, and physical education, rather than being creators of our own body of knowledge:

> Physical therapy has a soft underbelly because its science is in disarray. This disarray leaves it open to attacks against its inadequacies—attacks from medicine, attacks from government, challenges from fiscal agencies, and questions from the consuming public.[12(p1070)]

Hislop, who delivered this quote in her 1975 Mary McMillan Lecture (a prestigious lectureship offered annually by the American Physical Ther-

TABLE 1–1	Characteristics of a Profession*

Conceptual Characteristic
....
Establishment of a central mission

Performance Characteristics
....
Mastery of theoretical knowledge
Capacity to solve problems
Use of practical knowledge
Self-enhancement

Collective Identity Characteristics
....
Formal training
Credentialing
Creation of a subculture
Legal reinforcement
Public acceptance
Ethical practice
Penalties
Relations to other vocations
Relations to users of service

*List developed from Houle CO. *Continuing Learning in the Professions*. San Francisco, Calif: Jossey-Bass Publishers; 1981.

apy Association), proposed that *pathokinesiology*, the science of abnormal movement, should be the "distinguishing clinical science of physical therapy."[12(p1071)] An alternate view is that physical therapy is no different from other applied professions that borrow knowledge from the basic arts and sciences. This view is advanced by Carr and associates,[13] who believe that the multidisciplinary body of knowledge they refer to as *movement science* (a far broader concept than pathokinesiology or movement dysfunction) can be applied to form a foundation for physical therapy practice. It is through research that we can systematically develop a body of knowledge about physical therapy—irrespective of whether we believe this body of knowledge to be pathokinesiology, movement science, or some other amalgamation of the basic sciences applied to those with functional limitations.

Efficacy of Physical Therapy

The second major rationale for performing research in physical therapy relates to determining the efficacy of physical therapy treatments. When discussing this reason for doing research, physical therapists must be careful not to fall into an all-too-common line of reasoning identified by Hayes:

> Too often I hear physical therapists say that we need to do research to demonstrate that what we do works. This logic concerns me, because it is not the right attitude to carry into clinical research. We must study *whether* what we do works.[14(p12)]

A controversial report on the treatment of acute low back pain was issued by the Agency for Health Care Policy Research (AHCPR) of the US Public Health Service.[15] Similar in intent and scope to the Quebec Task Force referred to earlier in this chapter,[5] the AHCPR panel identified a variety of treatments for low back pain as either "recommended," "optional," or "not recommended" on the basis of research-based evidence. Of those treatments that are within the

scope of physical therapy practice, only patient education, spinal manipulation in certain circumstances, and conditioning exercises for trunk muscles were recommended. Treatments that were not recommended because of lack of evidence of effectiveness included physical agents administered by a health care practitioner, exercise with back-specific exercise machines, and exercises to stretch back muscles.

Physical therapists are understandably concerned that these guidelines will be used by insurers to deny coverage for the types of care that were not recommended by the panel. In a balanced critique of the guideline, Connolly concludes that "if the *Guideline* provides the spark to set research priorities, expand knowledge, and provoke clinicians to think critically and judiciously when selecting assessment and treatment methods for acute low back problems, it will play a major role in solving a major societal problem."[16(p97)] Reports such as those issued by the Quebec Task Force and the AHCPR make it clear that physical therapists have much work to do in determining whether what we do works.

Improvements in Patient Care

The third reason for research in physical therapy is perhaps the most important one, that of improving patient care. Research can improve care by helping clinicians make good decisions about the use of existing practices or by providing a systematic evaluation of the efficacy of new practices.

When we know what has or has not been supported by research we can make intelligent, evidence-based decisions about which clinical procedures to use with our clients. Within medicine, rates of surgeries such as hysterectomy, prostatectomy, and tonsillectomy vary widely from community to community.[17] This variation is thought, in part, to result from "conflicting information about whether a particular procedure will improve a patient's health or the quality of his life." [17(p126)] Clinical research about these procedures could provide additional evidence that would help physicians make informed decisions about recommending the procedures.

A group of Canadian practitioners recently hoped to determine whether there was enough scientific evidence to guide the selection of treatments for patients with lateral epicondylitis.[18] Studies that were reviewed included investigations of medical treatments such as oral nonsteroidal antiinflammatory drugs and steroid injections as well as treatments within the scope of physical therapy such as ultrasound, phonophoresis, iontophoresis, and friction massage. They concluded that "the poor quality and contradictory results of the randomised and controlled trials reported so far in the literature means that there is not enough *scientific* evidence to favour any particular type of treatment of acute lateral epicondylitis." [18(p650)] Clearly, research is needed to provide the evidence that is sought by health care practitioners who hope to conduct an evidence-based practice.

In addition to helping clinicians make judgments about the use of existing treatments, research can be used to test new procedures so that clinicians can make evidence-based decisions about whether to add them to their clinical arsenal. Harness-supported treadmill ambulation is one new treatment in need of such testing. In theory, harness-supported treadmill ambulation should enable patients to improve their ambulation function by training in a way that ensures safety, does not require hand-held assistive devices, uses relatively normal gait patterns, and has reduced energy demands when compared to unsupported walking. Hunter and colleagues published a study that evaluated one component (energy expenditure) of harness-supported treadmill ambulation for patients with transtibial amputation.[19] Therapists with a good knowledge base in research will be able to critique this article to determine whether they believe the results can be applied to the clinical situations in which they might

like to use harness-supported treadmill ambulation. Chapter 26 presents guidelines for evaluating research literature.

■ BARRIERS TO RESEARCH IN PHYSICAL THERAPY

Although most physical therapists recognize the importance of research, many obstacles to physical therapy research have been documented. Figure 1–2 shows the obstacles that were identified by more than 50% of the respondents in a 1980 study of California physical therapists.[20] These obstacles include lack of familiarity with research methodology, lack of statistical support, lack of funding, and lack of time. A 1990 study of occupational therapists documented similar barriers to research in this closely related rehabilitation profession.[21] An additional obstacle that has been identified relates to concerns for ethical use of animals or humans in research activities.

Lack of Familiarity with the Research Process

Research in physical therapy is sometimes viewed as a mysterious process that occupies the time of an elite group of physical therapists who do not deliver patient care and who may develop projects of little relevance to clinicians. The *PT Magazine* portrait of a day in the life of one physical therapy researcher presents a challenge to the "ivory tower" view of research by presenting a view of one researcher who is very much connected to the clinic and very committed to working with clinicians to develop research that helps them answer their questions.[22] Even when physical therapy research is grounded in clinical problems, the language of research and data analysis is still specialized, and those who have not acquired the vocabulary are understandably intimidated when it is spoken.

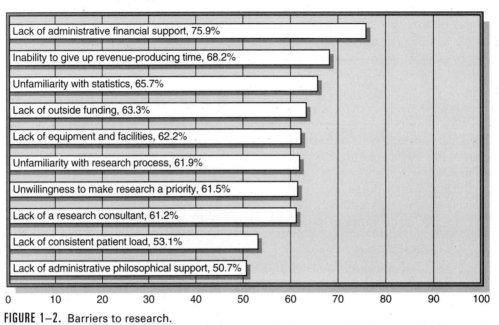

FIGURE 1–2. Barriers to research.
Compiled from data presented in Ballin AJ, Breslin WH, Wierenga KAS, Shepard KF. Research in physical therapy: philosophy, barriers to involvement, and use among California physical therapists. *Phys Ther.* 1980;60:888–895.

The goal of this book is to demystify the research process by clearly articulating the knowledge base needed to understand it.

Lack of Statistical Support for Research

The second major barrier to research is lack of statistical support. Section 6 (Chapters 20 to 24) of this book provides the reader with the conceptual background needed to understand most of the statistics reported in the physical therapy research literature.[23] A conceptual background does not, however, provide an adequate theoretical and mathematical basis for selection and computation of a given statistic on a particular occasion. Thus, most researchers will require the services of a statistician at some point in the research process. Guidelines for working with statisticians are provided in Chapter 27.

Lack of Funds for Research

A third barrier to research is lack of funding. Since research is not a revenue-producing activity like patient care or teaching, administrators find it difficult to provide clinicians or faculty members with the time needed to implement studies. In addition, research has many direct costs: equipment, computer time, statistical and engineering consultants, clerical time, production and travel for presentation of the research at conferences, and figure and photographic production for publication of the research. Funding sources for physical therapy research are discussed in Chapter 27.

Lack of Time

A fourth barrier to research in physical therapy is lack of time. Tasks with firm deadlines are given higher priority than research, which usually only has those deadlines that are self-imposed by researchers or specified by funding agencies. The immediate time pressures placed on physical therapy clinicians and academicians may lead to postponement or abandonment of research ideas. One solution to this problem is to design studies that are relatively easy to integrate into the daily routine of a physical therapy practice. Chapters 10, 12, and 15 present a variety of research designs particularly suitable for implementation in a clinical setting.

Ethical Concerns About Use of Human and Animal Subjects

The fifth barrier to research implementation is ethical concerns related to the use of either animals or humans as research subjects. Physical therapists who choose to study animal models should follow appropriate guidelines for the use, care, and humane destruction of animal subjects. Physical therapists who use human subjects in their research must pay close attention to balancing the risks of the research with potential benefits from the results. Chapter 3 examines ethical considerations in detail; Chapter 27 provides guidelines for working with the committees that oversee researchers to ensure that they protect the rights of research subjects.

Overcoming Barriers

Overcoming these barriers depends on leaders who are willing to commit time and money to research efforts and individuals who are willing to devote time and effort to improving their research knowledge and skills. Research is, however, rarely an individual effort. Therefore, one key to overcoming barriers to research is to develop productive research teams composed of individuals who, together, have all the diverse skills needed to plan, implement, analyze, and report research.

■ HISTORY OF RESEARCH IN PHYSICAL THERAPY

In 1960 Catherine Worthingham, a leader in physical therapy, called for physical therapists to give attention to developing the body of knowledge of physical therapy through research.[24] Eight years later Eugene Michels, a well-known physical therapy researcher, noted that the profession was in crucial need of more and better clinical research.[25] In 1975 Helen Hislop, in her prestigious Mary McMillan Lecture, spoke of one of the reasons that the clinical science of physical therapy is developing slowly:

> After fifty years, the science of physical therapy is entering its infancy. A great difficulty in developing the clinical science of physical therapy is that we treat individual persons, each of whom is made up of situations which are unique and, therefore, appear incompatible with the generalizations demanded by science.[12(p1076)]

In 1989 Rothstein, a physical therapist and editor of *Physical Therapy,* challenged physical therapists with the fact that we still know so little about the core techniques of the profession:

> Although we have begun to develop a body of research literature in physical therapy, we still lack a body of clinical literature. . . . We have no collective body of knowledge about how long it takes for even our simplest treatments to have a beneficial effect on some of the most straightforward conditions.[26(p796)]

And in 1995 Robertson reviewed 40 years of *Physical Therapy* citations in three thematic areas (knee, back, and electrical stimulation) to determine the extent of cohesion within the knowledge base related to these areas.[27] She found that "meager cumulation has occurred in the three thematic-based samples of physical therapy literature examined. Few articles in all three thematic areas cited papers from the same area, or even articles from the physical therapy literature. That is, few articles apparently used or extended existing findings published within the relevant areas of the literature of the discipline."[27(p227)]

These statements made over the past 4 decades might lead one to believe that no progress has been made in articulating and testing the body of knowledge of physical therapy. This is deceptive because part of the character of research is that when one question is answered, several more spring up in need of attention. Thus, the profession's appetite for research should be insatiable and apparently is, as indicated by the consistent cry for more research. As formidable as the barriers noted earlier are, and as true as the statements from the last 4 decades are, there is much to be proud of in the development of physical therapy research over the last 4 decades.

The history of research in physical therapy can be traced by examination of professional association goals, educational standards, development of publication vehicles for research reports, and support for research funding in the discipline. The object of the American Women's Physical Therapeutic Association (now the American Physical Therapy Association [APTA]), as defined in its first constitution of 1921 was "to establish and maintain a professional and scientific standard for those engaged in the profession . . . to disseminate information by the distribution of medical literature and articles of professional interest."[28(p5)] Today, one of the objects of the APTA is to "improve the art and science of physical therapy including practice, education, and research."[29(p907)] A portion of the mission statement for the Canadian Physiotherapy Association is to "foster excellence in education, practice, and research."[30]

As educational programs for physical therapists developed, the profession began to establish its own criteria for such educational programs. In 1974 the APTA House of Delegates adopted accreditation criteria for physical therapist education programs that required both that faculty be involved in scholarly pursuits and that students be able to use research principles to critically analyze research findings.[31] Current ac-

creditation criteria maintain the expectation that students be able to critically evaluate the literature and have added the expectation that students participate in scholarly activities.[32] The relatively recent development of Doctor of Philosophy (PhD) programs in physical therapy also points to the increased legitimacy of research in physical therapy.[33]

Scholarly publications in physical therapy have mirrored the increasing interest in research in physical therapy. The Chartered Society of Physiotherapists in Great Britain published its first volume of *Physiotherapy* in 1915. *Physical Therapy,* the journal of the APTA, was first published in 1921 as the *PT Review.* The 1980s saw the rise of various specialty journals in physical therapy, following the lead that medicine and nursing have provided for many years: the *Journal of Orthopaedic and Sports Physical Therapy* began in 1979; *Physical and Occupational Therapy in Pediatrics* was launched in 1980, and *Physical Therapy and Occupational Therapy in Geriatrics* followed shortly thereafter. The *Journal of Physical Therapy Education* was developed in 1986, in 1989 the *Journal of Pediatric Physical Therapy* was launched, and in 1992 *Issues in Aging,* formerly a newsletter of the Geriatrics Section of the APTA, changed its format to become a peer-reviewed journal.

Financial support of research is another indication of the value that is placed on research activities. The Foundation for Physical Therapy, founded in 1979, awarded almost $800,000 in research grants during 1997.[34] This is a marked increase from the $350,000 awarded in 1989/1990.[35] Physical therapists have also been successful in securing funds from corporate and government sources.

Though the refrains to increase and improve physical therapy research do not seem to change from one generation of therapists to the next, this review shows that professional associations and their components now place more emphasis on research than ever before, the educational standards for physical therapists include criteria related to research, doctoral programs in physical therapy exist, the number of journals related to physical therapy research has increased during the past two decades, and external funds for physical therapy research are available from several sources. Yes, the barriers to research are significant. Yes, identifying and using the available resources takes initiative and energy. However, the incentives to overcome these barriers are substantial, as the future of the profession within the health care system depends on our establishment of evidence on which to base our practice.

■ SUMMARY

Research is the creative process by which professionals systematically challenge their everyday practices. Developing a body of physical therapy knowledge, documenting the efficacy of physical therapy research, and improving patient care are reasons for conducting physical therapy research. Barriers to research are lack of familiarity with the research process, lack of statistical support, lack of funds, lack of time, and concern for the ethics of using animals and humans as research subjects. Growth in the importance of research to the profession of physical therapy is illustrated by the changing educational standards of the profession, expansion of research journals in physical therapy, and growth in funding for physical therapy research.

REFERENCES

1. Kettering CF. Cited in: Boyd TA. *Prophet of Progress.* New York, NY: EP Dutton and Co; 1961.
2. Payton OD. *Research: The Validation of Clinical Practice.* 3rd ed. Philadelphia, Pa: FA Davis Co; 1994.
3. Portney LG, Watkins MP. *Foundations of Clinical Research: Applications to Practice.* Norwalk, Conn: Appleton & Lange; 1993.
4. Polit DF, Hungler BP. *Nursing Research Principles and Methods.* 5th ed. Philadelphia, Pa: JB Lippincott Co; 1995.
5. Quebec Task Force on Spinal Disorders. Scientific approach to the assessment and management of activity-related spinal disorders: treatment of activity-related spinal disorders. *Spine.* 1987;12(suppl):S22–S30.
6. Delitto A, Cibulka MT, Erhard RE, Bowling RW, Tenhula JA. Evidence for use of an extension-mobilization category in acute low back syndrome: a prescriptive validation pilot study. *Phys Ther.* 1993;73:216–222.
7. Damiano DL, Kelly LE, Vaughn CL. Effects of quadriceps femoris muscle strengthening on crouch gait in children with spastic diplegia. *Phys Ther.* 1995;75:658–667.
8. Rothstein JM. Clinical literature [editorial]. *Phys Ther.* 1989;69:895.
9. Winter DA, Sienko SE. Biomechanics of below-knee amputee gait. *J Biomechanics.* 1988;21:361–367.
10. Currier DP. *Elements of Research in Physical Therapy.* 3rd ed. Baltimore, Md: Williams & Wilkins; 1990.
11. Houle CO. *Continuing Learning in the Professions.* San Francisco, Calif: Jossey-Bass Publishers; 1981.
12. Hislop HJ. The not-so-impossible dream. *Phys Ther.* 1975;55:1069–1080.
13. Carr JH, Shepherd RB, Gordon J, Gentile AM, Held JM. *Movement Science Foundations for Physical Therapy in Rehabilitation.* Rockville, Md: Aspen Publishers; 1987.
14. Hayes KW. Rose Excellence in Research Award recipient acceptance speech—February 11, 1995. *Orthop Pract.* 1995;7(2):12–13.
15. Rothstein JM, Delitto A, Scalzitti DA. *Understanding AHCPR Clinical Practice Guideline No. 14: Acute Low Back Problems in Adults.* Alexandria, Va: American Physical Therapy Association; 1995.
16. Connolly J. AHCPR Clinical Practice Guideline No. 14: Acute Low Back Problems in Adults: a commentary. *PT Magazine.* 1995;3:89–97.
17. Wennberg J, Gittelsohn A. Variations in medical care among small areas. *Sci Am.* 1982;246:120–134.
18. Labelle H, Guibert R, Joncas J, Newman N, Fallaha M, Rivard CH. Lack of scientific evidence for the treatment of lateral epicondylitis of the elbow. *J Bone Joint Surg Br.* 1992;74:646–651.
19. Hunter D, Smith Cole E, Murray JM, Murray TD. Energy expenditure of below-knee amputees during harness-supported treadmill ambulation. *J Orthop Sports Phys Ther.* 1995;21:268–276.
20. Ballin AJ, Breslin WH, Wierenga KAS, Shepard KF. Research in physical therapy: philosophy, barriers to involvement, and use among California physical therapists. *Phys Ther.* 1980;60:888–895.
21. Taylor E, Mitchell M. Research attitudes and activities of occupational therapy clinicians. *Am J Occup Ther.* 1990;44:350–355.
22. Reynolds JP. Statistical power: day in the life of a PT researcher. *PT Magazine.* 1995;3:32–39.
23. Zito M, Bohannon RW. Inferential statistics in physical therapy research: a recommended core. *J Phys Ther Educ.* 1990;4(1):13–16.
24. Worthingham C. The development of physical therapy as a profession through research and publication. *Phys Ther.* 1960;40:573–577.
25. Michels E. On closing the credibility gap. *Phys Ther.* 1968;48:1081–1082.
26. Rothstein JM. The Journal: past, present, and future [editorial]. *Phys Ther.* 1989;69:796.
27. Robertson VJ. Research and the cumulation of knowledge in physical therapy. *Phys Ther.* 1995;75:223–232.
28. American Women's Physical Therapeutic Association. Constitution. *Phys Ther.* 1921;1:5.

29. American Physical Therapy Association. Bylaws. *Phys Ther.* 1995;75:907.

30. Pepin J. CPA initiates fast action to tackle issues. *Physiotherapy Can.* 1995;47:229–230.

31. *Essentials of an Accredited Educational Program for the Physical Therapist.* Alexandria, Va: American Physical Therapy Association; 1974.

32. Commission on Accreditation in Physical Therapy Education. *Evaluative Criteria for Accreditation of Education Programs for the Preparation of Physical Therapists.* Alexandria, Va: American Physical Therapy Association; Effective January 1, 1998.

33. Soderberg GL. The future of physical therapy doctoral education. *J Phys Ther Educ.* 1989;3(1):15–19.

34. Foundation for Physical Therapy. Audited financial statements. Alexandria, Va: Foundation for Physical Therapy, December 31, 1997.

35. Foundation for Physical Therapy. 1989/90 Report. *Progress Report of the American Physical Therapy Association.* 1990;19(8):11.

Theory in Physical Therapy Research

Definitions of Theory
Level of Restrictiveness
Least Restrictive Definition
Moderately Restrictive Definition
Most Restrictive Definition
Tentativeness of Theory
Testability of Theory
Scope of Theory
Grand Theory

Middle-Range Theory
Muscle Strengthening with Electrical Stimulation
Etiology and Treatment of Chronic Ankle Instability
Relationship Between Theory, Research, and Practice

All of us have had ideas, and we may have dubbed some of these ideas theories. An instructor, after conducting an uninspired class on a beautiful spring day, may theorize that the level of interest in class discussion was inversely related to the outside environmental conditions. The students, on the other hand, may theorize that their interest in the outside conditions was inversely related to the enthusiasm and organization of the instructor!

When do ideas about the nature of the world become theories? What distinguishes theory from other modes of thought? Is theory important to an applied discipline such as physical therapy? The purpose of this chapter is to answer these questions by defining theory and some closely related terms, categorizing theories on the basis of scope, and examining the relationship between theory, practice, and research.

■ DEFINITIONS OF THEORY

Theories are, by nature, abstractions. Thus, the language of theory is abstract, and there are divergent definitions of theory and its components. Instead of presenting a single definition of theory, this section of the chapter examines three elements of various definitions of theory: level of restrictiveness, tentativeness, and testability.

Level of Restrictiveness

Definitions of theory differ in their level of restrictiveness, and the level of restrictiveness of the definition then has an impact on the purposes for which a theory can be used. To illustrate the differences between various levels of restrictiveness, a simplistic example about hemiplegia is developed throughout this section of the chapter. This example is not meant to be a well-developed theory; it is merely an illustration based on a clinical entity that most physical therapists should have encountered at some point in their professional education or practice. Table 2–1 summarizes the distinctions between the definitions and purposes of theories with different levels of restrictiveness.

LEAST RESTRICTIVE DEFINITION

The least restrictive form of theory is *descriptive theory,* defined by Fawcett as theories that "describe or name specific characteristics of individuals, groups, situations, or events."[1(p19)] This definition is least restrictive because it requires only description—and not prediction or explanation—of phenomena. Thus, following this definition of descriptive theory, the statement "Patients with hemiplegia have difficulty ambulating, eating, and reading" is a simple form of theory because it characterizes (difficulty ambulating, eating, and reading) a phenomenon (patients with hemiplegia).

Descriptive theories may be further classified as either *ad hoc theories* or *categorical theories.* The statement "Patients with hemiplegia have difficulty ambulating, eating, and reading" presents an ad hoc collection of characteristics of patients with hemiplegia. An ad hoc list is not exhaustive; it is merely a list of possible characteristics. The statement about difficulty ambulating, eating, and reading in no way implies that these traits are the only difficulties experienced by patients with hemiplegia. Contrast the ad hoc list with the statement "The deficits experienced by patients with hemiplegia may be motor, sensory, or functional." This is an example of a categorical descriptive theory since it implies that all the deficits experienced by a patient with hemiplegia can be classified into one of these three categories. In the ad hoc example, discovery of another type of difficulty (e.g., speaking) would not invalidate the theoretical statement since the list was not meant to be exhaustive. In the categorical example, discovery of another classification of deficits (e.g., cognitive) would require revision of the theory because the categories listed were meant to be exhaustive.

MODERATELY RESTRICTIVE DEFINITION

Kerlinger has advanced a more restrictive definition of theory: "A theory is a set of interrelated constructs (concepts), definitions, and propositions that present a systematic view of phenomena by specifying relations among variables, with the purpose of explaining and predicting the phenomena."[2(p9)] Several terms used by Kerlinger to define theory need definition themselves.

First, although the definition implies that constructs and concepts are similar, Kerlinger and others distinguish between the two. A *concept* has been defined as a "word or phrase that describes an abstract idea or mental image of some phenomenon."[3(p16)] Concepts are generally

TABLE 2-1	**Level of Restrictiveness in Theory Definitions**		
	Level of Restrictiveness		
	Least	*Moderate*	*Most*
Definition	Account for or characterize phenomena	Specify relationships between constructs	Specify relationships and form a deductive system
Purpose	Description	Prediction	Explanation
Comments	Subdivided into ad hoc and categorical theories	Sometimes referred to as conceptual frameworks or models	Can take the form of if-then statements

thought to be observable. Thus, "joint range of motion" is a concept that can be observed by measuring joint motion with a goniometer. A *construct* "refers to a property that is neither directly nor indirectly observed"[3(p21)] and has been "deliberately and consciously invented or adopted for a special scientific purpose."[2(p27)] Thus, according to this definition, constructs are more abstract than concepts. "Motivation" and "social support" are examples of constructs; direct measurement of the constructs themselves is impossible since levels of motivation and social support can only be inferred from individual and family behaviors.

Although the aforementioned authors recognize a distinction between concepts and constructs, many others use the terms interchangeably. Even those who make the distinction recognize that the boundaries between concept and construct are not clear. Given the blurred distinction between them, the two terms will be used interchangeably within this text.

Second, a *proposition* is "a statement about a concept or the relationship between concepts."[3(p16)] The term *hypothesis* is sometimes used interchangeably with proposition, as in Kerlinger's definition that a hypothesis is "a conjectural statement of the relation between two or more variables."[2(p17)] The hallmark of Kerlinger's definition of theory, then, is that it must specify relationships between concepts.

The earlier statement about patients with hemiplegia would need to be developed considerably before Kerlinger would consider it to be theory. Such a developed theory might read like this: "The extent to which hemiplegic patients will have difficulty ambulating is directly related to the presence of flaccid paralysis, cognitive deficits, and balance deficits and inversely related to prior ambulation status." This is no longer a simple description of several characteristics of hemiplegia; it is a statement of relationships between concepts.

Researchers who prefer the most restrictive definition of theory may consider descriptions at this moderately restrictive level to be *conceptual frameworks* or *models*. Polit and Hungler, for example, are careful to distinguish between theory and less well articulated conceptual frameworks in nursing.[4]

Theory that meets Kerlinger's definition is known as *predictive theory* since it can be used to make predictions based on the relationships between variables. If the four factors in this hypothetical theory about hemiplegic gait were found to be good predictors of eventual ambulation outcome, therapists might be able to use information gathered at admission to predict long-term ambulation status.

MOST RESTRICTIVE DEFINITION

The most restrictive view of theory is that "theories involve a series of propositions regarding the interrelationships among concepts, from which a large number of empirical observations can be deduced."[4(p96)] This is the most restrictive definition because it requires both relationships between variables and a deductive system.

Deductive reasoning goes from the general to the specific and can take the form of if-then statements. To make the hypothetical theory of hemiplegic gait meet this definition we would need to add a general gait component to the theory. This general statement might read: "Human gait characteristics are dependent on muscle power, skeletal stability, proprioceptive feedback, balance, motor planning, and learned patterns." The specific deduction from this general theory of gait is the statement: "In patients with hemiplegia, the critical components that lead to difficulty ambulating independently are presence of flaccidity (muscle power), impaired sensation (proprioceptive feedback), impaired perception of verticality (balance), cognitive difficulties (motor planning), and prior ambulation status (learned patterns). In an if-then format, this theory might read as follows:

1. *If* normal gait depends on intact muscle power, skeletal stability, proprioceptive feedback, balance, motor planning, and learned patterns, and

2. *if* hemiplegic gait is not normal,

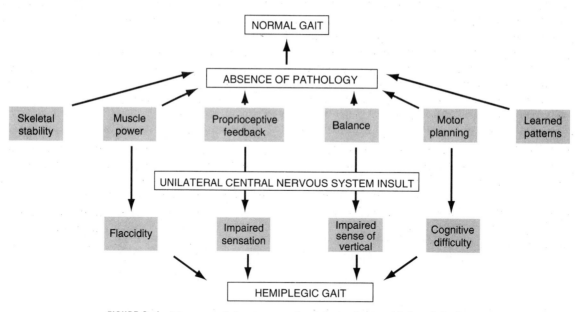

FIGURE 2–1. Diagram of the theory of gait in patients with hemiplegia.

3. *then* patients with hemiplegia must have deficits in one or more of the following areas: muscle power, skeletal stability, proprioceptive feedback, balance, motor planning, and learned patterns.

This theory, then, forms a deductive system by advancing a general theory for the performance of normal gait activities, and then examining the elements that are affected in hemiplegic patients. Figure 2–1 presents this theory schematically. The six elements in the theory are central to the figure. In the absence of pathology, normal gait occurs, as shown above the central elements; in the presence of pathology, the elements are altered and an abnormal gait results, as shown below the gait elements.

With a deductive system in place, theory can begin to be used to explain natural phenomena. *Explanatory theory* looks at the why and how questions that undergird a problem, generally in more explicit terms than illustrated in Figure 2–2. The hypothetical explanatory theory about gait begins to explain ambulation difficulty in terms of six elements needed for normal gait.

Tentativeness of Theory

The second element of the definition of theory is its tentativeness. The tentative nature of theory is emphasized by Portney and Watkins:

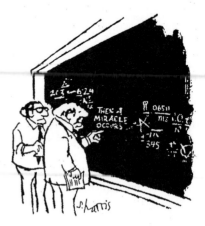

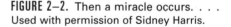
"I THINK YOU SHOULD BE MORE EXPLICIT HERE IN STEP TWO."

FIGURE 2–2. Then a miracle occurs. . . .
Used with permission of Sidney Harris.

A theory is only a tentative explanation of phenomena. . . . Theories reflect the present state of knowledge and must adapt to changes in that knowledge as technology and scientific evidence improve. . . . Many theories that are accepted today will be discarded tomorrow.[5(p22)]

Thus, theory is not absolute; rather, it is a view that is acceptable, at the time, to the scientists studying the phenomenon. For example, the idea that the sun revolved around the earth (geocentric theory) suited its time. It was also a useful theory:

> It described the heavens precisely as they looked and fitted the observations and calculations made with the naked eye; . . . it fitted the available facts, was a reasonably satisfactory device for prediction, and harmonized with the accepted view of the rest of nature. . . . Even for the adventurous sailor and the navigator it served well enough.[6(p295)]

However, the small discrepancies between the geocentric theory and the yearly calendar were troublesome to Renaissance astronomers and led to the development of the heliocentric theory, the one we still believe, that the earth revolves around the sun. Perhaps a later generation of scientists will develop different models of the universe that better explain the natural phenomena of the changing of days and seasons. Natural scientists do not assume an unchangeable objective reality that will ultimately be explained by the perfect theory; there is no reason for physical therapy researchers to assume that their world is any more certain or ultimately explainable than the natural world.

Testability of Theory

Krebs and Harris[7] believe that testability is the sine qua non (an indispensable condition) of theory. Thus, they believe that theory needs to be formulated in ways that allow the theory to be tested. However, theories cannot be proved true because one can never test them under all the conditions under which they might be applied. Even if testing shows that the world behaves in the manner predicted by a theory, this testing does not prove that the theory is true; other rival theories might provide equally accurate predictions. Theories can, however, be proved false by instances in which the predictions of the theory are not borne out.

For example, if one can accurately predict the discharge ambulation status of patients with hemiplegia based on tone, sensation, perception, and cognition, then the theory is consistent with the data. However, rival theories might predict discharge ambulation status just as well. A behaviorally oriented therapist might develop a theory that predicts discharge ambulation status as a function of the level of motivation of the patient and the extent to which the therapist provides immediate rewards for gait activities. If the behavioral theory accurately predicts discharge ambulation status of patients with hemiplegia as well as the other theory does, it would also be consistent with the data. Neither theory can be proved in the sense that it is true and all others are false; both theories can, however, be shown to be consistent with available information.

■ SCOPE OF THEORY

Theories have been classified by different researchers in terms of their scope. Fawcett and Downs[3(p62)] classify theories as either grand or middle-range theories. To illustrate what is meant by these two different scopes, examples of each type are described.

Grand Theory

Grand theories provide broad conceptualizations of phenomena. The grand theory level is far better represented in the nursing literature than in the physical therapy literature. Thus, one example from nursing and one example from physical therapy are used to illustrate grand theory.

One of several grand theories in nursing is the Roy Adaptation Model, which was developed from several psychological and sociological frameworks. This model assumes that people are biopsychosocial beings who adapt to stimuli using one of four subsystems, or adaptive modes: physiological needs, self-concept, role function, and interdependence.[8] The goal of nursing is to facilitate the adaptation process along the health-illness dimension of life.[9] Recognize that this description of the Roy Adaptation Model is skeletal and is presented for illustrative purposes only; in-depth discussions of this model can be found in the references cited. Figure 2–3 presents a simplified schematic of the Roy Adaptation Model.[10] The activities of a nurse who is caring for a man who has just undergone a transtibial amputation can be used to illustrate the application of this theory to practice. The nurse might elevate the patient's residual limb to control edema (a physiological factor); discuss his altered body image (a self-concept factor); discuss how the amputation may affect his

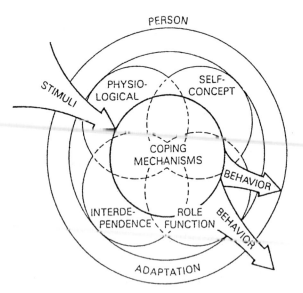

FIGURE 2–3. Simplified diagram of the Roy Adaptation Model of nursing.
From Andrews HA, Roy C. *Essentials of the Roy Adaptation Model.* Norwalk, Conn: Appleton-Century-Crofts; 1986:44. Reprinted by permission of Prentice-Hall, Inc., Upper Saddle River, NJ.

leisure activities (a role function factor); and facilitate discussion about his being willing to accept assistance with lawn care (an interdependence factor).

Hislop's[11] conceptual model of pathokinesiology and movement dysfunction as the basis for physical therapy is one of few works in physical therapy that can be classified as grand theory. This model looks at physical therapy using the overarching phenomena of movement disorders (others have modified the term from disorders to dysfunction) and pathokinesiology (the application of anatomy and physiology to the study of abnormal human movement). Figure 2–4 is an interpretation of Hislop's formulation of the pathokinesiological basis for physical therapy. Physical therapy is viewed as a triangle with a base of service values supplemented by science, focusing on treatment of motion disorders through therapeutic exercise based on the principles of pathokinesiology. In this theory, physical therapy is viewed as affecting motion disorders related to four of six components of a hierarchy of systems ranging from the family to the cellular level of the body. The goals of physical therapy are either to restore motion homeostasis or to enhance adaptation to permanent impairment.

An alternate conceptualization of physical therapy might be termed the functional framework for physical therapy. Figure 2–5 presents a schematic conceptualization of such a functional framework. The first three elements of the seven-tiered triangle are identical to those of Hislop, and the goals of restoring normal motion or adapting to permanent impairment are also the same as hers.[11] This conceptualization differs from Hislop's in that it emphasizes that it is the functional consequences of movement disorders that precipitate the need for physical therapy, recognizes therapeutic exercise as only one of several types of interventions, and recognizes function as a higher level goal than motion. A named science such as pathokinesiology is not created; this model accepts that professions may legitimately base themselves on the applications of existing sciences.

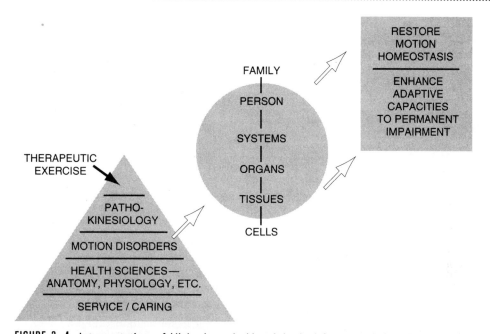

FIGURE 2–4. Interpretation of Hislop's pathokinesiological framework for physical therapy. The triangle represents the structure of physical therapy, the circle a hierarchy of systems affected by physical therapy, and the square the goals of physical therapy. Adapted from Hislop HJ. The not-so-impossible dream. *Phys Ther.* 1975;55:1073, 1075. Reprinted from *Physical Therapy* with the permission of the American Physical Therapy Association.

Which grand theory of physical therapy is correct: Hislop's pathokinesiology model or the functional framework introduced here? The answer is that neither needs to be correct but each

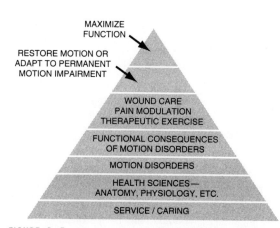

FIGURE 2–5. Model of a functional framework for physical therapy.

must be useful. The purpose of grand theory is to provide broad conceptualizations of a phenomenon, in this case physical therapy. Each theory should be critically evaluated in terms of the extent to which it accurately describes physical therapy and provides a framework for study of phenomena within physical therapy. Different researchers will find that one or the other theory provides a better framework for the questions they wish to ask about physical therapy. Stevens wrote of the folly of adhering to one correct nursing theory:

> The next obstacle to understanding and developing nursing theory . . . is the great press for a universal, unitary nursing theory. . . . Imagine what we would think of the field of psychology were it to dictate that each of its practitioners be Freudian. Indeed, it is the conflict and diversity among theories that account for much of the progress in any discipline. A search for conformity is an attempt to stultify the growth of a profession.[12(ppxii–xiii)]

Physical therapists need not choose between pathokinesiological, functional, or other frameworks. What they must do is analyze, develop, and use these theories to enhance their understanding of physical therapy.

Middle-Range Theory

Middle-range theories are more specific than grand theories; they address individual problems and issues, rather than trying to place an entire discipline into a single theoretical context. Two examples of middle-range theory in physical therapy are presented: theories of muscle strength augmentation with electrical muscle stimulation and a model of the etiology and treatment of chronic ankle instability.

MUSCLE STRENGTHENING WITH ELECTRICAL STIMULATION

Delitto and Snyder-Mackler[13] have presented two middle-range theories about muscle strengthening with percutaneous electrical stimulation. The two theories were developed to explain the results of research relating to muscle strengthening with electrical stimulation. Based on research reports documenting the effectiveness of neuromuscular electrical stimulation, Delitto and Snyder-

Mackler sought to explain the mechanism for the increases in strength. Two opposing theories were advanced: overload and differential recruitment. They then proposed how these two theories could be tested and the types of results that would be found if either theory were operating.

Figure 2–6 is a schematic presentation of research results that would support each theory. The overload theory predicts that muscle performance improvements with electrical stimulation or exercise should parallel each other at all training intensities because electrical stimulation and voluntary exercise both place similar functional overloads on muscles. The differential recruitment theory predicts that muscle performance improvement differences between high-intensity electrical stimulation and high-intensity exercise will be small, but that muscle performance improvement differences between low-intensity electrical stimulation and low-intensity exercise will be great. The physiological basis that is advanced to explain this difference is differential recruitment of muscle fibers in voluntary and electrically elicited contractions. At low intensities, slow-twitch fibers are recruited volitionally. At high intensities, both slow-twitch and fast-twitch fibers are recruited volitionally. With electrically elicited contractions, fast-twitch fibers are recruited first, regardless of intensity of training. Thus, high-intensity electrically simulated con-

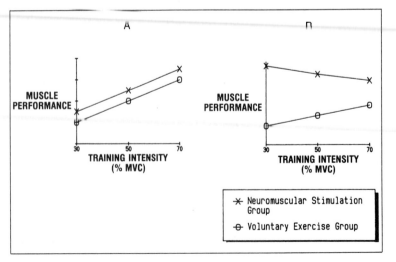

FIGURE 2–6. Competing theories of muscle strength augmentation using percutaneous electrical stimulation.
From Delitto A, Snyder-Mackler L. Two theories of muscle strength augmentation using percutaneous electrical stimulation. *Phys Ther.* 1990;70:163. Reprinted from *Physical Therapy* with the permission of the American Physical Therapy Association.

tractions and high-intensity volitional contractions are similar in that they both involve recruitment of fast-twitch fibers. At low intensities, the two types of contractions are quite different in that the volitional low-intensity contraction will recruit slow-twitch fibers, and the electrically elicited contraction will recruit fast-twitch fibers. Hence, the supposition is that differences between volitional and electrically induced contractions will be greatest at lower training intensities.

These two muscle strengthening theories fit the most restrictive definition of theory. They both describe relationships between concepts, the primary concepts being muscle performance, training intensity, and type of exercise. Each of the strengthening theories has a deductive system that moves from the general (patterns of fiber recruitment) to the specific (improvements in muscle performance). Each theory can be stated in if-then language: *If* muscle strengthening in the two modes works through a general overload principle, *then* the following results will be seen. The theories are obviously explanatory; they provide physiological rationales for differences between strength increases with each exercise type. These two theories can be tested as suggested by Figure 2–6; they can also provide a framework for further studies of neuromuscular electrical stimulation. In fact, Snyder-Mackler, Delitto, and colleagues have implemented research studies that test portions of these theories. Their aggregate results,[14–16] shown in Figure 2–7, demonstrate a need for further refinement of their theories of muscle strengthening. That is, the lines representing voluntary exercise and electrical stimulation at differing intensities are neither parallel (as predicted by the overload theory) nor do they demonstrate greater differences at low intensities (as predicted by the differential recruitment theory).

ETIOLOGY AND TREATMENT OF CHRONIC ANKLE INSTABILITY

Lentell and associates[17] reported the results of a study with the primary purpose of determining whether peroneal muscle weakness and clinically detectable balance deficits were present in

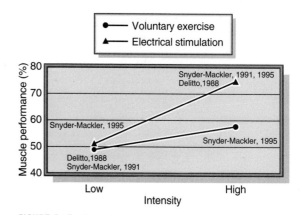

FIGURE 2–7. Results of studies testing the theories of muscle strengthening with electrical stimulation. Data are from the following sources: Delitto A, Rose SJ, McKowen JM, et al. Electrical stimulation versus voluntary exercise in strengthening thigh musculature after anterior cruciate ligament surgery. *Phys Ther.* 1988; 68:660–663. Reprinted with permission of the American Physical Therapy Association; Snyder-Mackler L, Ladin Z, Schepsis AA, Young JC. Electrical stimulation of the thigh muscles after reconstruction of the anterior cruciate ligament. *J Bone Joint Surg Am.* 1991;73: 1025–1036; and Snyder-Mackler L, Delitto A, Bailey SL, Stralka SW. Strength of the quadriceps femoris muscle and functional recovery after reconstruction of the anterior cruciate ligament. *J Bone Joint Surg Am.* 1995;77: 1166–1173.

individuals with chronic ankle instability. A secondary purpose was to determine the extent to which peroneal muscle weakness and balance deficits were related in individuals with chronic ankle instability. The background information cited by the authors indicated that three causative factors are frequently given for chronic ankle instability: anatomical instability, peroneal muscle weakness, and proprioceptive deficits. In the discussion section of the article, the authors noted that there are three mechanisms of support for any joint: osseous configuration, ligamentous restraints, and muscular restraints.

Figure 2–8 presents two schematic drawings, with differing levels of complexity, of how the general support mechanisms can be applied to the ankle and how treatment might proceed based on identified deficits. The question marks in Figure 2–8A illustrate the portions of the the-

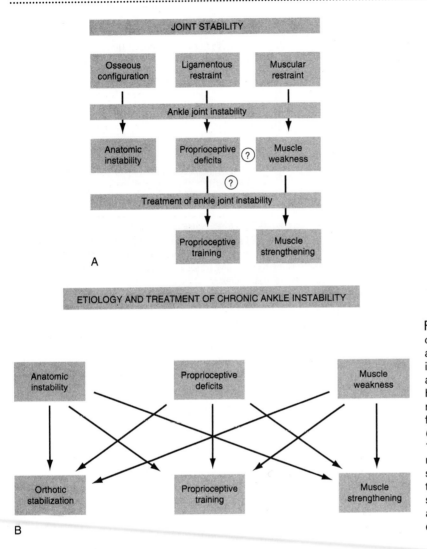

FIGURE 2–8. Diagram of the theory that underlies the etiology and treatment of chronic ankle instability. **A.** A simple theory as extracted from Lentell GL, Katzman LL, Walters MR. The relationship between muscle function and ankle stability. *J Orthop Sports Phys Ther.* 1990;11:605–611. The question marks on the diagram represent the relationships tested in that study. **B.** A detailed expansion of the lower portion of **A,** as suggested by the missing elements in **A.**

ory tested in the research report: (1) Are proprioceptive deficits and muscle weakness characteristic of unstable ankles, and (2) Are muscle weakness and proprioceptive deficits related in chronically unstable ankles? This conceptualization meets the most restrictive definition of theory in that it has a deductive system: if all joints depend on bony, ligamentous, and muscular restraints for stability, and if loss of one or more of these supports causes instability, then loss of one or more of these supports in the ankle should cause ankle instability.

The benefit of a theoretical framework is that it suggests areas for further research in a way that an isolated study cannot. A schematic diagram of a theory may also make gaps in one's thinking visually apparent. When developing the figures based on information presented in the article, it became apparent that there was initially no proposed treatment factor that directly corresponded to the anatomical instability factor (Fig. 2–8A); orthotic stabilization was therefore added (Fig. 2–8B). In addition, straight lines from problems to treatments seemed limited. Perhaps, for example, strength can contribute to functional stability in the absence of anatomical stability. This idea of compensatory treatment led to the additions of the diagonal arrows in Figure 2–8B.

Table 2–2 presents a range of possible study topics suggested by the elaboration of a theory about chronic ankle instability. An entire research career could be built around testing the elements of this theory. Each subsequent project would either confirm portions of the theory or lead to refinements of the hypothesized relationships. In fact, Lentell has continued to use this theoretical framework to study the contributions of proprioceptive deficits, muscle function, and anatomical laxity to functional instability of the ankle.[18]

TABLE 2–2	**Research Suggested by the Ankle Instability Model**

Anatomic instability
- What are the bony relationships of the unstable ankle in weight bearing?
- Are heel-off and push-off different for normal ankles and unstable ankles?

Proprioceptive deficits
- Does proprioception differ between once-sprained ankles and chronically unstable ankles?
- Do unstable ankles show deficits on multiple measures of proprioception?
- Do unstable ankles have both open- and closed-chain proprioceptive deficits?

Muscle weakness
- Can muscle weakness of unstable ankles be demonstrated in closed-chain testing?
- How do unstable ankles perform on functional muscle strength tests?
- Do muscles other than peroneals contribute to ankle instability?

Relationships among support factors
- Are anatomical stability and proprioceptive deficits related?
- Are anatomical stability and muscle weakness related?
- To what extent are strength and proprioceptive deficits related?

Treatment questions
- Can orthotic stabilization substitute for any of the three support factors?
- Can strengthening, in the absence of weakness, aid stability?
- Does proprioceptive training decrease the frequency of giving way?

■ RELATIONSHIP BETWEEN THEORY, RESEARCH, AND PRACTICE

Theory is important because it allows researchers to place questions into logically related clusters and provides a basis for developing ongoing lines of inquiry, as illustrated in the examples used in this chapter. Figure 2–9 presents a schematic drawing showing the relationship between theory, research, and clinical practice. Theory is either developed through clinical observations and experiences (e.g., "It seems to me that patients who pay for their own therapy more often follow home exercise instructions than do those whose insurance companies cover the cost") or logical speculation (e.g., "If pain is related to the accumulation of metabolic byproducts in the tissues, then modalities that increase local blood flow should help reduce pain").[19]

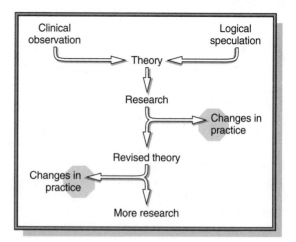

FIGURE 2–9. Relationship between theory, research, and practice.

Theory is then tested formally through research. Based on the research results, the theory is either confirmed or modified, as are clinical practices based on the theory. If the research itself was conducted with a clinical population and types of treatments that can be easily implemented in actual practice were used, then clinicians may change their practices based on the research results themselves. If the research was conducted with animals, with normal human subjects, or with techniques not directly applicable to the clinic, then the results will not be directly applicable to the clinical setting. Instead, the research results may lead to modification of the theory, and modification of the theory may in turn lead clinicians to rethink the ways in which they treat their patients.

■ SUMMARY

Theory in physical therapy can be defined according to levels of restrictiveness, tentativeness, and testability. The different levels of theory are used for description, prediction, and explanation. Theories are also differentiated on the basis of scope. Grand theories attempt to place a large body of work into a unified framework and are represented by Roy's Adaptation Model of nursing[8] and Hislop's pathokinesiological framework for physical therapy.[11] Middle-range theories address specific problems and are represented by Delitto and Snyder-Mackler's[13] theories of electrically stimulated muscle strength augmentation and Lentell's[17,18] theory of the etiology and treatment of chronic ankle instability. Theory, research, and practice are related through theories that are developed through clinical observation or logical speculation, through research that tests theories, and through revisions of theory and clinical practice based on research results.

REFERENCES

1. Fawcett J. *Analysis and Evaluation of Nursing Theories.* Philadelphia, Pa: FA Davis Co; 1993.
2. Kerlinger FN. *Foundations of Behavioral Research.* 3rd ed. Fort Worth, Tex: Holt, Rinehart & Winston Inc.; 1986.
3. Fawcett J, Downs FS. *The Relationship of Theory and Research.* 2nd ed. Philadelphia, Pa: FA Davis Co; 1992.
4. Polit DF, Hungler BP. *Nursing Research: Principles and Methods.* 5th ed. Philadelphia, Pa: JB Lippincott Co; 1995.
5. Portney LG, Watkins MP. *Foundations of Clinical Research: Applications to Practice.* Norwalk, Conn: Appleton & Lange; 1993.
6. Boorstin DJ. *The Discoverers: A History of Man's Search to Know His World and Himself.* New York, NY: Harry N Abrams; 1991.
7. Krebs DE, Harris SR. Elements of theory presentations in *Physical Therapy. Phys Ther.* 1988;68:690–693.
8. Roy C. The Roy Adaptation Model. In: Riehl-Sisca JP, ed. *Conceptual Models for Nursing Practice.* 3rd ed. Norwalk, Conn: Appleton & Lange; 1989:105–114.
9. Phillips KD, Blue CL, Brubaker KM, et al. Sister Callista Roy: Adaptation Model. In: Marriner-Tomey A, Alligood MR, eds. *Nursing Theorists and Their Work.* 4th ed. St. Louis, Mo: CV Mosby Co; 1997:243–266.
10. Andrews HA, Roy C. *Essentials of the Roy Adaptation Model.* Norwalk, Conn: Appleton-Century-Crofts; 1986: 44.
11. Hislop HJ. The not-so-impossible dream. *Phys Ther.* 1975; 55:1069–1080.
12. Stevens BJ. *Nursing Theory: Analysis, Application, Evaluation.* 2nd ed. Boston, Mass: Little, Brown & Co; 1984.
13. Delitto A, Snyder-Mackler L. Two theories of muscle strength augmentation using percutaneous electrical stimulation. *Phys Ther.* 1990;70:158–164.
14. Delitto A, Rose SJ, McKowen JM, Lehman RC, Thomas JA, Shively RA. Electrical stimulation versus voluntary exercise in strengthening thigh musculature after anterior cruciate ligament surgery. *Phys Ther.* 1988;68:660–663.
15. Snyder-Mackler L, Ladin Z, Schepsis AA, Young JC. Electrical stimulation of the thigh muscles after reconstruction of the anterior cruciate ligament. *J Bone Joint Surg Am.* 1991;73:1025–1036.
16. Snyder-Mackler L, Delitto A, Bailey SL, Stralka SW. Strength of the quadriceps femoris muscle and functional recovery after reconstruction of the anterior cruciate ligament. *J Bone Joint Surg Am.* 1995;77:1166–1173.
17. Lentell GL, Katzman LL, Walters MR. The relationship between muscle function and ankle stability. *J Orthop Sports Phys Ther.* 1990;11:605–611.
18. Lentell G, Baas B, Lopez D, et al. The contributions of proprioceptive deficits, muscle function, and anatomic laxity to functional instability of the ankle. *J Orthop Sports Phys Ther.* 1995;21:206–215.
19. Tammivaara J, Shepard KF. Theory: the guide to clinical practice and research. *Phys Ther.* 1990:70:578–582.

3

Research Ethics

Boundaries Between Practice and Research

Moral Principles of Action
The Principle of Nonmaleficence
The Principle of Beneficence
The Principle of Utility
The Principle of Autonomy

Informed Consent

Research Codes of Ethics
Informed Consent
Design Justifies Study

Avoidance of Suffering and Injury
Risk Is Commensurate with
    Potential Benefit
Independent Review
Publication Integrity
Explicit Attention to Ethics

Research Risks
Physical Risks
Psychological Risks
Social Risks
Economic Risks

Ethical principles provide a basis for making decisions about personal and professional conduct. Professional groups often formalize ethical principles into codes of ethics that apply general ethical principles to specific practices of professionals. For example, the American Physical Therapy Association (APTA) *Code of Ethics* for the physical therapist provides guidelines for therapist-patient interactions, for interprofessional relations, and for relationships with external parties such as health care insurers and equipment manufacturers.[1] In addition to codes of ethics relating to practice, various organizations have developed more specific ethical guidelines for the conduct of research.[2–5]

The existence of these specialized guidelines indicates that there are fundamental differences between practice and research, and that these differences have ethical implications. The purpose of this chapter is to articulate ethical principles of importance to the conduct of research. First, attention is given to determining the boundaries between practice and research. Second, basic moral principles of action are presented. Examples of these moral principles in action are given for occurrences in everyday life, for treatment situations, and for research settings. Third, a special case of the moral principle of autonomy—informed consent—is examined in detail. Fourth, the application of the moral principles to research is illustrated through analysis of several widely used research codes of ethics. Finally, a categorization of research risks is presented.

■ BOUNDARIES BETWEEN PRACTICE AND RESEARCH

Every physical therapist–patient relationship is predicated on the principle that the physical therapist can render services that are likely to benefit the patient. The roles, relationships, and goals found in the treatment milieu are vastly different from those in the research setting. In the research setting the physical therapist becomes an investigator rather than a practitioner; the patient becomes a subject. The patient seeks out a practitioner who may or may not decide to accept the patient for treatment; the investigator seeks out potential subjects who may or may not agree to participate in the proposed research. The patient's goal is improvement; the investigator's goal is development of knowledge.

When accepted physical therapy care is delivered in the context of physical therapist–patient interaction, it is clear that the intent of the episode is therapeutic. When an innovative treatment technique is tested on a group of normal volunteers, it is clear that the intent of the episode is knowledge development. However, when a new technique is administered to a clinical population, the distinction between treatment and research becomes blurred. If the physical therapist views each participant as a patient, then individualized treatment modifications based on each patient's response would be expected. Alternately, if the physical therapist views each participant as a subject, then standardization of treatment protocols is often desirable. Protecting subjects from the risks of participating in research requires that one be able to distinguish research from practice. The National Commission for the Protection of Human Subjects of Biomedical and Behavioral Research, in its *Belmont Report,* developed a definition of research that makes such a distinction:

> Research (involving humans) is any manipulation, observation, or other study of a human being . . . done with the intent of developing new knowledge and which differs in any way from customary medical (or other professional) practice. . . .

Research may usually be identified by virtue of the fact that [it] is conducted according to a plan.[6(pp6,7)]

Three main elements of this definition warrant careful consideration: intent, innovation, and plan.

The Belmont definition recognizes that a fundamental difference between practice and research is that the two entities have different intents. Practice goals relate to individual patients. Research goals relate to the development of new knowledge. Because of these disparate goals, different levels of protection from risk are needed for patients and subjects.

Health care rendered to an individual is always presumed to have some probability of benefit. When deciding whether to undergo a particular treatment, a patient will evaluate its risks against its potential benefits. In contrast, research on human subjects is often of no benefit to the individual who assumes the risk of participation; rather, subsequent patients benefit from the application of the new knowledge. Some projects fall in a gray zone between research and practice. In this zone, innovative therapies with potential benefits are tested, providing both potential individual benefits and new knowledge.[6]

The second element of the Belmont definition is that the procedure differs in some way from customary practice. Simply reporting the treatment results of a series of patients who have undergone standard shoulder reconstruction rehabilitation would not be considered research. Because the treatment given is not innovative, the patients do not need special protection; the risk of being a patient whose results happen to be reported is no different than the risk associated with the treatment. Note, however, that if standard treatment calls for isokinetic testing every 4 weeks, but the group in the series is tested every week, this would now be classified as research. The risks of repeated isokinetic testing, however minimal, are different than the risks of standard treatment alone. An implication of this component of the Belmont definition is that innovative therapies should be considered research, and conducted with appropriate research safeguards, until they can be shown to be effective and are adopted as accepted or customary practice.

The third element of the Belmont definition that distinguishes research from practice is that research generally is conducted according to a plan. This implies a level of control and uniformity that is usually absent from clinical practice.

■ MORAL PRINCIPLES OF ACTION

All professionals, including physical therapists, deal with complex, specialized issues for which the correct course of action may not be clear. Thus, professionals tend to be guided not by a rigid set of rules, but by general principles that demand that each practitioner assess a given situation in light of those principles, and make decisions accordingly.

Although the content of the decisions one makes as a professional differs from one's personal decisions, the underlying principles that should guide these decisions are the same. This is also the case whether one is acting as a practitioner seeing a patient or as an investigator studying a subject: the content of practice and research decisions may differ, but the underlying principles remain the same. Before presenting ethical principles for the conduct of research, it is therefore appropriate to lay a common groundwork of moral principles of action. Four major principles are discussed: nonmaleficence, beneficence, utility, and autonomy. Examples from daily life, practice, and research are used to illustrate these principles.

The Principle of Nonmaleficence

The principle of nonmaleficence states that "we ought to act in ways that do not cause need-less harm or injury to others."[7(p32)] In addition, the principle implies that we should not expose others to unnecessary risk. In daily life this means that one should not rob people at knife point in the subway nor should one drive while intoxicated. People with backyard pools need to have them fenced properly to protect curious children from accidental drowning. Society levels civil and criminal penalties against members who violate the principle of nonmaleficence.

For physical therapy clinicians nonmaleficence means that one should neither intentionally harm one's patients nor cause unintentional harm through carelessness. Suppose that a therapist is seeing a frustrating patient—one who demands much of the therapist but does not comply with home exercises to increase shoulder range of motion. The therapist decides to "teach the patient a lesson," being deliberately vigorous in mobilization techniques to make the patient "pay" for not following directions. This action would violate the principle of nonmaleficence; the regimen was intentionally sadistic, not therapeutic.

The practice of physical therapy does, however, require that we expose patients to various risks in order to achieve treatment goals. We cannot guarantee that no harm will come to patients in the course of treatment: they may fall, they may become sore, their skin may become irritated. However, fulfilling the principle of nonmaleficence means that we have to exercise due care in the practice of our profession. Due care requires the availability of adequate personnel during gait activities, planned progression of exercise intensity, and monitoring of skin condition during procedures.

In the conduct of research we also must avoid exposing subjects to unnecessary risk. Detailed delineation of the risks of research are presented later in this chapter. In general, though, the principle of nonmaleficence requires that we refrain from research that uses techniques we know to be harmful and that research be terminated if harm becomes evident. Though the risks of harm as a consequence of research can be great, there is also harm associated with *not* conducting research. If research is not performed to assess the effects of physical therapy, then patients may be exposed to time-consuming, expensive, or painful treatments that may be ineffective or harmful. When the effects of a treatment are unknown, it is necessary to place someone at risk to systematically assess those effects. The researcher's job is to minimize these necessary risks.

The Principle of Beneficence

The principle of beneficence states that "we should act in ways that promote the welfare of other people."[7(p34)] Not only should we not harm them, but we should attempt to help them. A daily example of the principle of beneficence is the person who goes grocery shopping for a homebound neighbor.

The professional-client relationship is based on the principle of beneficence. Patients would not come to a physical therapist unless they believed the therapist could help them. The extent of beneficence required is not always clear, however. Occasionally working beyond one's usual hours to provide transfer training to a family member who cannot attend during normal clinic hours is a reasonable expectation of a professional. Never taking a vacation out of a sense of duty to one's patients is an unreasonable expectation.

The principle of beneficence presents conflicts for researchers. As noted previously, the individual subject who assumes the risks of the research may not receive any benefits from the research project. Individuals who agree to be in a vigorous early movement group following anterior cruciate ligament surgery take the risk that the reconstructed ligament may stretch or tear. They may, however, benefit from a shorter rehabilitation time if the new regimen does not lead to failure. The researcher-subject relationship puts immediate beneficence aside for the sake of new knowledge that should allow clinicians to establish beneficent relationships with future patients.

The Principle of Utility

The principle of utility states that "we should act in such a way as to bring about the greatest benefit and the least harm."[7(p36)] If a family has limited financial resources, they need to make utility decisions. Should funds be spent on health insurance or life insurance? Which is potentially more devastating financially, an enormous hospital bill or loss of the primary earner's income? The answer that would bring about the most potential benefit and the least risk of harm would vary from family to family. If a clinic cannot accommodate all the patients that desire appointments on a given day, decisions about who receives an appointment should focus on who will benefit most from immediate treatment, and who will be harmed least by delayed treatment. Health services researchers may frame health care funding debates in terms of utility. For example, what will bring about the greatest benefit and the least harm: funding for prenatal care or funding for neonatal intensive care treatment for premature infants?

In the conduct of research the principle of utility can guide the development of research agendas. Which projects will contribute most to the advancement of patient care in physical therapy? Which projects involve risks that are disproportional to the amount of beneficial information that can be gained? Should a funding agency support a project that would assess the effects of different stretching techniques on later injury in recreational athletes, or a project that would develop new movement initiation techniques for patients with Parkinson's disease? The former project has the potential to reduce lost workdays for large numbers of full-time employees; the latter has the potential to prevent or delay the institutionalization of small numbers of patients with the disease. Knowing about the principle of utility does not make allocation decisions easy!

The Principle of Autonomy

The principle of autonomy states that "rational individuals should be permitted to be self-determining."[7(p40)] Suppose that your elderly mother owns and lives alone in a house that badly needs a new roof. She indicates that it doesn't rain often, that it only leaks in the formal dining room, and that she won't live long enough to get her money's worth out of a new roof. Your respect for her autonomy indicates that you should respect her decision to determine whether her roof will be repaired. However, you may believe that since the house is your mother's primary financial asset and may be used to pay for eventual health care for her, she will benefit from the preservation of the structural stability of that asset, even if you must violate her autonomy by hiring a roofer yourself. This violation of the principle of autonomy "for someone's own good" is known as paternalism.

Autonomy issues in patient treatment and research revolve around the concept of informed consent. Informed consent is an essential component of the research process and is therefore discussed in detail in the following section.

▮ INFORMED CONSENT

Informed consent requires that patients or subjects give permission for treatment or testing, and that they be given adequate information in order to make educated decisions about undergoing the treatment or test. Four components are required for true autonomy in making either health care or research participation decisions: disclosure, comprehension, voluntariness, and competence.[8]

Information about treatment or research is needed before a patient or subject can make an informed decision from among several treatment options. Disclosure of treatment details should include the nature of the condition, the long-term effects of the condition, the effects of not treating the condition, the nature of available treatment procedures, anticipated benefits of any procedures, the probability of actually achieving these benefits, and potential risks of undergoing the procedure. Time commitments related to the treatment should be detailed, as should cost of the treatment. For patients, providing this information may be verbal or written. The therapist explains the evaluative procedures to the patient, proceeds with an evaluation if the patient agrees, and then outlines the planned course of treatment to the patient. The patient may determine that the time needed for treatment is not worth the anticipated benefit and may not proceed with treatment.

Disclosure of research details involves many of the same information items, depending on the nature of the research. Because research is usually not for the immediate benefit of the participant, more formal protection of the research subject is required than is needed for the patient. Thus, information about research risks and potential benefits must be written.

However, disclosing information is not enough. The practitioner or researcher must ensure that the patient or subject comprehends the information given. Physical therapists who are sensitive to the comprehension issue describe procedures in lay language, prepare written materials that are visually appealing, provide ample time for explanation of procedures and for answering questions, and allow ample time before requiring a participation decision.

The clinician or researcher also needs to ensure the voluntariness, or freedom from coercion, of consent. If free health care is offered in exchange for participation in a research study, will a poor family's decision to participate be truly voluntary? When a physical therapist requests that a man who is a patient participate in a study, and ensures him that his care will not suffer if he chooses not to participate, is it unreasonable for the patient to feel coerced based on the presumption that there might be subtle consequences of not participating? Practitioners and researchers need to be sensitive to real or perceived coercive influences faced by their patients or subjects.

Competence is the final component of informed consent. One must determine whether potential patients or subjects are legally empowered to make decisions for themselves. Consent from the legal guardian must be sought for minor children. If a legal guardian has been appointed for individuals who are mentally ill, mentally retarded, or incompetent, then consent must be sought from this party. When conducting research with populations in whom "proxy" consent is required, the researcher should also consider the views of the subjects themselves. This should be done especially if it appears that they can make informed decisions about participation even though they do not have the legal power to do so.[9] Suppose that a physical therapist wishes to study the differences between in-class and out-of-class therapy for public school children with cerebral palsy. If out-of-class therapy has been the norm, a boy who voices a preference for out-of-class treatment should not be required to be a member of the in-class group even though his parents have given permission for him to be assigned to either group.

The opposite problem occurs when a group is legally empowered to make decisions, but the characteristics of the group make informed consent difficult or impossible. For example, at state institutions for developmentally disabled adults, many of the residents may be their own legal guardians, with the legal ability to make their own decisions about participation in many activities. They might, however, be unable to comprehend the risks and potential benefits of participation in a research project, and therefore any consent they gave would not be informed.

■ RESEARCH CODES OF ETHICS

The general moral principles of action discussed earlier become formalized when they are developed into codes of ethics to guide the practice of

various professionals. There are four codes of ethics that can provide physical therapy researchers with guidance on ethical issues. The first of these is the Nuremberg Code developed in 1949 as a reaction to Nazi atrocities in the name of research.[3] The second is the World Medical Association's Declaration of Helsinki developed in 1964 and modified in 1975.[4] The third is the US federal government's Department of Health and Human Services (DHHS) regulations which govern research conducted or funded by the department.[5] The fourth document is the *Integrity in Physical Therapy Research* document adopted by the APTA in 1987 and under revision in 1998.[2] The Nuremberg, Helsinki, and DHHS documents are reproduced in their entirety in Levine's *Ethics and Regulation of Clinical Research.*[10]

Seven distinct ethical themes can be gleaned from these documents; most are present in at least two of the four documents. The themes are informed consent, whether the research design justifies the study, avoidance of suffering and injury, risks commensurate with potential benefit, independent review of research protocols, integrity in publication, and explicit attention to ethics.

Informed Consent

One principle common to all the documents is that of voluntary consent of the individual participating in the research. The responsibility for ensuring the quality of consent is with the individual who "initiates, directs, or engages in"[3(p426)] the experiment. This means that the very important issues of consent should be handled by an involved researcher. Using clerical staff to distribute and collect informed consent forms does not meet this requirement. In addition to securing the consent of their human research participants, researchers should treat animal subjects humanely[2] and respect the environment[4] in the course of their research. Box 3–1 highlights the Tuskegee Syphilis Study, an

Tuskegee Syphilis Study[11]

The Tuskegee Syphilis Study, spanning 40 years from 1932 to 1972, is one of the most infamous cases of ethical abuses in health care research within the United States. The study was conducted by the US Public Health Service in cooperation with a variety of other agencies, including the Alabama State Department of Health, the Macon County Health Department, and the Tuskegee Institute. The basic fact of the case is that approximately 400 black men with syphilis were left untreated for 40 years to study the "natural history" of the disease. Participants did not realize that they were being studied, did not know that they were being tested for syphilis, were not informed of the results of testing, and were not aware that treatment was being withheld.

Miss Eunice Rivers, a young black nurse, coordinated data collection within the study. She played a critical role by establishing credibility with participants and providing continuity throughout the extended study. The study itself involved physical examination of the men, radiographs, lumbar punctures, minimal treatment for the syphilis, and a variety of "perks" for participants, including free aspirin and tonics, burial funds, and some health care for their families. Therefore, Nurse Rivers both coordinated the nontreatment study and also played an important public health role within the rural black community in Macon County.

There were several points at which it might have been "natural" to discontinue the study. The first was in the early 1940s when penicillin became available. If the researchers could justify the early years of the study because of the equivocal effectiveness of the then-available treatments for syphilis, they could no longer use this justification once penicillin became a known treatment. A second natural opportunity to stop the study and provide treatment to participants also occurred during the early 1940s when many participants received draft notices for World War II. If a man who was drafted was found to have syphilis, protocol indicated that he should receive treatment for the disease. However, special exceptions to this protocol were made for members of the Tuskegee study, who were neither inducted into service nor treated for their syphilis.

The problems with the study were exposed in 1972, nearly 40 years after its initiation. Hearings about the study resulted in the development of revised procedures for federally sponsored human experimentation. Contemporary guidelines under which most institutional review boards operate today are based on these post-Tuskegee regulations. Ultimately, surviving participants were provided with comprehensive medical care and cash settlements and the heirs of deceased participants received cash settlements.

The Tuskegee experiment inspired the play *Miss Evers' Boys*,[12] which reminds us that responsible scientific inquiry rests on the moral choices of individual researchers:

Miss Evers [representing Nurse Rivers]: There was no treatment. Nothing to my mind that would have helped more than it hurt.

Caleb [representing a participant]: Maybe not in '33. But what about '46 and that penicillin. That leaves every year, every month, every day, every second right up to today to make a choice. It only takes a second to make a choice.

important historical example documented in both a book[11] and a play,[12] in which the informed consent process was violated in a particularly egregious way.

Design Justifies Study

A link exists between research methodology and research ethics: "The experiment should be so designed . . . that the anticipated results will justify the performance of the experiment."[3(p426)] The implication is that it is not appropriate to expose humans to risks for a study that is so poorly designed that the stated purposes of the research cannot be achieved. This, then, is essentially a utility issue: Why expose people to risk if the probability of benefit is low?

Avoidance of Suffering and Injury

Avoidance of suffering and injury is a nonmaleficence concern. Risks can be avoided through careful consideration during the design of a study, and by careful protection of physical safety and avoidance of mental duress during the implementation of the study. A safety concern in the design phase of a study might occur for researchers deciding how to quantify the effects of exercise on the quadriceps femoris muscle. They might consider using various histologic, strength, radiologic, or girth measures to document change. The final decision about which measures to use would depend both on the specific research questions and on which measures are likely to cause the least amount of suffering or injury.

Safety issues during research implementation would arise if one were evaluating the gait of patients with hemiplegia when walking on a treadmill. Adequate personnel to act as spotters would be needed, as would someone to monitor blood pressure and electrocardiographic changes.

Privacy during evaluation and treatment, and confidentiality of results can also be considered here as an issue of prevention of mental suffering. Seemingly innocuous portions of the research protocol may be stressful to the subject. For example, a protocol that requires documentation of weight may be acceptable to a subject if the measure is taken and recorded by only one researcher. The same subject may be extremely uncomfortable with a protocol in which the body weight is recorded on a data sheet that ac-

companies the subject to five different measurement stations for viewing by five separate researchers.

A final component of the safety issue is that the researcher must terminate the study, or an individual's participation in the study, if injury or harm becomes apparent. A relatively recent tragic drug trial was halted after five patients died of liver failure and two patients survived only after receiving liver transplants after taking long-term doses of the drug fialuridine to treat hepatitis B.[13] Although the injury or harm that may occur in physical therapy research is less dramatic than liver failure and death, researchers must still conduct their trials in ways that allow them to identify safety concerns in a timely fashion.

Risk Is Commensurate with Potential Benefit

High-risk activities can only be justified if the potential for benefit is also great. Levine noted that researchers are usually quick to identify potential benefits of their research, without always considering carefully all the potential risks to participants.[6] Because of the subtle nature of many risks, and the duty of researchers to minimize and consider all risks, the last section of this chapter presents an analysis of risks associated with research.

Independent Review

Adequate protection of human subjects requires that a body independent of the researcher review the protocol and assess the level of protection afforded to the human subjects. The generic name for such an independent body is an *institutional review board* (IRB). The IRB's charge is to examine research proposals to ensure that there is adequate protection of human subjects in terms of safety and confidentiality, that the elements of informed consent are present, and that the risks of the study are commensurate with the potential benefits. Specific information about the nature of these committees and the procedures for putting the principles of informed consent into action are covered in Chapter 27.

Publication Integrity

Researchers need to ensure the accuracy of reports of their work, should not present other's work as their own, and should acknowledge any financial support or other assistance received during the conduct of a research study. Chapter 28 provides specific guidelines for determining who should be listed as a study author, and how to acknowledge the participation of those who are not authors.

Explicit Attention to Ethics

Researchers need to give explicit attention to ethical principles when they design, implement, and report their research. Researchers should act to change research projects for which they are responsible if ethical problems arise, or should dissociate themselves from projects if they have no control over unethical acts.[2] For example, assume that a physical therapist is collecting data in a study that is under the direction of a physician. If the therapist believes that patient consent is being coerced, he or she should seek to change the consent procedure with the physician directly, discuss his or her concerns with the institutional review board that approved the study, or refuse to participate further if no change occurs.

■ RESEARCH RISKS

Much of the discussion in this chapter has been related in some way to risk-benefit analysis. The risks of research can be categorized as physical, psychological, social, and economic.[6] Each category is described, and examples from the physical therapy literature are presented when available.

Physical Risks

The physical risk associated with some research is well-known. When a particular risk is known, subjects should be informed of its likelihood, severity, duration, and reversibility. Methods for treating the physical harm should also be discussed if appropriate. If a strengthening study uses isokinetic equipment to provide an eccentric overload stimulus to hamstring musculature, participants need to know that almost all will develop delayed muscle soreness, that it appears within 2 days after exercise, and typically lasts up to 8 days.[14] A higher-risk procedure, such as an invasive muscle biopsy, might include the risk of infection. Participants should receive information about signs and symptoms of infection, and procedures to follow if infection occurs.

A more subtle form of physical risk is the effect of not receiving treatment. Subjects who agree to receive an experimental treatment may be asked to discontinue a treatment of known effectiveness in favor of a treatment with unknown benefits and risks. Subjects who are placed in a control group are often deprived of the benefits of the accepted treatment for the condition in question. A report by Snyder-Mackler and colleagues provides an example of a study in which discontinuance of accepted treatment was not considered acceptable by the institutional review board of one of the hospitals at which the study took place. This was resolved by having the control group receive traditional physical therapy and the experimental group receive both traditional physical therapy and the helium-neon laser irradiation that was the modality under study.[15]

Risks of research may be population specific. For example, treatments such as the use of ultrasound over epiphyseal plates are relatively low risk in adults but may have high risks for children.[16] When delineating the risks of participation in a given study, researchers must consider whether the procedures they are using pose special risks to the population they are studying.

Physical risks of an intervention are not always known or may not become apparent for long periods of time. For example, the use of "twister" cables in the treatment of rotational hip deformities is now thought to cause femoral anteversion; this risk was not known when twisters were originally used.[17] Researchers must always consider whether the potential benefit of a study is proportional to its long-term or hidden risks.

Psychological Risks

Although physical therapy researchers naturally focus on the physical risks of their research, they must also consider psychological risks. Subject selection that requires normality can cause psychological harm to those identified as abnormal. Subjects receiving an experimental treatment may lie awake nights wondering what untoward effects they may experience. Subjects in the hypothetical anterior cruciate ligament study described earlier in this chapter may experience guilt if their reconstruction fails and the need for a second reconstruction disrupts family or work life. Subjects in studies that investigate sensitive topics may have emotional reactions to data collection efforts.[18] Researchers must carefully consider ways to minimize the psychological risks to participants in their studies.

Social Risks

The major social risk to individual research subjects is the breach of confidentiality. For example, a participant in a work-hardening study that classified test results as valid (subjects exerting full effort) or invalid (subject not exerting full effort) might have difficulty gaining future employment if labeled a malingerer.

Another confidentiality concern relates to the manner in which subjects are identified for the research. Patients who received a mailed questionnaire from a researcher not connected with their care might understandably wonder how the investigator received their name, and whether their name and address will be put to other uses.

Economic Risks

When research has a combined knowledge and treatment effect, at least some portion of the payment for the research will be the responsibility of subjects or the subjects' health care insurers. Even if the treatment in question is not experimental, the participant may incur additional costs through lost work hours, baby-sitting fees while undergoing treatment, and transportation costs to and from the research facility.

A major source of economic risk associated with research involves the cost of care related to negative outcomes of research. Levine indicates that current ethical thought is that researchers should provide compensation for untoward effects of their research. He notes, though, that few centers have taken the initiative to develop a system for accomplishing this compensation.[10]

■ SUMMARY

The differences between practice and research demand that the participants in research receive special protection from the risks associated with research. The general moral principles of nonmaleficence, beneficence, utility, and autonomy form the base on which research codes of ethics are built. Informed consent requires that participation be a voluntary action taken by a competent individual who comprehends the risks and benefits of research participation as disclosed by the researcher. In addition to securing the informed consent of their subjects, researchers must ensure that the design of a study justifies its conduct, that procedures are designed to minimize risk, that risk is commensurate with potential benefits, that an independent review body has approved the conduct of the research, that integrity is maintained in publication of the research, and that careful consideration is given to all ethical concerns related to the study. The risks associated with research may be physical, psychological, social, and economic.

REFERENCES

1. American Physical Therapy Association. Code of Ethics. *Phys Ther.* 1998;78:107–110.
2. American Physical Therapy Association. *Integrity in Physical Therapy Research.* Alexandria, Va: American Physical Therapy Association; 1987.
3. The Nuremberg Code. Trials of War Criminals before the Nuremberg Military Tribunals under Control Council Law No. 10, Vol 2. Washington, DC: US Government Printing Office; 1949:181–182. In: Levine RJ, ed. *Ethics and Regulation of Clinical Research.* 2nd ed. New Haven, Conn: Yale University Press; 1988:425–426.
4. World Medical Association. Declaration of Helsinki: Recommendations Guiding Medical Doctors in Biomedical Research Involving Human Subjects. Tokyo, Japan: 29th World Assembly; 1975. In: Levine RJ, ed. *Ethics and Regulation of Clinical Research.* 2nd ed. New Haven, Conn: Yale University Press; 1988:427–429.
5. Department of Health and Human Services Rules and Regulations, 45 CFR 46. Federal Register, March 8, 1983. In: Levine RJ, ed. *Ethics and Regulation of Clinical Research.* 2nd ed. New Haven, Conn: Yale University Press; 1988:393–412.
6. Levine RJ. The boundaries between biomedical or behavioral research and the accepted and routine practice of medicine. In: The National Commission for the Protection of Human Subjects of Biomedical and Behavioral Research. *The Belmont Report: Ethical Principles and Guidelines for the Protection of Human Subjects of Research, Appendix Volume I.* Washington, DC: US Government Printing Office; 1975. DHEW Publication OS 78-0013.
7. Munson R. *Intervention and Reflection: Basic Issues in Medical Ethics.* 5th ed. Belmont, Calif: Wadsworth Publishing Co; 1996.
8. Sim J. Informed consent: ethical implications for physiotherapy. *Physiotherapy.* 1986;72:584–587.
9. Thurber FW, Deatrick JA, Grey M. Children's participation in research: their right to consent. *J Pediatr Nurs.* 1992;7:165–170.
10. Levine RJ. *Ethics and Regulation of Clinical Research.* 2nd ed. New Haven, Conn: Yale University Press; 1988: 159.
11. Jones JH. *Bad Blood: The Tuskegee Syphilis Experiment.* New and expanded ed. New York, NY: Maxwell McMillan International; 1993.
12. Feldshuh D. *Miss Evers' Boys.* Acting ed. New York, NY: Dramatists Play Service; 1995.
13. Thompson L. The cure that killed. *Discover.* 1994;15: 56,58,60–62.
14. Kellis E, Baltzopoulos V. Isokinetic eccentric exercise. *Sports Med.* 1995;19:202–222.
15. Snyder-Mackler L, Barry AJ, Perkins AI, Soucek MD. Effects of helium-neon laser irradiation on skin resistance and pain in patients with trigger points in the neck or back. *Phys Ther.* 1989;69:336–341.
16. McDiarmid T, Ziskin MC, Michlovitz SL. Therapeutic US. In: Michlovitz SL, ed. *Thermal Agents in Rehabilitation.* 3rd ed. Philadelphia, Pa: FA Davis Co; 1996:168–212.
17. Rose GK. *Orthotics: Principles and Practice.* London: William Heinemann Medical Books; 1986:52.
18. Cowles KV. Issues in qualitative research on sensitive topics. *West J Nurs Res.* 1988;10:163–179.

Research Design

4

Research Problems, Questions, and Hypotheses

Developing Answerable Research Questions

Topic Identification and Selection

Problem Identification and Selection

Action-Knowledge Conflict

Knowledge-Knowledge Conflict

Policy-Action Conflict

Knowledge Void

Theoretical Framework Identification and Selection

Question Identification and Selection

Research Methods Identification and Selection

Criteria for Evaluating Research Problems

Study Is Feasible

Problem Is Interesting

Problem Is Novel

Problem Can Be Studied Ethically

Question Is Relevant

The first step in any research venture is to define the problem that is to be studied. The clarity with which a researcher views the problem at hand will greatly influence each and every subsequent step of the research process. Researchers should therefore devote a great deal of intellectual energy to developing their research problems. The purpose of this chapter is to present strategies to facilitate problem and question development and to advance criteria for determining whether a question has promise as a basis for research.

■ DEVELOPING ANSWERABLE RESEARCH PROBLEMS

"The challenge in searching for a research question is not a shortage of uncertainties in the universe; it is the difficulty of finding an *important* one that can be transformed into a *feasible* and valid **study plan** [emphasis in original]."[1(p12)] Novice researchers usually have little difficulty identifying a general topic of interest: "I want to do something with the knee" or "My interest is in children with cerebral palsy." From these general statements of interest, novice researchers often take a giant leap directly into asking research questions: "What is the relationship between hamstring strength and knee stability in patients with anterior cruciate ligament tears?" "Does use of ice massage improve hip range of motion in children with spastic diplegia?"

The answers to these questions may well be important to advancing the body of knowledge in physical therapy. Moving directly from topic to question, however, does not establish that the questions are relevant to problems within the profession. This leap also fails to place the research question in a theoretical context. At the inception of a research project, researchers need to focus on broad *problems* within the profession, rather than on narrow questions they would like to answer. By focusing on problems, researchers are more likely to develop relevant questions, and their research is more likely to benefit both the researcher and the profession. The process of moving from a general topic to a specific research question involves four sets of ideas: topic identification and selection, problem identification and selection, theoretical framework identification and selection, and question identification and selection. A fifth step, determining the research methods, flows from the development of the ideas in previous four steps. For each step in the process researchers must first be creative enough to generate many ideas, and then must be selective enough to focus on a limited number of ideas for further study. Figure 4–1 shows this process. Each diamond represents an expansion and contraction of ideas; the ovals represent the idea selected for further development; and each row of the figure represents one expansion-contraction cycle. The background of the figure (shaded rectangle) is the professional literature, which guides the entire problem development process.

Topic Identification and Selection

As noted earlier, selection of a general topic is usually not a problem for researchers. For those

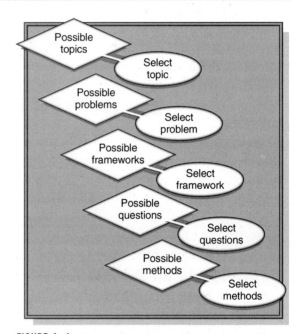

FIGURE 4–1. Research problem development. The diamonds represent the expansion and contraction of ideas; the ovals represent selection of an idea for further development; and the shaded rectangle in the background represents the professional literature that is the foundation on which all problems are built.

who cannot identify a general area of interest, direction should come from reading widely in the literature and discussing problems with colleagues until a spark of interest is found. From all the possible topics considered by a researcher, one is selected for further study. For example, a therapist who begins a new job at a work conditioning center might quickly identify several areas of possible study: the role of cardiovascular conditioning in return to work, the use of back belts on the job, or the concept of injury legitimacy. Note that while focused on one area of practice, all of the topics are relatively broad because the therapist does not yet know what is and is not known about each topic. Finding out more about each will allow the therapist to determine which topics seem most likely to yield interesting and feasible research possibilities. The therapist in this example chooses to study the use of back belts on the job, thereby completing the first of the four cycles of expansion (identification of many possible topics) and contraction (selection of a single topic from the many) of ideas that takes place during the development of a research question.

Problem Identification and Selection

After a topic is selected, it is the job of the researcher to articulate important problems related to that topic area. Problems, whether in daily life or in research, are perplexing situations without clear solutions. The purpose of research in physical therapy is to shed light on the perplexing situations of the profession.

One way of articulating research problems is to develop a series of logical statements that can be thought of as "givens," "howevers," and "therefores." The "given" is a statement of information that is generally accepted as true. The "however" contradicts or casts doubt on the "given." The conflict between the "givens" and the "howevers" creates the perplexing situation that is the research problem. The perplexing situation leads, "therefore," to the development of a research question. The conflicts that lead to research questions may be between actions, policies, or knowledge, as articulated by Clark.[2] In the following quotes from published research studies the terms "given," "however," and "therefore" are inserted to allow the reader to see how the authors have used this logical process to identify their problems of interest.

ACTION-KNOWLEDGE CONFLICT. These conflicts arise when practitioners act in ways that are not consistent with the formal knowledge of the profession:

> [GIVEN:] Back supports or back belts recently have been marketed as a significant aid in the prevention of low back pain. [HOWEVER,] the scientific literature does not confirm their benefit. [THEREFORE,] more substantial work in this area is needed before the approach can be considered acceptable.[3(p1271)]

> [GIVEN:] According to conventional physical therapy practice, therapeutic ultrasound (US) should not be used on patients with cancer because of the possibility of exacerbating tumor growth. [HOWEVER,] this contention is not adequately supported in the scientific literature. . . . [THEREFORE,] the purpose of our study was to determine whether the application of continuous therapeutic US would alter the growth or metastasis of [a sarcoma] in mice.[4(pp3,5)]

KNOWLEDGE-KNOWLEDGE CONFLICT. The conflict here is between different types of knowledge, in this example, between experiential knowledge and scientifically based knowledge:

> [GIVEN:] The scheme of selective tension testing proposed by Cyriax is a clinical system of diagnosis of painful problems of soft tissues. . . . The validity of the scheme is grounded in theory and extensive clinical observation. [HOWEVER,] it has not been studied objectively or empirically. . . . [THEREFORE,] the primary purpose of our study was to begin the examination of the construct validity of the Cyriax system of soft tissue diagnosis.[5(pp697,699)]

POLICY-ACTION CONFLICT. This type of conflict examines the relationship between professional actions and internal or external rules:

> [GIVEN:] [There are] reports of widespread use of physical therapy aides to deliver patient treatment. . . . [HOWEVER,] controversy surround[s] this practice. [THEREFORE,] we wished to obtain a baseline of information about the practices and opinions of physical therapists within our state relative to utilization of on-the-job-trained support personnel.[6(p422)]

KNOWLEDGE VOID. This type of problem is generated because of a void, rather than a conflict:

> [GIVEN:] Several studies have demonstrated that mobilization of the cervical spine can aid or reduce the occurrence of cervical headaches. [HOWEVER,] few studies have isolated treatment to just the upper cervical joints. [THEREFORE,] the purpose of this study was to examine the effect of mobilization of the upper cervical spine on frequency, duration, and intensity of cervical headaches.[7(p186)]

[GIVEN:] The most common complications after hip arthroplasty surgery are dislocation of the prosthesis, local infection, and loosening. . . . Many studies have reported on the rate of hip dislocation in acute hospitals. [HOWEVER,] there have been no studies reporting on the incidence of dislocation in rehabilitation hospitals. . . . [THEREFORE,] this study was undertaken as a first step toward understanding hip dislocation in the rehabilitation setting."[8(p444)]

As shown by the examples just presented, a problem cannot be defined until the researcher understands what is or is not known (the "givens" and "howevers") about the topic area of interest. Any given topic will yield many potentially researchable conflicts. Identifying and then selecting from among these potential problems is the second of the series of expansion and contraction of ideas that must occur before a research study is designed. The conflicts and voids that form the basis for research problems can be identified through a review of the professional literature. Details about finding relevant literature and synthesizing the results are presented in Chapters 25 and 26.

Theoretical Framework Identification and Selection

Once a problem is selected, it needs to be placed into a theoretical framework that will allow it to be viewed in relation to other research. The literature review that was conducted to establish the problem was likely to be fairly narrowly focused on the topic at hand. In contrast, the theoretical grounding provides a much broader perspective from which to view the problem. Defining and selecting a theoretical framework for the study is the third cycle of expansion (identification of possible frameworks) and contraction (selection of a framework) of ideas within the problem development process. Sometimes a researcher will be drawn to a particular framework based on previous interests or education; other times the researcher will need to read widely in several areas in order to settle

on a framework that seems most promising for further study.

One of the example problems presented earlier was based on the conflict between the popular use of back supports to prevent low back pain and the lack of scientific evidence of their effectiveness.[3] One theoretical framework for thinking about the use and effectiveness of back supports might be thought of as a biomechanical framework, presented schematically in Figure 4–2. In this framework, back supports are viewed as biomechanical devices that increase intraabdominal pressure and decrease compressive load on the spine. Studying back supports from this biomechanical perspective would involve defining variables related to the framework. For example, if back supports decrease compressive loads on the spine, then demands on back extensor muscles should be reduced. If demands on back extensors are reduced when wearing a back support, then endurance of back extensors should be enhanced. This approach to the study of the effect of back supports was used by Ciriello and Snook.[3] Choosing a biomechanical framework had several implications for their study. First, the back support they studied needed to be a rigid enclosure belt that would provide the type of abdominal compression indicated in the model. Flexible supports that provide a reminder to lift carefully, but do not offer a great

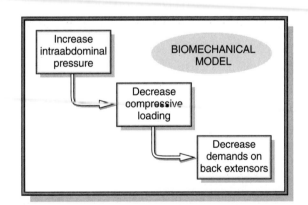

FIGURE 4–2. Biomechanical framework for studying back supports.

deal of abdominal compression, would not be appropriate for study using this biomechanical framework. Second, the measured variables within the study needed to represent back extensor endurance. Variables such as injury rates and time lost to back injuries when using back supports may be interesting—but they are not relevant when viewing back supports from this biomechanical framework.

This biomechanical approach to the study of the use and effectiveness of back supports is not, however, the only way to conceptualize this topic. For example, other researchers might prefer to work from a health promotion framework, shown in Figure 4–3. In such a framework, use of back supports would be viewed through a lens that looks at health promotion behaviors in the workplace as the result of the convergence of a complex set of cognitive factors (for example, the perceived level of control

that workers have over health in the workplace) and modifying factors (e.g., situational factors such as the consequences of violating company policies about the use of safety equipment on the job).[9] Researchers who use this framework for thinking about the use and effectiveness of back supports would likely measure worker behaviors and beliefs, rather than physical factors such as endurance of back extensors. While the biomechanical framework may show the physiological effects of the back support, the health promotion model may shed light on factors that would increase usage of the device among workers.

Adopting a theoretical framework, then, is a way of choosing a lens through which one views the problem of interest. The framework helps the researcher define what will and will not be studied and helps the researcher select appropriate variables for study.

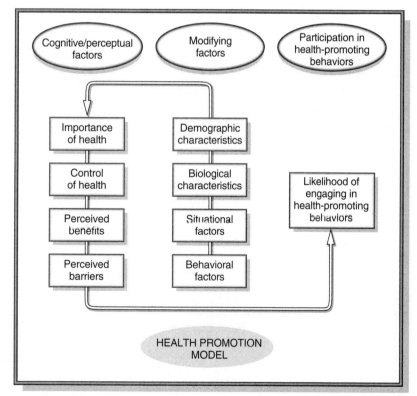

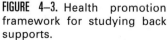 **FIGURE 4–3.** Health promotion framework for studying back supports.

Question Identification and Selection

Once the problem is identified and placed in a theoretical perspective, the researcher must develop the specific questions that will be studied. This is done through the fourth cycle of expansion (identification of many possible questions) and contraction (selection of a limited number of questions for study) of ideas within the problem development process. The biomechanical framework for studying the use and effectiveness of back supports might yield the following research questions:

1. Do back supports increase intraabdominal pressure?
2. How well do different back supports unload the spine?
3. Are the strength and endurance characteristics of back extensor muscles different for workers who do and do not wear back supports on the job?
4. Do back supports preserve the endurance characteristics of back extensor muscles?

Others could be generated, but four are enough to demonstrate the types of questions suggested by the framework. Some researchers prefer to state the purpose of their study as a question, others prefer to state their purpose as an objective, which takes the form of a declarative sentence. Ciriello and Snook studied question 3, above, but stated their purpose as an objective: "The study investigated whether back supports preserve the endurance characteristics of the back extensors, indirectly indicating decreased loading."[3(p1271)]

After stating their purpose as either a question or an objective, many researchers advance a *research hypothesis*. The research hypothesis is the researchers' educated guess about the outcome of the study. This educated guess is generally based on the theoretical grounding for the study, previous research results, or on the clinical experiences of the researchers. Ciriello and Snook advanced the following hypothesis in their study of back supports: "It was hypothe-

sized that there would be significant differences in the [endurance of back extensor muscles] as a result of wearing the back belt."[3(p1272)] Having such a hypothesis enables researchers to place their results into the context of the theory or experience that led them to conduct the study. Research hypotheses should not be confused with the statistical hypotheses within a study. The statistical hypotheses, subdivided into *null* and *alternate* hypotheses, are essentially given once a particular type of statistical analysis is selected. Statistical hypotheses are discussed in greater detail in Chapters 20 and 21.

Research Methods Identification and Selection

Only after the research question is determined can the investigator begin to consider which research methods are appropriate to answer the question. Research methods are discussed in detail in Chapters 5 through 16.

■ CRITERIA FOR EVALUATING RESEARCH PROBLEMS

While proceeding through the steps of research problem development, the researcher is faced with several selection decisions. Which topic, problem, or question should be studied? Which research approach to the question should be adopted? Cummings and associates[1(p14)] believe that a good research problem is feasible, interesting, novel, ethical, and relevant; the acronym FINER can be used to remember these five characteristics.

Study Is Feasible

Feasibility should be assessed in terms of subjects, equipment and technical expertise, time, and money. For example, if therapists wish to study differences between two electrical stimulation bicycle ergometry programs for patients with spinal cord injuries, they need to have access to adequate numbers of patients who will be willing to participate in a lengthy study. If the phenomenon of delayed muscle soreness is to be studied, subjects who are willing to experience soreness must be found.

Physical therapy researchers need to be realistic about the technical resources available to them. If a therapist wishes to study hindfoot movement during ambulation in different types of footwear, then motion analysis equipment is required. If the proper equipment is not available, then another problem should be selected for study.

The time needed to complete a research study is often underestimated. As noted in Chapter 1, lack of time is a significant impediment for clinical researchers. Therefore, clinicians need to develop research questions that can be answered within the time constraints of their clinics. Chapters on case reports (Chapter 12), single-system designs (Chapter 10), and outcomes research (Chapter 15) introduce research methods that may fit well within the context of a busy clinical practice.

Financial resources needed to conduct research must also be considered. Direct costs such as equipment, postage, and printing must be met. Personnel costs may include salaries and benefits for the primary investigator, data collectors, secretaries, statisticians, engineers, and photographers. If there are no funds for statisticians and engineering consultants, then complex experimental designs with highly technical measures should not be attempted.

Problem Is Interesting

The research question must be of interest to the investigator. Because physical therapy is a broad profession that is just beginning to articulate its research base, a wide range of interesting unanswered questions exists. All physical therapists should therefore be able to identify several questions that whet their intellectual appetites. The discovery that accompanies research is exciting—but several steps along the way are tedious and time-consuming. Thus, interest in the topic must be high to motivate the researcher to move through the drudgery to reach the discovery.

Problem Is Novel

Good research is novel in that it adds to knowledge. However, novice researchers are often unrealistic in their desire to be totally original in what they do. Novelty can be found in projects that confirm or refute previous findings, extend previous findings, or provide new findings.[1(p14)] Because many aspects of physical therapy are not well-documented, novel research ideas abound.

Problem Can Be Studied Ethically

An ethical study is one in which the elements of informed consent can be met and the risks of the research are in proportion to the potential benefits of the research, as described in Chapter 3. In the rehabilitation literature, for example, there are no experimental studies that compare a comprehensive rehabilitation program for patients who have had cerebral vascular accidents to a program consisting of no rehabilitation services. Such a protocol would be considered unethical because a totally untreated control group would be at risk for developing complications of bed rest or requiring extended care. Researchers overcome this ethical concern by comparing different levels of rehabilitation services, rather than completely depriving some patients of such care.

Question Is Relevant

When developing research questions, physical therapists need to answer an important relevancy question: "Who cares?" If the first phase of the problem development process was taken seriously, the researcher should be able to provide a ready answer to that question. If the researcher skipped that phase, and generated a research question without knowing how it related to a problem within the profession, then the question may not be relevant to physical therapy practice. Relevant physical therapy research questions are grounded in day-to-day problems faced by physical therapists.

■ SUMMARY

The research problem development process involves selection of a topic of interest, a problem within the profession, a theoretical framework for the study, and one or more specific questions related to the problem as conceptualized through the theoretical framework. The research hypothesis articulates the researchers' educated guess about the outcome of the study. Good research problems are feasible, interesting, novel, ethical, and relevant.

REFERENCES

1. Cummings SR, Browner WS, Hulley SB. Conceiving the research question. In: Hulley SB, Cummings SR, eds. *Designing Clinical Research*. Baltimore, Md: Williams & Wilkins; 1988.
2. Clark DL. Worksheet A—Statement of the Problem. Unpublished material. Charlottesville, Va: School of Education, University of Virginia; 1990.
3. Ciriello VM, Snook SH. The effect of back belts on lumbar muscle fatigue. *Spine*. 1995;20:1271–1278.
4. Sicard-Rosenbaum L, Lord D, Danoff JV, Thom AK, Eckhaus MA. Effects of continuous therapeutic ultrasound on growth and metastasis of subcutaneous murine tumors. *Phys Ther*. 1995;75:3–13.
5. Hayes KW, Petersen C, Falconer J. An examination of Cyriax's passive motion tests with patients having osteoarthritis of the knee. *Phys Ther*. 1994;74:697–709.
6. Bashi HL, Domholdt E. Use of support personnel for physical therapy treatment. *Phys Ther*. 1993;73:421–436.
7. Schoensee SK, Jensen G, Nicholson G, Gossman M, Katholi C. The effects of mobilization on cervical headaches. *J Orthop Sports Phys Ther*. 1995;21:184–196.
8. Krotenberg R, Stitik T, Johnston MV. Incidence of dislocation following hip arthroplasty for patients in the rehabilitation setting. *Am J Phys Med Rehabil*. 1995;74:444–447.
9. Pender NJ, Walker SN, Sechrist KR, Frank-Stromborg M. Predicting health-promoting lifestyles in the workplace. *Nurs Res*. 1990;39:326–332.

5

Research Paradigms

Quantitative Paradigm
  Assumptions of the Quantitative
    Paradigm
  Assumption 1
  Assumption 2
  Assumption 3
  Assumption 4
  Assumption 5
  Quantitative Methods
  Theory
  Selection
  Measurement
  Manipulation
  Control
Qualitative Paradigm
  Assumptions of the Qualitative
    Paradigm
  Assumption 1
  Assumption 2

Assumption 3
Assumption 4
Assumption 5
Qualitative Methods
Theory
Selection
Measurement
Manipulation and Control
Single-System Paradigm
  Assumptions of the Single-System
    Paradigm
  Single-System Methods
  Theory
  Selection
  Measurement
  Manipulation and Control
**Relationships Among the Research
Paradigms**

Knowledge is continually evolving. What was believed to be true yesterday may be doubted today, scorned tomorrow, and resurrected in the future. Just as knowledge itself evolves, beliefs about how to create knowledge also evolve. Our beliefs about the methods of obtaining knowledge constitute *research paradigms.*[1(p15)] The beliefs that constitute a paradigm are often so entrenched that researchers themselves do not question the assumptions that undergird the re-

search methodology they use. Although the details of the various research methods are presented in later chapters, this chapter is presented first to provide readers with a broad framework for thinking about the research paradigms that support those methods.

The dominant research paradigm within physical therapy is the quantitative paradigm. Two competing paradigms of importance to physical therapy are the qualitative and single-system paradigms. The study of competing research paradigms in physical therapy is important for two reasons. First, research based on the competing paradigms is reported in the physical therapy literature, so consumers of the literature need to be familiar with the assumptions that undergird these paradigms. Second, competing research paradigms in any discipline emerge because of the inability of the dominant paradigm to answer all the important questions of the discipline. Researchers therefore need to consider competing paradigm research not only in terms of the specific research questions addressed but also in terms of what the research implies about the limitations of the dominant paradigm.

The purpose of this chapter is to develop these three research paradigms for consideration. This is done by first emphasizing differences between the paradigms and later examining relationships among the paradigms. The quantitative paradigm is discussed first. This paradigm focuses on the study of groups whose treatment is often manipulated by the investigator. The qualitative paradigm is then discussed. This paradigm focuses on broad description and understanding of phenomena without direct manipulation. The final paradigm to be analyzed is the single-system paradigm, which focuses on individual responses to manipulation.

Deciding on the terminology to use for the different research paradigms is difficult. The paradigms are sometimes described in philosophical terms, sometimes in terms of components of the paradigm, and sometimes in terms of the methods that usually follow from the philosophical underpinnings of the paradigm. Table 5–1 presents the various names that have been used to identify what are being labeled in this chapter as quantitative, qualitative, and single-system paradigms. Accurate use of the different philosophical labels requires a strong background in the history and philosophy of science, backgrounds that most physical therapists do not have. To avoid imprecise use of the language of philosophy, the more "methodological" terms are used in this text rather than the more "philosophical" terms. This choice may, however, lead to the

TABLE 5–1	Alternate Names for the Three Research Paradigms	
Quantitative Paradigm	**Qualitative Paradigm**	**Single-System Paradigm**
Positivist	Naturalistic	Idiographic
Received view	Phenomeno-	N = 1
Logical	logical	Single-subject
positivist	Ethnographic	
Nomothetic	Idiographic	
Empiricist	Postpositivist	
	New paradigm	

misconception that paradigms and methods are interchangeable. They are not. A paradigm is defined by the assumptions and beliefs that guide researchers. A method is defined by the actions taken by investigators as they implement research. Adoption of a paradigm implies the use of certain methods but does not necessarily limit the researcher to those methods. Thus, research designs are specific ways of organizing methods within a study. The presentation of the assumptions of each paradigm is followed by general methodological implications of the paradigm. Later chapters present specific designs associated with these paradigms.

QUANTITATIVE PARADIGM

The quantitative paradigm is what has become known as the traditional method of science. The term *quantitative* comes from the emphasis on measurement that characterizes this paradigm. The paradigm has its roots in the 1600s with the development of Newtonian physics.[2,3] In the early 1900s the French philosopher Auguste Comte and a group of scientists in Vienna became proponents of related philosophical positions often labeled *positivism* or *logical positivism.*[4] This positivist philosophy is so labeled because of the central idea that one can only be certain, or positive, of knowledge that is verifiable through measurement and observation.

Assumptions of the Quantitative Paradigm

Just as there are multiple terms for each paradigm, there are multiple views about the critical components of each paradigm. Lincoln and Guba use five basic axioms to differentiate what they refer to as positivist and naturalistic paradigms.[1(p37)] Their five axioms are presented here as the basis of the quantitative paradigm. The qualitative and single-system paradigms are developed by retaining or replacing these with alternate axioms. Table 5–2 summarizes the assumptions of the three paradigms.

ASSUMPTION 1. The first assumption of the quantitative paradigm is that there is a single objective reality. One goal of quantitative research is to determine the nature of this reality through measurement and observation of the phenomena of interest. This reliance on observation is sometimes termed *empiricism.* A second goal of quantitative research is to predict or control reality. After all, if researchers can empirically determine laws that regulate reality in some predictable way, then they should be able to use this knowledge to attempt to influence that reality in equally predictable ways.

ASSUMPTION 2. The second basic assumption of the quantitative paradigm is that the investigator and subject, or object of inquiry, can be independent of one another. In other words, it is assumed that the investigator can be an unobtrusive observer of a reality that does not change by virtue of the fact that it is being studied. Researchers who adopt the quantitative paradigm do, however, recognize that it is sometimes difficult to achieve this independence. Rosenthal,[5] in his text on experimenter effects in behavioral research, related a classic story about "Clever Hans," a horse who could purportedly tap out the correct response to mathematical problems by tapping his hoof. Hans's skills intrigued a researcher, Pfungst, who tested Hans's abilities under different controlled conditions. Pfungst found that Hans could tap out the correct answer only when his questioner was a literate individual who knew the answer to the question. He found that knowledgeable questioners unconsciously raised their eyebrows, flared their nostrils, or raised their heads as Hans was coming up to the correct number of taps. Rosenthal notes:

> Hans' amazing talents . . . serve to illustrate further the power of self-fulfilling prophecy. Hans' questioners, even skeptical ones, expected Hans to give the correct answers to their queries. Their expectation was reflected in their unwitting signal to Hans that the time had come for him to stop his tapping. The signal cued Hans to stop, and the questioner's expectation became the reason for Hans' being, once again, correct.[5(p138)]

Despite the recognition of the difficulty of achieving the independence of the investigator and subject, the assumption of the quantitative paradigm is that it is possible and desirable to do so through a variety of procedures that isolate

TABLE 5–2 **Assumptions of the Three Research Paradigms**

	Paradigm		
Assumption	*Quantitative*	*Qualitative*	*Single-System*
Reality	Single, objective	Multiple, constructed	Single, objective
Relationship between investigator and subject	Independent	Dependent	Independent
Generalizability of findings	Desirable and possible	Situation specific	System specific
Cause-and-effect relationships	Causal	Noncausal	Causal
Values	Value free	Value bound	Value free

subjects and researchers from information that might influence their behavior. Ways to maximize this independence are presented in Chapter 6.

ASSUMPTION 3. The third basic assumption of the quantitative paradigm is that the goal of research is to develop generalizable characterizations of reality. The generalizability of a piece of research refers to its applicability to other subjects, times, and settings. The concept of generalizability leads to the classification of qualitative research as *nomothetic,* or relating to general or universal principles. Quantitative researchers recognize the limits of generalizability as threats to the validity (discussed in greater detail in Chapter 7) of a study; however, they believe that generalizability is an achievable aim and that research which fails to be reasonably generalizable is flawed.

ASSUMPTION 4. The fourth basic assumption of the quantitative paradigm is that causes and effects can be determined and differentiated from one another. Quantitative researchers are careful to differentiate experimental research from nonexperimental research on the basis that causal inferences can only be drawn if the researcher is able to manipulate an independent variable (the "presumed cause") in a controlled fashion while observing the effect of the manipulation on a dependent variable ("the presumed effect"). Quantitative researchers attempt to eliminate or control extraneous factors that might interfere with

the relationship between the independent and dependent variables (see Chapters 9 and 11 for more information on experimental and nonexperimental research).

ASSUMPTION 5. The final assumption of the quantitative paradigm is that research is value free. The controlled, objective nature of quantitative research is assumed to eliminate the influence of investigator opinions and societal norms on the facts that are discovered. Inquiry is seen as the objective discovery of truths and the investigator the impartial discoverer of these truths.

Quantitative Methods

The adoption of these quantitative assumptions has major implications for the methods of quantitative research. Five methodological issues are discussed in relation to the assumptions that underlie the quantitative paradigm: theory, selection, measurement, manipulation, and control. These issues are summarized in Table 5–3. Quotes from a single quantitative piece of research are used to illustrate the way in which each of these methodological issues is handled within the quantitative paradigm.

THEORY. The first methodological issue relates to the role of theory within a study. Qualitative researchers are expected to articulate an a priori theory, that is, theory developed in advance of the conduct of the research. The purpose of the

---

TABLE 5-3 Methods of the Three Research Paradigms			
	Paradigm		
Method	*Quantitative*	*Qualitative*	*Single-System*
Theory	A priori	Grounded	A priori
Number and selection of subjects	Groups, random	Small number, purposive	One, purposive
Measurement tools	Instruments	Human	Instruments
Type of data	Numerical	Language	Numerical
Manipulation	Present	Absent	Present
Control	Maximized	Minimized	Flexible

research is then to determine whether the components of the theory can be confirmed. This top-down notion of theory development was presented in Chapter 2 on theory and Chapter 4 on problem development. Delitto and associates'[6] comparison of the effectiveness of matched and unmatched treatments for acute low back syndrome is an experimental study in the quantitative tradition. As such, an a priori theoretical perspective guided the study:

> Many researchers and practitioners encourage classifying patients with LBS (low back syndrome) according to signs and symptoms. . . . A classification system can only be justified if (1) a clinician can examine and reliably assign the patient to a classification that directs care and (2) implementing the assigned treatment results in more efficacious management of patients than comparative, nonspecific management strategies.[6(p217)]

The elements of this informal theory are (1) that low back syndromes can be classified, and (2) that if treatments that match the classification can be implemented, then matched treatments should be more effective than the unmatched ones. The purpose of the study is to test the elements of this a priori theory.

SELECTION. The second methodological issue relates to the generalizability of the research. The elaborate sampling and assignment procedures adopted by Delitto and colleagues are expressions of the quantitative belief in the importance of generalizability:

> A subject had to improve in at least two extension movements and worsen with at least one flexion movement to be placed in the extension category. . . . To place a patient in a manipulation category we use a composite of three of four positive tests. Once the patients were placed in the extension-mobilization group, they were randomly assigned to either an experimental group (n = 14, matched and specifically directed) or a comparison group (n = 10, unmatched and nonspecific).[6(p218)]

When quantitative researchers cannot control the nature of their subjects as well as they might like, they (or their critics) usually express this concern as an unfortunate limitation of the research:

> In view of the significant differences between the treatment groups for age, and the obvious (although nonsignificant) differences in days since onset, we would have expected the authors [Delitto and colleagues] to control for these potential biases . . .[7(p223)]

MEASUREMENT. The third methodological issue relates to a desire for a high level of precision in measurements as an expression of the belief in an objective reality. A critic of Delitto and colleagues' study expressed his preference for more precise measures than the low back pain questionnaire used within the study:

> Movement testing and the pain response to movement testing are key elements to the authors' classification system. . . . Various goniometric devices are available for measuring flexion/extension quickly and reliably and thus provide for objective data to document any changes related to the two treatments tested.[8(p225)]

Measurement theory, presented later in this text, is largely based on the concept that researchers use imperfect measurement tools to estimate the "true" characteristics of a phenomenon of interest, and that the best measures are those that come closest to this "truth" on a consistent basis.

MANIPULATION. The fourth methodological issue is related to the role of manipulation within a study. Quantitative researchers believe that the best research is that which allows one to determine causes and effects in response to controlled manipulations of the experimenter. Although Delitto and colleagues do not use the words cause and effect in describing their results, the causal implication is clear:

> The results of this study support our hypothesis that a priori classification of certain patients with LBS followed by a matched, specifically defined conservative management strategy may result in a more effective outcome when compared with an unmatched, nonspecific treatment.[6(p220)]

Thus, they believe that the difference in outcome between their groups was caused by their manipulation of the treatment that was delivered to each group.

CONTROL. The fifth and final methodological issue is related to the control of extraneous factors within the research design. Delitto and colleagues, for example, attempted to control the extraneous factor of acuity by eliminating patients with chronic low back pain from their study. In addition, they controlled the frequency and timing of treatment within the study, requiring that patients return for retreatment and reevaluation at as close to 3-day and 5-day intervals as was possible. Because of this tight control, the types of patients studied by Delitto and colleagues, as well as the frequency and timing of the treatment provided, may not resemble the patients and treatment variables typically seen by clinicians. Researchers who adopt the quantitative paradigm generally believe that control of extraneous variables is critical to establishment of cause-and-effect relationships, even when such control leads to the implementation of experimental procedures that may not be fully representative of typical clinical practices.

These then, are examples of how five methodological issues—theory, selection and assignment, measurement, manipulation, and control—are handled by researchers who work within the framework of the quantitative paradigm.

QUALITATIVE PARADIGM

Just as the mechanistic view of Newtonian physics provided the roots for the development of the quantitative paradigm, the relativistic view of quantum mechanics provided the roots for the development of the qualitative paradigm. Zukav contrasted the "old," Newtonian physics with the "new," quantum physics:

The old physics assumes that there is an external world which exists apart from us. It further assumes that we can observe, measure, and speculate about the external world without changing it. . . . The new physics, quantum mechanics, tells us clearly that it is not possible to observe reality without changing it. If we observe a certain particle collision experiment, not only do we have no way of proving that the results would have been the same if we have not been watching it, all that we know indicates that it would not have been the same, because the results that we got were affected by the fact that we were looking for it.[2(pp30-31)]

Since the quantitative paradigm has proved inadequate even for the discipline of physics, a "hard" science, qualitative researchers argue that there is little justification for continuing to apply it to the "soft" sciences in which human behavior is studied.

Assumptions of the Qualitative Paradigm

The assumptions that form the basis for the qualitative paradigm are antithetical to the assumptions of the quantitative paradigm. Once again Lincoln and Guba's[1] concepts, but not their terminology, form the basis for this section of the chapter. What Lincoln and Guba label the *naturalistic paradigm* will be referred to in this text as the *qualitative paradigm*. Table 5–2 provides an overview of the assumptions of the qualitative paradigm.

ASSUMPTION 1. The first assumption of the qualitative paradigm is that the world consists of multiple constructed realities. "Multiple" means that there are always several versions of reality. "Constructed" means that participants attach meaning to events that occur within their lives, and that this meaning is an inseparable component of the events themselves. Refer to Box 5–1 for a simple test of the phenomenon of multiple constructed realities. It is easy to demonstrate how multiple constructed realities may be present within physical therapist–patient interactions. For example, if one man states that his therapist is cold and

---

BOX 5-1

Instructions: Count the number of "F"s in the quote below:

"FABULOUS FITNESS FOLLOWS FROM YEARS OF FREQUENT WORKOUTS COMBINED WITH FOCUSED FOOD CHOICES."

See solution at the end of the chapter.

---

unfeeling, that is his reality. If a woman states that the same therapist is professional and candid, that is her reality. The notion of a single, objective reality is rejected. Researchers who adopt the qualitative paradigm believe that it is fruitless to try to determine the therapist's "true" manner because the therapist's demeanor does not exist apart from how it is perceived by different patients.

ASSUMPTION 2. The second assumption of the qualitative paradigm is that investigator and subject are interdependent, that is, the process of inquiry itself changes both the investigator and the subject. While quantitative paradigm researchers seek to eliminate what is viewed as undesirable interdependence of investigator and subject, qualitative paradigm researchers accept this interdependence as inevitable and even desirable. For example, a qualitative researcher would recognize that a therapist who agrees to participate in a study of therapist demeanor is likely to change, at least in subtle ways, his or her demeanor during the period that he or she is observed.

ASSUMPTION 3. The third assumption of the qualitative paradigm is that knowledge is time and context dependent. Qualitative paradigm researchers reject the nomothetic approach and its concept of generalizability. In this sense, then, qualitative research is *idiographic,* meaning that it pertains to a particular case in a particular time and context. The goal of qualitative research is a deep understanding of the particular. Re-searchers who adopt the qualitative paradigm hope that this particular understanding may lead to insights about similar situations. While not generalizable in the quantitative tradition, themes or concepts found consistently in qualitative research with a small number of subjects may represent essential components of phenomena that, with further investigation, would also be found in larger samples.

ASSUMPTION 4. The fourth assumption of the qualitative paradigm is that it is impossible to distinguish causes from effects. The whole notion of cause is tied to the idea of prediction, control, and an objective reality. Researchers who adopt the qualitative paradigm believe it is more useful to describe and interpret events than it is to attempt to control them to establish oversimplified causes and effects. In the therapist demeanor example, qualitative researchers believe that it would be impossible to determine whether a certain therapist demeanor caused better patient outcomes or whether certain patient outcomes caused different therapist demeanors. Because of their belief in the inability to separate causes from effects, qualitative researchers would focus on describing the multiple forces that shape therapist-patient interactions.

ASSUMPTION 5. The fifth assumption of the qualitative paradigm is that inquiry is value bound. This value-ladenness is exemplified in the type of questions that are asked, the way in which constructs are defined and measured, and the interpretation of the results of research. The traditional view of scientists is that they are capable of "dispassionate judgment and unbiased inquiry."[9(p109)] Qualitative researchers, however, believe that all research is influenced by the values of the scientists who conduct research and the sources that fund research. The status of research about breast cancer provides one example of the value-ladenness of the research enterprise. During the late 1980s and early 1990s a study of pharmaceutical prevention of breast cancer was undertaken by the National Cancer Institute (Breast Cancer Prevention Trial). In an editorial, the president of the American Public Health Association eloquently expressed that association's concern about the values driving the study:

> I was dismayed that chemopreventive trials with their likely support from pharmaceuticals and other commercial interests, and seductive offer of quicker results may drive the research agenda. In our warranted zeal to decrease disability and death by cancer we may be unduly reluctant to pursue environmental and behavioral approaches. They may take longer to give results, but may ultimately provide the only applicable solutions.[10(p2)]

When the large-sample study showed promising results earlier than expected, the trial was discontinued, ostensibly to enable women beyond those in the study population to begin to reap the benefits of the treatment.[11] Cynics might wonder whether the "pharmaceutical and other commercial interests" played any role in influencing an early end to the study to enable earlier commercial production of the drug. Researchers who adopt the qualitative paradigm recognize that they are unable to separate values from inquiry. They do not believe that it is productive to pretend that science is objective, particularly in light of controversies such as that cited in the foregoing example.

Qualitative Methods

These five assumptions have an enormous impact on the conduct of qualitative paradigm re-

search. The roles of theory, selection, measurement, manipulation, and control are all vastly different in qualitative research than in quantitative research, as summarized in Table 5–3. Jensen and associates[12] used the qualitative paradigm to structure their study of the nature of therapist-patient interactions of novice and experienced clinicians. This study is used to provide examples of the methods that flow from adoption of the beliefs of the paradigm.

THEORY. The first methodological issue relates to the role of theory. Because researchers who adopt the qualitative paradigm accept the concept of multiple constructed realities, they do not begin their inquiry with a researcher-developed theoretical framework. They begin the research with an idea of what concepts or constructs may be important to an understanding of a certain phenomenon, but they recognize that the participants in the inquiry will define other versions of what is important. A rigid theoretical framework of the researcher would constrain the direction of the inquiry and might provide a less than full description of the phenomenon of interest. Jensen and colleagues express this need for flexible exploration in terms of a "black box":

> We call the therapeutic intervention the black box because we know so little about what happens between therapist and patient. The focus . . . was to begin to look at the black box and explore what actually happens during the time the patient is in the physical therapy clinical setting. . . . We anticipate that our original conceptual model [developed during the study being cited] will be altered many times as we gain in our knowledge of the work of the physical therapists.[12(pp315,322)]

SELECTION. The second methodological issue relates to the way in which subjects are selected. Rather than selecting a randomized group of individuals, qualitative researchers purposely select individuals who they believe will be able to lend insight to the research problem. Jensen and colleagues describe just such a method:

> A purposive sample was used. . . . We selected therapists on the basis of experience as a practic-

ing physical therapist. . . . At this initial level of investigation, our observations were of highly experienced and less experienced clinicians working with similar patient populations. These therapists were selected so that a variety of orthopedic outpatient settings were represented.[12(pp315,322)]

In this example, purposive sampling procedures led to the selection of only eight therapists from four settings. Most traditional quantitative researchers would find this sample to be insufficient because it would not likely be representative of a larger group and because small samples do not lend themselves to statistical analysis. These are not considered problems in qualitative research since representativeness and statistical analysis are not the goals of the inquiry.

MEASUREMENT. The third methodological issue relates to the primary measurement tool of qualitative research, the "human instrument." Because of the complexity of the multiple realities the qualitative researcher is seeking to describe, a reactive, thinking instrument is needed, as noted by Jensen and associates:

> We collected data through nonparticipant observation, recording of field notes, and audiotaping of each treatment session. . . . The field notes also included a rough sketch of the physical environment and a record of nonverbal activities including eye and hand contact between the therapist and the patient.[12(p316)]

The data collected in qualitative studies is usually not numerical, but, rather, is verbal and consists of feelings and perceptions rather than presumed facts. Researchers gather a great deal of descriptive data about the particular situation they are studying so that they can provide a "rich" or "thick" description of the situation. Since interpretation of the information is dependent on the time and context of the study, it is important that time and context information be well articulated.

MANIPULATION AND CONTROL. Fourth and fifth, the qualitative researcher does not manipulate or control the research setting. Rather, the setting is manipulated in unpredictable ways by the interaction between the investigator and the subjects. The mere fact that the researcher is present or asks certain questions is bound to influence the subjects and their perception of the situation.

The natural setting is used for research. Because everything is time and context dependent, researchers who adopt the qualitative paradigm believe there is little to be gained—and much to be lost—from creating an artificial study situation, as noted by Jensen and colleagues:

> We still have much to learn about professional practice, particularly investigations conducted within the natural practice environment. The wealth of knowledge embedded in the clinical actions of physical therapy practitioners is poorly understood.[12(p315)]

This belief about the importance of studying practice in a natural environment led Jensen and her colleagues to study therapist-patient pairs during the course of a routine day. These researchers would likely agree that their observation of treatment sessions changed the therapist-patient interactions in some ways. However, think of how much less natural the interactions would have been if the researchers had created an artificial environment in which each therapist had to deal with only one patient, free from the interruptions of the telephone, other patients, and colleagues. Researchers guided by the quantitative paradigm would generally try to create an artificial environment so that they could control these extraneous factors and focus on the interactions. These researchers, guided by the qualitative paradigm, viewed these factors as integral to patient-therapist interactions and described rather than controlled them:

> The more experienced therapists were observed to handle interruptions and tasks outside of direct treatment efficiently without disrupting the treatment session. . . . The novices we observed reacted quickly to most environmental stimuli such as intercom interruptions and patient scheduling tasks, often losing focus on direct patient care activities.[12(p320)]

It is clear from this example that these five methodological issues—theory, selection and assignment, measurement, manipulation, and control—are handled very differently within a qualitative framework compared to a quantitative one. Theory unfolds during the study instead of directing the study. Participants are selected for their unique contributions rather than for representativeness. Measurement is done with a "human instrument" who can react and redirect the data gathering process rather than being done with a standardized measurement protocol. The object of the study is observed rather than manipulated. And, finally, the setting for data collection is natural and uncontrolled rather than artificial and tightly controlled.

■ SINGLE-SYSTEM PARADIGM

The single-system paradigm developed out of a concern that the use of traditional group research methods focused away from the unit of clinical interest: the individual. Assume that a group study of the effectiveness of a particular gait training technique on gait velocity is implemented with 30 patients who have undergone transtibial amputation. If gait velocity improves for 10 patients, remains the same for 10 patients, and declines for 10 patients, then the average velocity for the group will not change very much and the group conclusion is likely to be that the treatment had no effect. This group conclusion ignores the fact that the treatment was effective for 10 patients but detrimental for 10 other patients. A clinically relevant conclusion might be that the treatment has the potential to improve velocity but that clinicians should also recognize that the opposite effect is also seen in some patients. An appropriate focus for future research would be the identification of those types of patients for whom this technique is effective. Unfortunately, this type of subgroup analysis rarely occurs, and practitioners are left with the general group conclusion that the new technique is not effective. Single-system research eliminates the group conclusion and focuses on treatment effects for individuals.

Table 5–1 lists several different names for single-system research. Ottenbacher[13(p45)] uses the term *single-system* rather than the more common *single-subject* because there are some instances in which the single unit of interest would itself be a group rather than an individual. For example, a physical therapy administrator might wish to study departmental productivity before and after a reorganization. If the concern was not with changes in individual therapist productivity, but only with the productivity of the department as a whole, then the effect of the reorganization could be studied as a single system. Because single system is a more inclusive term, it will be used throughout this text.

Assumptions of the Single-System Paradigm

The basic assumption of the single-system paradigm is that the effectiveness of treatment is subject and setting dependent. Single-system researchers believe that research should reflect the idiographic nature of practice by focusing on the study of individuals. With the exception of this focus on individuals rather than groups, the rest of the assumptions of the single-system paradigm are those of the quantitative paradigm, as shown in Table 5–2. In fact, the single-system paradigm focuses exclusively on experimental problems in which there is active manipulation of the individual under study.

The single-system paradigm is sometimes confused with the clinical case report or case study. The two are very different. The case report or case study is a description, very often a retrospective description, of a course of treatment of an individual (see Chapter 12). Single-system research, on the other hand, uses a systematic process of introduction and withdrawal of treatments to allow for controlled assessment of the effects of a treatment (see Chapter 10).

Single-System Methods

Because many assumptions are shared between the quantitative and single-system paradigms, many methods are shared as well, as shown in Table 5–3. Diamond and Ottenbacher's[14] study of the effect of a tone-inhibiting dynamic ankle-foot orthosis on stride characteristics of an adult with hemiparesis is used to illustrate these methods in practice. In this study, three walking conditions were compared: barefoot walking, a traditional plastic ankle-foot orthosis (AFO), and a tone-inhibiting ankle-foot orthosis (TIAFO).

THEORY. First, single-system paradigm research generally operates from an a priori theoretical foundation, as illustrated by a quote from Diamond and Ottenbacher:

> Based on available literature and clinical experience, we hypothesized that the TIAFO would be associated with the most normal stride.[14(p424)]

SELECTION. Second, selection of the individual for study is purposive. In the AFO study, the subject had discontinued use of a traditional AFO but continued to have gait difficulties. Thus, the TIAFO was prescribed as an alternative to an orthosis that had not met all of the subject's gait needs. Single-system researchers would not choose to study someone for whom they did not believe the intervention was uniquely appropriate. This is in contrast to the group approach in which 30 subjects who had had cerebral vascular accidents might all be studied with the TIAFO and the traditional AFO. How likely is it that all 30 of these subjects would have problems with the traditional AFO that would require trial of the TIAFO? If the TIAFO in such a study was not shown to be more effective than a traditional AFO, it might be because the group needs did not warrant the use of the TIAFO. The single-system paradigm requires that the individuals studied have a specific need for the treatment implemented.

MEASUREMENT. Third, precise measurement is an integral part of the single-system paradigm. Repeated measures taken during baseline and treatment phases are compared. Thus, measurement accuracy and reliability are critical to the ability to draw conclusions about the effects of treatment. This measurement focus is apparent in Diamond and Ottenbacher's study:

> Walking velocity (in meters per second) was measured by timing the subject with a stopwatch as he walked 11 m. Reliability of the velocity measurement was assessed by having two therapists record the time for the subject to ambulate a distance of 11 m during baseline trials.[14(p426)]

MANIPULATION AND CONTROL. Fourth, experimental manipulation is part of the definition of single-system research. This is illustrated in Diamond and Ottenbacher's[14] study by their manipulation of the conditions under which the subject walked: barefoot, with an AFO, and with a TIAFO. Finally, control of extraneous factors is important in the conduct of single-system research, as it was with quantitative research. Diamond and Ottenbacher[14] controlled the experimental setting by randomizing the presentation of the three gait conditions, and controlling the frequency of measurement sessions. Table 5–3 indicates, however, that the control in single-system paradigm research may be more flexible than that of traditional group designs. In group designs researchers usually attempt to control the nature of the treatment administered so that all individuals within the group receive approximately the same treatment. With the single-system designs, the treatment can be administered as it would be in the clinic. Thus, the intervention can be tailored to accommodate scheduling changes, status changes, or varying patient moods. Chapter 10 presents several designs that use the general methods associated with the single-system paradigm.

■ RELATIONSHIPS AMONG THE RESEARCH PARADIGMS

There are those who believe that the paradigms are mutually exclusive, that in adopting the assumptions of one paradigm the assumptions of the others must be forsaken. Lincoln and Guba make a case for the separateness of the quantitative and qualitative paradigms:

> Postpositivism is an entirely new paradigm, *not* reconcilable with the old. . . . We are dealing with an entirely new system of ideas based on fundamentally *different*—indeed sharply contrasting— assumptions. . . . What is needed is a transformation, not an add-on. That the world is round cannot be added to the idea that the world is flat [emphasis in original].[1(p33)]

A more moderate view is that the assumptions underlying the different paradigms are relative rather than absolute. Relative assumptions need not be applied to every situation; they can be applied when appropriate to a given research problem. Many authors believe that one paradigm is useful for some forms of study and other paradigms are useful for other forms of study.[15–17] This text adopts the moderate view that all forms of study have the potential to add to knowledge and understanding. The contrasting assumptions of the paradigms can be managed as we all manage many belief-action clashes on a daily basis. For example, many people believe that the world is round. However, in daily activities they act as if the world is flat by using flat maps to get from place to place, and by visualizing the part of the world they are most familiar with as flat. They hold one belief, but find it useful to suspend that belief in their daily activities.

Likewise, a belief in multiple constructed realities need not prevent one from studying a certain problem from the perspective of a single objective reality. A belief that it is impossible to study any phenomenon without affecting it in some way need not prevent one from attempting to minimize these effects through the design control methods developed in Chapters 6 through 16. The potential contributions of the different research paradigms are best realized when investigators recognize the assumptions that undergird their methods and make explicit the limitations of their methods.

This moderate view also implies that the paradigms can be mixed within a study to address different aspects of a research problem. For example, Emery's[18] study of the impact of prospective payment on the nature and practice of clinical education combined quantitative and qualitative methods. All subjects completed several survey instruments that quantified constructs such as capacity for change and social climate. In addition, qualitative information was generated from interviews with each subject.

Relationships among the paradigms therefore range from lack of recognition of competing paradigms, to separation of paradigms for different purposes, to combination of paradigms within research studies. Leininger provides some useful advice to researchers struggling with which of these views to adopt:

> I hold that the researcher needs to be clear why he or she is choosing the method, the purposes of the research, and the paradigmatic views that come from each method. . . . Rather than "mix and match" for popular or peaceful coexistence reasons, thought needs to be given [to] the question: What are the purposes and reasons for combining or separating the . . . methods? . . . To quickly embrace one method over the other, or to combine methods *without* knowing the reasons seems highly questionable.[17(p21)]

■ SUMMARY

Research paradigms are the beliefs that underlie the conduct of inquiry. The dominant paradigm in physical therapy research is currently the quantitative paradigm, which emphasizes generalizable measurement of a single objective reality with groups of subjects that are often manipulated by the investigator. The competing qualitative paradigm emphasizes the study of multiple constructed realities through in-depth study of particular settings, with an emphasis on determining underlying meanings within a particular context. The competing single-system paradigm includes many of the beliefs of the quantitative paradigm with the important exception of the concept of generalizability; single-system studies look at changes in individuals, since the individual is the unit of interest within a discipline such as physical therapy. Some researchers believe that adoption of one paradigm precludes the use of other paradigms; other researchers believe that all three paradigms are useful when applied to appropriate questions.

REFERENCES

1. Lincoln YS, Guba EG. *Naturalistic Inquiry.* Beverly Hills, Calif: Sage Publications; 1985.
2. Zukav G. *The Dancing Wu Li Masters: An Overview of the New Physics.* New York, NY: Bantam Books; 1979.
3. Irby DM. Shifting paradigms of research in medical education. *Acad Med.* 1990;65:622–623.
4. Phillips DC. After the wake: postpositivistic educational thought. *Edu Res.* 1983;12(5):4–12.
5. Rosenthal R. *Experimenter Effects in Behavioral Research.* Enlarged ed. New York, NY: Irvington Publishers; 1976.
6. Delitto A, Cibulka MT, Erhard RE, Bowling RW, Tenhula JA. Evidence for use of an extension-mobilization category in acute low back syndrome: a descriptive validation pilot study. *Phys Ther.* 1993;73:216–228.
7. Williams M, McKenzie RA. Commentary to Delitto A, Cibulka MT, Erhard RE, Bowling RW, Tenhula JA. Evidence for use of an extension-mobilization category in acute low back syndrome: a descriptive validation pilot study. *Phys Ther.* 1993;73:216–228. *Phys Ther.* 1993; 73:223.
8. Farrell JP. Commentary to Delitto A, Cibulka MT, Erhard RE, Bowling RW, Tenhula JA. Evidence for use of an extension-mobilization category in acute low back syndrome: a descriptive validation pilot study. *Phys Ther.* 1993;73:216–228. *Phys Ther.* 1993;73:224–226.
9. Mahoney MJ. *Scientist as Subject: The Psychological Imperative.* Cambridge, Mass: Ballinger Publishing Co; 1976.
10. Make public health our research priority. *Nation's Health.* 1993;23(4):2.
11. Breast cancer trial stopped early. *BMJ.* 1998;316:1187.
12. Jensen GM, Shepard KF, Hack LM. The novice versus the experienced clinician: insights into the work of the physical therapist. *Phys Ther.* 1990;70:314–323.
13. Ottenbacher KJ. *Evaluating Clinical Change: Strategies for Occupational and Physical Therapists.* Baltimore, Md: Williams & Wilkins; 1986.
14. Diamond MF, Ottenbacher KJ. Effect of a tone-inhibiting dynamic ankle-foot orthosis on stride characteristics of an adult with hemiparesis. *Phys Ther.* 1990;70: 423–430.
15. Morse JM, Field PA. *Qualitative Research Methods for Health Professionals.* 2nd ed. Thousand Oaks, Calif: Sage Publications; 1995:3.
16. Shepard KF. Qualitative and quantitative research in clinical practice. *Phys Ther.* 1987;67:1891–1894.
17. Leininger MM. Nature, rationale, and importance of qualitative research methods in nursing. In: Leininger MM, ed. *Qualitative Research Methods in Nursing.* Orlando, Fla: Grune & Stratton; 1985.
18. Emery MJ. The impact of the prospective payment system: perceived changes in the nature of practice and clinical education. *Phys Ther.* 1993;73:11–25.

BOX 5-1 **(continued from page 55)**

Solution: If you are like most adults, you counted 7 "F"s in the sample. Read it again:
"FABULOUS FITNESS FOLLOWS FROM YEARS OF FREQUENT WORKOUTS COMBINED WITH FOCUSED FOOD CHOICES."
There are 7 "F" sounds (fabulous, fitness, follows, from, frequent, focused, food), but 8 "Fs" (of). People who understand the relationship between letters and sounds intuitively search for the "F" sound when doing this exercise. In doing so, the task that is completed is different than the task that was assigned. If it is possible to interpret even a simple letter-counting exercise in different ways, think of the difficulty in developing "objective" measures that are more complicated! Qualitative researchers believe that such attempts are futile and instead embrace the depth of understanding that accompanies different ways of seeing the world.

6

Design Overview

Identification of Variables
Analysis of Research Titles
Levels and Types of Independent
Variables
Dependent Variables

Design Dimensions
Research Purposes
Timing of Data Collection
Manipulation
Manipulation Is Retrospective
The Variable Is Nonmanipulable
The Researcher Chooses Not to Manipulate
*The Independent Variable Is a Component of
the Dependent Variable*
*Interpretation Based on Controlled
Manipulation*

Control
Implementation of the Independent
Variable
Selection and Assignment of
Subjects
Extraneous Variables in the Setting
Extraneous Variables Related to
Subjects
Measurement Variation
Information Received by the
Subject and Researcher
Incomplete Information
Subject Blinding
Researcher Blinding

Research design is a creative process during which the investigators determine how they can best answer their research questions. A prerequisite to understanding research design is the ability to identify the different types of variables within the design. Once the variables are defined, research designs can be analyzed based on three basic dimensions: the purpose of the research, the timing of the data collection, and the extent to which the researcher manipulates subjects. Once these dimensions are determined, researchers use a variety of techniques to control various aspects of the research process. This chapter analyzes the variables within research studies, presents a matrix of research types, and outlines ways in which controls are implemented within research designs. Even though this chapter on design is presented separately from earlier chapters on problem development and later chapters on data analysis, recognize that these phases of the research process are, in fact, inseparable. The research problem influences the design, which in turn influences the analysis.

■ IDENTIFICATION OF VARIABLES

A *variable* is some characteristic that takes different forms within a study. In contrast, a *constant* takes only one form within a study. If differences between range-of-motion values for men and women are studied, then sex is a variable. If range-of-motion values for women only are studied, sex is a constant. When research is used to describe phenomena or relationships, then researchers do not need to differentiate among different types of variables. When the purpose of research is to analyze differences among groups or treatments, then it is important to differentiate between *independent* and *dependent* variables within the study. According to Kerlinger, "an *independent variable* is the *presumed* cause of the *dependent variable,* the *presumed* effect."[1(p32)] An independent variable is also sometimes called a *factor.* Unfortunately, authors do not always explicitly identify the number and character of the variables within their studies. Three examples are presented here to illustrate a process by which readers can discern the often complicated sets of variables within research studies.

Analysis of Research Titles

The article title of a published research study presents preliminary information about the independent and dependent variables. Preliminary identification of the independent and dependent variables in the three research reports we are examining in this chapter is presented in Table 6–1, based solely on the information contained in the title of each article.[2–4]

Levels and Types of Independent Variables

A full description of each independent variable includes the *levels* of the independent variable. The levels of the independent variable are the forms that the independent variable takes within the study. The three articles whose titles are listed in Table 6–1 are used to demonstrate what is meant by levels of the independent variable. As you will see, the studies are more complex than their titles alone indicate.

Identification of the independent variable in the first example, Crawford and Snaith's research on therapeutic ultrasound, is straightforward.[2] The design is diagrammed in Figure 6–1. There was one independent variable, which could be titled "group" or "ultrasound." There were two levels of group: true ultrasound, which was the experimental treatment, and sham ultrasound, which was the control treatment. Patients rated their heel pain on a 10-cm visual analogue scale (VAS) at their first and last visits. The dependent variable was "reduction of pain" as measured by the differences between the VAS scores at the

TABLE 6–1	Independent and Dependent Variables in Three Research Article Titles	
Title	**Independent Variable(s)**	**Dependent Variable**
"How effective is therapeutic ultrasound in the treatment of heel pain?"[2]	Ultrasound	Heel pain
"Effect of high-voltage pulsed current and alternating current on macromolecular leakage in hamster cheek pouch microcirculation"[3]	Current	Macromolecular leakage
"Effects of positioning and exercise on intracranial pressure in a neurosurgical intensive care unit"[4]	Positioning and exercise	Intracranial pressure

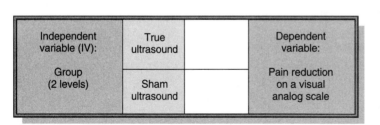

FIGURE 6–1. Study of the effect of ultrasound on heel pain. One independent variable, "group," was used. Although measures of heel pain were recorded at the beginning and at the end of the series of treatments, the authors took the difference between these measures to form the dependent variable, "pain reduction."
Design presented in Crawford F, Snaith M. How effective is therapeutic ultrasound in the treatment of heel pain? *Ann Rheum Dis.* 1996;55:265–267.

beginning and end of treatment. Concisely stated, the purpose of the study was to determine whether there was a difference in pain reduction between the true ultrasound and the sham ultrasound groups. The levels of the independent variable in this study represent different groups of subjects. Therefore, the term for this type of independent variable is a *between-groups* independent variable, or an independent variable with "independent levels."

The second example, a study of the effect of electrical stimulation on the microcirculation of hamster cheek pouches, is considerably more complex than the ultrasound study. As diagrammed in Figure 6–2, Taylor and associates examined seven different groups of hamsters, each receiving a different form of electrical stimulation, across three different time periods.[3] The first independent variable, therefore, was "group" with seven levels: control, cathodal high-voltage pulsed current (HVPC) at 90% of visible motor threshold (VMT), cathodal HVPC at

		Independent variable: Time (3 levels)				
		3 min	4 min	5 min		
Independent variable: Group (7 levels)	Histamine-only control group				Dependent variables:	
	Cathodal HVPC at 90% VMT				Number of leaks Areas of leaks Brightness of leaks	
	Cathodal HVPC at 50% VMT					
	Cathodal HVPC at 10% VMT					
	Anodal HVPC at 90% VMT					
	Anodal HVPC at 50% VMT					
	Anodal HVPC at 10% VMT					

FIGURE 6–2. Study of the effect of current on macromolecular leakage. Two independent variables were used: "group" with 7 levels and "time" with 3 levels. Although the leakage variables were actually measured four times, the first measurement was not directly compared with the other measures; rather, it was used as a baseline that was subtracted from the measures collected at each of the other times. HVPC = high-voltage pulsed current; VMT = visible motor threshold.
Design presented in Taylor K, Mendel FC, Fish DR, Hard R, Burton HW. Effect of high-voltage pulsed current and alternating current on macromolecular leakage in hamster cheek pouch microcirculation. *Phys Ther.* 1997; 77:1729–1740.

50% of VMT, cathodal HVPC at 10% of VMT, anodal HVPC at 90% of VMT, anodal HVPC at 50% of VMT, and alternating current at 90% of VMT. The dependent variables were derived from histological images that allowed counting of the number of leakage sites in the microcirculation, the area of the leakage, and the brightness of the leakage. The images were collected at 1.5, 3.0, 4.0, and 5.0 minutes after the start of treatment, with the 1.5-minute data being used as a baseline against which to compare the other three times. Thus, time was a second independent variable, with three levels: 3 minutes, 4 minutes, and 5 minutes after treatment. The "group" variable in this study, like that in the ultrasound study, is a between-groups variable, or a variable with independent levels. With a between-groups independent variable, each subject appears in only one level of the variable. The time variable is a different type of independent variable because each subject appears in each level of the independent variable. This type of independent variable is known as a *within-group* variable, or a variable with dependent levels.

In the third example, Brimioulle and colleagues examined the effects of positioning and exercise on intracranial pressure in a neurosurgical intensive care unit.[4] Their study design adds another layer of complexity to the identification of independent variables, as diagrammed in Figure 6–3. Patients with high or low intracranial pressure underwent either passive or active exercise in up to three different positions. The dependent variables of heart rate, systemic arterial pressure, intracranial pressure (ICP), and cerebral perfusion pressure were measured at rest and during various motions. On first analysis, then, it appears that there might be four independent variables within this study: group (high vs. normal intracranial pressure), exercise type (active vs. passive), position (supine, 30-degrees head-up, 45-degrees head-up), and activity (rest vs. motion). On closer examination of the study, one finds that the authors never compare the high pressure to the normal pressure groups, nor do they compare the active to the passive groups. Rather than dealing with these group-

ings as independent variables, the authors, in effect, conducted four "mini-studies": one with patients with high ICP who received passive exercise, one with patients with normal ICP who received passive exercise, one with patients with high ICP who received active exercise, and one with patients with normal ICP who received active exercise. This leaves two potential independent variables for each of the mini-studies: position and activity.

For the two mini-studies of patients with normal intracranial pressure, the authors tested each patient at rest and in motion in each of the three positions. Therefore, these studies had two independent variables, position and activity. Each of the variables had dependent levels because each patient was represented at each level of each variable. Thus, both of these independent variables would be considered "within-group" variables.

For the two mini-studies of patients with high ICP, the authors tested each patient at rest and in motion at only one position, the 30-degree head-up position. The position variable was not investigated for these groups because the other positions may be contraindicated for patients with elevated intracranial pressure. Thus, for the patients with high intracranial pressure, the studies had only one independent variable, "activity," with dependent levels.

From the examples presented in this section of the chapter, readers should now understand how to identify the names and levels of the independent variables within the studies. This identification process involves making some preliminary judgments about possible variables on the basis of the article title, purpose statement, and methods. Final determination of the variables and their levels depends on determining which comparisons the authors actually make within the study. Sometimes entire variables "disappear" because no comparisons are made. In Brimioulle and associates'[4] study of patients in neurosurgical intensive care units, for example, "pressure" was not a variable because there was no comparison between patients with high and normal ICP. Sometimes entire variables disap-

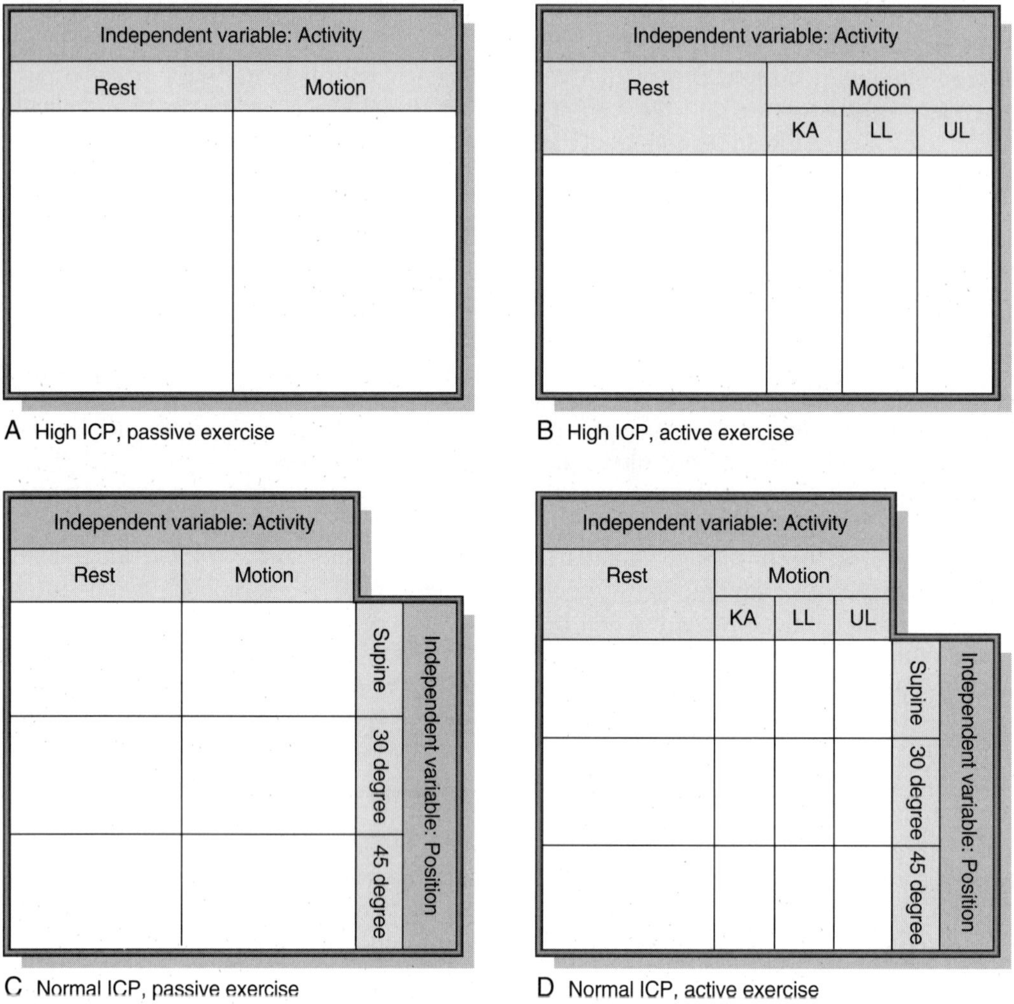

Independent variable: Activity	
Rest	Motion

A High ICP, passive exercise

Independent variable: Activity			
Rest	Motion		
	KA	LL	UL

B High ICP, active exercise

Independent variable: Activity		Independent variable: Position
Rest	Motion	
		Supine
		30 degree
		45 degree

C Normal ICP, passive exercise

Independent variable: Activity				Independent variable: Position
Rest	Motion			
	KA	LL	UL	
				Supine
				30 degree
				45 degree

D Normal ICP, active exercise

FIGURE 6–3. Study of the effect of exercise and position on intracranial pressure. This article presents a complex design that is actually four mini-studies in one. **A** and **B.** For patients with high intracranial pressure (ICP) only the effect of exercise was examined. **C** and **D.** For patients with normal ICP, the impact of both exercise and position was examined. **A** and **C.** For the passive groups, only rest and motion phases were compared for the activity variable. **B** and **D.** For the active groups, comparisons for the activity variable were made between rest phases and three different motion phases (knee adduction [KA], lower limb activity [LL], and upper limb activity [UL]). **C** and **D.** For the normal ICP groups the position variable was examined at three levels: supine, with the head up 30 degrees, and with the head up 45 degrees.
Design presented in Brimioulle S, Moraine J-J, Norrenberg D, Kahn RJ. Effects of positioning and exercise on intracranial pressure in a neurosurgical intensive care unit. *Phys Ther.* 1997;77:1682–1689.

pear because the levels are combined mathematically for analysis: In Crawford and Snaith's[2] study the apparent "time" variable was eliminated when posttreatment scores were sub-

tracted from pretreatment scores. Finally, levels of variables sometimes disappear because one level is used to normalize the other levels (e.g., in the electrical stimulation study of Taylor and colleagues[3] the data collection that occurred at 1.5 minutes into treatment was not a level in and of itself, but was used as a baseline against which to compare the other levels).

Dependent Variables

Dependent variables (DVs), as the presumed "effects" within a study, are "dependent" on the differences in the levels of the independent variables. If the independent variables can be thought of as the "grouping" factors, then the dependent variables can be thought of as the "measured" factors. Unlike independent variables, the different values that DVs take within a study are not described as levels.

When identifying DVs, it is often useful to differentiate between the "conceptual" dependent variable and the "operational" dependent variable. In the ultrasound study of Crawford and Snaith[2] the conceptual DV is "pain reduction" and the operational DV is "pain reduction as measured on a visual analogue scale." In the electrical stimulation study of Taylor and colleagues[3] the conceptual dependent variable is "macromolecular leakage" and the operational DVs are number of leaks, area of the leakage, and brightness of the leakage as seen through histological analysis. Describing the DVs in both conceptual and operational terms provides a framework for analyzing articles from both theoretical and technical viewpoints.

■ DESIGN DIMENSIONS

The interplay among three research design dimensions is shown in a matrix of research types in Figure 6–4. There are three broad purposes of research: *description, analysis of relationships,* and *analysis of differences* between groups or treatments. There are two levels to the time dimension: *retrospective,* in which the researcher uses data collected before the research question was developed, and *prospective,* in which the researcher completes data collection after the re-

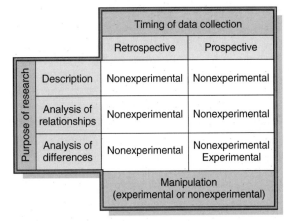

FIGURE 6–4. Matrix of research types showing three design dimensions: purpose of the research (rows), timing of data collection (columns), and manipulation (cells).

search question is developed.[5] There are also two basic levels of the manipulation dimension: *experimental* research involves controlled manipulation of subjects; *nonexperimental* research does not.

Research Purposes

To illustrate what is meant by the three different purposes of research, imagine that you are interested in studying the broad topic of functional recovery after total knee arthroplasty (TKA). One purpose for research about this topic would be to *describe* the functional status of patients at various intervals after TKA. A second purpose would be to *analyze the relationships* among various preoperative factors (such as gait velocity and quadriceps femoris strength) and functional status at intervals after TKA surgery. A third purpose would be to *analyze the differences* in functional recovery after TKA between, for example, one group of patients who received individualized postoperative exercise instructions and another group who participated in a group exercise program. Although each of these examples presents an approach to studying the topic of functional recovery after TKA, each project serves a very different purpose. Data from the first project would enable therapists to describe typical recovery patterns to their patients; data from the second study would enable therapists to predict which patients might be at risk for a poor recovery; and data from the third study would help therapists determine preferred patterns of care for patients after TKA. Because each of these hypothetical projects fulfills a need for information related to the topic, one of the projects is not inherently superior to any of the others.

Timing of Data Collection

The timing of data collection with respect to development of the research problem is the second important dimension of research design. There are two levels to the time dimension: *retrospective,* in which the researcher uses data collected before the research question was developed, and *prospective,* in which the researcher completes data collection after the research question is developed.[5]

All three of the general research purposes can be accomplished with either prospective or retrospective designs. One could describe the functional status of patients at various intervals after TKA either by extracting functional recovery data from existing medical records (retrospective) or by setting up a data collection protocol to gather systematic functional recovery data at specified intervals after surgery (prospective). One could analyze relationships among preoperative factors and functional status after TKA surgery either by extracting both the preoperative and functional data from the medical records of patients who have completed their rehabilitation after TKA (retrospective) or by collecting both the preoperative and functional data under controlled conditions designed to answer a specific question (prospective). One could also analyze differences in functional recovery after TKA between patients receiving individual or group therapy either by comparing discharge data of patients who happened to receive indi-

vidualized therapy to those who happened to receive group therapy (retrospective) or by randomly assigning new patients to individual or group therapy groups and then tracking their functional progress during recovery (prospective).

There are two notable twists to the use of the terms retrospective and prospective. First, in practice, research projects may combine retrospective and prospective elements, as previously defined. For example, a researcher might analyze relationships between preoperative factors and postoperative recovery by first extracting preoperative data from the medical record (retrospective) and then collecting new data on functional outcomes after surgery (prospective).

Second, an alternate set of definitions focuses on the sequence of cause-and-effect determinations, rather than on timing of data collection. Imagine that a researcher wishes to determine the effect of activity on development of osteoarthritis of the knee. The alternate definition for retrospective research is research in which the researcher works backwards from effect (osteoarthritis) to cause (activity). Doing such a study would first involve identifying groups of older patients with and without osteoarthritis. Next, the researcher would ask those patients to complete a lifelong activity questionnaire that might quantify "activity" through items about physical activity at work, during activities of daily living, and through participation in exercise and sports. Although the activity data are "prospective" according to our original definition (they were collected for the purpose of this particular study), the study involves a "retrospective" look, according to the alternate definition, at possible causes for osteoarthritis.

The alternate definition for prospective research is research in which the researcher works forward from cause to effect. Studying the link between activity and osteoarthritis from such a "prospective" viewpoint would involve identifying a group of young people without osteoarthritis, tracking their activity levels throughout their lives, determining which of the original subjects actually developed osteoarthritis, and then analyzing the data to determine whether activity levels are related to the development of osteoarthritis.

The common element of both the original and the alternate definitions relates to the level of control within the study. With either set of definitions, researchers have less control over the variables within retrospective studies than they do the variables in prospective ones. Methods for controlling variables are covered later in this chapter.

Manipulation

There are two basic levels of the manipulation dimension: *experimental* research involves controlled manipulation of subjects; *nonexperimental* research does not. Figure 6–4 illustrates the relationship of the manipulation dimension to the purpose and time dimensions. Research that describes phenomena or analyzes relationships among variables is nonexperimental, regardless of whether the data are collected prospectively or retrospectively. Research that analyzes differences retrospectively is also nonexperimental. Research that analyzes differences prospectively may be either experimental or nonexperimental. This illustrates that experimental research is but one of many different types of research that a clinician may encounter during a career of reading the literature or participating in research studies.

Many authors divide experimental research into *true experimental* and *quasiexperimental* subcategories based on the level of control present in the study. True experiments are characterized by high levels of control. This control takes the form of at least two separate groups of subjects, with random assignment of subjects to groups. The term *randomized clinical trial* is used frequently to describe health care research that is truly experimental in nature.[6]

Quasiexperimental research is characterized by less control than true experimental research, and this lesser degree of control of the experimental situation is achieved either with a single subject group, whereby subjects act as their own controls, or by using multiple groups to which subjects are not randomly assigned. Some authors believe that quasiexperimental studies are inferior designs that should only be used when a true experimental study is not feasible.[7,8] Some authors even classify quasiexperimental designs as nonexperimental research.[6]

There are two problems with such strong differentiation between true experimental and quasiexperimental research. First, the value of quasiexperimental research designs in which subjects are used as their own controls is underestimated. There are many clinical research questions for which single-group, quasiexperimental designs are ideal; several are presented in later chapters. Second, the ability of true experimental designs to capture the complexity of the clinical situation is overestimated. True experiments are far more controlled than the daily practice of physical therapy, and the results of such experiments may apply only to similarly controlled situations.[9] In this text, then, the term *experimental research* is used to refer to both truly experimental and quasiexperimental designs.

The specification that manipulation be controlled distinguishes experimental designs from nonexperimental. However, determination of whether controlled manipulation has occurred is more complicated than might be imagined. In some experiments, controlled manipulation is obvious. For example, Crawford and Snaith measured pain levels before and after true ultrasound or sham ultrasound in two groups of patients with episodes of heel pain.[2] Treatment with either true or sham ultrasound was the manipulation. Random assignment to treatment group and standardization of the ultrasound variables lent a great deal of control to the experiment.

However, some nonexperimental research studies appear to be experimental because an independent variable takes several values within the study. Closer examination reveals that although an independent variable is present, it has not been manipulated in a controlled manner by the researcher. There are four general categories of nonmanipulated independent variables: (1) the manipulation was retrospective, (2) the variable is inherently nonmanipulable, (3) the variable could have been manipulated but was not, and (4) the independent variable is an integral part of the measurement of the dependent variable.

MANIPULATION IS RETROSPECTIVE. Consider a case in which a therapist reviews the initial and discharge range-of-motion measurements reported in the clinical records of his or her last 20 patients with low back pain who received heat and exercise. This type of study is retrospective because the researcher seeks to answer a question by examining data that were collected before the question was developed. When the data are collected before the question is developed the researcher has little or no control over the actual implementation of the treatment, the outside activities of the patients, or the technique of measuring range of motion. Even though the heat and exercise are manipulations, this example docs not meet the controlled-manipulation criterion and is considered a nonexperimental study.

THE VARIABLE IS NONMANIPULABLE. A common example of a nonmanipulable independent variable is subject age. Researchers cannot change the age of subjects who present themselves for study; they can only group subjects according to age. Rantanen and coworkers did this when they studied the relationship of knee extension strength and stair-climbing ability in 75- and 80-year-old men and women.[10] Their analyses included a determination of whether there were differences in the two variables between the older (80-year-olds) and younger (75-year-olds) subjects. This type of nonmanipulated independent variable is called an *attribute* or a *classification* variable. When a grouping is made on the basis of some attribute, and not through random assignment, it is called a *block*.

THE RESEARCHER CHOOSES NOT TO MANIPULATE. Sometimes a variable can be manipulated but is not. The study of Rantanen and coworkers, described earlier, provides an example of knee extension strength as a nonmanipulated variable.[10] It is possible to manipulate knee extension strength with a progressive resistive exercise program. A study that tested stair-climbing ability after an effective knee extension exercise program would be an experimental study of the effect of knee extension strengthening on stair-climbing ability. Rantanen and coworkers, however, did not *manipulate* knee extension strength. They merely *measured* knee extension strength and stair-climbing ability and examined the relationships among these variables. Despite the potential for manipulation of the variable knee extension strength, the researchers chose to study the problem nonexperimentally, without manipulation.

THE INDEPENDENT VARIABLE IS A COMPONENT OF THE DEPENDENT VARIABLE. Sometimes an inherent part of the measurement of a dependent variable is treated as an independent variable. With the increasing sophistication of measurement tools in physical therapy comes the ability to vary aspects of the measurement itself. For example, isokinetic testing can occur at varying speeds, anterior-posterior displacement of the tibia on the femur can be measured under different stress levels, and grip strength can be measured at different handle positions on a dynamometer.

An example of this form of nonmanipulation of an independent variable is found in Ninos and colleagues' study of electromyographic (EMG) analysis of the squat performed in two different foot positions.[11] The data analysis procedure for this study included four different independent variables: knee flexion angle (5 levels between 10 and 60 degrees of knee flexion), direction of movement (2 levels, ascending and descending phases of the squat), muscle (4 levels: vastus medialis, vastus lateralis, semimembranosus and semitendinosus, and biceps femoris), and foot placement (neutral and 30 degrees turned out).

The first three of these variables are inherent components of doing a squat. The knees move through different angles, there are ascending and descending phases, and muscles on both sides of the knees are active. Certainly the researchers "manipulated" the subjects by having them do squats. However, the three variables that are inherent in doing any squat would be part of any descriptive study of EMG activity during squats. The final variable, foot placement, appears to be the only element of this study that can be considered experimental. The varied foot placement represents the researchers' manipulation of the way in which squats are done.

When the only manipulation that occurs is an inherent part of the measurement of the dependent variable, the research should be considered nonexperimental. However, an important distinction must be made between testing versus training. Knee flexion angle in the Ninos and associates' study was a nonmanipulated component of doing the squats within the study. If they had done a study in which they compared knee extensor strength following "deep-squat" versus "shallow-squat" exercise programs, then the independent variable becomes knee angle. Manipulating the knee angle in this way during a squat would be an experimental approach; recording EMG activity during the angles normally occurring during a squat is a nonexperimental, descriptive approach.

INTERPRETATION BASED ON CONTROLLED MANIPULATION. Experimental research occurs when the researcher manipulates a variable or variables in a controlled fashion. Nonexperimental research describes existing phenomena, without alteration through manipulation. Although one type of research is not inherently superior to the other, interpretation of research results differs depending on the methods of study. Thus, it is important that readers of the literature be able to distinguish between experimental and nonexperimental studies.

In particular, the presence of controlled manipulation enables researchers to draw *causal conclusions* about the variable under study, although the strength of the conclusions depends on the level of control in the research study. For example, Wolfson and associates studied the ef-

fects of balance and strength training on various functional measures in older adults.[12] In one component of this complex study they assigned each subject to one of four groups (control, balance training, strength training, combined balance and strength training). The training proceeded for 3 months, after which balance, strength, and gait measures were taken. They found, in part, that the groups that received balance training exhibited significant improvements in some of the balance variables. The controlled manipulation of the training program allowed them to conclude that the balance activities caused the changes in balance performance.

In contrast, Lynn and coworkers implemented a nonexperimental study comparing balance characteristics of women with and without osteoporosis.[13] They found that the women with osteoporosis exhibited different balance strategies than the women without osteoporosis. Because there was no controlled manipulation of the bone density variable, it cannot be said that the presence or absence of osteoporosis *caused* the balance changes—any more than it can be said that different balance strategies *caused* the osteoporosis.

■ CONTROL

In any type of study, some level of control must be present. Six types of control are common: control of implementation of the independent variable, control of subject selection and assignment, control of extraneous variables related to the setting, control of extraneous variables related to the subjects, control of measurement of the dependent variable, and control of information given to subjects and researchers.

Implementation of the Independent Variable

In controlling the independent variable, the investigator must develop a rationale to govern the implementation of the variable and a mechanism to monitor the implementation. In a study of the effect of heat and exercise on range of motion of the low back, the implementation of the heat and exercise would need to be systematized in some way. Does "heat" mean hot pack, ultrasound, or diathermy? If a hot pack is used, should packs of the same size be used on all patients, or should there be flexibility to accommodate patients of different sizes? Should heating continue until a certain skin temperature has been reached or for a defined period of time?

Feinstein described two general research philosophies that influence how these implementation decisions are made: fastidiousness and pragmatism.[9] Fastidious researchers seek precise control over all aspects of implementation, believing that the ability to draw causal conclusions is jeopardized by variations in treatment implementation. Pragmatic researchers seek closer simulation of clinical environments, believing that research results are most useful when the setting reflects the vagaries of the clinical setting. Both approaches are acceptable, but the limitations of both approaches need to be acknowledged by researchers. Fastidious researchers must acknowledge the limited clinical applicability of their work; pragmatic researchers must acknowledge their limited ability to draw causal conclusions from their work.

Selection and Assignment of Subjects

The second control component is control over the selection of subjects for the study and assignment of subjects to groups within the study. First, criteria for selection of individuals to be included in the study must be determined. In our hypothetical study of low back range of motion, many subject selection questions would arise. Should both men and women be studied? What age groups are appropriate for study? Does it make any difference whether the patient is being seen for a first episode of back pain or for a chronic condition that has recently flared up? Those who prefer fastidious designs tend to define selection criteria narrowly and therefore study relatively homogeneous groups. Those who prefer pragmatic designs develop broader selection criteria and therefore study relatively heterogeneous groups.

Once the criteria for admission to the study are determined, actual admission of individuals to the study must proceed. Random selection of a limited number of subjects from a larger subject pool is generally considered the best way to control for a variety of subject factors by maximizing the probability that any extraneous factors in the sample are present in the proportions actually found in the overall population. An in-depth discussion of sampling is presented in Chapter 8.

Extraneous Variables in the Setting

The third component of control is control over the setting. *Extraneous,* or *confounding,* variables are factors other than the independent variables that may influence the dependent variables. Control of extraneous variables includes, for example, keeping the temperature, lighting, time of day of testing, and the like constant to rule out differences in these factors as possible explanations for any changes in the dependent variable.

Extraneous Variables Related to Subjects

Control of extraneous variables related to the subject is the fourth means of control within research design. Researchers usually attempt to hold factors other than the independent variable constant for all subjects or groups. In this way, extraneous variables are controlled because they will affect all subjects or groups equally. In our hypothetical study of low back range of motion, one extraneous variable might be the level of analgesic, antiinflammatory, or antispasmodic medication being taken by subjects. A fastidious approach to the research problem would require tight control over medication; a pragmatic approach would permit greater variability from subject to subject.

The use of a randomly assigned control group, in and of itself, is a powerful tool that balances extraneous variables throughout the groups. If a randomly assigned, untreated control group is used in the study of low back range of motion, controlling the medications taken by subjects may not be necessary. The process of randomization increases the chance (but does not guarantee) that any medication effects will be balanced across the treatment and control groups.

In studies with only one group, control of extraneous variables must be achieved through means other than a control group. If one were to study a single group of patients after cerebral vascular accident to determine the effect of body-weight supported ambulation on gait velocity, it would be important to establish that changes were the result of treatment and not the normal healing process (maturation). One way to control for the effect of maturation would be to take weekly velocity measurements of all patients and admit into the study only those who had several weeks of stable velocity measures.

A second common way to control extraneous variables is to use the same subjects for all levels of the independent variable. This only works if the effect the researcher is measuring is thought to be short-lived. Brooks and associates studied the effect of electrode alignment (longitudinal vs. horizontal) on quadriceps femoris muscle torque generated during electrical stimulation [14] Because the short-term application of electrical stimulation should not cause permanent alterations in torque-generating capacity, an ideal way to control extraneous subject factors is to use a *repeated measures,* or *repeated treatment,* design, whereby subjects act as their own controls and receive all experimental conditions. In addition, repeated treatment designs require fewer subjects and may require less time for setup and preparation because the number of subjects is reduced.

The repeated measures design, however, introduces its own set of extraneous variables related to the administration of multiple treatments. If one of the electrode placements is always given last, fatigue may reduce the torque generated by that placement. Conversely, familiarity with the electrical stimulation unit may lead to greater relaxation of antagonist muscles and greater torque production by the agonist during the second placement. One way to control the effects of familiarization with equipment or procedures is to schedule one or more training sessions with subjects prior to actual data collection.

Another way to control fatigue and learning in a repeated measures design is by randomizing, or *counterbalancing*, the order of presentation of the experimental conditions (i.e., half the subjects get the longitudinal placement first and half get the horizontal placement first). This becomes problematic when more than two levels of treatment are present. If there are 3 levels (A, B, and C) of the independent variable, there are six possible presentation orders (3!—i.e., 3 factorial, or $3 \times 2 \times 1 = 6$): ABC, ACB, BAC, BCA, CAB, and CBA. With 4 levels, the number of permutations increases to 24 (4!—$4 \times 3 \times 2 \times 1 = 24$). With 6 levels, there are 720 possible orders (6!—$6 \times 5 \times 4 \times 3 \times 2 \times 1 = 720$). Random assignment of subjects to all available orders in a study with 6 levels of an independent variable would require a minimum of 720 subjects. To obviate the need for so many subjects, a sampling of orders can be used.

There are two basic strategies for selecting treatment orders in a repeated measures design with several levels of the independent variable. These two strategies can be illustrated by a hypothetical study of gait characteristics with four different foot units in a transtibial prosthesis: a solid-ankle-cushion-heel foot (SC), a single-axis foot (SA), a multiaxial foot (MA), and a dynamic response foot (DR). The first strategy is to randomly select an order and then rotate the starting position, as shown in Figure 6–5A. In a *random start with rotation,* each condition appears at each position in the rotation equally often. One fourth of the subjects would be randomly

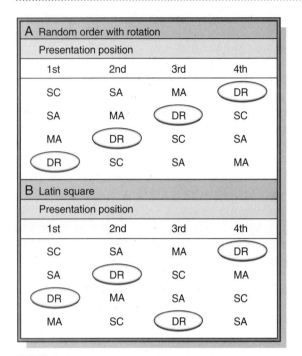

A Random order with rotation

Presentation position			
1st	2nd	3rd	4th
SC	SA	MA	(DR)
SA	MA	(DR)	SC
MA	(DR)	SC	SA
(DR)	SC	SA	MA

B Latin square

Presentation position			
1st	2nd	3rd	4th
SC	SA	MA	(DR)
SA	(DR)	SC	MA
(DR)	MA	SA	SC
MA	SC	(DR)	SA

FIGURE 6–5. Selection of presentation orders from many possibilities. With four levels of the independent variable (SC = solid ankle cushion heel; SA = single axis; MA = multiaxial; DR = dynamic response), there are 24 (4!) possible orders. **A.** Selection of four orders through random ordering of the first row, and through rotation of orders for the remaining rows. The highlighted condition, DR, illustrates that each level is represented at each presentation position in a systematic way through rotation. **B.** Selection of four orders through generation of a Latin square. The highlighted condition, DR, illustrates that each level is represented at each presentation position in a random way that also ensures that each condition precedes and follows each other condition only once.

assigned the order in the first row; one fourth, the order in the second row; and so on.

The second strategy is to use a *Latin square* technique. The Latin square technique ensures not only that each condition appears at each position equally often, but also that each condition precedes and follows every other condition equally often. Thus, a Latin square has a greater level of randomization than does a random start with rotation. A sample Latin square is shown in

Figure 6–5B. Rules for the formation of a Latin square can be found in several texts.[15–17]

Measurement Variation

The fifth component of control is control of the measurement techniques used to provide data for the experiment. Reliability and validity of measurements used in experiments are critical to the ability to draw conclusions from the data. Sound design includes pilot testing of the measures to be used to ensure that each measure is reproducible. If multiple raters are used in the study, a pilot study to ensure the interrater reliability of measures is essential. Chapters 17 through 19 are devoted to measurement theory, research designs that evaluate reliability and validity of measurement tools, and examination of measures commonly employed in physical therapy research.

Information Received by the Subject and Researcher

The final means of control in designs is control of the information given to the subject and the researcher during the course of the study. Placebo effects, subject expectations, and researcher expectations may all result in changes in the dependent variable that are unrelated to the implementation of the independent variable. Three means of information control are commonly used to limit these effects: incomplete information, subject blinding, and researcher blinding.

INCOMPLETE INFORMATION. Sometimes subjects are given incomplete information about the purpose of the study to control any effects that their expectations about the results would cause. For example, Gahimer studied patient education behaviors of therapists in outpatient orthopedic settings, but did not want the therapists in the study to know the specific variable of interest.[18] She assumed that if therapists knew the specific purpose of the study they might change their teaching behaviors during the observation period. When Gahimer obtained informed consent from participants, she stated only that she wished to study patient-therapist interaction. In this way she was truthful, but incomplete, as the specific measure of interest was disguised from the therapists.

With an innocuous study involving documentation of patient education behaviors, there is no ethical problem in withholding the specific purpose of the study. However, study of higher-risk procedures requires complete disclosure of purposes and risks so that subjects can make an informed decision about participation.

SUBJECT BLINDING. A second means of controlling information is to withhold information about which of several treatments a patient is receiving. In many procedures in physical therapy, patient blinding is not possible because of the nature of the procedures themselves. Subjects in our hypothetical low back range-of-motion study would obviously be able to distinguish between a heat/exercise program and a manual therapy approach to treatment of low back pain.

When the treatment is a physical modality, subjects may be partially blinded to which physical modalities they are receiving. For example, subjects may be told that they may or may not feel a heat sensation with ultrasound treatment; the control group may then receive placebo or sham ultrasound, whereby the machine is not plugged in or the intensity is not turned on. This approach was used by Crawford and Snaith[2] in their study, presented earlier in the chapter, of the treatment of heel pain with ultrasound. Ethical treatment of research subjects requires that they be informed of the possibility of receiving a placebo treatment.

RESEARCHER BLINDING. A third means of controlling information is to blind the researcher to the group membership of, or treatment received by, the subjects. In this way any expectations that the experimenter may have about the outcome

of the study are not inadvertently communicated to subjects.

Researcher blinding was implemented in the Crawford and Snaith study.[2] An assistant set up the equipment, draping the machine so that the investigator treating the patients would not be able to view the dials and know whether true or sham ultrasound was being given. If the treatment is such that the therapist cannot be blinded to the treatment (e.g., a study of two different forms of manual therapy), then an independent investigator would need to take the measures of interest in the study, without knowing which patients had received which treatment.

A study in which either the subject or the researcher is blind to the treatment administered is termed a *single-blind* study. A study in which both subject and researcher are blinded is termed a *double-blind* study. Unfortunately, research designs that attempt to blind either researchers or subjects may not be as effective as hoped. Deyo and associates studied the effectiveness of blinding techniques with transcutaneous electrical nerve stimulation.[19] After completion of a double-blind study, they asked subjects to indicate whether they believed their units were working properly and asked researchers to indicate which subjects they believed had functioning units. They found that both subjects and researchers guessed correctly more often than would have been predicted by chance, indicating only partial success of the blinding procedure. They hypothesized that the lack of full blinding was due to sensory differences between real and sham therapy and to unintended communication between the subjects and researchers.

Implementation of the treatment, extraneous variables in the setting, extraneous subject variables, selection and assignment of subjects, measurement techniques, and information given to subjects and researchers must all be controlled in an experimental design. In Chapters 7 and 8, additional design considerations—validity and sampling—are presented. After these general design considerations are presented, Sections 3 and

4 provide a more detailed look at different types of experimental and nonexperimental designs.

■ SUMMARY

Variables within studies are often classified as independent (the "grouping" variable) or dependent (the "measured" variable). Independent variables, in turn, have levels that are compared to one another with respect to the dependent variables. Research types can be defined according to three dimensions: purpose (description, analysis of relationships, analysis of differences), timing (retrospective or prospective data collection), and manipulation (experimental, nonexperimental). Researchers can achieve control by uniformly implementing the independent variable, selecting and assigning subjects randomly, eliminating extraneous variables from the setting, limiting extraneous variables related to subjects, ensuring the reliability of measurements of the dependent variable, and limiting the information provided to themselves and to subjects.

REFERENCES

1. Kerlinger FN. *Foundations of Behavioral Research.* 3rd ed. Fort Worth, Tex: Holt, Rinehart & Winston; 1986.
2. Crawford F, Snaith M. How effective is therapeutic ultrasound in the treatment of heel pain? *Ann Rheum Dis.* 1996;55:265–267.
3. Taylor K, Mendel FC, Fish DR, Hard R, Burton HW. Effect of high-voltage pulsed current and alternating current on macromolecular leakage in hamster cheek pouch microcirculation. *Phys Ther.* 1997;77:1729–1740.
4. Brimioulle S, Moraine J-J, Norrenberg D, Kahn RJ. Effects of positioning and exercise on intracranial pressure in a neurosurgical intensive care unit. *Phys Ther.* 1997;77: 1682–1689.
5. Tietjen GL. *A Topical Dictionary of Statistics.* New York, NY: Chapman & Hall; 1986:125.
6. Norton BJ, Strube MJ. Making decisions based on group designs and meta-analysis. *Phys Ther.* 1989;69:594–600.
7. Campbell DT, Stanley JC. *Experimental and Quasi-Experimental Designs for Research.* Chicago, III: Rand McNally College Publishing Co; 1963.
8. Oyster CK, Hanten WP, Llorens LA. *Introduction to Research: A Guide for the Health Science Professional.* Philadelphia, Pa: JB Lippincott Co; 1987:70.
9. Feinstein AR. An additional basic science for clinical medicine, II: limitations of randomized trials. *Ann Intern Med.* 1983;99:544–550.
10. Rantanen T, Era P, Heikkinen E. Maximal isometric knee extension strength and stair-mounting ability in 75- and 80-year-old men and women. *Scand J Rehabil Med.* 1996;28:89–93.
11. Ninos JC, Irrgang JJ, Burdett R, Weiss JR. Electromyographic analysis of the squat performed in self-selected lower extremity neutral rotation and 30° of lower extremity turn-out from the self-selected neutral position. *J Orthop Sports Phys Ther.* 1997;25:307–315.
12. Wolfson L, Whipple R, Derby C, et al. Balance and strength training in older adults: intervention gains and Tai Chi maintenance. *J Am Geriatr Soc.* 1996;44:498–506.
13. Lynn SG, Sinaki M, Westerlind KC. Balance characteristics of persons with osteoporosis. *Arch Phys Med Rehabil.* 1997;78:273–277.
14. Brooks ME, Smith EM, Currier DP. Effect of longitudinal versus transverse electrode placement on torque production by the quadriceps femoris muscle during neuromuscular electrical stimulation. *J Orthop Sports Phys Ther.* 1990;11:530–534.
15. Shaughnessy JJ, Zechmeister EB. *Research Methods in Psychology.* 2nd ed. New York, NY: McGraw-Hill Publishing Co; 1990:217.
16. Winer BJ. *Statistical Principles in Expeimental Design.* 2nd ed. New York, NY: McGraw-Hill Publishing Co; 1971:685–691.
17. Kirk RE. *Experimental Design: Procedures for the Behavioral Sciences.* Belmont, Calif: Wadsworth Publishing Co; 1968.
18. Gahimer JE, Domholdt E. Amount of perceived education in physical therapy practice and perceived effects. *Phys Ther.* 1996;76:1089–1096.
19. Deyo RA, Walsh NE, Schoenfeld LS, Ramamurthy S. Can trials of physical treatments be blinded? The example of transcutaneous electrical nerve stimulation for chronic pain. *Am J Phys Med Rehabil.* 1990;69:6–10.

Research Validity

Internal Validity
  History
  Maturation
  Testing
  Instrumentation
  Statistical Regression to the Mean
  Assignment
  Mortality
  Interactions Between Assignment
    and Maturation, History, or
    Instrumentation
  Diffusion or Imitation of Treatments
  Compensatory Equalization of
    Treatments
  Compensatory Rivalry or Resentful
    Demoralization

Construct Validity
  Construct Underrepresentation
  Experimenter Expectancies
  Interaction Between Different
    Treatments
  Interaction Between Testing and
    Treatment

External Validity
  Selection
  Setting
  Time

**Relationship Among Types of
Validity**

The validity of a piece of research is the extent to which the conclusions of that research are believable and useful. Cook and Campbell have outlined four types of validity, and this chapter relies to a great extent on their work.[1] When determining the value of a piece of research, readers need to ask four basic questions about the research:

1. Is the research designed so that there are few alternative explanations for changes in the dependent variable other than the effect of the independent variable? Factors other than the independent variables that could be related to changes in the dependent variable are threats to *internal validity*.

2. Are the research constructs defined and used in such a way that the research can be placed in the framework of other research within the field of study? Poor definition of constructs or inconsistent use of constructs is a threat to *construct validity*.

3. To whom can the results of this research be applied? Sampling and design factors

that lead to limited generalizability are threats to *external validity*.

4. Are statistical tools used correctly to analyze the data? Irregularities in the use of statistics are threats to *statistical conclusion validity*.

The purpose of this chapter is to provide a discussion of the first three types of validity. Understanding statistical conclusion validity requires some background in statistical reasoning. Threats to statistical conclusion validity are therefore covered in Chapter 20 when statistical reasoning is introduced. Each of the remaining three types of validity has several identifiable threats that can be illustrated either in examples from the physical therapy literature or in examples of hypothetical research in physical therapy. For each of these threats, at least one example is presented and mechanisms for controlling the threat suggested. The chapter ends with an examination of the interrelationships between the types of validity.

■ INTERNAL VALIDITY

Internal validity is the extent to which the results of a study demonstrate that a causal relationship exists between the independent and dependent variables. In experimental research, the central question about internal validity is whether the treatments (or the various levels of the independent variable) caused the observed changes in the dependent variable. In nonexperimental research designed to delineate differences between groups in the absence of controlled manipulation by the researcher, the question becomes whether the independent variable is a plausible explanation of group differences on the dependent variable.

The general strategy that researchers use to increase internal validity is to maximize their control over all aspects of the research project. Eliminating extraneous variables through control of the experimental setting removes them as plausible causes of changes in the dependent variable. Randomized assignment of subjects to treatment groups maximizes the probability that extraneous subject characteristics will be evenly distributed across groups. To check randomization, the researcher can collect information about patient characteristics that threaten internal validity to determine whether the characteristics in question were equally represented across groups.

When developing research proposals, investigators should carefully carefully consider each threat to internal validity to determine whether their design is vulnerable to that threat. If it is, the researchers must decide whether to institute additional controls to minimize the threat, collect additional information to document whether the threat materialized, or accept the threat as an unavoidable design flaw. There is no perfect research design, and high levels of internal validity may compromise construct or external validity, as discussed at the end of the chapter. Eleven of Cook and Campbell's threats to internal validity are important for physical therapy researchers and are discussed below.[1]

History

History is a threat to internal validity when events unrelated to the treatment of interest occur during the course of the study and may plausibly change the dependent variable. Amundsen and associates studied the effect of a group exercise program on the mean aerobic power of elderly women living in a high-rise apartment complex.[2] They used a nonrandom method to assign subjects to the experimental group and the control group. The experimental group was made up of women who participated consistently in the group exercise program, and the control group was made up of women whose schedules did not permit their attendance at the exercise sessions. Several historical events could reduce the internal validity of this, or any, study. Consider the effect on the study of an elevator malfunction in the building that required all individuals in the study to walk up at least two flights of stairs to get to their apartments during the last 3 weeks of the study. This hypothetical historical event, which is not under the researchers' control, would introduce another aerobic training stimulus into the study. In the absence of control, the researchers should gather information to determine how much of an effect stair climbing may have had on the results of the study.

Researchers could ask subjects to estimate the number of times per day that they climbed the stairs during the interruption in elevator service. If experimental and control subjects used the stairs with equal frequency, then the effect of the stair climbing would be uniform across the

two groups, and some separation of the effects of the stair climbing versus the effects of the group exercise program could be accomplished, as shown in Figure 7–1. The hypothetical data in this figure show that the groups began the study with the same average fitness level, that the control group improved slightly, and that the experimental group improved markedly. The conclusion drawn from this data might be written in a journal article as follows:

The control group showed a 0.5 metabolic equivalent (MET) improvement in mean aerobic power at the posttest, presumably because of the unintended training stimulus of stair climbing during the last 3

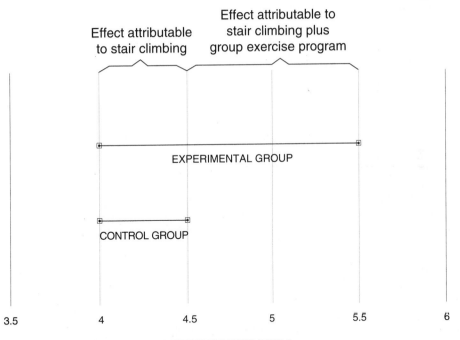

FIGURE 7–1. Separation of the effects of stair climbing from the effects of a group exercise program in a test of aerobic power. Both the control and experimental groups participated in stair climbing; only the experimental group participated in a group exercise program. Both groups had mean pretest scores of 4.0 metabolic equivalents (METs); the control group had a mean posttest score of 4.5 METs, and the experimental group had a mean posttest score of 5.5 METs. For the control group, any changes in aerobic power can be attributed to the stair climbing. For the experimental group, part of the change seen can be attributed to the stair climbing; the change above that seen in the control group can be attributed to the added effect of the group exercise program.

weeks of the study. The experimental group, who also received the unintended stimulus of stair climbing, showed three times the mean aerobic power improvement of the control group. We assume that the experimental group results represent an approximately 0.5 MET improvement related to stair climbing and a 1.0 MET improvement attributable to the group exercise program.

Researchers can use three strategies to minimize the effects of history: planning, use of a randomly selected control group, and description of unavoidable historical events. In experimental studies, careful planning by the researcher can minimize the chances that historical events will influence the study. If a geographical region is usually snowed in during February, a study that requires subject attendance at treatment sessions 5 days per week should probably be scheduled at another time of year. If testing of subjects requires a full day with half-hour rests between measurements, it might be wise to isolate subjects and researchers from radios and televisions so that news that happens to occur on the day of testing will not influence subject or researcher performance.

Use of a control group provides the researcher with some ability to separate the effects of history from the effects of the treatment. Use of a control group in this manner was illustrated by the hypothetical example of the elevator malfunction, in which the effect of stair climbing by the control group was separated from the combined effect of stair climbing and exercise group participation by the experimental group. Random assignment of subjects to groups is the best way to minimize the effects of history, because the different groups will likely be affected equally by the historical event.

In some instances, historical events that cannot be avoided may occur. In retrospective nonexperimental studies, control of history is impossible because the historical events have already occurred. If an uncontrolled historical event that may cause changes in the dependent variable does occur, it is important to collect and present information about the event. Emery[3] did a retrospective study of the impact of the implementation of Medicare's prospective payment system on physical therapy practice and clinical education in teaching hospitals. Since the number and degree level of physical therapy education programs was changing during the time period he studied, it is difficult to know which of the clinical education changes might be related to changes in the payment system versus changes in the educational system. When unable to control a threat, researchers have a responsibility to present information about the threat so that readers may form an opinion about its seriousness.

Maturation

Maturation, changes within a subject due to the passage of time, is a threat to internal validity when it occurs during the course of a study and may plausibly cause changes in the dependent variable. Subjects get older, more experienced, or bored during the course of a study. Patients with neurological deficits may experience spontaneous improvement in their conditions; subjects with orthopedic injuries may become less edematous, have less pain, and be able to bear more weight with time.

As was the case with historical threats to internal validity, single-group studies do not provide a basis from which the researcher may separate the effects of maturation from the effects of treatment. Yarkony and associates used a single-group design to document the functional improvement of paraplegic patients completing an inpatient rehabilitation program.[4] The maturation threat in this study is that, with experience, young people with paraplegia may demonstrate increased skill in managing their injury even in the absence of a formal rehabilitation program.

Maturation effects can be controlled in several ways. The first is through use of a control group, preferably with random assignment of subjects to either the control or the experimental group. Use of the control group allows the effects of maturation alone to be observed in the control group.

The treatment effects are then evaluated in terms of how much the treatment group improved in comparison with the control group.

A second way to control for the effects of maturation is to take multiple baseline measures of subjects before implementing the treatment. Suppose that you have a group of patients with ankle sprains who have persistent edema despite protected weight bearing, compression bandage wrap, elevation when possible, and use of ice packs three times daily. Documentation of baseline volume over a period of several days or weeks would provide appropriate comparison measures against which the effects of a compression and cryotherapy pump regimen could be evaluated. Figure 7–2 shows three patterns of baseline measurements: stable, irregular, and steadily progressing. Results after the intervention are interpreted in light of the baseline pattern documented before the intervention. Pa-

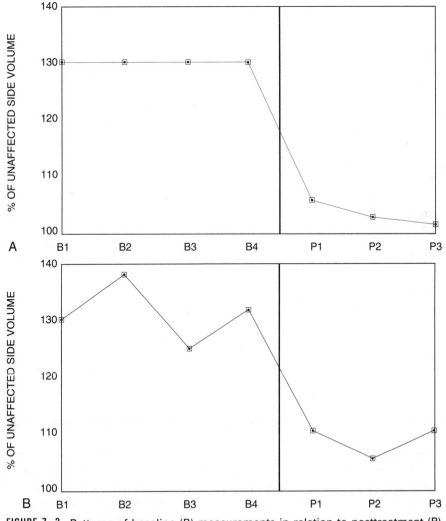

FIGURE 7–2. Patterns of baseline (B) measurements in relation to posttreatment (P) measurements. **A.** Stable baseline. **B.** Irregular baseline.

Illustration continued on following page

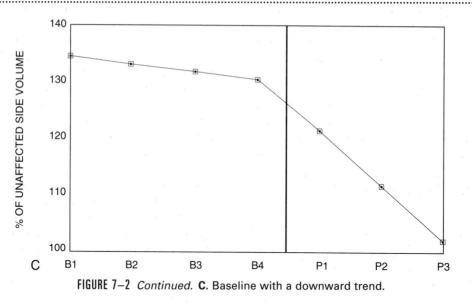

FIGURE 7–2 *Continued.* **C.** Baseline with a downward trend.

tients in Figure 7–2A had no change in the weeks before intervention but showed dramatic improvements after treatment. Patients in Figure 7–2B had weekly fluctuations in edema before treatment and marked improvement after treatment. Patients in Figure 7–2C showed consistent, but slow, improvement in the weeks before treatment and more rapid improvement after treatment.

Maturation effects may be seen in repeated treatment research designs. Any time patients receive more than one treatment, they may respond differently to later treatments than to earlier treatments. Performance on the dependent variable may improve for later treatments because of increased experience with the treatment, or performance may decline because of fatigue or boredom. In Brooks and associates' repeated treatment study of the torque produced by electrical stimulation of the quadriceps femoris muscle with horizontal or longitudinal electrode placement, subjects may have felt more accustomed to the electrical stimulation with time, improving performance during the second electrode placement pattern.[5] Conversely, their quadriceps femoris muscles may have fatigued during the course of the study, demonstrating decreased performance during

the second electrode placement pattern. The authors controlled for these possible effects by randomizing the order in which they presented the treatments to subjects.

Testing

Testing is a threat to internal validity when repeated testing itself is likely to result in changes in the dependent variable. For example, on the first day of treatment, a male patient with a painful shoulder who is unfamiliar with the therapist and with the procedure for taking range-of-motion measurements may be unable to relax his shoulder girdle musculature to provide an accurate measure of his passive range of motion. Improved measurements on subsequent days may reflect familiarization with the testing procedure and more effective relaxation during testing, rather than effectiveness of the treatment.

Three basic design strategies can be used to minimize testing effects. The first is to use randomly selected experimental and control groups so that the effects of testing in the control group can be removed by comparison with the effects of testing and treatment in the experimental group. This is analogous to the removal of the effects of history and maturation through use of a control group.

The second strategy is to eliminate multiple testing through use of a posttest-only design. However, in the absence of a pretest to establish that control and experimental groups were the same at the start of the experiment, posttest-only studies must have effective random assignment of subjects to groups.

The third design strategy is to conduct familiarization sessions with the testing equipment so that the effects of learning are accounted for before the independent variable is manipulated. To determine the extent of familiarization needed, the researcher should conduct a pilot study to determine how much time or how many sessions are needed before performance is stable. One drawback of multiple testing is the possibility that the familiarization process will itself constitute a "treatment." For example, if subjects familiarize themselves with a strength testing protocol once a week for 4 weeks, they may have exercised enough during familiarization to show a training response.

Instrumentation

Instrumentation is a threat to internal validity when changes in measuring tools themselves are responsible for observed changes in the dependent variable. Many tools that record physical measurements need to be calibrated with each testing session. Calibration is a process by which the measuring tool is compared with standard measures to determine its accuracy. If inaccurate, some tools can be adjusted until they are accurate. If a tool has limited adjustability, the researcher may need to apply a mathematical correction factor to convert inaccurate raw scores into accurate transformed scores. If temperature or humidity influences measurement, this factor must be controlled, preferably through testing under constant conditions or, alternatively, through mathematical adjustment for the differences in physical environment.

Researchers themselves are measuring tools ("human instruments"). An example of the variability in the human instrument has surely been felt by almost any student: It is almost impossible for an instructor to apply exactly the same criteria to each paper in a large stack. Maybe the instructor starts out lenient but cracks down as he or she proceeds through the stack. Maybe the instructor who is a stickler at first adopts a more permissive attitude when the end of the stack is in sight. Maybe a middling paper is graded harshly if it follows an exemplary paper; the same paper might be graded favorably if it follows an abysmal example. A variety of observational clinical measures, such as identification of gait deviations, functional levels, or abnormal tone, may suffer from similar problems. Measurement issues in physical therapy research are addressed in detail in Section 5, Measurement.

Statistical Regression to the Mean

Statistical regression is a threat to internal validity when subjects are selected on the basis of extreme scores on a single administration of a test. A hypothetical example illustrates the mathematical principle behind statistical regression to the mean: We have three recreational runners, each of whom has completed ten 10-km runs in an average time of 50 minutes, and a range of times from 40 to 60 minutes. The distribution in Figure 7–3A represents the race times of the three runners.

Suppose we wish to test a new training regimen designed to decrease race times to see if the regimen is equally effective with runners at different skill levels. We place runners into categories based on a single qualifying race time, have them try the training regimen for 1 month, and record their times at an evaluation race completed at the end of the 1-month training period. At the qualifying race, we place runners into one of three speed categories based on their time in that race: Subjects in the fast group finished in less than 45 minutes, subjects in the average group finished between and including 45 and 55

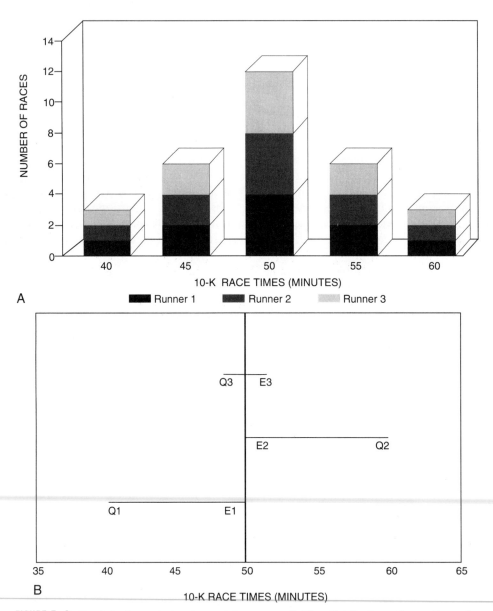

FIGURE 7–3. Statistical regression toward the mean. **A.** The distribution of race times for three runners, as shown by the different shading patterns on the bars. All three runners have an average race time of 50 minutes. **B.** The effect of statistical regression toward the mean if the runners are placed into different groups based on qualifying times at a single race. Q represents qualifying times for each runner; E represents the runners' evaluation times at a subsequent race. Runner 1 appears to have slowed from 40 to 50 minutes, Runner 2 appears to have speeded up from 60 to 50 minutes, and Runner 3 stayed approximately the same.

minutes, and subjects in the slow group finished in greater than 55 minutes.

The times marked with a Q in Figure 7–3B show that Runner 1 performed much better than average on the day of the qualifying race (40 minutes), Runner 2 performed much worse than usual on the qualifying day (60 minutes), and Runner 3 gave an average performance (49 minutes). Runners 1 and 2 gave atypical performances on the qualifying day and in subsequent races would be expected to perform closer to their "true" running speed. Thus, even without intervention, Runner 1 would likely run the next race slower and Runner 2 would likely run the next race faster. Runner 3, who gave a typical performance, is likely to give another typical performance at the next race. In other words, the extreme scores will tend to "regress toward the mean." This regression toward the mean for the evaluation race is represented by the times marked with an E in Figure 7–3B. If we do not consider the effects of statistical regression, we might conclude that the training program has no effect on average runners, speeds up the slow runners, and slows down the fast runners.

In general, the way to control for statistical regression toward the mean is to select subjects for groups on the basis of reliable, stable measures. If the measures used to form groups are inherently variable, then subjects are best assigned to groups on the basis of a distribution of scores collected over time, rather than by a single score that might not reflect true ability.

Assignment

Assignment to groups is a threat to internal validity when groups of subjects are different from one another on some variable that is related to the dependent variable of interest. Cook and Campbell labeled this particular threat "selection."[1] The term *assignment* is more precise and differentiates between the internal validity threat related to group assignment and the external validity threat, presented later, of subject selection.

Assignment threatens internal validity most often in designs in which subjects are not randomly assigned to groups or in nonexperimental designs in which study group membership cannot be manipulated by the investigator. For example, Mäenpää and Lehto used a retrospective nonexperimental design to determine the relative success of three different nonoperative ways to manage patellar dislocation.[6] The three different groups were immobilized as follows: plaster cast, posterior splint, and bandage/brace. Because the treatment received was based on physician preference, there is no way to determine why individual patients were treated with a particular immobilization method, and no randomization process to increase the likelihood that the groups would be similar on important extraneous variables. For example, the bandage/brace group consisted of proportionately more women than the other groups. Since women tend to have more predisposing anatomical factors for patellar dislocation than men, perhaps the higher redislocation rate for the bandage/brace group is related to the higher proportion of women, rather than to the type of immobilization.

Control of assignment threats is most effectively accomplished through random assignment to groups within a study (see Chapter 8). When random assignment to groups is not possible, researchers may use statistical methods to "equalize" groups (see Chapter 22).

Mortality

Mortality is a threat to internal validity when subjects are lost from the different study groups at different rates or for different reasons. Despite the best efforts of the researcher to begin the study with randomly selected groups who are equivalent on all important factors, differential mortality can leave the researcher with very different groups by the end of the study. Assume that a researcher has designed a strengthening study in which one group of 50 subjects participates in a combined concentric and eccentric program of moderate intensity and another group of 50 participates in a largely eccentric program of higher intensity. Forty-five of the subjects in the moderate group complete the program, with an average increase in strength of 20%. Fifteen of the subjects in the high-intensity group complete the program, with an average increase in strength of 40%. Concluding that the high-intensity program was superior to the moderate-intensity program would ignore the differential mortality of subjects from the two groups. This problem of mortality might be written up as follows in a journal article:

Subjects who completed the high-intensity program showed greater strength increases than did subjects who completed the moderate-intensity program. Note, however, that there was differential loss of subjects from the two groups. Ninety percent of the moderate-intensity group completed the program. The 5 subjects who dropped out did so because of time constraints that prevented regular participation in the exercise program. Only 30% of the high-intensity group completed the program. Of the 35 subjects who dropped out of the study, 5 did so because of time constraints and 30 did so because they were unable to tolerate the delayed muscle soreness associated with this exercise program. We conclude that the moderate-intensity program provides moderate strength gains and is tolerated by a majority of subjects. The high-intensity program provides impressive strength gains for the few who can tolerate the discomfort associated with the program.

An example from the literature is Amundsen and associates' study of the effect of group exercise on the aerobic power of elderly women, in which 36 women initially volunteered to participate in the exercise group.[2] Fourteen completed more than half the exercise sessions and constituted the exercise group; 15 completed less than half the exercise sessions and were not used in the data analysis; 2 could not tolerate the testing procedure; and 5 did not participate and constituted the control group. The exercise group, therefore, consisted of less than half the women who started the program. The conclusion that the exercise regimen was effective needs to be

tempered by the fact that less than half of the participants completed it.

Researchers can control experimental mortality by planning to minimize possible mortality and collecting information about the lost subjects and about reasons for the loss of subjects. Researchers need to make compliance with an experimental routine as easy as possible for subjects, while maintaining the intent of the experiment. Administering treatments at a place of work or at a clinic where patients are already being treated will likely lead to higher compliance than if patients have to drive across town to participate in the study. Developing protocols that minimize discomfort are likely to lead to higher levels of retention within a study. Testing and treating on a single day will avoid the loss of subjects that inevitably accompanies a protocol that requires several days of participation.

When answering the research question requires longer-term participation and its attendant loss of subjects, researchers can document the characteristics of the subjects who drop out of the study to determine if they are similar to those who remain in the study. If the dropouts have characteristics similar to those of subjects who remain in the study, and if the rate and character of dropouts are similar across study groups, then differential mortality has not occurred. Such a loss of subjects is random and affects the study groups equally.

Interactions Between Assignment and Maturation, History, or Instrumentation

Assignment effects can interact with maturation, history, or instrumentation to either obscure or exaggerate treatment effects. These interactions occur when maturation, history, or instrumentation effects act differently on treatment and control groups.

A hypothetical example of an Assignment × History interaction would be seen in Amundsen and associates' study if only one of the groups of elderly women was affected by the interruption in elevator service in the high-rise apartment.[2] If the groups used the stairs at different rates, then the study results would need to be interpreted in view of the differential effect of history on the groups. Assume that the members of the control group with the conflicting schedules went out more than the experimental group and used the stairs at least once a day to go outside to catch the bus. Members of the experimental group tended to stay home and did not use the stairs at all if the elevator was not working. In this scenario, the historical event of an elevator malfunction changed the study from a comparison of a control group versus an experimental group to a comparison of stair climbing versus group exercise. This problem might be described as follows in a journal article:

During the course of the study, an elevator malfunction occurred that affected the control group but not the experimental group. Rather than comparing an exercising experimental group with a nonexercising control as originally planned, the comparison was between a group who participated in an 8-week group exercise program and a group who participated in a 3-week stair-climbing program.

In this scenario, the hypothetical threat of an Assignment × History interaction to internal validity was uncontrollable but explainable. Such threats can be explained only if researchers remain alert to possible threats and collect information about the extent to which subjects were affected by the threat.

An interaction between assignment and maturation occurs when different groups are maturing at different rates. If a study of the effectiveness of a rehabilitation program for patients who have had a cerebral vascular accident (CVA) used one group of patients 6 months after their CVA and another group 2 months after their CVA, the group with the more recent CVA would be expected to show greater spontaneous improvement.

An Assignment × Instrumentation interaction occurs when an instrument is more or less sensitive to change in the range at which one of the treatment groups is located. For example, assume that a researcher seeks to determine which of two methods of instruction, lecture or self-study through a course offered on the Internet, results in superior student achievement in kinesiology. The students in the different instructional groups take a pretest that has a maximum score of 100 points. The group being taught by the lecture method has an average pretest score of 60; the group being taught via the Internet has an average pretest score of 20. The traditional group can improve only 40 points; the Internet group can improve up to 80 points. Thus, the interaction between assignment and instrumentation exaggerates the differences in gain scores between the two groups by suppressing the gain of the group who started at 60 points. When scores "top out" and an instrument cannot register greater gains, this is termed a *ceiling effect*; when scores "bottom out" and an instrument cannot register greater declines, this is termed a *basement* or *floor effect*.

Control of interactions with assignment is accomplished through the same means that assignment, history, maturation, and instrumentation are controlled individually: random assignment to groups, careful planning, and collection of relevant information when uncontrolled threats occur. As is the case with assignment threats alone, mathematical equalization of groups can sometimes compensate for interactions between assignment and history, maturation, or instrumentation.

Diffusion or Imitation of Treatments

Diffusion of treatments is a threat to internal validity when subjects in treatment and control groups share information about their respective treatments. Assume that an experiment that evaluates the relative effectiveness of open- and closed-chain exercise in restoring quadriceps torque in patients who have undergone anterior cruciate ligament reconstruction is implemented in a single clinic. Can't you picture a member of the open-chain group and a member of the closed-chain group discussing their respective programs while icing their knees down after treatment? Perhaps a man in the open-chain group decides that stair climbing is just the thing he needs to speed his rehabilitation program along, and a man in the closed-chain group decides to buy a cuff weight and add some leg lifts to his program. If this treatment diffusion occurs, the difference between the intended treatments will be blurred.

Researchers can control treatment diffusion by minimizing contact between participants in the different groups, blinding subjects when possible, and orienting participants to the importance of sticking to the rehabilitation program to which they are assigned. Sometimes researchers will offer subjects the opportunity to participate in the alternate treatment after the study is completed if it proves to be the more effective treatment. This offer should make subjects less tempted to try the alternate treatment during the study period.

Compensatory Equalization of Treatments

Compensatory equalization of treatment is a threat to internal validity when a researcher with preconceived notions about which treatment is more desirable showers attention on subjects who are receiving the treatment the researcher perceives to be less desirable. This extra attention may alter scores on the dependent variable if the attention leads to increased compliance with treatment, increased effort during testing, or even increased self-esteem leading to a general sense of well-being.

Researchers should control compensatory equalization of treatment by avoiding topics about which they are biased or by designing studies in which their bias is controlled through researcher blinding. In addition, if a researcher has a strong sense that one treatment is more desirable than the other, he or she needs to consider whether it is ethical to contrast the two treatments in an experimental setting.

Compensatory Rivalry or Resentful Demoralization

Rivalry and demoralization are threats to internal validity when members of one group react to the perception that they are receiving a less desirable treatment than other groups. This reaction can take two forms: compensatory rivalry (a "we'll show them" attitude) and resentful demoralization (a "why bother" attitude). Compensatory rivalry tends to mask differences between control and treatment groups; resentful demoralization tends to exaggerate differences between control and experimental groups. Researchers can control rivalry and resentment by controlling the information given to subjects, blinding themselves and subjects to group membership, and having a positive attitude toward all groups.

■ CONSTRUCT VALIDITY

Construct validity is concerned with the meaning of variables within a study. One of the central questions related to construct validity is whether the researcher is studying a "construct as labeled" or a "construct as implemented." An example of the difference between these two constructs is illustrated by a hypothetical example wherein a researcher uses active range of motion as a dependent measure of shoulder function. The construct as labeled is "function"; the construct as implemented is "active range of motion." Some readers might consider active range of motion to be a good indicator of function, but others might consider it an incomplete indicator of function. Those who are critical of the use of active range of motion as a functional indicator are questioning the construct validity of the dependent variable.

Cook and Campbell described 10 separate

threats to construct validity. Their list is collapsed into the four threats described in the following sections. The general strategy for controlling threats to construct validity is to develop research problems and designs through a thoughtful process that draws on the literature and theory of the discipline.

Construct Underrepresentation

Construct underrepresentation is a threat to construct validity when constructs are not fully developed within a study. In Manfroy and associates' study of the effect of exercise, prewrap, and athletic tape on resistance to ankle inversion, the independent variable construct "exercise" was not developed fully.[7] This variable had two levels: "before exercise" and "after 40 minutes of exercise." As the authors note,

> A point of practical interest concerns the time point when the tape lost its effectiveness: was it after 5, 10, 20, or 30 minutes of exercise? . . . Because the two measurement points were more than 40 minutes apart in the present study, we could not resolve the time course of any short-term changes in resistance.[7(p161)]

Fuller explication of the construct of exercise would require more than two measures across time—perhaps at 5, 10, 20, and 40 minutes of exercise.

Construct underrepresentation may also be a concern related to the dependent variables within a study. For example, Powers and associates[8] studied the locomotor function of individuals with patellofemoral pain (PFP). Each subject's gait was analyzed during free-speed and fast walking, ascending and descending stairs, and ascending and descending ramps. McClay, in an invited commentary to the article, noted that

> The activities tested . . . may not have been painful for these subjects. . . . The authors' assumption was that the subjects with PFP would exhibit a compensatory pattern. However, if the

activity does not cause pain, mechanics are not likely to be altered.[9(p1076)]

In this example, the concern is that the construct of "locomotion" has been underrepresented by selecting low-level activities that do not elicit pain.

Construct underrepresentation can also apply to the intensity of a construct. Kluzik and colleagues studied the effect of a neurodevelopmental treatment on reaching in children with spastic cerebral palsy.[10] They analyzed reaching motions before and after a single neurodevelopmental treatment. In an invited commentary accompanying publication of Kluzik and associates' article, Scholz noted the following:

> Something, albeit subtle, has resulted from the intervention. Expecting a more dramatic improvement in the reaching performance of this population following only one treatment is probably too much to ask in the first place. Future work should focus on the evaluation of long-term effects.[11(p77)]

Scholz thus recognized that the construct has been underrepresented because it was applied only once and recommended future work with a more intense representation of the construct. It should be noted that two of the original authors, Fetters and Kluzik, have now published follow-up work that addresses this concern by comparing the impact of 5 days of neurodevelopmental treatment with 5 days of practice of reaching tasks.[12]

Experimenter Expectancies

Experimenter expectancy is a threat to construct validity when the subjects are able to guess the ways in which the experimenter wishes them to respond. In Chapter 5, "Clever Hans" was introduced during the discussion of whether it is possible to have independence of the investigator and subject. Recall that Clever Hans was a horse who could provide the correct response to mathematical problems by tapping his foot the correct number of times. His talents could be explained by the fact that questioners apparently unconsciously raised their eyebrows, flared their nostrils, or raised their heads as Hans was coming up to the correct number of taps. Rosenthal, who wrote about Hans, framed the issue in terms of the expectation of the examiner:

> Hans' questioners, even skeptical ones, expected Hans to give the correct answers to their queries. Their expectation was reflected in their unwitting signal to Hans that the time had come for him to stop his tapping. The signal cued Hans to stop, and the questioner's expectation became the reason for Hans' being, once again, correct.[13(p138)]

In the story of Clever Hans, the construct as labeled was "ability to do mathematics." The construct as implemented, however, was "ability to respond to experimenter cues."

Brodzka and associates' study of long-term function of persons with bilateral below-knee amputations is an example of a study in which experimenter expectancy may have been a threat to construct validity.[14] In this study, physical therapists and occupational therapists from a rehabilitation center went to the homes of patients with bilateral below-knee amputations who had undergone postoperative rehabilitation at the center to determine their level of function in the home and community. It can be assumed that the therapists hoped to find patients who were functioning well in the face of their physical impairments. It can also be assumed that the subjects knew of the therapists' expectations. Given this, it is easy to imagine that patients might have exaggerated their abilities and that therapists might have been all too willing to believe in the exaggerated abilities. The construct as labeled was "function in the home and community"; however, the construct as implemented probably was "function in the home and community as described to a therapist who has reason to hope for high levels of function."

Researchers can control experimenter ex-

pectancy effects by limiting information given to subjects and themselves, by having different researchers who bring different expectations to the experimental setting replicate their study, and by selecting topics from which they can maintain an objective distance.

Interaction Between Different Treatments

Interaction between different treatments is a threat to construct validity when treatments other than the one of interest are administered to subjects. McIntosh and colleagues[15] studied facilitation of gait patterns in patients with Parkinson's disease with different forms of rhythmic auditory stimulation. Some of the patients with Parkinson's disease were taking dopaminergic medications on their regular dosing schedule and some had discontinued their medication 24 hours in advance of the study. If the authors had put all of the patients with Parkinson's disease into a single group, it would have been impossible for them to separate the effects of the stimulation from the effect of being on medication. In fact, the authors had a specific theoretical reason for examining patients on and off of medication (to determine the contribution of the basal ganglia in responding to rhythmic stimulation) and therefore analyzed each group separately.

In some instances, control of interaction between different treatments is often difficult to achieve because of ethical considerations in clinical research. For example, if it would be unsafe for patients with Parkinson's disease to be off their medication temporarily, then McIntosh and colleagues would have had no choice but to study the combined impact of stimulation and medication. However, researchers can document who receives additional treatment and can analyze data by subgroups if not all subjects are exposed to the additional treatments. If all subjects are exposed to multiple treatments, researchers need to carefully label the treatments to make this obvious.

Interaction Between Testing and Treatment

Interaction between testing and treatment is a threat to construct validity when a test itself can be considered an additional treatment. As discussed in the section on testing as a threat to internal validity, controlling for the threat to internal validity made by familiarization with the test may sometimes constitute an additional treatment. In the case of strength testing, repeated familiarization sessions with the equipment may constitute a training stimulus. The treatment as labeled may be "nine strength training sessions"; the treatment as implemented may be "nine strength training sessions and three strength testing sessions."

One way to control for interaction between testing and treatment is to compare a treatment group who was pretested, a treatment group who was not pretested, a control group who was pretested, and a control group who was not pretested. This allows the researcher to compare the effects of the test and treatment combined with the effects of treatment alone, the test alone, and neither the test nor the treatment. No examples of this design (known as a Solomon four-group design) were found in the physical therapy literature, presumably because of the large number of subjects that would be required to form all four groups. In addition, researchers can control for interaction between testing and treatment by limiting testing to the end of the study.

■ EXTERNAL VALIDITY

External validity is concerned with the issue of to whom, in what settings, and at what times the results of research can be generalized. Cook and Campbell distinguished between generalizing *across* groups, settings, or times and generalizing *to* particular persons, settings, or times.[1] One can generalize to groups, settings, or times similar to the one studied. One can generalize across groups, settings, or times if one has studied multiple subgroups of people, settings, or times. If researchers study the effect of a progressive resistive exercise technique on the biceps strength of elderly women, they can generalize their results only to elderly women. If they study the same question with a diverse group of men and women with an average age of 35 years, they can generalize their results to other diverse groups with an average age of 35. Even though the researchers have tested men and women of different age groups in the second example, they cannot generalize across age groups or sexes unless they analyze the diverse group according to subgroups. In this example, the overall group might show an increase in strength even if the elderly individuals in the group showed no change.

The question of generalizability of research results is equally applicable to descriptive research, relationship analysis, or difference analysis. Controlling the threats to external validity requires thoughtful consideration of the population to whom the results of the study can be applied, combined with practical considerations of the availability of subjects for study.

Selection

Selection is a threat to external validity when the selection process is biased in that it yields subjects who are in some manner different from the population to which the researchers hope to generalize their results. Researchers must accept that subjects who are willing to participate as research subjects may differ from the general population. As stated by Cook and Campbell, "Even when respondents belong to a target class of interest, systematic recruitment factors lead to findings that are only applicable to volunteers, exhibitionists, hypochondriacs, scientific do-gooders, those who have nothing else to do, and so forth."[1(p73)]

Amundsen and associates' study of a group exercise program for elderly women suffers from this threat to external validity.[2] First, subjects volunteered to participate in the program; presumably, this group of women differed in some way from those who did not volunteer. Maybe they had more positive attitudes toward exercise, had less to do, or were more adventuresome than those who did not volunteer. In a second self-selection process, some of the women who had originally volunteered for the study did not participate regularly. Presumably, the volunteers who participated regularly were different in some way from the volunteers who did not participate regularly. Thus, the group to which the study results can be generalized is elderly women who volunteer for and participate regularly in an exercise program. Taking a similar program and making it a mandatory part of the daily routine at a retirement center might yield disappointing results if the treatment is administered to a group who has little interest in the exercise program.

A study by Hanke and colleagues illustrates the threat of selection to external validity in a descriptive research report.[16] The purpose of the study was to determine the reliability of measurements of body center-of-mass momentum of healthy adults while rising from sitting to standing. Subjects were 19 healthy adults between the ages of 25 and 38 years. In an invited commentary accompanying the research article, DiFabio noted that

> . . . the use of subjects without known impairments to establish criterion standards for evaluating clinical impairment must be analyzed carefully. Measures of motor performance in nondisabled subjects do not have automatic validity, and studies done exclusively with nondisabled subjects need to establish the relevancy and usefulness of the measure intended for clinical use.[17(p115)]

The authors responded to this concern by noting that:

> If the expertise of a physical therapist resides in the evaluation and enhancement of human movement function, then knowledge of how movement is generated by healthy persons across the lifespan should equip the practitioner with valuable tools and insights for solving problems displayed by persons with disorders of movement function.[16(p117)]

This useful intellectual exchange illustrates that different readers may have differing opinions about the seriousness of validity concerns within a piece of research.

Researchers can control selection as a threat to external validity by carefully considering the target population to whom they wish to generalize results, selecting subjects accordingly, and carefully writing their research conclusions to avoid making inferences to groups or across subgroups who have not been studied.

Setting

Setting is a threat to external validity when peculiarities of the setting in which the research was conducted make it difficult to generalize the results to other settings. In a study of leg movements of preterm infants, Heriza videotaped leg movements in an effort to sample spontaneous leg movements of each infant.[18] To meet the requirements of her data analysis system, she had to stabilize the infants in some way during taping; she did so by using one hand to support the head and the other hand to maintain the trunk in a midline position. This level of interference with the child is certainly less than, for example, using a pinprick as a stimulus to begin kicking. However, the researcher and the reader still must consider the possibility that an infant's kicking behavior while he or she is supported by a human touch may differ from the infant's kicking behavior in the absence of support. In a later study, Heriza and her colleagues were able to reduce this threat to external validity by using a taping system that recorded spontaneous kicks without physical support from the investigators.[19]

Control of threats to external validity posed by setting requires that researchers simulate as closely as possible the setting to which they hope to generalize their results. Researchers who hope their studies will have clinical applicability must try to duplicate the complexities of the clinical setting within their studies. Researchers who wish to describe subjects or settings as they exist naturally must make the research process as unobtrusive as possible.

Time

Time is a threat to external validity when the results of a study are applicable to limited time frames. For example, Emery's study of the impact of the prospective payment system on physical therapy practice and clinical education is somewhat time limited.[3] The study examined the 4 years (1984 to 1988) following the implementation of a new method of paying for hospital services delivered to patients covered by Medicare. If the data were collected in 1989 and analyzed in 1990, the submission of the article to the journal in 1991 is relatively timely. The delay of 18 months from initial submission to publication is fairly typical for a journal that employs a peer review process that often involves one or two cycles of revision and reevaluation. Even though publication was fairly timely, dramatic changes in health care payment systems during the late 1980s and 1990s have extended far beyond patients covered by Medicare. Readers, then, must take into account this change as they determine the usefulness of Emery's data to their practice.

Time threats to external validity can be managed by authors through timely submission of research results for publication and by description of known changes that make the research results less applicable than when the data were collected. In addition, when articles are used some years after their publication date, readers have the responsibility to incorporate contemporary knowledge into their own review of the usefulness of the results to current practice.

■ RELATIONSHIP AMONG TYPES OF VALIDITY

Eighteen different threats to validity have been presented. These threats are not, however, independent entities that can be controlled one by one until the perfect research design is created. The relationship between the validity threats can be either cumulative or reciprocal.

Cumulative relationships occur when a change that influences one of the threats influences other threats in the same way. For example, researchers may initially think to use a randomly assigned control group in a study because they want to control for the effects of maturation. By controlling for maturation in this way they also control for history, assignment, testing, and so on.

Reciprocal threats occur when controlling a threat to one type of validity leads to realization of a different threat to validity. For instance, if a researcher wants to achieve the highest level of internal validity possible, he or she will standardize the experimental treatment so that there are few extraneous variables that could account for changes in the dependent measures. However, this standardization compromises external validity because the results can be applied only to settings in which the treatment would be equally well controlled.

The reciprocal relationship between validity threats is illustrated in Mäenpää and Lehto's study of conservative care of patients with patellar dislocation.[6] As noted earlier in the chapter, one of the groups of patients seemed to have a higher proportion of women patients than the other two groups. This represents an assignment threat to internal validity. To eliminate this threat from this retrospective study, the authors could have chosen to study only men or only women. In doing so, they would have reduced external validity by narrowing the group to whom the results of the study could be generalized. Mäenpää and Lehto couldn't win. If they studied men and women they had to cope with a possible threat to internal validity. Conversely, if they studied only men, they would have limited external validity.

■ SUMMARY

Threats to the believability and utility of research can be classified as threats to internal, construct, or external validity. Internal validity concerns whether the treatment caused the effect; construct validity concerns the meaning attached to concepts used within the study; and external validity concerns the persons, settings, or times to which or across which the results can be generalized. Many of the threats to validity are reciprocal because controlling one leads to problems with another.

REFERENCES

1. Cook T, Campbell D. *Quasi-Experimentation: Design and Analysis Issues for Field Settings.* Chicago, Ill: Rand McNally & Co; 1979:37–94.
2. Amundsen LR, DeVahl JM, Ellingham CT. Evaluation of a group exercise program for elderly women. *Phys Ther.* 1989;69:475–483.
3. Emery MJ. The impact of the prospective payment system: perceived changes in the nature of practice and clinical education. *Phys Ther.* 1993;73:11–25.
4. Yarkony GM, Roth EJ, Meyer PR, et al. Rehabilitation outcomes in patients with complete thoracic spinal cord injury. *Am J Phys Med Rehabil.* 1990;69:23–27.
5. Brooks ME, Smith EM, Currier DP. Effect of longitudinal versus transverse electrode placement on torque production by the quadriceps femoris muscle during neuromuscular electrical stimulation. *J Orthop Sports Phys Ther.* 1990;11:530–534.
6. Mäenpää H, Lehto MUK. Patellar dislocation: the long-term results of nonoperative management in 100 patients. *Am J Sports Med.* 1997;25:213–217.
7. Manfroy PP, Ashton-Miller JA, Wojtys EM. The effect of exercise, prewrap, and athletic tape on the maximal active and passive ankle resistance to ankle inversion. *Am J Sports Med.* 1997;25:156–163.
8. Powers CM, Perry J, Hsu A, Hislop HJ. Are patellofemoral pain and quadriceps femoris muscle torque associated with locomotor function? *Phys Ther.* 1997;77:1063–1078.
9. McClay IS. Invited commentary. *Phys Ther.* 1997;77:1075–1076.
10. Kluzik J, Fetters L, Coryell J. Quantification of control: a preliminary study of effects of neurodevelopmental treatment on reaching in children with spastic cerebral palsy. *Phys Ther.* 1990;70:65–76.
11. Scholz JP. Commentary. *Phys Ther.* 1990;70:76–78.
12. Fetters L, Kluzik J. The effects of neurodevelopmental treatment versus practice on the reaching of children with spastic cerebral palsy. *Phys Ther.* 1996;76:346–358.
13. Rosenthal R. *Experimenter Effects in Behavioral Research.* Enlarged ed. New York, NY: Irvington Publishers; 1976:138.
14. Brodzka WK, Thornhill HL, Zarapkar SE, et al. Long-term function of persons with atherosclerotic bilateral below-knee amputation living in the inner city. *Arch Phys Med Rehabil.* 1990;71:895–900.
15. McIntosh GC, Brown SH, Rice RR, Thaut MH. Rhythmic auditory-motor facilitation of gait patterns in patients with Parkinson's disease. *J Neurol Neurosurg Psychiatry.* 1997;62:22–26.
16. Hanke TA, Pai Y-C, Rogers MW. Reliability of measurements of body center-of-mass momentum during sit-to-stand in healthy adults. *Phys Ther.* 1995;75:105–118.
17. DiFabio RP. Invited commentary. *Phys Ther.* 1995;75:113–115.
18. Heriza CB. Organization of leg movements in preterm infants. *Phys Ther.* 1988;68:1340–1346.
19. Geerdink JJ, Hopkins B, Beek WJ, Heriza CB. The organization of leg movements in preterm and full-term infants after term age. *Dev Psychobiol.* 1996;29:335–351.

Selection and Assignment of Subjects

Significance of Sampling and Assignment

Populations and Samples

Probability Sampling
  Simple Random Sampling
  Systematic Sampling
  Stratified Sampling
  Cluster Sampling

Nonprobability Sampling
  Samples of Convenience
  Snowball Sampling
  Purposive Sampling

Assignment to Groups
  Random Assignment by Individual
  Random Assignment by Block
  Systematic Assignment
  Matched Assignment
  Consecutive Assignment
  Deciding on an Assignment
    Method

Sample Size

Researchers rarely have the opportunity to study all the individuals who possess the characteristics of interest within a study. Fiscal and time constraints often limit researchers' ability to study large groups of subjects. In addition, the study of very large groups may be undesirable because it takes time and resources away from improving other components of the research design.[1(p3)] *Sampling* is the process by which a subgroup of subjects is selected for study from a larger group of potential subjects. *Assignment* is the process by which subjects in the sample are assigned to groups within the study. This chapter acquaints readers with the major methods of selecting subjects and assigning them to groups.

■ SIGNIFICANCE OF SAMPLING AND ASSIGNMENT

If a group of physical therapists is interested in studying, for example, rehabilitation outcomes in patients who have undergone total knee arthroplasty (TKA), they must somehow determine which of thousands of possible subjects will be studied. The way in which subjects are identified for study, and for groups within the study, has a profound impact on the validity of the study.

Sampling methods influence the characteristics of the sample, which in turn influence the generalizability, or external validity, of a piece of research. If, for example, a sample of patients

95

with TKA includes only subjects older than 75 years, the research results cannot be generalized to younger patient groups.

The method by which subjects are assigned to groups within the study influences the characteristics of subjects within each group, which in turn influences the internal validity of the study. Assume that we design an experiment on the effect of continuous passive range of motion (CPM) on knee range of motion after TKA. We use a design that includes one experimental group (routine rehabilitation plus CPM) and one control group (routine rehabilitation only). The threats to internal validity posed by history, maturation, testing, and assignment can all be controlled by assignment procedures that yield groups of patients with similar ages, medical problems, preoperative ambulation status, and the like.

■ POPULATIONS AND SAMPLES

The distinction between a population and a sample is an important one. A *population* is the total group of interest. A *sample* is a subgroup of the group of interest. *Sampling* is the procedure by which a sample of *units* or *elements* is selected from a population. In clinical research, the sampling unit may be the individual or a group of related individuals, such as graduating classes of therapists or patients treated at particular clinics.

Defining the population of interest is not a simple matter. There are generally two types of populations who are considered in research, the target population and the accessible population. The *target population* is the group to whom researchers hope to generalize their findings. The *accessible population* is the group of potential research subjects who are actually available for a given study.

Hulley and colleagues listed four types of characteristics that define populations: clinical, demographic, geographical, and temporal.[2(p18)] Clinical and demographic characteristics define the target population. The target population for our TKA study might be defined as individuals who have undergone a unilateral TKA and were at least 60 years of age at the time of the surgery. Geographical and temporal characteristics define the accessible population. The accessible population for our TKA study might consist of individuals with the aforementioned clinical and demographic characteristics who underwent surgery in any one of eight Indianapolis hospitals during the 5-year period from 1995 to 1999. Table 8–1 presents a hypothetical distribution of patients at the eight hospitals during this time period. This accessible population of 3000 patients provides the basis for many of the examples in this chapter.

Once the researcher has defined the accessi-

TABLE 8-1	Hypothetical Sample of Patients Who Underwent Total Knee Arthroplasty by Hospital and Year					
Hospital	*1995*	*1996*	*1997*	*1998*	*1999*	*Total*
A	22	25	28	26	24	125
B	50	55	60	40	45	250
C	48	49	52	51	50	250
D	80	78	75	71	71	375
E	72	72	77	77	77	375
F	95	107	98	97	103	500
G	100	103	95	100	102	500
H	120	130	130	122	123	625
Total	587	619	615	584	595	3000

ble population in a general way, he or she needs to develop more specific *inclusion* and *exclusion* characteristics. We already know that patients aged 60 years or older who underwent unilateral TKA at one of eight hospitals from 1995 to 1999 are included in our accessible population. Some patients who fit this description should, nevertheless, be excluded from participation in the study. For example, we need to decide whether to exclude patients who experienced postoperative infection, surgical revision, or rehospitalization soon after the TKA.

The decision to include or exclude subjects with certain characteristics must be made in light of the purpose of the research. If the purpose of our study is to provide a description of functional outcomes after TKA, then excluding cases with complications would artificially improve group outcomes by eliminating those likely to have a poor outcome. In contrast, if the purpose of a study is to describe the functional outcomes that can be expected after completion of a particular rehabilitation regimen, then exclusion of patients who could not complete therapy seems reasonable.

After the researcher specifies inclusion and exclusion criteria, he or she needs a sampling frame from which to select subjects. A *sampling frame* is a listing of the elements in the accessible population. In our TKA study, we would ask that someone in the medical records department in each of the eight hospitals create a sampling frame by developing a list of patients aged 60 years or older who underwent a TKA from 1995 to 1999.

Existing sampling frames are available for some populations. If we wish to study physical therapists' opinions on appropriate use of support personnel in delivering rehabilitation services, we could use either a professional association membership list or a state physical therapy licensing board list as our sampling frame. Use of an existing sampling frame necessarily defines the target population for the research. If we use the professional association membership list, we can generalize only to other professional association members; if we use the licensing board list,

we can generalize to licensed physical therapists regardless of whether they belong to the professional association.

The most basic distinction between sampling methods is between *probabilistic* and *nonprobabilistic* methods. Generation of probability samples involves randomization at some point in the process; generation of nonprobability samples does not. Probability samples are preferable when the researcher hopes to generalize from an accessible population to a target population. This is because probability samples tend to have less sampling error than nonprobability samples. *Sampling error* "refers to the fact that the vagaries of chance will nearly always ensure that one sample will differ from another, even if the two samples are drawn from exactly the same target population in exactly the same random way."[3(pp45,46)] Probability samples tend to be less variable and better approximations of the population than nonprobability samples.

PROBABILITY SAMPLING

Four types of probability sampling are presented in this section. As required by definition, all involve randomization at some point in the sampling process. The extent of randomization, however, differs from technique to technique.

Simple Random Sampling

Simple random sampling is a procedure in which each member of the population has an equal chance of being selected for the sample, and selection of each subject is independent of selection of other subjects. Assume that we wish to draw a random sample of 300 subjects from the accessible population of 3000 patients in Table 8–1. To literally "draw" the sample, we would write each patient's name on a slip of paper, put the 3000 slips of paper in a rotating cage, mix the slips thoroughly, and draw out 300 of the slips. This is an example of sampling *without replacement,* because each slip of paper is not replaced in the cage after it is drawn. It is also possible to sample with replacement, in which case the selected unit is placed back in the population so that it may be drawn again. In clinical research it is not feasible to use the same person more than once for a sample, so sampling without replacement is the norm.

Drawing a sample from a cage, or even from a hat, may work fairly well when the accessible population is small. With larger populations, it becomes difficult to mix the units thoroughly. This apparently happened in the 1970 US draft lottery, when troops were being deployed to Vietnam. Capsules representing days of the year were placed in a cage for selection to determine the order in which young men would be drafted into the armed forces. Days from the later months of the year were selected considerably earlier than days from months earlier in the year. Presumably, the capsules were not mixed well, leading to a higher rate of induction among men with birthdays later in the year.[3(pp5-7)]

The preferred method for generating a simple random sample is to use random numbers that are provided in a table or generated by a computer. Table 8–2 shows a portion of the random numbers table reproduced in Appendix A.[4] Before consulting the table, the researcher numbers the units in the sampling frame. In our TKA study, the patients would be numbered from 0001 to 3000. Starting in a random place on the table, and moving in either a horizontal or vertical direction, we would include in our sample any four-digit numbers from 0001 to 3000 that we encounter. Any four-digit numbers greater than 3000 are ignored, as are duplicate numbers. The process is continued until the required number of units is selected. From within the boldface portion of Table 8–2 in Column 7, Rows 76 through 80, the following numbers, which correspond to individual subjects, would be selected for our TKA sample: 1945, 2757, and 2305.

Simple random sampling is easy to comprehend, but it is sometimes difficult to implement. If the population is large, the process of assigning a number to each population unit becomes extremely time-consuming. The other probability

sampling techniques are easier to implement than simple random sampling and may control sampling error as well as simple random sampling. Therefore, the following three probability sampling procedures are used more frequently than simple random sampling.

Systematic Sampling

Systematic sampling is a process by which the researcher selects every nth person on a list. To generate a systematic sample of 300 subjects from the TKA population of 3000, we would select every 10th person. The list of 3000 patients might be ordered by patient number, social security number, date of surgery, or birth date. To begin the systematic sampling procedure, a random start within the list of 3000 patients is necessary. To get a random start we can, for example, point to a number on a random numbers table, observe four digits of the license plate number on a car in the parking lot, reverse the last four digits of the accession number of a library book, or ask four different people to select numbers between zero and nine and combine them to form a starting number. There are endless ways to select the random starting number for a systematic sample. If the random starting number for a systematic sample of our TKA population is 1786, and the sampling interval is 10, then the first four subjects selected would be the 1786th, 1796th, 1806th, and 1816th individuals on the list.

Systematic sampling is an efficient alternative to simple random sampling, and it often generates samples that are as representative of their populations as simple random sampling.[5] The exception to this is if the ordering system used somehow introduces a systematic error into the sample. Assume that we use dates of surgery to order our TKA sample, and that for most weeks during the 5-year period there were 10 surgeries performed. Because the sampling interval is 10, and there were usually 10 surgeries performed per week, systematic sampling would tend to overrepresent patients who had surgery on a

TABLE 8-2 Segment of a Random Numbers Table[*]

Column

Row	1	2	3	4	5	6	7	8	9	10	11	12	13	14
71	91227	21199	31935	27022	84067	05462	35216	14486	29891	68607	41867	14951	91696	85065
72	50001	38140	66321	19924	72163	09538	12151	06878	91903	18749	34405	56087	82790	70925
73	65390	05224	72958	28609	81406	39147	25549	48542	42627	45233	57202	94617	23772	07896
74	27504	96131	83944	41575	10573	08619	64482	73923	36152	05184	94142	25299	84347	34925
75	37169	94851	39177	89632	00959	16487	65536	49071	39782	17095	02330	74301	00275	48280
76	11508	70225	51111	38351	19444	66499	71945	05442	13442	78675	48081	66938	93654	59894
77	37449	30362	06694	54690	04052	53115	62757	95348	78662	11163	81651	50245	34971	52924
78	46515	70331	85922	38379	57015	15765	97161	17869	45349	61796	66345	81073	49106	79860
79	30986	81223	42416	58353	21532	30502	32305	86482	05174	07901	54339	58861	74818	46942
80	63798	64995	46583	09765	44160	78128	83991	42865	92520	83531	80377	35909	81250	54238

* Complete table appears in Appendix A.
From Beyer WH, ed. *Standard Mathematical Tables.* 27th ed. Boca Raton, Fla: CRC Press; 1984.

certain day of the week. Table 8–3 shows an example of how patients with surgery on Monday might be overrepresented in the systematic sample; the boldface entries indicate the units chosen for the sample. If certain surgeons usually perform their TKAs on Tuesday, their patients would be underrepresented in the sample. If patients who are scheduled for surgery on Monday typically have fewer medical complications than those scheduled for surgery later in the week, this will also bias the sample. It is unlikely that the assumptions made to produce this hypothetical bias would operate so systematically in real life—the number of cases per week is likely more variable than presented here, and surgeons likely perform TKAs on more than one day of the week. However, possible systematic biases such as this should be considered when one is deciding how to order the population for systematic sampling.

Stratified Sampling

Stratified sampling is used when certain subgroups must be represented in adequate num-

bers within the sample or when it is important to preserve the proportions of subgroups in the population within the sample. In our TKA study, if we hope to make generalizations across the eight hospitals within the study, we need to be sure there are enough patients from each hospital in the sample to provide a reasonable basis for making statements about the outcomes of TKA at each hospital. On the other hand, if we want to generalize results to the "average" patient undergoing a TKA, then we need to have proportional representation of subjects from the eight hospitals.

Table 8–4 contrasts *proportional* and *nonproportional* stratified sampling. In proportional sampling, the percentage of subjects from each hospital is the same in the population and the sample (with minor deviations because subjects cannot be divided in half; compare Columns 3 and 5). However, the actual number of subjects from each hospital in the sample ranges from 12 to 62 (Column 4). In nonproportional sampling, the percentage of subjects from each hospital is different for the population and the sample (compare Columns 3 and 7). However, the actual number of subjects from each hospital is the same (Column 6, with minor deviations because subjects cannot be divided in half).

Stratified sampling from the accessible population is implemented in several steps. First, all units in the accessible population are identified according to the stratification criteria. Second, the appropriate number of subjects is selected from each stratum. Subjects may be selected from each stratum through simple random sampling or systematic sampling. More than one stratum may be identified. For instance, we might want to ensure that each of the eight hospitals and each of the 5 years of the study period are equally represented in the sample. In this case, we first stratify the accessible population into eight groups by hospital, then stratify each hospital into five groups by year, and finally draw a random sample from each of the 40 Hospital × Year subgroups.

Stratified sampling is easy to accomplish if the stratifying characteristic is known for each

TABLE 8–3	Systematic Bias in a Systematic Sample

Subject	Date of Surgery	Surgeon
1786	**1–8–99 (Monday)**	**A***
1787	1–8–99 (Monday)	A
1788	1–9–99 (Tuesday)	B
1789	1–9–99 (Tuesday)	B
1790	1–10–99 (Wednesday)	C
1791	1–10–99 (Wednesday)	C
1792	1–11–99 (Thursday)	D
1793	1–11–99 (Thursday)	D
1794	1–12–99 (Friday)	E
1795	1–12–99 (Friday)	E
1796	**1–15–99 (Monday)**	**A**
1797	1–15–99 (Monday)	A

* Boldface rows indicate the patients selected for the study. If the sampling interval is 10, and approximately 10 surgeries are performed per week, patients of Surgeon A, who usually performs total knee arthroplasties on Monday, will be overrepresented in the sample.

TABLE 8-4 **Proportional and Nonproportional Stratified Sampling of Patients at Eight Hospitals**

Hospital	Population Distribution		Proportional Sample		Nonproportional Sample	
	N	%	N	%	N	%
A	125	4.1	12	4.0	37	12.3
B	250	8.3	25	8.3	37	12.3
C	250	8.3	25	8.3	37	12.3
D	375	12.5	38	12.7	37	12.3
E	375	12.5	38	12.7	38	12.7
F	500	16.7	50	16.7	38	12.7
G	500	16.7	50	16.7	38	12.7
H	625	20.8	62	20.6	38	12.7
Total	3000	100.0	300	100.0	300	100.0

sampling unit. In our TKA study, both the hospital and year of surgery are known for all elements in the sampling frame. In fact, those characteristics were required for placement of subjects into the accessible population. A much different situation exists, however, if we decide that it is important to ensure that certain knee replacement models are represented in the sample in adequate numbers. Stratifying according to this characteristic would require that someone read all 3000 medical charts to determine which knee model was used for each subject. Because of the inordinate amount of time it would take to determine the knee model for each potential subject, we should consider whether simple random or systematic sampling would likely result in a good representation of each knee model.

Another difficulty with stratification is that some strata require that the researcher set classification boundaries. The strata discussed so far (hospital, year, and knee model) are discrete categories of items. Consider, though, the dilemma that would occur if we wanted to stratify on a variable such as "amount of inpatient physical therapy." If we wanted to ensure that differing levels of physical therapy are represented in the sample, we would need to decide what constitutes low, medium, and high amounts of inpatient physical therapy. Not only would we have

to determine the boundaries between groups, we would also have to obtain the information on all 3000 individuals in the accessible population. Once again, we should consider whether random or systematic sampling would likely result in an adequate distribution of the amount of physical therapy received by patients in the sample.

In summary, stratified sampling is useful when a researcher believes it is imperative to ensure that certain characteristics are represented in a sample in specified numbers. Stratifying on some variables will prove to be too costly and must therefore be left to chance. In many cases, simple random or systematic sampling will result in an adequate distribution of the variable in question.

Cluster Sampling

Cluster sampling is the use of naturally occurring groups as the sampling units. It is used when an appropriate sampling frame does not exist or when logistical constraints limit the researcher's ability to travel widely. There are often several stages to a cluster sampling procedure. For example, if we wanted to conduct a nationwide study on outcomes after TKA, we could not use simple random sampling because the entire population of patients with TKA is not enumerated—that is, a nationwide sampling frame does not exist. In addition, we do not have the funds to travel to all the states and cities that would be represented if a nationwide random sample were selected. To generate a nationwide cluster sample of patients who have undergone a TKA, therefore, we could first sample states, then cities within each selected state, then hospitals within each selected city, and then patients within each selected hospital. Sampling frames for all of these clusters exist: The 50 states are known, various references list cities and populations within each state,[6] and other references list hospitals by city and size.[7]

Each step of the cluster sampling procedure can be implemented through simple random, systematic, or stratified sampling. Assume that we have the money and time to study patients in six states. To select these six states, we might stratify according to region and then randomly select one state from each region. From each of the six states selected, we might develop a list of all cities with populations greater than 50,000 and randomly select two cities from this list. The selection could be random or could be stratified according to city size so that one larger and one smaller city within each state are selected. From each city, we might select two hospitals for study. Within each hospital, patients who underwent TKA in the appropriate time frame would be selected randomly, systematically, or according to specified strata. Figure 8–1 shows the cluster sampling procedure with all steps illustrated for one state, city, and hospital. The same process would occur in the other selected states, cities, and hospitals.

Cluster sampling can save time and money compared with simple random sampling be-

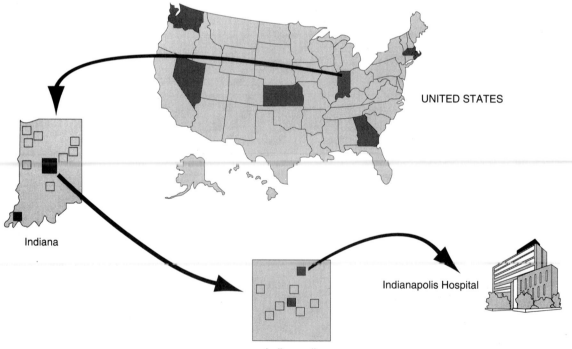

UNITED STATES

Indiana

Indianapolis

Indianapolis Hospital

FIGURE 8–1. Partial example of cluster sampling. Six of 50 states are selected, two cities are selected in each state, and two hospitals are selected from each city. Selected units are shaded; only one state, city, and hospital is illustrated.

cause subjects are clustered in locations. A simple random sample of patients after TKA would likely take us into 50 states and hundreds of cities. The cluster sampling procedure just described would limit the study to 12 cities in six states.

Cluster sampling can occur on a smaller scale as well. Assume that some researchers wish to study the effectiveness of a new electrotherapy modality on patients with chronic pain, and the accessible population consists of patients with chronic pain who seek physical therapy care in a single city. This example is well suited to cluster sampling because a sampling frame of this population does not exist. In addition, it would be difficult to train all therapists within the city to use the new modality with their patients, and there is probably a limited number of machines available for use. Cluster sampling of a few physical therapy departments or practices, and then a few therapists within each department or practice, would be efficient use of the researcher's time for both identifying appropriate patients and training therapists with the new modality.

Cluster sampling may also be necessitated by administrative constraints. Assume that researchers wish to determine the relative effectiveness of two educational approaches to third graders' developing awareness of individuals with physical disabilities: In one approach children simulate disabilities themselves, and in the other approach individuals with disabilities make presentations to the students. A superintendent is unlikely to allow the study to take place if it requires a random sampling of third graders across the school system with disruption of classrooms. Since third graders exist in clusters, it seems natural to use schools or classrooms as the sampling unit, rather than the individual pupil.

■ NONPROBABILITY SAMPLING

Nonprobability sampling is widely used in physical therapy research and is distinguished from probability sampling by the absence of randomization. One reason for the predominance of nonprobability sampling in physical therapy research is limited funding. Because many studies are self-funded, subject selection is confined to a single setting with a limited number of available patients, so the researcher often chooses to study the entire accessible population. Three forms of nonprobability sampling are discussed: convenience, snowball, and purposive sampling.

Samples of Convenience

Samples of convenience involve the use of readily available subjects. Physical therapy researchers commonly use samples of convenience of patients in certain diagnostic categories at a single clinic. If we conducted our study of patients after TKA by using all patients who underwent the surgery from 1995 to 1999 at a given hospital, this would represent a sample of convenience. If patients who undergo TKA at this hospital are different in some way from the overall population of patients who have this surgery, then our study would have little generalizability beyond that facility.

The term "sample of convenience" seems to give the negative implication that the researcher has not worked hard enough at the task of sampling. In addition, we already know that probability samples tend to have less sampling error than nonprobability samples. But before one totally discounts the validity of samples of convenience, it should be pointed out that the accessible populations discussed earlier in the chapter can also be viewed as large samples of convenience. An accessible population that consists of "patients post-TKA who are 60 years old or older and had the surgery at one of eight hospitals in Indianapolis from 1995 to 1999" is technically a large sample of convenience from the population of all the individuals in the world who have undergone TKA. Figure 8–2 shows the distinctions among a target population, an accessible population, a random sample, and a sample of convenience.

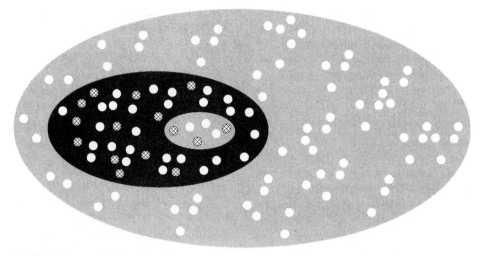

FIGURE 8–2. Distinctions among target populations, accessible populations, samples of convenience, and random samples. The white dots represent elements within the population. The large gray ellipse represents the target population. The black ellipse represents the accessible population. The small gray ellipse represents a sample of convenience. The cross-hatched dots represent a random sample from the accessible population.

Consecutive sampling is a form of convenience sampling. Consecutive samples are used in a prospective study in which the population does not exist at the beginning of the study; in other words, a sampling frame does not exist. If researchers plan a 2-year prospective study of the outcomes of TKA at a particular hospital beginning January 1, 1999, the population of interest does not begin to exist until the first patient has surgery in 1999. In a consecutive sample, all patients who meet the criteria are placed into the study as they are identified. This continues until a specified number of patients is collected, a specified time frame has passed, or certain statistical outcomes are seen.

Snowball Sampling

A snowball sample may be used when the potential members of the sample are difficult to identify. In a snowball sample researchers identify a few subjects who are then asked to identify other potential members of the sample. If a team of researchers wishes to study patients who

return to sports activities earlier than recommended after ligament reconstruction surgery, snowball sampling is one way to generate a sufficient sample. The investigators will neither be able to purchase a mailing list of such patients, nor will they be able to determine return-to-sport dates reliably from medical records since many patients will not disclose their early return to the health care providers who advised against it. However, if the researchers can use personal contacts to identify a few subjects who returned early, it is likely that those subjects will be able to identify other potential subjects from among their teammates or workout partners.

Purposive Sampling

Purposive sampling is used when a researcher has a specific reason for selecting particular subjects for study. Whereas convenience sampling uses whatever units are readily available, purposive sampling uses handpicked units that meet the researcher's needs. Random, convenience, and purposive samples can be distinguished if we return to the hypothetical study of different educational modes for teaching children about physical disabilities. If there are 40 elementary schools in a district and the researchers randomly select two of them for study, this is clearly a random sample of schools from the accessible population of a single school district. If the researchers select two schools in close proximity to their place of work, this constitutes a sample of convenience. If the researchers pick the first school because it is large and students are from families with high median incomes and pick the second school because it is small and draws students from families with modest median incomes, this constitutes a purposive sample. Rather than selecting for a representative group of subjects, the researchers deliberately pick subjects who illustrate different levels of variables they believe may be important to the question at hand. Purposive sampling is more often used by qualitative researchers, who are interested in developing an in-depth understanding of a particular situation, than by quantitative researchers, who wish to develop a generalizable understanding of the phenomenon of interest.

■ ASSIGNMENT TO GROUPS

When a study requires more than one group, the researchers need a method for assigning subjects to groups. Random assignment to groups is preferred and is appropriate even when the original selection procedure was nonrandom. Thus, many studies in the physical therapy literature use a sample of convenience combined with random assignment to groups. The goal of group assignment is to create groups that are equally representative of the entire sample. Because many statistical techniques require equal group sizes, a secondary goal of the assignment process is often to develop groups of equal size.

There are four basic ways to randomly assign subjects to groups within a study. These methods can be illustrated by a hypothetical sample of 32 patients who have undergone TKA; age and sex are listed for each patient in Table 8–5.

TABLE 8–5	Existing Sample Characteristics: Case Number, Sex, and Age*		
1. F, 70	9. F, 62	17. M, 70	25. M, 76
2. M, 60	10. F, 78	18. F, 63	26. F, 72
3. M, 71	11. F, 68	19. M, 71	27. F, 77
4. F, 64	12. M, 81	20. F, 76	28. F, 67
5. F, 65	13. F, 69	21. F, 61	29. F, 69
6. F, 68	14. F, 60	22. M, 67	30. M, 67
7. M, 68	15. M, 66	23. M, 65	31. M, 65
8. M, 69	16. M, 66	24. M, 63	32. M, 62

* Mean age is 68 years; 50% of sample is female.

The sample has a mean age of 68 years and consists of 50% women and 50% men. Each of the four assignment techniques was applied to this sample; the processes are described in the following four sections, and the results are presented in Tables 8–6 to 8–9.

The design of our hypothetical study calls for four groups of patients, each undergoing a different post-TKA rehabilitation program. The four programs are variations based on two techniques for increasing range of motion (continuous passive motion [CPM] and manual stretching) and two techniques for restoring muscular function (open- and closed-chain exercise). Range-of-motion technique is one independent variable, and strengthening technique is the second independent variable. One group receives open-chain exercise and manual stretching, one group receives open-chain exercise and CPM, one group receives closed-chain exercise and manual stretching, and the final group receives closed-chain exercise and CPM.

Random Assignment by Individual

The first method of random assignment is to randomly assign each individual in the sample to one of the four groups. This could be done with a roll of a die, ignoring rolls of 5 and 6. When this assignment technique was applied to the hypothetical sample in Table 8–5, the open-chain/manual treatment was represented by a

TABLE 8-6	Random Assignment by Individual		
Group 1*: Open Chain/Manual	**Group 2†:** Open Chain/CPM‖	**Group 3‡:** Closed Chain/Manual	**Group 4§:** Closed Chain/CPM
5. F, 65	4. F, 64	1. F, 70	6. F, 68
9. F, 62	14. F, 60	2. M, 60	7. M, 68
17. M, 70	15. M, 66	3. M, 71	8. M, 69
21. F, 61	20. F, 76	10. F, 78	14. F, 60
	24. M, 63	12. M, 81	18. F, 63
	28. F, 67	13. F, 69	19. M, 71
	30. M, 67	16. M, 66	22. M, 67
	31. M, 65		23. M, 65
	32. M, 62		25. M, 76
			26. F, 72
			27. F, 77
			29. F, 69

* $n = 4$, mean age = 64.5 years, women = 75.0%.
† $n = 9$, mean age = 65.5 years, women = 44.4%.
‡ $n = 7$, mean age = 70.7 years, women = 42.8%.
§ $n = 12$, mean age = 68.8 years, women = 50.0%.
‖ Continuous passive motion.

roll of 1, the open-chain/CPM condition by a roll of 2, the closed-chain/manual treatment by a roll of 3, and the closed-chain/CPM treatment by a roll of 4. The results of the procedure are shown in Table 8–6. Note that the group sizes range from four to 12 subjects.

The advantage of assignment by individual is that it is easy to do. The main disadvantage is that with a small sample size, the resulting group sizes are not likely to be equal. With a larger sample size, the probability that group sizes will be nearly equal is greater.

TABLE 8-7	Random Assignment by Block		
Group 1*: Open Chain/Manual	**Group 2†:** Open Chain/CPM‖	**Group 3‡:** Closed Chain/Manual	**Group 4§:** Closed Chain/CPM
1. F, 70	2. M, 60	8. M, 69	10. F, 78
3. M, 71	4. F, 64	11. F, 68	12. M, 81
7. M, 68	5. F, 65	15. M, 66	13. F, 69
16. M, 66	6. F, 68	18. F, 63	14. F, 60
21. F, 61	9. F, 62	19. M, 71	20. F, 76
22. M, 67	17. M, 70	23. M, 65	26. F, 72
24. M, 63	25. M, 76	30. M, 67	28. F, 67
27. F, 77	31. M, 65	32. M, 62	29. F, 69

* Mean age = 67.9 years, women = 37.5%.
† Mean age = 66.3 years, women = 50.0%.
‡ Mean age = 66.3 years, women = 25.0%.
§ Mean age = 71.5 years, women = 87.5%.
‖ Continuous passive motion.

TABLE 8-8 Systematic Assignment

Group 1[*]: Open Chain/Manual	Group 2[†]: Open Chain/CPM[∥]	Group 3[‡]: Closed Chain/Manual	Group 4[§]: Closed Chain/CPM
1. F, 70	2. M, 60	3. M, 71	4. F, 64
5. F, 65	6. F, 68	7. M, 68	8. M, 69
9. F, 62	10. F, 78	11. F, 68	12. M, 81
13. F, 69	14. F, 60	15. M, 66	16. M, 66
17. M, 70	18. F, 63	19. M, 71	20. F, 76
21. F, 61	22. M, 67	23. M, 65	24. M, 63
25. M, 76	26. F, 72	27. F, 77	28. F, 67
29. F, 67	30. M, 67	31. M, 65	32. M, 62

[*] Mean age = 67.5 years, women = 75.0%.
[†] Mean age = 66.9 years, women = 62.5%.
[‡] Mean age = 68.9 years, women = 25.0%.
[§] Mean age = 68.5 years, women = 37.5%.
[∥] Continuous passive motion.

Random Assignment by Block

The second assignment method uses blocks of subjects to ensure equal group sizes. Say that in our sample of patients who underwent TKA, we wish to have four groups of eight subjects. To assign by block, we can use a random numbers table to select eight numbers for the first group, eight for the second group, and so on. Looking at the last two digits in each column and proceeding from left to right beginning in Column 1 of Row 71 of the random numbers table (Table 8–2), the numbers between 01 and 32 are boldface and italic, skipping any duplicates. The first eight subjects who correspond to the first eight numbers constitute the first group. The next eight numbers constitute the second group, and so on. The complete results of this assignment

TABLE 8-9 Matched Assignment

Group 1[*]: Open Chain/Manual	Group 2[†]: Open Chain/CPM[∥]	Group 3[‡]: Closed Chain/Manual	Group 4[§]: Closed Chain/CPM
14. F, 60	21. F, 61	9. F, 62	18. F, 63
31. M, 65	24. M, 63	32. M, 62	2. M, 60
28. F, 67	4. F, 64	5. F, 65	6. F, 68
15. M, 66	22. M, 67	16. M, 66	23. M, 65
1. F, 70	29. F, 69	11. F, 68	13. F, 69
30. M, 67	7. M, 68	17. M, 70	8. M, 69
10. F, 78	27. F, 77	20. F, 76	26. F, 72
3. M, 71	19. M, 71	25. M, 76	12. M, 81

[*] Mean age = 68.0 years, women = 50.0%.
[†] Mean age = 67.5 years, women = 50.0%.
[‡] Mean age = 68.1 years, women = 50.0%.
[§] Mean age = 68.4 years, women = 50.0%.
[∥] Continuous passive motion.

procedure are shown in Table 8–7. Random assignment to groups by block can become time-consuming with large samples.

Systematic Assignment

The process of systematic assignment is familiar to anyone who has taken a physical education class where teams were formed by "counting off." Researchers count off by using a list of the sample and systematically placing subsequent subjects into subsequent groups. Table 8–8 shows the groups generated by systematic assignment for this example. The first person was assigned to the open-chain/manual group, the second person to the open-chain/CPM group, the third person to the closed-chain/manual group, the fourth person to the closed-chain/CPM group, the fifth person to the open-chain/manual group, and so on.

Matched Assignment

In matched assignment, subjects are matched on important characteristics and these subgroups are randomly assigned to study groups. In our sample of TKA patients, subjects were matched on both age and sex. The four youngest women in the sample were placed in a subgroup and then were randomly assigned to study groups. To randomly assign the matched subjects to groups, four different-colored poker chips, each representing a study group, were placed into a container. As shown in Table 8–9, the first chip drawn placed the youngest woman into the open-chain/manual group; the second chip drawn placed the next youngest woman into the open-chain/CPM group, and so on. The four youngest men were then placed into a subgroup and were assigned randomly to study groups. This procedure continued for the next youngest subgroups until all subjects were assigned to groups.

The matched assignment procedure is somewhat analogous to stratified sampling and has some of the same disadvantages as stratified sampling. First, it ensures relatively equal distributions only on the variables that are matched. The possibility that other characteristics may not be evenly distributed across the groups may be forgotten in light of the homogeneity on the matched variables. In addition, the information needed for matching on some variables is difficult and expensive to obtain. If we wanted to match groups according to range of motion and knee function before surgery, we would have had to collect this data ourselves or depend on potentially unreliable retrospective data.

Consecutive Assignment

The four assignment methods presented thus far are used when an existing sample is available for assignment to groups. This is not the case when consecutive sampling is being used, for example, to identify patients as they undergo surgery or enter a health care facility. When a consecutive sample is used, then assignment to groups needs to be consecutive as well. The basic strategy used for consecutive assignment is the development of an ordered list with group assignments made in advance. As subjects enter the study they are given consecutive numbers and assigned to the group indicated for each number.

Deciding on an Assignment Method

The best assignment method ensures that group sizes are equal, group characteristics are similar, and group characteristics approximate the overall sample characteristics. Assignment by individuals leads to a situation in which group sizes are not necessarily equal; this is more of a problem with small group studies than with large group studies. Matched assignment obviously often leads to the least variability between groups on the matched variables, but it may not randomize other extraneous factors. In addition, it may be expensive and time-consuming to collect the information on which subjects will be matched.

The choice between block assignment and systematic assignment is probably arbitrary unless the researcher suspects some regularly recurring pattern in subjects. In this case, block assignment should be used. With large samples, and in the absence of a regularly recurring pattern in the subject listing, systematic assignment provides an effective and efficient way to place subjects into groups.

SAMPLE SIZE

The preceding discussion of sampling and assignment was based on one major assumption—that the researcher knows how many subjects should be in the sample and in each group. In the real world, researchers must make decisions about sample size, and these decisions have a great deal of impact on the validity of the statistical conclusions of a piece of research. A complete discussion of the determination of sample size is deferred until the statistical foundation of the text is laid, but one general principle of sample size determination is presented here.

This general principle is that larger samples tend to be more representative of their parent populations than smaller samples. To illustrate this principle, consider our hypothetical sample of 32 patients who underwent TKA as an accessible population from which we shall draw even smaller samples. From the population of 32 subjects, four independent samples of 2 subjects and four independent samples of 8 subjects are selected. An independent sample is drawn, recorded, and replaced into the population before the next sample is drawn.

Tables 8–10 and 8–11 show the results of the sampling, and Figure 8–3 plots the distribution of the average age of subjects in the different-sized samples. Note that average ages for the samples of eight subjects are clustered more closely around the actual population age than are the average ages for the smaller samples. This, then, is a visual demonstration of the principle that large samples tend to be more representative of their parent populations. In addition, this clus-

TABLE 8–10 Characteristics with Sample Sizes of 2

Sample 1	Sample 2	Sample 3	Sample 4
7. M, 68	27. F, 77	21. F, 61	10. F, 78
17. M, 70	11. F, 68	4. F, 64	25. F, 76

Note: In Samples 1 through 4, the mean ages are 69.0, 72.5, 62.5, and 77.0 years, respectively. The percentage of women in each sample ranges from 0.0% to 100.0%.

tering of sample characteristics close to the population characteristics means that there is less variability from sample to sample with the larger sample sizes.

For experimental research, group sizes of about 30 participants are often considered the minimum size needed to make valid generalizations to a larger population and to meet the assumptions of certain statistical tests.[1,8] For descriptive research, the precision of the description depends on the size of the sample. For example, a survey of 100 respondents shows that 60% prefer Brand X hand-held dynamometer and 40% prefer Brand Y. Without going into any of the statistical theories underlying how researchers determine the precision of their results, with this result with 100 subjects we could be 95% certain that the true preference for Brand X is between 50.2% and 69.8%. With 1000 sub-

TABLE 8–11 Characteristics with Sample Sizes of 8

Sample 1	Sample 2	Sample 3	Sample 4
1. F, 70	1. F, 70	3. M, 71	3. M, 71
3. M, 71	6. F, 68	4. F, 64	5. F, 65
6. F, 68	7. M, 68	5. F, 65	6. F, 68
14. F, 60	17. M, 70	6. F, 68	9. F, 62
15. M, 66	22. M, 67	7. M, 68	16. M, 66
29. F, 69	25. M, 76	14. F, 60	17. M, 70
30. M, 67	27. F, 77	24. M, 63	26. F, 72
32. M, 62	30. M, 67	27. F, 77	32. M, 72

Note: In Samples 1 through 4, the mean ages are 66.6, 70.4, 67.0, and 68.3 years, respectively. The percentage of women in each sample ranges from 37.5% to 68.3%.

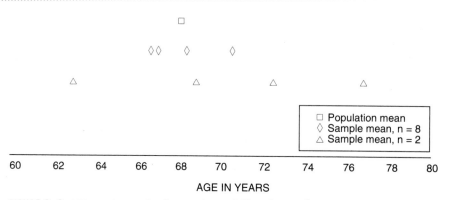

FIGURE 8–3. Effect of sample size on the stability of sample mean age.

jects we could be 95% certain that the true preference for Brand X is between 56.9% and 63.1%. With 2000 subjects we could be 95% certain that the true preference for Brand X is between 57.8% and 62.2%. As a researcher, one has to determine whether the increase in precision from 100 to 1000 to 2000 subjects is worth the additional time and money associated with the larger samples.

When deciding on sample size, researchers should always account for anticipated experimental mortality. If a subject's participation is required on only one day, then retention of selected subjects should be relatively high. If participation requires a commitment of a great deal of time, over a longer time period, researchers should expect that experimental mortality will be high.

Sometimes researchers are glibly advised to "get as many subjects as you can." If only 20 subjects are available, it is good advice—the researcher should try to use them all. However, if several hundred subjects are available, such advice may be inappropriate. First, recommending that sample sizes be as large as possible is ethically questionable, because this means large numbers of individuals are exposed to procedures with unknown benefits. Second, very large samples can create administrative problems that detract from other aspects of the research process. Third, sometimes the results of research on very large groups produce statistical distinc-

tions that are trivial in practice, as is discussed in greater detail in Chapter 20.

■ SUMMARY

Selection and assignment of subjects influence the internal, external, and statistical conclusion validity of research. Populations are total groups of interest; samples are subgroups of populations. Probability samples use some degree of randomization to select subjects from the population. Common methods of probability sampling are simple random, systematic, stratified, and cluster sampling. Nonprobability samples do not rely on randomization. Common methods of nonprobability sampling are convenience and purposive sampling. Assignment to groups within a study can be accomplished randomly regardless of whether or not the method used to select the sample was random. Common forms of random assignment are individual, block, systematic, and matched assignment. A general principle in determining an appropriate sample size is that larger samples tend to be more representative of their parent populations than smaller samples.

REFERENCES

1. Fink A. *How to Sample in Surveys.* Thousand Oaks, Calif: Sage Publications; 1995.
2. Hulley SB, Gove S, Browner WS, Cummings SR. Choosing the study subjects: specification and sampling. In: Hulley

SB, Cummings SR, eds. *Designing Clinical Research.* Baltimore, Md: Williams & Wilkins; 1988.

3. Williams B. *A Sampler on Sampling.* New York, NY: John Wiley & Sons; 1978.

4. Beyer WH, ed. *Standard Mathematical Tables.* 27th ed. Boca Raton, Fla: CRC Press; 1984.

5. Floyd JA. Systematic sampling: theory and clinical methods. *Nurs Res.* 1993;42:290–293.

6. *Commercial Atlas and Marketing Guide.* 130th ed. Chicago, Ill: Rand McNally & Co; 1999.

7. *American Hospital Association Guide to the Health Care Field, 1997–98.* Chicago, Ill: American Hospital Association; 1997.

8. Kraemer HC, Thiemann S. *How Many Subjects? Statistical Power Analysis in Research.* Newbury Park, Calif: Sage Publications; 1987:27.

Experimental Designs

Group Designs

Single-Factor Experimental Designs	Multiple-Factor Experimental Designs
Pretest-Posttest Control-Group Design	Questions That Lead to a Multiple-Factor Design
Posttest-Only Control-Group Design	Factorial Versus Nested Designs
Single-Group Pretest-Posttest Design	Completely Randomized Versus Randomized-Block Designs
Nonequivalent Control-Group Design	Between-Subjects, Within-Subject, and Mixed Designs
Time Series Design	
Repeated Measures or Repeated Treatment Designs	

Experimental research, as defined in Chapter 6, is characterized by controlled manipulation of variables by researchers. This controlled manipulation can be used with groups of subjects or with individuals. In this chapter, experimental designs for groups of subjects are described in detail. These group designs are subdivided into single-factor and multiple-factor research designs according to the number of independent variables used in the design.

◼ SINGLE-FACTOR EXPERIMENTAL DESIGNS

Single-factor experimental designs have one independent variable. Although multiple-factor ex-

perimental designs, which have more than one independent variable, are becoming increasingly common, single-factor designs remain an important part of the physical therapy literature. In 1963 Campbell and Stanley published what was to become a classic work on single-factor experimental design: *Experimental and Quasi-Experimental Designs for Research.*[1] Their slim volume diagrammed 16 different experimental designs and outlined the strengths and weaknesses of each. Such a comprehensive catalogue of single-factor designs cannot be repeated here, but several of the more commonly observed designs are illustrated by studies from the physical therapy literature. It should be noted that some of the studies presented included secondary purposes that involved an additional independent variable. If readers go to the research reports themselves, they will find that some of the studies are more complex than would be assumed from reading this chapter.

Pretest-Posttest Control-Group Design

The first design example is the pretest-posttest control-group design. This design is also referred to as a *randomized clinical trial* or *randomized controlled trial* (RCT). In addition, this is an example of a *between-subjects design* because the differences of interest are those differences that occur between subject groups. The Campbell and Stanley notation for the pretest-posttest control-group design is as follows[1(p13)]:

R   O   X   O
R   O   O

The Os represent observation, or measurement. The X represents an intervention, or manipulation. The Rs indicate that subjects were assigned randomly to the two groups.

In clinical research, the pretest-posttest control-group design is often altered slightly, as follows:

R   O X_1 O
R   O X_2 O

This alteration is often made in order to deal with clinical populations ethically. If the researcher does not wish to withhold treatment altogether, one group receives a typical treatment, and the other group receives the experimental treatment.

Dean and Shepherd performed an experiment using a pretest-posttest control-group design that contrasted the effect of reaching tasks with control tasks.[2] Twenty subjects were randomly assigned to either the reaching group or the control group. The strongest evidence for the effectiveness of the experimental treatment is when the experimental group changes in the desired direction and the control group remains the same. In the Dean and Shepherd study this ideal pattern of results was seen; the experimental subjects improved their scores on the reaching tasks while the control subjects did not.[2]

Variations on the pretest-posttest control-group design include taking more than two measurements and using more than two treatment groups. An example of both variations is found in Griffin and associates' study of reduction of chronic posttraumatic hand edema with high-voltage pulsed current, intermittent pneumatic compression, or placebo treatments.[3] The notation for this design would be as follows:

R   O   O X_1 O
R   O   O X_2 O
R   O   O   O

Patients were randomly assigned to the stimulation, compression, or placebo group. The placebo group received sham high-voltage stimulation. The first measure (pretest) was taken when the patient arrived at the clinic. The second measure (posttest) was taken after subjects rested for 10 minutes with their arm positioned at the level of the heart. This rest period was used to control for the possible effects of varied hand positions prior to coming to the clinic for treatment. The third measure (posttreatment) was taken after the conclusion of treatment.

Posttest-Only Control-Group Design

A second design is the posttest-only control-group design. Researchers use this design when they are not able to take pretest measurements, and therefore the posttest is the only basis on which to make judgments about the effect of the independent variable on the dependent variable. This design is also a between-subjects design.

The Campbell and Stanley notation for this design is as follows[1(p25)]:

R   X   O

R   O

An example of this design is found in Arciero and colleagues' study of tourniquet use in anterior cruciate ligament (ACL) surgery.[4] They compared a variety of measures—including quadriceps and hamstring muscle strength and hopping tests—between a group of patients who had a tourniquet during ACL reconstruction surgery and a group that had not had a tourniquet during the procedure. In this study, preoperative and immediate postoperative measures of strength and hopping ability would not be accurate because of the pain and dysfunction associated with either an injured or acutely reconstructed knee. Therefore, only postprocedure measures were taken. Because subjects were randomly assigned to groups, it is assumed (but not guaranteed) that the randomization procedure balanced any extraneous variables across the two groups.

Single-Group Pretest-Posttest Design

The Campbell and Stanley notation for the single-group pretest-posttest design is as follows[1(p7)]:

O   X   O

A slight variation on this design is seen in Harada and associates' study of the effectiveness of an individualized physical therapy program on balance and gait speed of older people in residential care facilities.[5] In this study, almost 30 patients with balance and functional impairments were treated with an individualized physical therapy program for 4 to 5 weeks. The independent variable was physical therapy, with three levels: baseline, immedi-

ately after intervention, and 1 month after intervention. The dependent variables were two different balance scores and gait speed. Patients showed significant improvements on the balance variables at both follow-up periods. This design did not control for the possibility that patients would make similar gains without a formal rehabilitation program. To control for this possibility, a study comparing physical therapy with no physical therapy would need to be conducted.

Nonequivalent Control-Group Design

The nonequivalent control-group design is used when a nonrandom control group is available for comparison. The Campbell and Stanley notation for this design is as follows[1(p47)]:

O   X   O

O   O

The dotted line between groups indicates that subjects were not randomly assigned to groups. Amundsen and colleagues studied the effects of a group exercise program on various physiological variables in elderly women.[6] Five women completed pretests and posttests but were unable to participate in the training sessions, 19 attended fewer than half of the twice-weekly sessions, and 14 completed at least half of the sessions. Comparisons were made between the 14 regular attendees (exercise group) and the 5 untrained women (control group). This nonrandom assignment to groups did not control for extraneous factors that might explain different results between the two groups.

Another approach to the nonequivalent control-group design is the use of cohorts for the experimental groups. The term *cohort* is generally used to refer to any group; a more specific use of the term refers to groups of individuals who follow each other in time. A cohort approach would be a convenient way to study the effects of a planned curriculum change on entry-level job performance of recent physical therapy graduates. The last class, or cohort, who studied under the old curriculum would form the control group; the class, or cohort, who were exposed to the curricular innovation would form the experimental group.

Time Series Design

The time series design is used to establish a baseline of measurements before initiation of treatment to either a group or an individual. When a comparison group is not available, it becomes important to either establish the stability of a measure before implementation of treatment or document the extent to which the measure is changing solely as a function of time. The Campbell and Stanley notation for the time series design is as follows[1(p37)]:

O   O   O   O   X   O   O   O   O

The number of measurements taken before, after, or even during the intervention varies depending on the nature of the study. If it is important to assess changes over many time intervals, any of the two or more group designs can be modified by use of additional measurements before or after treatment.

Ulione used a time series approach to study the impact of a health promotion and injury prevention program at a child development center.[7] Data on the upper respiratory illnesses, diarrhea, and injuries of the children in the development center were collected once a week for 4 weeks prior to and after the health promotion program. The four measurements taken before and after the intervention provide a fuller picture of the health status of the children than would single pretest and posttest measures. Although the time series approach can be applied to group designs, as it was in the Ulione article, in physical therapy research it is commonly used with a single-system approach, which is considered in detail in Chapter 10.

Repeated Measures or Repeated Treatment Designs

Repeated measures designs are widely used in health science research. The term *repeated measures* means that the same subjects are measured under all the levels of the independent variable. In this sense, any of the pretest-posttest designs can be considered a repeated measures design because each subject is measured at both levels (before and after treatment) of a possible independent variable. The *repeated treatment* design is a type of repeated measures design in which each subject receives more than one actual treatment. The repeated measures designs are also referred to as *within-subject* designs because the effect of the independent variable is seen within subjects in a single group rather than between the groups.

Scudds and associates studied the effect of transcutaneous electrical nerve stimulation (TENS) on skin temperature in asymptomatic subjects.[8] Their independent variable, "stimulation," had three levels: high-frequency TENS, low-frequency TENS, and sham TENS. The 24 subjects each received all three of these levels, with treatments 24 hours apart. Although repeated treatment designs ensure that subject characteristics such as age and sex remain constant across the levels of the independent variable, they create a new set of extraneous factors related to familiarization with the experimental procedures. These factors should be controlled by counterbalancing the order of administration of the treatments, as Scudds and colleagues did when they randomized the order of treatments with a Latin square (see Chapter 6).

■ MULTIPLE-FACTOR EXPERIMENTAL DESIGNS

Multiple-factor experimental designs are used frequently in physical therapy research. Because of their widespread use, it is essential that physical therapists have command of the language and concepts related to multiple-factor designs. This section of the chapter is divided into several subsections. After a discussion of the basic research questions that would prompt a researcher to develop a multiple-factor design, some common multiple-factor designs are presented.

Questions That Lead to a Multiple-Factor Design

Researchers usually design multiple-factor experiments because they are interested not only in the individual effects of the multiple factors on the dependent variable, but also in the effects of the interaction between the multiple factors on the dependent variable. For example, say we wished to conduct a study to determine the effects of different physical therapy programs (heat/exercise, manual therapy, and home program) on low back range of motion in patients with low back pain. We could start by selecting 60 patients for study and randomly assigning them to one of the three groups. The first independent variable would be type of treatment, or group. Say two therapists are going to provide the treatments. We might wonder whether one therapist might simply get better results than the other therapist, regardless of the type of treatment provided. A second independent variable, then, is therapist. If therapist is added as a second independent variable, a third question must also be asked in this design: Is one therapist more effective with one type of treatment and the other therapist more effective with another type of treatment? In other words, is there an interaction between type of treatment and therapist? It is the study of interaction that clearly differentiates a multiple-factor experimental design from a single-factor design.

Factorial Versus Nested Designs

The Type of Treatment × Therapist design developed previously is a factorial design. In a *factorial design,* the factors are crossed, meaning

that each level of one factor is combined with each level of each other factor. This simply means that each treatment group has members who are exposed to each therapist, and each therapist is exposed to members of each treatment group. This design is diagrammed in Figure 9–1. Group is one variable, with three levels: heat/exercise, manual therapy, and home program. Therapist is the second variable, with two levels: A and B. There are six cells in the design, formed by crossing the two factors. In this example, assume there is an equal number, say 20, of subjects in each cell. The assigned therapists measure lumbar flexion at 2 weeks postinjury, implement the appropriate program to each subject, and measure lumbar flexion at 6 weeks postinjury. The dependent variable is the difference in range of motion from 2 weeks to 6 weeks postinjury.

Figure 9–2 shows a hypothetical set of data and a graph of the data. Figure 9–2A shows that Therapist A is superior overall to Therapist B (the overall mean for Therapist A is a 40-degree improvement in range of motion; the overall mean for Therapist B is 30 degrees), regardless of the type of treatment being delivered. The

	INDEPENDENT VARIABLE: THERAPIST	
	A	B
Heat/exercise	HA	HB
Manual therapy	MA	MB
Home program	PA	PB

(INDEPENDENT VARIABLE: GROUP)

FIGURE 9–1. Two-factor, 3 × 2 factorial design. The notation within each cell shows the combination of the two independent variables. For example, HA indicates that individuals within this cell received the heat/exercise treatment from Therapist A.

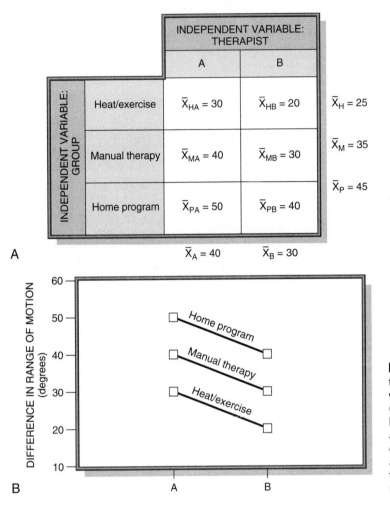

A

B

FIGURE 9–2. Example with no interaction. **A.** Sample data. The notations within the cells represent the mean ($\overline{X}$) scores for subjects for each combination. The means in the margins are the overall means for the column or row. **B.** Graph of sample data. Parallel lines indicate that there is no interaction between therapist and treatment.

home program (overall mean is 45 degrees) is superior overall to the manual therapy and heat/exercise programs (overall means are 35 degrees and 25 degrees, respectively), regardless of which therapist was delivering the treatment. In this example, there is no interaction between treatment and therapist. The home program is the superior treatment, regardless of therapist, and Therapist A gets superior results, regardless of the treatment given. This lack of interaction is shown graphically by the parallel lines in Figure 9–2B between therapists for the three treatments. A concise way to summarize these results is to say there are *main effects* for both type of treat-

ment and therapist, but no interaction between type of treatment and therapist.

Figure 9–3 presents a different set of data. In this instance, Figure 9–3A shows that there are no overall differences in treatment (mean improvement for each treatment, regardless of therapist, is 30 degrees) and no overall differences in therapist results (mean improvement for each therapist, regardless of treatment, is 30 degrees). However, there is a significant interaction between treatment and therapist. In Figure 9–3B Therapist A achieved better results using a home program and Therapist B achieved better results using heat/exercise. Both obtained intermediate

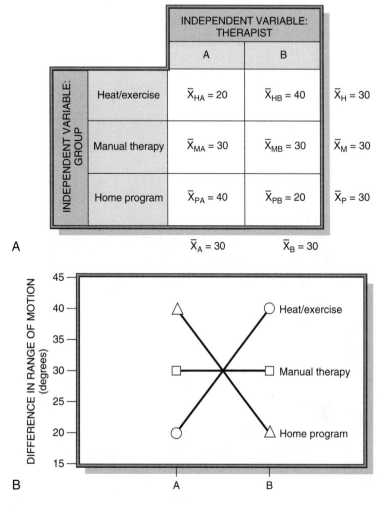

FIGURE 9–3. Example with interaction. **A.** Sample data. The notations within the cells represent the mean ($\bar{X}$) scores for subjects for each combination. The means in the margins are the overall means for the column or row. **B.** Graph of sample data. Nonparallel lines indicate an interaction between therapist and treatment.

results using manual therapy. A concise way of summarizing these results is to say there are no main effects for either type of treatment or therapist, but there is an interaction between type of treatment and therapist. If we had studied only the different treatment types without examining the second factor, therapists, we would have concluded that there were no differences between these treatments. The two-factor study allows us to come to a more sophisticated conclusion: Even though there are no overall differences between the treatments and therapists studied, certain therapists are considerably more effective when using certain treatments.

Nested designs occur when not all the factors cross one another. For example, we could make the earlier example more complex by adding some additional therapists and an additional clinic. The treatment variable remains the same: It has three levels—heat/exercise, manual therapy, and home program. Perhaps there are two competing clinics in town—one has a clientele with varied diagnoses, and the other specializes in spine disorders. This is a second independent variable, with two levels: general and specialty clinics. One research question might be whether patient outcomes at the two clinics are different. The research question of whether different therapists achieve different results remains. This could be studied by using three different therapists at each clinic. Because there are different therapists at each clinic, the therapist variable is nested within the clinic variable. Figure 9–4 presents a schematic view of this hypothetical design in which treatment and clinic are crossed and therapist is nested within clinic.

Completely Randomized Versus Randomized-Block Designs

The Treatment × Therapist example just presented could also be termed a *completely randomized design* because type of treatment and therapist assignment were both manipulable variables and subjects were assigned randomly to both treatment group and therapist.

Sometimes a *randomized-block design* is used, in which one of the factors of interest is not manipulable. If, for example, we had wanted to look at the factors sex and treatment, then sex would have been a classification or attribute

variable. Subjects would be placed into blocks on the basis of sex and then randomly assigned to treatments.

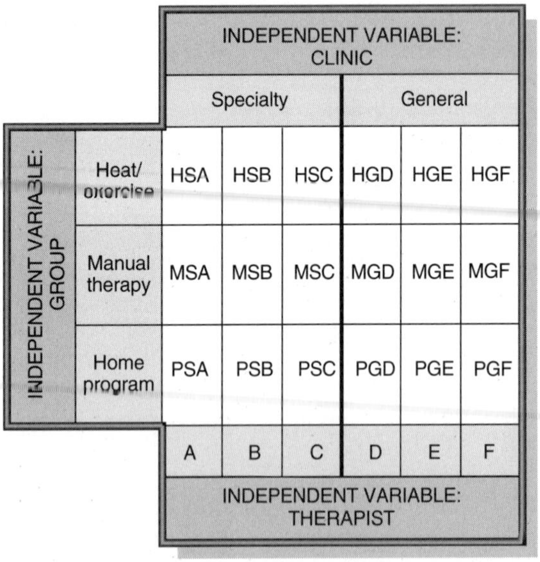

Between-Subjects, Within-Subject, and Mixed Designs

The Treatment × Therapist example could also be termed a *between-subjects* design for both factors. Different subjects were placed into each of the six cells of the design. The research questions related to differences between groups who received different treatments and between groups who had different therapists.

In a *within-subject* design, one group of subjects receives all levels of the independent variable. Taylor and colleagues used a within-subject design to study the effect of stretching with or without heat or cold application on hamstring muscle length.[9] There were two independent variables: treatment (three levels: static stretch with heat, static stretch with cold, and static stretch alone) and time (two levels: pretreatment and posttreatment). Each subject was measured before and after the application of each of the treatments, which were separated in time by about a week. Thus, both independent variables in this study were repeated measures factors, making this a within-subject design.

A *mixed*, or *split-plot*, design contains a combination of between-subjects and within-subject factors. Bandy and Irion studied hamstring stretching with such a design.[10] Subjects were randomly assigned to one of four stretching groups (group with four levels: 15-second stretches, 30-second stretches, 60-second stretches, and a control group that did not stretch) and measured before and after 6 weeks of stretching (time with two levels: pretreatment and posttreatment). In this study, a common mixed design, the familiar single-factor, pretest-posttest, control-group design is treated as a two-factor design. However, readers should realize that this type of study can also be treated as a one-factor design. Figure 9–5 shows the two different ways of treating this design. The left-

		INDEPENDENT VARIABLE: CLINIC					
		Specialty			General		
INDEPENDENT VARIABLE: GROUP	Heat/ exercise	HSA	HSB	HSC	HGD	HGE	HGF
	Manual therapy	MSA	MSB	MSC	MGD	MGE	MGF
	Home program	PSA	PSB	PSC	PGD	PGE	PGF
		A	B	C	D	E	F
		INDEPENDENT VARIABLE: THERAPIST					

FIGURE 9–4. Schematic diagram of three-factor, nested design. Treatment (H, M, P) and clinic (S, G) are crossed factors. Therapist (A–F) is nested within clinic.

FIGURE 9–5. One- and two-factor approaches to the pretest-posttest control-group design. The one-factor approach, on the right, using group as the independent variable and range-of-motion difference scores as the dependent variable. The two-factor approach, on the left, using group and time as independent variables and range-of-motion scores as the dependent variable.
Sample data, with cell and margin means, are included from Bandy WD, Irion JM. The effect of time on static stretch on the flexibility of the hamstring muscles. *Phys Ther.*1994;74:845–852.

Independent variable: Group	Independent variable: Timing of data collection		Data reduction
	Pretreatment	Posttreatment	Pretreatment minus posttreatment
15-second stretches	15-pre $\bar{X} = 50.14$	15-post $\bar{X} = 46.36$	15-diff $\bar{X} = 3.78$
30-second stretches	30-pre $\bar{X} = 51.64$	30-post $\bar{X} = 39.14$	30-diff $\bar{X} = 12.50$
60-second stretches	60-pre $\bar{X} = 50.07$	60-post $\bar{X} = 39.21$	60-diff $\bar{X} = 10.86$
Control no stretching	Control-pre $\bar{X} = 45.47$	Control-post $\bar{X} = 45.20$	Control-diff $\bar{X} = 0.27$

hand grid shows the two-factor approach, with "group" as one independent variable and "time" as the second independent variable. Analyzing the design as a two-factor study requires that one determine whether the pattern of change across time is consistent between the groups. Figure 9–6 graphs eight average data points (four

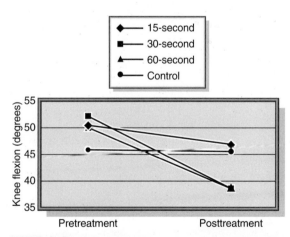

FIGURE 9–6. Interaction with two-factor approach. Nonparallel lines between treatment and control groups indicate a group × time interaction.
Data from Bandy WD, Irion JM. The effect of time on static stretch on the flexibility of the hamstring muscles. *Phys Ther.* 1994;74:845–852.

groups at two times), clearly showing that the control group has a different pattern than the other groups, and that the 30-second and 60-second groups have very similar patterns of change across time.

The right-hand grid of Figure 9–5 shows how the "time" variable can be eliminated by reducing each group's average from two data points (pretreatment and posttreatment) to one data point (pretreatment-posttreatment difference). Analyzing the design as a one-factor study would involve comparing the four average differences to determine whether they are different from one another. Whether a study is analyzed as a one-factor or a two-factor design depends on a variety of mathematical assumptions that will be discussed later in the text (see Chapters 20 through 22).

■ SUMMARY

Experimental research is characterized by controlled manipulation of variables by the researcher. Single-factor experimental designs are those in which the researcher manipulates only one variable. Common single-factor designs include the pretest-posttest control-group design, the posttest-only control-group design, the single-group pretest-posttest design, the nonequivalent control-group design, the time series design, and the repeated treatment design. Multiple-factor research designs are those in which the researcher studies more than one variable and is interested in the interactions among variables. Common forms of multiple-factor designs include factorial and nested designs; completely randomized and randomized block designs; and between-subjects, within-subjects, and mixed designs.

REFERENCES

1. Campbell DT, Stanley JC. *Experimental and Quasi-Experimental Designs for Research*. Chicago, Ill: Rand McNally College Publishing Co; 1963.
2. Dean CM, Shepherd RB. Task-related training improves performance of seated reaching tasks after stroke. *Stroke*. 1997;28:722–728.
3. Griffin JW, Newsome LS, Stralka SW, Wright PE. Reduction of chronic posttraumatic hand edema: a comparison of high voltage pulsed current, intermittent pneumatic compression, and placebo treatments. *Phys Ther*. 1990;70:279–286.
4. Arciero RA, Scoville CR, Hayda RA, Snyder RJ. The effect of tourniquet use in anterior cruciate ligament reconstruction. *Am J Sports Med*. 1996;24:758–764.
5. Harada N, Chui V, Fowler E, Lee M, Reuben DB. Physical therapy to improve functioning of older people in residential care facilities. *Phys Ther*. 1995;75:830–839.
6. Amundsen LR, DeVahl JM, Ellingham CT. Evaluation of a group exercise program for elderly women. *Phys Ther*. 1989;69:475–483.
7. Ulione MS. Health promotion and injury prevention in a child development center. *J Pediatr Nurs*. 1997;12:148–154.
8. Scudds RJ, Helewa A, Scudds RA. The effects of transcutaneous electrical nerve stimulation on skin temperature in asymptomatic subjects. *Phys Ther*. 1995;75:621–628.
9. Taylor BF, Waring CA, Brashear TA. The effects of therapeutic application of heat or cold followed by static stretch on hamstring muscle length. *J Orthop Sports Phys Ther*. 1995;21:283–286.
10. Bandy WD, Irion JM. The effect of time on static stretch on the flexibility of the hamstring muscles. *Phys Ther*. 1994;74:845–852.

Single-System Design

Problems with Group Designs

Characteristics of Single-System
Designs

Single-System Designs
A-B Designs
Withdrawal Designs

Multiple-Baseline Designs
Alternating-Treatment Designs
Interaction Designs

Limitations of Single-System
Designs

A great difficulty in developing the clinical science of physical therapy is that we treat individual persons, each of whom is made up of situations which are unique and, therefore, appear incompatible with the generalizations demanded of science.[1(p1076)]

This quote, from Helen Hislop's 1975 Mary McMillan Lecture to the American Physical Therapy Association, elegantly frames the basic argument in favor of studying individuals rather than groups. As noted in Chapter 5, the limitations of traditional group designs have led to the creation of a new research paradigm—the single-system paradigm—that focuses on the effectiveness of treatment in the context of a specific subject in a specific setting. In addition to this basic philosophical argument in favor of single-system designs, advocates of this paradigm also cite many practical disadvantages of group designs in rehabilitation research.

■ PROBLEMS WITH GROUP DESIGNS

First, it is often difficult to structure powerful group designs in rehabilitation settings. Although a complete discussion of statistical power is deferred until Chapter 20, for now it is enough to know that powerful designs are those in which the data have the mathematical characteristics that make it likely that any true differences between groups will be detected by the statistical tools used to analyze the data. These mathematical characteristics include large sample sizes, subjects who have similar values on the dependent variable at the beginning of the study, and large differences between groups at the conclusion of the study. Imagine that you work in an outpatient orthopedic setting and wish to compare the effects of exercise alone versus exercise and joint mobilization combined on the shoulder function of patients with adhesive capsulitis. To create a powerful design, you should probably have 30 patients in each group, you should specify that each patient must start treatment with a shoulder function score within a certain narrow range, and you should follow patients for a complete course of treatment. If your clinic sees one new patient per week with a diagnosis of adhesive capsulitis, and if half of those patients have shoulder function scores within the range needed to be included in the study, it would take 120 weeks to recruit the 60 subjects needed to implement a powerful group design! Since most clinics do not have the resources needed to mount a 2-year study, the result is that many group studies without adequate power are implemented. Such studies often have few subjects in each group, include heterogeneous subjects who vary greatly on the dependent variable at the beginning of the study, and study subjects for only a few visits rather than across a full course of treatment. When a study lacks power and no difference between groups is identified, it is difficult to determine whether there is, in fact, no benefit to the experimental treatment or whether there is, in fact, a real benefit that was not detected because the design did not create the mathematical conditions needed to identify a difference. Advocates of single-system research believe that carefully crafted single-system designs provide clinicians with more useful information than do poorly crafted group designs.

Second, group designs typically only call for measurement of subjects a few times within the study. When subjects are only measured at the beginning and end of a study, the researcher is unable to determine the typical pattern of fluctuation in the dependent variable in the absence of an experimental manipulation. A difference from pretest to posttest may be part of a pattern of natural fluctuation, rather than a difference related to the independent variable. As will be shown later in the chapter, single-system designs are characterized by extended baselines that establish the extent of natural fluc-

tuation on the variables of interest within the study.

Third, group designs often have problems with external validity. Because of the need to standardize treatment across subjects within the study, there may be a mismatch between some subjects and the intervention that is planned. On average, the treatment may be appropriate for the subjects within the group, but it may not be ideal for each subject. In addition, the standardization that is typical of group designs means that treatment is controlled in ways that may not be typical of the clinic. When a statistical advantage is found in an experimental group compared to a control group, clinicians know that the treatment, when applied to groups similar to the one that was studied, is likely to be effective for the group as a whole. The group design, however, usually provides little information about which subgroups responded best—or did not respond at all. This means that the results of group designs often provide clinicians little guidance on whether a treatment is likely to be effective with a particular patient with particular characteristics. The generalizability of results from group studies can be described as "sample-to-population" generalizability.

In contrast, single-system designs are characterized by experimental treatments that are tailored to the needs of the specific subject being studied. In addition, the subject is usually described in detail. This means that clinicians can determine the similarity of one of their patients to the single subject under study and make an educated clinical judgment about the applicability of the treatment to their patient. Sim refers to this as "case-to-case generalizability," and believes that this kind of generalizability is important to clinicians trying to make evidence-based judgments about how to treat their patients.[2]

■ CHARACTERISTICS OF SINGLE-SYSTEM DESIGNS

Single-system designs are often confused with clinical case reports or case studies. The two are very different. The case report or case study is a description, very often a retrospective description, of a course of treatment of an individual. The case study is therefore a nonexperimental form of inquiry, which is covered in more detail in Chapter 12. Single-system designs, in contrast, include controlled manipulation of an independent variable and are conducted prospectively. Sim defines single-system research as:

> A quasi-experimental, prospective design utilising a sample of one, involving the sequential introduction and withdrawal (or modification) of an intervention (the predictor variable), to determine its effect on one or more outcome variables, through repeated measurement.[2(p263)]

The important elements of this definition are that single-system designs are experimental, involve repeated measurements, and are prospective.

The experimental nature of single-system designs is shown by the controlled way in which the independent variable is implemented and the dependent variables are measured. All single-system designs have at least two levels of the independent variable, typically a baseline phase and an intervention phase. The patient serves as his or her own control through the collection of an extended series of baseline measurements, which are contrasted to a series of measurements taken during the intervention phase. These dependent measures are collected with standardized procedures at defined intervals.

The prospective nature of single-system designs is illustrated by the deliberate, planned intervention. Even though the researcher may deviate from the original treatment plan to accommodate the specific needs of the patient, these changes are carefully documented and recorded. Because of the planned nature of the study, researchers go through standard institutional review board processes to obtain approval to do the study, and they seek formal informed consent from the patients who participate in the research.

■ SINGLE-SYSTEM DESIGNS

Several authors have categorized single-system designs in different ways.[3,4] For the purpose of this chapter, a slight modification of Backman and associates' classification will be used.[4] To their scheme of four basic variations (A-B designs, withdrawal designs, multiple-baseline designs, and alternating-treatment designs) is added a fifth (interaction designs). Each of these designs is described in the rest of this chapter. Readers who wish a more complete enumeration of examples of the different designs should consult the review article of Backman and associates,[4] which describes 40 single-system designs related to rehabilitation that were published between 1985 and 1995.

A-B Designs

A-B designs have been described as the foundation of single-system research. By convention, A represents baseline phases, and B represents treatment phases. An A-B design represents a baseline phase followed by a treatment phase. The researcher collects multiple measures over time during the baseline phase to document the patient's status prior to implementation of the treatment. When the treatment is initiated, the measurements continue, and the pattern of change during the treatment phase is compared to the pattern established during the baseline. One weakness of the design is that it does not control for events or extraneous factors that might act simultaneously with the implementation of the treatment. If present, such factors, rather than the treatment, might be the cause of any changes seen in the dependent variables.

An A-B design was used by Goodman and Bazyk[5] to evaluate the effects of a short thumb opponens splint on hand function in a 4-year-old girl with cerebral palsy. Baseline measures of hand function were collected twice a week for 4 weeks. Then the child was treated for 4 weeks by wearing the splint for 6 hours during the day and all night. Hand function measures, while the child was not wearing the splint, were collected twice a week during the 4 weeks of the treatment. Thus, for each variable the researchers had eight points of treatment data to compare to eight points of baseline data. Significant improvements in most of the hand function measures were found. The authors note that a stronger, withdrawal design (described in the following section) could not be implemented because of time constraints. Thus, these results are open to historical influences, such as a change in spasticity medications or entry into a preschool program that emphasized manual activities, that might have influenced hand function during the study.

A slight variation on the A-B design was used by Mulcahey and colleagues[6] to evaluate outcomes of tendon transfer surgery and occupational therapy in a child with tetraplegia secondary to spinal cord injury. Ten or more measures of various hand function tests were taken during the A phase, before surgery. After surgery, the patient participated in standard postoperative care, including occupational therapy, for 4 weeks. Thus, the intervention for this study was the combination of the surgery and the postoperative care. The B phase in this study was subdivided into three follow-up phases at $2\frac{1}{2}$ months, 6 months, and 12 months after surgery. During each of the three follow-up phases, at least nine measures of each variable were taken over a 2-week period. This extended follow-up phase permits the researchers to draw conclusions about both the short-term and long-term impact of the tendon transfer surgery.

Withdrawal Designs

Withdrawal designs, sometimes referred to generically as A-B-A designs, are characterized by implementation and withdrawal of treatment over the course of the study. In an A-B-A design a baseline is followed by treatment and then by another baseline. Other variants either reverse the order of treatments and baselines (B-A-B) or have multiple cycles of application and withdrawal of treatment (A-B-A-B). When studying a phenomenon that is expected to change as the intervention is implemented and withdrawn, these designs provide good control of extraneous factors by enabling the researcher to see if the hypothesized change occurs each time the treatment is applied or withdrawn.

One potential difficulty with withdrawal designs is that the researcher must consider the ethical implications of withdrawing a treatment that appears to be successful. A second potential difficulty with withdrawal designs is that the expected pattern of change in the dependent variable with each new phase of the study will occur only if the changes are reversible. For example, if one is studying gait characteristics with and without an ankle-foot orthosis, the gait changes would be expected to come and go with the application and withdrawal of the orthosis. If this happens, this is considered good evidence that the treatment, and not some extraneous factor, is the cause of the changes in the dependent variables. On the other hand, if one is studying the effect of a particular physical therapy program on gait characteristics of a patient using a prosthesis after transfemoral amputation, one hopes that improvements are maintained after the therapy has ended. If the second baseline phase remains the same as the treatment phase, some might interpret this to mean that some factor other than the treatment might have caused the sustained change. Others might argue that such a pattern of evidence, rather than providing weak evidence of treatment effectiveness, provides strong support for the long-term impact of the treatment. Thus, it is difficult to interpret the results of A-B-A designs with variables that are not expected to change when the intervention is removed.

Gardner and colleagues[7] conducted an A-B-A single-subject design to study the effect of partial body weight support with treadmill locomotion on gait after incomplete spinal cord injury. First, temporal-distance measures of gait were collected once a week for 6 weeks during the first baseline phase (AI). Second, gait training with the partial body weight support system and treadmill was implemented three times per week for 6 weeks and gait measures were collected once a week (B). Finally, the gait measures were collected once a week for 3 weeks during the second baseline (AII). In general, improvements were seen from phase AI to B, but were not seen from phase B to AII. Because the gait improvements persisted into the AII phase, the authors needed to advance arguments to support their contention that the changes from AI to B were the result of their intervention and not from an extraneous factor.

Multiple-Baseline Designs

There are several variations of the multiple-baseline designs. However, they all share the same purpose, to control for threats to internal validity without requiring that treatment be withdrawn.[4] The general format for the multiple-baseline study is to conduct several single-system studies, with baselines at different times or for different durations. An example of this design is Dekker and associates' study of the effects of intraarticular triamcinolone acetonide on pain, range of motion, and function of the painful shoulders of patients with hemiplegia.[8] Nine inpatients from the same rehabilitation center were identified over the course of a 12-month period and were randomly assigned to baselines of either 2 weeks or 3 weeks. Thus, this design included both ways of varying the baselines—by having baselines occur at different times and for different durations. To illustrate the benefit of having baselines at different times, assume that a historical threat to internal validity occurred during the second half of the 12-month period. For example, if the nursing staff implemented a protected positioning and transfer program during months 6 through 12 of the study, decreases in pain for the last several patients might be because of this program, rather than due to the effect of the steroid injections. If only one case was used, it would be impossible to separate the effects of the staffing change from the effect of the injections.

To illustrate the benefit of having baselines of different durations, assume that shoulder dysfunction in hemiplegia remits as patients experience less inadvertent shoulder trauma as they require less assistance with transfers, gait, and activities of daily living. If this recovery pattern tends to kick in after about 2 weeks of inpatient rehabilitation, and if the baseline is 2 weeks long for all patients, then changes in the dependent variables might be because of this natural progression rather than because of the effects of the injections. By having varied baselines of 2 and 3 weeks, any natural improvement at 2 weeks would be observable in those patients with the longer baseline. Figure 10–1 shows hypothetical scores that assume that pain decreases are related to natural history and not to the effect of the injections. The addition of the other patients allows the researcher to see that all subjects had stable baselines for the first 2 weeks and all subjects had decreases in pain after 2 weeks, irrespective of when the injections were started.

Alternating-Treatment Designs

Alternating-treatment designs include the use of different treatments, each administered independently of the other. In describing such designs, the letters B, C, D, E, and so on are used to represent the different treatments; A continues to represent the baseline phase or phases. This design is well-suited to treatments that are expected to have short-lived effects. For example, a straightforward study of gait velocity of a patient wearing different ankle-foot orthoses might be represented by the notation A-B-A-C-A. This would mean that a baseline with no orthosis was established (A); this baseline phase was followed by gait assessments while the patient wore one orthosis, perhaps a solid-ankle plastic ankle-foot orthosis (B); followed by a second baseline phase (A); followed by gait assessments while

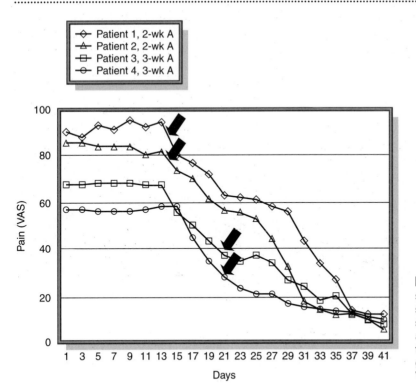

FIGURE 10–1. Hypothetical data presentation for a multiple-baseline study. Note that all baselines are stable until approximately 2 weeks and show a decreasing trend thereafter, irrespective of the beginning of treatment (*arrows*). VAS = visual analog scale.

the patient wore the second orthosis, perhaps an articulating-ankle plastic ankle-foot orthosis (C); and the study concluded with a final baseline phase (A). In this hypothetical case, the alternate treatments are administered in different phases of the study.

Diamond and Ottenbacher investigated this general topic using a different variation of the alternating-treatment design.[9] Subjects walked barefoot during the baseline phase, and walked barefoot and with two different orthoses in an alternating fashion within one intervention phase. Notation for this study might be A-A, B, C-A. The commas indicate that the three conditions (A, B, and C) were alternated within a single phase. The actual sequence of measurement was as follows: (1) The first baseline phase consisted of five measurement sessions in the barefoot condition; (2) the intervention phase consisted of 12 measurement sessions, and each of the three conditions was evaluated within each

session, with the order of presentation randomized within each session; (3) the second baseline phase consisted of four measurement sessions with the barefoot condition. Figure 10–2 shows the fairly consistent superiority of the tone-inhibiting dynamic ankle-foot orthosis during each measurement session on the dependent measure of gait velocity. This design works particularly well when patients are experiencing overall improvements irrespective of the treatment. The alternating design lets the researcher evaluate each condition in light of the velocity that the patient exhibits on a given day. For instance, the 10th measurement session shows high velocities in all conditions and the 11th session shows a return to a more typical level for all conditions. Thus, day-to-day variability is controlled because the measure of interest is not absolute velocity, but rather the difference in velocity between conditions for a given day.

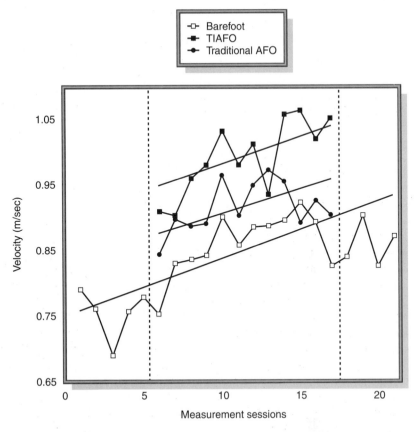

FIGURE 10–2. Example of data presentation for an alternating-treatment study. The study tested ambulation velocity in meters per second of one hemiparetic subject across three conditions (barefoot ambulation, ambulation with a prefabricated ankle-foot orthosis [AFO], and ambulation with a tone-inhibiting dynamic ankle-foot orthosis [TIAFO]) over 21 measurement sessions. From Diamond MF, Ottenbacher KJ. Effect of a tone-inhibiting dynamic ankle-foot orthosis on stride characteristics of an adult with hemiparesis. *Phys Ther.* 1990;70:423–430. Reprinted from *Physical Therapy* with permission of the American Physical Therapy Association.

One specific form of an alternating-treatment design is sometimes referred to as an N of 1 randomized controlled trial (RCT).[10] In such a trial, two different treatments are randomly implemented during different phases of a study. The usual purpose of an N of 1 RCT is to determine which of two or more competing treatments is more effective for a given patient.

Interaction Designs

Interaction designs are used to evaluate the effect of different combinations of treatments. Assume that a comprehensive pain control program has been designed and includes the use of electroanalgesia (B) and relaxation (C). Re-

searchers might wish to differentiate the effects of these components to determine whether a single component or the combination of components is most effective. The following design could separate these effects A-B-A-C-A-BC-A. That is, baseline phases separate an electroanalgesia phase, a relaxation phase, and a combined-treatment phase.

An example of this design is Embrey and associates' examination of the effects of neurodevelopmental treatment and orthoses on knee flexion during gait.[11] The design of this study is A-B-A-BC-A, with neurodevelopmental treatment as the B intervention and orthoses as the C treatment. In this study, the researchers apparently were not interested in the effect of the orthoses alone, hence the absence of an isolated C treatment.

■ LIMITATIONS OF SINGLE-SYSTEM DESIGNS

Although many authors and researchers are enthusiastic about the information that can be gleaned from carefully constructed single-system designs, others are sharply critical of this form of inquiry for at least four reasons.[12,13] First, the designs may create ethical dilemmas because the need for an extended baseline leads to a delay in treatment, because researchers may withdraw effective treatments during the course of the study, and because of the increased cost of care related to data collection during baseline and withdrawal phases.

Second, the weaker single-system designs are subject to internal validity threats because they do not adequately control for extraneous factors, such as history or maturation, that might be responsible for changes in the dependent variables. In addition, there is the possibility that apparent improvements may reflect either familiarity with, or a treatment effect from, the repeated testing.

Third, generalizability may be low. Because the interventions may change during the course of the study to meet the individual needs of the patient, these designs are difficult to replicate. Because patients and interventions are carefully matched, therapists may have difficulty determining whether patients they are seeing are good matches for the treatments described in the study. Researchers who advance these generalizability concerns are not persuaded that case-to-case generalizability, as described by Sim,[2] is as valid as the sample-to-population generalizability that characterizes group designs.

Finally, the theory and practice of statistical analysis of single-system designs is in its infancy. Some authors believe that the common methods of analysis that are reported in the literature frequently violate a variety of statistical tenets. A more complete discussion of statistical analysis of single-system designs is presented in Chapter 22.

■ SUMMARY

Group research designs are often limited because too few subjects are available for powerful statistical analysis and because the impact of the treatment on individuals is obscured by the group results. Single-system designs overcome these limitations with controlled initiation and withdrawal of individualized treatments for a single subject, with repeated measurements of the dependent variables across time, and by analysis methods designed for use with data from only one subject. Broad categories of single-system designs include A-B designs, withdrawal designs, multiple-baseline designs, alternating-treatment designs, and interaction designs. Despite the advantages of single-system designs, some find them to be limited because of ethical concerns, lack of control of extraneous variables, limited generalizability, and violation of statistical assumptions.

REFERENCES

1. Hislop HJ. The not-so-impossible dream. *Phys Ther.* 1975;55:1069–1080.
2. Sim J. The external validity of group comparative and single system studies. *Physiotherapy.* 1995;81:263–270.
3. Ottenbacher KJ. *Evaluating Clinical Change: Strategies for Occupational and Physical Therapists.* Baltimore, Md: Williams & Wilkins; 1986.
4. Backman CL, Harris SR, Chisholm J-AM, Monette AD. Single-subject research in rehabilitation: a review of studies using AB, withdrawal, multiple baseline, and alternating treatments designs. *Arch Phys Med Rehabil.* 1997;78:1145–1153.
5. Goodman G, Bazyk S. The effects of a short thumb opponens splint on hand function in cerebral palsy: a single-subject study. *Am J Occup Ther.* 1991;45: 726–731.
6. Mulcahey MJ, Smith BT, Betz RR, Weiss AA. Outcomes of tendon transfer surgery and occupational therapy in a child with tetraplegia secondary to spinal cord injury. *Am J Occup Ther.* 1995;49:607–617.
7. Gardner MB, Holden MK, Leikauskas JM, Richard RL. Partial body weight support with treadmill locomotion to improve gait after incomplete spinal cord injury: a single-subject experimental design. *Phys Ther.* 1998;78: 361–374.
8. Dekker JHM, Wagenaar RC, Lankhorst GJ, de Jong BA. The painful hemiplegic shoulder: effects of intra-articular triamcinolone acetonide. *Am J Phys Med Rehabil.* 1997;76:43–48.

9. Diamond MF, Ottenbacher KJ. Effect of a tone-inhibiting dynamic ankle-foot orthosis on stride characteristics of an adult with hemiparesis. *Phys Ther.* 1990;70:423–430.

10. Backman CL, Harris SR. Case studies, single subject research and N of 1 randomized trials: comparisons and contrasts. *Am J Phys Med Rehabil.* 1999;78:170–176.

11. Embrey DG, Yates L, Mott DH. Effects of neuro-developmental treatment and orthoses on knee flexion during gait: a single-subject design. *Phys Ther.* 1990;70:626–637.

12. Bithell C. Single subject experimental design: a case for concern? *Physiotherapy.* 1994;80:85–87.

13. Reboussin DM, Morgan TM. Statistical considerations in the use and analysis of single-subject designs. *Med Sci Sports Exerc.* 1996;28:639–644.

Nonexperimental Designs

Overview of Nonexperimental Research

Description
  Retrospective Descriptive Research
  Prospective Descriptive Research
  Observation
  Examination
  Interview
  Questionnaire
Analysis of Relationships
  Retrospective Analysis of
    Relationships

Prospective Analysis of
  Relationships
Analysis of Differences
  Retrospective Analysis of
    Differences
  Prospective Analysis of Differences

In contrast to experimental research, nonexperimental research does not involve manipulation of variables. Kerlinger noted that "in the nonexperimental research situation, . . . control of the independent variables is not possible. Investigators must take things as they are and try to disentangle them." [1(p349)] In nonexperimental studies, then, the researcher examines records of past phenomena, documents existing phenomena, or observes new phenomena unfolding. The label "*non*experimental" may imply an unfavorable comparison with research that meets the controlled-manipulation criterion for "experimental" research. This is an unfortunate implication. Nonexperimental research is exceedingly important within the physical therapy literature. A review of selected articles in *Physical Therapy* shows that from 1984 to 1995 over half of the articles were reports of nonexperimental work.[2]

The purpose of this chapter is to provide the reader with an overview of the diversity of nonexperimental research designs. Because nonexperimental research does not have to fit a rigid definition of controlled manipulation, the variety of nonexperimental designs is greater than that of experimental designs. In fact, there are nonexperimental research designs to fit every research type in the design matrix introduced in Chapter 6 and reproduced here as Figure 11–1. Therefore, this chapter is organized by providing examples of nonexperimental research articles that fit into each of the six cells of the matrix of research types. As in earlier chapters, the pertinent portion of each study is reviewed; readers who go to the literature will find that some of the articles are more involved than would be assumed just from reading this chapter. A factor that complicates discussion of nonexperimental

		Timing of data collection	
		Retrospective	Prospective
Purpose of research	Description	Nonexperimental	Nonexperimental
	Analysis of relationships	Nonexperimental	Nonexperimental
	Analysis of differences	Nonexperimental	Nonexperimental Experimental
		Manipulation (experimental or nonexperimental)	

FIGURE 11–1. Matrix of research types showing three design dimensions: purpose of the research (rows), timing of data collection (columns), and manipulation (cells).

research is that there are many different terms that are used to describe certain types of nonexperimental studies. Table 11–1 provides a brief description of these forms of research. Because some of these forms of nonexperimental research are extremely important within the physical therapy literature, they are presented in more detail in later chapters: case reports (Chapter 12), qualitative research (Chapter 13), epidemiological research (Chapter 14), outcomes research (Chapter 15), survey research (Chapter 16), and methodological research (Chapters 17 and 18).

■ DESCRIPTION

The purpose of descriptive research is to document the nature of a phenomenon through the systematic collection of data. In this text, a study is considered descriptive if it either provides a snapshot view of a single sample measured once or involves measurement and description of a sample several times over an extended period of time. The former approach is said to be *cross-sectional;* the latter is referred to as *longitudinal.*

In most descriptive studies, many different variables are documented. For the most part,

though, there is no presumption of cause or effect. Thus the distinction between independent and dependent variables is not usually made in reports of descriptive research. As is the case with all three research purposes that make up the matrix of research types, a distinction can be made between prospective and retrospective descriptive research designs.

Retrospective Descriptive Research

The purpose of retrospective descriptive research is to document the past. The description of the past may be of inherent interest, may be used to evaluate the present against the past, or may be used to make decisions in the present based on information from the past. The common denominator among research studies of this type is the reliance on archival data. *Archives* are "records of documents recounting the activities of individuals or of institutions, governments, and other groups." [3(p130)] Archival data may be found in medical records, voter registration rosters, newspapers and magazines, telephone directories, meeting minutes, television news programs, and a host of other sources. The information found in archival records must be systematically analyzed for its relevance by the researcher. *Content analysis* is the painstaking process that involves applying operational definitions and decision rules to the records to extract the data of interest.

Examples of the decisions that might need to be made can be seen in Roach and associates' study in which they used medical record data to study the relationship between duration of physical therapy services and change in functional status in patients with lower-extremity orthopedic problems.[4] One criterion for including cases in the study was that the subjects have a primary diagnosis of a lower-extremity problem. Would a patient with lower-extremity reflex sympathetic dystrophy (RSD) fit this criterion? RSD often begins with an orthopedic problem but presents as a neurovascular phenomenon. The operational definition would need to specify whether RSD

TABLE 11-1	Types of Nonexperimental Research
Term	**Definition**
Case report	Systematic documentation of a well-defined unit; usually a description of an episode of care for an individual, but sometimes an administrative, educational, or other unit
Correlational research	Research conducted for the purpose of determining the interrelationships among variables
Developmental research	Research in which observations are made over time to document the natural history of the phenomenon of interest
Epidemiological research	Research that documents the incidence of a disease or injury, determines causes for the disease or injury, or develops mechanisms to control the disease or injury
Evaluation research	Research conducted to determine the effectiveness of a program or policy
Historical research	Research in which past events are documented because they are of inherent interest or because they provide a perspective that can guide decision making in the present
Meta-analysis	Research process by which the results of several studies are synthesized in a quantitative way
Methodological research	Research conducted to determine the reliability and validity of clinical and research measurements
Normative research	Research that uses large, representative samples to generate norms on measures of interest
Policy research	Research that is conducted to inform policy making and implementation
Qualitative research	Research conducted to develop a deep understanding of the particular, usually using interview and observation
Secondary analysis	Research that reanalyzes data collected for one purpose to answer new research questions
Survey research	Research in which the data are collected by having subjects complete questionnaires or respond to interview questions

cases were included or excluded. Cases that were included in the analysis were then described by their primary diagnosis. If a patient entered the hospital because of a hip fracture, which was treated with total hip arthroplasty, would the primary diagnosis be "fracture of hip or pelvis" or "total hip arthroplasty?" Decision rules would be established to enable the researchers to consistently determine the primary diagnosis for patients who received a total hip arthroplasty for a hip fracture. Because it is difficult to anticipate every possible variation within the medical records, the operational definitions are usually established with the help of a pilot data extraction project. On the basis of the pilot study, definitive decision rules and operational definitions are made before the study itself is begun.[5]

Medical record data is not the only type of retrospective work that may be of interest to the profession of physical therapy. For example, Chevan and Chevan used US Bureau of the Census data to generate a statistical profile of physical therapists in 1980 and 1990.[6] Because they were doing a *secondary analysis* of data collected for another purpose, they had to do a considerable amount of data filtering to maximize the accuracy and usefulness of the data. For example, the census data did not distinguish between physical therapists and physical therapist assistants. Therefore, they used educational level as a "proxy" to distinguish between PTs and PTAs. Only those identified as PTs *and* as having at least 4 years of college were selected for the sample. Although this procedure likely rejected a few retirement-aged PTs who obtained licenses before a 4-year degree was required and included a few PTAs who had 4-year degrees in addition to the 2-year degree needed to practice as a PTA, it nevertheless appeared to be the best way to filter the data to obtain a high proportion of PTs and a low proportion of PTAs.

Evaluation research is another type of non-experimental research that is typically conducted retrospectively. Sometimes evaluation research looks at the outcomes of a program at a single facility, as was the case with Bohannon and Cooper's[7] evaluation of rehabilitation after total knee arthroplasty at a single hospital. Other times, evaluation research looks at the processes involved in delivering a service to large groups of patients across many facilities. This was the case with Jette and associates' study of the quality of home health care services.[8]

Another possible retrospective approach is *epidemiological research*. Epidemiology is the study of disease, injury, and health in a population, and epidemiological research encompasses a broad range of methods (not all of them retrospective) that are used to study population-based health issues. Lu-Yao and coworkers used retrospective methods to study the treatment of elderly Americans with hip fractures.[9] In this study, a sample of the Medicare claims database was used to determine the characteristics of patients with hip fracture, the surgical procedure used to repair the fracture, and the survival rate up to 3 years after the fracture. The very large sample size—26,434 cases—which is likely to be representative of the larger population of elderly Americans with hip fractures, is one thing that differentiates epidemiological research from smaller studies that use samples of convenience from one or just a few hospitals. Additional information on epidemiological research can be found in Chapter 14.

Another research approach that uses retrospective descriptive methods is *historical research*. The purpose of historical research is to document past events because they are of inherent interest or because they provide a perspective that can guide decision making in the present. An example of historical research in physical therapy is the study of direct access legislation patterns by Taylor and Domholdt.[10] These patterns were determined by obtaining records from several archival sources: the laws themselves, state records that documented the sequence of events surrounding attempts to pass direct access legislation, and newsletters from different states. In addition to the retrospective data, information was requested from individuals who were active in the states when direct access legislation was being pursued. Thus, this study combined retrospective and prospective data collection to develop a fuller description of the phenomenon under study. This study is an example of *policy research* since it was conducted to "inform people who create or implement policies . . . affecting large groups of people."[11(p649)]

Another form of research that usually rests on retrospective description is the *case report* or *case study*. Although the terms are sometimes used interchangeably, they are often differentiated. When they are, the case report is described as the less controlled, less systematic of the two forms of inquiry.[12] One example of a retrospective case report is Jones and Erhard's[13] report of their work with a patient who entered therapy with a misdiagnosis of trochanteric bursitis. The purpose of the case was to describe the signs and symptoms that alerted the therapist to the misdiagnosis, as well as the process that led to the correct diagnosis of femoral neck stress fracture. Case reports and case studies are covered in more detail in Chapters 12 and 13.

Prospective Descriptive Research

Prospective descriptive research enables the researcher to control the data that are collected for the purpose of describing a phenomenon. The prospective nature of data collection often makes the results of such research more believable than the results of purely retrospective studies. There are four basic methods of data collection in prospective descriptive research: observation, examination, interview, and questionnaire.

OBSERVATION. An example of the observational method is a study by Geerdink and colleagues, who studied the development of kicking movements in pre-term and full-term infants by videotaping them and analyzing kicking frequency and angular motions.[14] They collected data at three different periods of time: when the infants were 6, 12, and 18 weeks of age. Another term for this type of research is *developmental,* meaning that the infants were described at more than one point in time to document the effects of the passage of time. This study, then, included both descriptive components (to describe movement patterns at the different times for each group) and analytical components (comparing the movement patterns across times and groups).

EXAMINATION. An example of prospective descriptive research that includes examination of patients is Plancher and coworkers'[15] study of reconstruction of the anterior cruciate ligament (ACL) in patients who were at least 40 years old. In this study, 40- to 60-year-old patients who had an ACL reconstruction were examined at an average of 55 months after surgery. The examination included, among other things, Lachman testing, knee laxity measurements, range-of-motion measures, and tests for crepitation. The patients in this study were identified through medical records review, but the data for the study were collected prospectively to answer the question about the status of the knees at follow-up.

Another variation on prospective descriptive research is seen in the *methodological study* of Rosa and associates,[16] who examined the ability of therapeutic touch practitioners to detect the human energy fields they claim to be able to detect and manipulate. The goals of methodological research are to document and improve the reliability and validity of clinical and research measures. This study, published in *JAMA* (the Journal of the American Medical Association),

was received with a great deal of interest because a portion of the article reported on the fourth-grade science project of one of the authors. To determine the ability of the practitioners to detect a human energy field, each practitioner placed his or her hands palm-up through a screen that kept the practitioner from seeing the experimenter. The experimenter then conducted 10 trials with each practitioner in which the experimenter hovered one of her hands over one of the hands of the practitioner. The practitioner was asked to indicate which of his or her hands was closest to the examiner's hands for each trial. Most practitioners were not able to reliably detect the correct hand. More detail about methodological research is presented in Chapters 17 and 18.

INTERVIEW. The interview method of data collection was used by Mack and colleagues to study the perceived risks to independent living of older, community-dwelling adults.[17] Data were collected by interviewing more than 100 community-dwelling elders about the importance of remaining within their homes, the factors enabling them to remain independent, the situations that might jeopardize their independence, and the resources that would help them remain independent. The interview method was ideal for this study since older adults may have visual problems that would make reading a questionnaire difficult, and some elders may have had little education, resulting in difficulties in both reading questionnaires and writing answers. In addition, the researchers were interested in these individuals' perceptions about risks to their independence; answers to a questionnaire item about such a complex notion as "risks to independence" would likely lack the depth and breadth of answers obtained in an interview. The interview method is not without hazards, however. Without the anonymity of a mailed questionnaire, participants may give what they believe to be socially acceptable answers. In this study, they might have exaggerated the importance of remaining independent if they felt that the interviewers themselves placed a great deal of importance on independence. This style of open-ended questioning, which is analyzed later for content themes, fits some definitions of qualitative research and is covered in more detail in Chapter 13.

QUESTIONNAIRE. The questionnaire method was used by Ingram to survey the opinions of physical therapy education program directors on essential functions of physical therapist students.[18] The respondents were entry-level physical therapy program directors, by definition a well-educated group whose reading and writing skills should be sufficient to respond to a questionnaire. In addition, the national sample that was desired made mailing the questionnaire far more efficient and less expensive than conducting interviews with subjects. Another advantage of a mailed questionnaire is that it can maintain the anonymity of the respondent. The particular type of survey used by Ingram was the *Delphi technique.* This technique uses a series of questionnaires to elicit a consensus from a group of experts. Each round of questionnaires builds on information collected in the previous round, and generally asks participants to indicate their levels of agreement or disagreement with group opinions from the previous round. Chapter 16 provides guidelines for survey research.

■ ANALYSIS OF RELATIONSHIPS

The second major group of nonexperimental research consists of the designs in which the primary purpose is the analysis of relationships among variables. The general format for this research is that one group of subjects is tested on several different variables and the mathematical interrelationships among the variables are studied. This type of research is sometimes called *correlational research.* The term *correlation* also refers to a specific statistical technique. Therefore, there is a temptation to consider as correlational research only those studies in which the

statistical correlation technique is used. As is seen in the examples, however, analysis of relationships entails more than just statistical correlation techniques. For example, epidemiological researchers often use a variety of ratios to express the association between subject characteristics and the presence or absence of disease. Therefore, in this text, the term *correlation* is reserved for the specific statistical analysis, and the longer, but more accurate, *analysis of relationships* is used to describe a general type of research.

There are several reasons why one would want to identify relationships among variables. The first is that establishing relationships among variables without researcher manipulation may suggest fruitful areas for future experimental study. Research of this type is said to have *heuristic* value, meaning that the purpose of the study is to discover or reveal relationships that may lead to further enlightenment. The value of such heuristic research is not necessarily in its immediate results, but in the direction in which it moves the researcher.

The second specific purpose for the analysis of relationships among variables is that it allows scores on one variable to be predicted on the basis of scores on another variable. In clinical practice, a strong relationship between certain admission and discharge characteristics in a group of patients who recently completed their course of treatment might allow better prediction of discharge status for future patients.

The third specific purpose of the analysis of relationships is to determine the reliability of measurement tools. Reliability is the extent to which measurements are repeatable. In clinical practice, we plan treatment on the basis of certain measurements or observations. If a therapist evaluates the length of a new prosthesis for a patient who has had an amputation and cannot reliably determine whether the pelvis is level, she might recommend to the prosthetist that he shorten the prosthesis on Monday, lengthen the prosthesis on Tuesday, and leave it alone on Wednesday! The statistical determination of the reliability of measurements provides an indication of the amount of confidence that should be placed in such measures.

A fourth reason to analyze relationships among variables is to determine the validity of a measure. By comparing scores on a new test with those on a well-established, or criterion, test, the extent to which the tests are in agreement can be established. Reliability and validity of measurements are discussed in detail in Chapters 17 and 18.

Retrospective Analysis of Relationships

Relationships can be analyzed retrospectively through use of medical records or through secondary analysis of data collected for other purposes. Guccione and colleagues[19] used data from the Framingham Study to determine the effects of specific medical conditions on the functional limitations of elders. The Framingham Study collected a variety of health status measures on residents of this Massachusetts town every 2 years beginning in 1948. The data used in this study were collected on 1826 individuals during the 18th biennial examination from 1983 to 1985. Among other things, the researchers calculated an odds ratio to show the "odds of functional dependence in performing a functional task among subjects with a specific medical condition divided by the odds of dependence in that task among all subjects." [19(p353)] Compared to the total sample, those with stroke were 2.82 times as likely to be dependent in stair climbing and those with knee osteoarthritis were 1.98 times as likely to be dependent in stair climbing.

Prospective Analysis of Relationships

Analysis of relationships is often accomplished prospectively, with concomitant control over selection of subjects and administration of the measuring tools. A typical example of research in which relationships are analyzed prospec-

tively is Powers and associates' study of the relationship between muscle force and temporal-spatial gait characteristics for patients with transtibial amputation.[20] Some of the findings were that hip extensor strength on the amputated side was correlated to gait speed, that hip abduction strength on the sound side was correlated with cadence, and that knee extensor strength on both sides was correlated with stride length. Although determining the extent of the relationship among these factors is of interest to clinicians who treat patients after transtibial amputation, identifying the relationships does not imply that manipulation of one variable will influence the others. From these results we may be tempted to conclude that an exercise program that improves hip extensor, hip abductor, and knee extensor strength will cause an increase in gait speed, cadence, and stride length. However, because the variables in this study were not subjected to controlled manipulation, such causal inferences are not justified.

Prospective analysis of relationships was also used to establish the validity of physical examination for the diagnosis of sprained ankles. To test the value of delayed physical examination versus arthrography in detecting ruptured lateral ankle ligaments, van Dijk and associates[21] performed delayed physical examinations and ankle arthrography on 160 consecutive patients who presented to the emergency room with a history of an acute injury to the lateral ankle. The arthrography was considered to be the criterion measure, or "gold standard," against which the physical examination was compared. Van Dijk and associates evaluated the relationship between the physical examination result and the arthrography with the traditional epidemiological concepts of sensitivity, specificity, positive predictive value, and negative predictive value. They concluded that "physical examination gives information of diagnostic quality which is equal to that of arthrography, and causes little discomfort to the patient." [21(p958)] These epidemiological concepts are presented in more detail in Chapter 14.

Normative research is another form of descriptive research. In normative studies large, representative groups are examined to determine typical values on the variables of interest. Andrews and associates[22] characterized their descriptive work on muscle force measurements with hand-held dynamometers as "normative." They studied 156 individuals in all, with at least 50 people in each of three age groups, and at least 25 men and 25 women within each age group. Twenty-five people in each subgroup seems small for a normative study, but given the paucity of data, this information is probably as "normative" as is available at this time.

ANALYSIS OF DIFFERENCES

The general purpose of research in which differences are analyzed is to focus on whether groups or treatments are different in some reliable way. Although analysis of differences is often accomplished experimentally, there have been many nonexperimental studies in which differences were analyzed. Nonexperimental analysis of differences among groups or treatments is called *ex post facto* or *causal-comparative* research. The independent variables in such studies are not manipulated but are the presumed cause of differences in the dependent variable. The *ex post facto* (after the fact) designation refers to the fact that assignment to groups is not under the control of the investigator, but rather is determined by existing characteristics of the individuals within the study. Note that ex post facto does not mean questions are developed after data collection; ex post facto designs may use either retrospective or prospective data collection.

Retrospective Analysis of Differences

Medical records provide a vast source of information about patient treatment and outcomes. When groups of patients can be identified from the medical records as having undergone certain

courses of treatments, it is possible to study the relationship of treatment to outcome in a retrospective manner. Three articles illustrate three different ways of developing groups in the retrospective ex post facto designs.

The first, by Timm, is a large retrospective study of postsurgical knee rehabilitation.[23] The medical charts of more than 5000 patients who had undergone surgery in one calendar year were reviewed. Four groups of patients who had completed knee rehabilitation were identified by the type of program they had completed, as documented in the medical chart: no exercise, home exercise, isotonic exercise, or isokinetic exercise. Thus the groups constituted patients treated in the same time frame, but with different rehabilitation protocols. This large group, retrospective study focusing on global outcomes of treatment could be described with the contemporary term, *outcomes research*. More detail about outcomes research is presented in Chapter 15.

One disadvantage of retrospective designs such as this is that nonrandom placement into groups makes it impossible to determine why a particular patient was placed in a particular rehabilitation group. For example, did those who wanted to return to athletic competition get placed in the isokinetic group, thereby giving it a bias toward motivated patients? Unless the medical records contain information about patient goals and motivation, there is no way to determine whether or not this bias occurred.

In a second retrospective ex post facto study, successive cohorts were studied to determine whether the Medicare prospective payment system affected use of physical therapy services by the hospitalized elderly. Holt and Winograd studied the medical records of certain patients aged 75 years or older for a period of 6 years.[24] The first 4 years of records were from patients treated before implementation of the prospective payment system; the last 2 years were from patients treated after implementation of the prospective payment system. The difference in patient selection between this study and Timm's study of postperative knee rehabilitation is that answering this study question required sampling of patients from two different points in time; Timm's rehabilitation study is strengthened by its use of patients treated in a single time frame.

The third example of subject grouping within the retrospective ex post facto designs followed what is called the *case-control* design. In this design, a group of patients with the desired effect is identified, and then a group without the effect is identified. Presumed causes for the effects are then sought, and the proportions of patients with the causes in the two groups are compared. One example of a case-control design is Morris and associates' study of the effect of preexisting conditions on mortality in trauma patients.[25] In this study patients who died after trauma (the cases) were compared with age- and injury-matched patients who survived trauma (the controls). The incidence in both groups of 11 preexisting chronic conditions that were thought to influence survival rate after trauma was then established. The confidence that can be placed in case-control research depends in large part on the criteria used to define the case and control groups.[26,27]

A final example of retrospective analysis of differences among groups is a specialized research technique called *meta-analysis*. This technique provides a means to synthesize research results across several different studies.[28–30] Meta-analysis is usually undertaken when a body of research about the effectiveness of a given technique provides discrepant results. Narrative reviews of the literature are subject to the biases of the author, as noted rather humorously, but perhaps truthfully, by Glass:

> A common method of integrating several studies with inconsistent findings is to carp on the design or analysis deficiencies of all but a few studies— those remaining frequently being one's own work or that of one's students and friends—and then advance the one or two "acceptable" studies as the truth of the matter.[31(p7)]

Meta-analytical methods provide a quantitative way of synthesizing the results of different research studies on the same topic. A relevant example of meta-analysis is Moreland and colleagues'[32] study of the effectiveness of electromyographic biofeedback to improve lower-extremity function after stroke. Only eight of 79 relevant studies on electromyographic biofeedback met the inclusion criteria and contained the necessary statistical information to be included in the meta-analysis. The independent variable in all studies was "treatment," with biofeedback (alone or combined with conventional therapy) compared to conventional therapy. The dependent variables differed from study to study, but all included some measures of lower-extremity function. The basic concept behind meta-analysis is that the size of the differences between treatment groups (the effect size) is mathematically standardized so that it can be compared between studies with different, but conceptually related, dependent variables.

Prospective Analysis of Differences

Prospective analysis of differences is the final cell of the six-cell matrix of research types. It is the only cell that is shared between the experimental and nonexperimental designs. By definition, the experimental designs must be prospective, and their purpose is to determine the effects of some intervention on a dependent variable by analyzing the differences in groups who were and were not exposed to a manipulation or the differences within a single group exposed to more than one experimental treatment. Differences between groups or within a group can also be analyzed in the absence of controlled manipulation.

An example of a nonexperimental study in which the independent variable could have been manipulated but was not is Jansen and Minerbo's comparison of early dynamic mobilization with immobilization after flexor tendon repair in the hand.[33] To make this comparison, the researchers selected subjects retrospectively by reviewing their medical records to determine who had been immobilized postoperatively and who had received early dynamic splinting.

Even though the division into treatment groups was accomplished before question development, the researchers collected data themselves at $4\frac{1}{2}$ months after surgery. As was the case with our other comparisons between retrospective and prospective studies, we can place more confidence in this study because prospective data analysis allowed the researchers to standardize the measures used in the study. If the study had been completely retrospective, with group assignment and dependent measures drawn from the medical chart, the uniformity of the measures would be questioned. If the study had been completely prospective, with random group assignment, treatment, and then measurement, it no longer would have been a nonexperimental study because the manipulation would have been under the control of the investigators.

There are many clinical examples of nonexperimental analyses of differences in which the independent variable was inherently nonmanipulable. Walsh and associates[34] compared the physical impairments and functional limitations of individuals with total knee arthroplasty to those without knee problems 1 year after surgery. The individuals with total knee arthroplasty were identified first, and the control subjects without knee problems were then selected so that they would match the age and gender distribution of the cases. Similarly, Wiley and Damiano compared lower-extremity strength profiles between children with spastic cerebral palsy and their age-matched peers without cerebral palsy.[35] These studies illustrate the importance of nonexperimental research when the question involves a variable that cannot be manipulated.

■ SUMMARY

Unlike experimental research, nonexperimental research does not require controlled manipulation of variables. Because of this permissive definition, there is a great variety of nonexperimental research designs. Descriptive studies use retrospective or prospective data collection to characterize a phenomenon of interest. In studies that involve the analysis of relationships, researchers use prospective or retrospective data collection to measure variables, which they then analyze to make predictions, establish odds, or determine reliability or validity of the measures. Nonexperimental analysis of differences, or ex post facto research, is accomplished when a nonmanipulated variable, such as diagnosis, sex, or age, is the only independent variable being studied.

REFERENCES

1. Kerlinger FN. *Foundations of Behavioral Research*. 3rd ed. Fort Worth, Tex: Holt, Rinehart & Winston; 1986:349.
2. Robertson VJ. A quantitative analysis of research in *Physical Therapy*. *Phys Ther*. 1995;75:313–327.
3. Shaugnessey JJ, Zechmeister EB. *Research Methods in Psychology*. 2nd ed. New York, NY: McGraw-Hill Publishing Co; 1990:130.
4. Roach KE, Ally D, Finnerty B, et al. The relationship between duration of physical therapy services in the acute care setting and change in functional status in patients with lower-extremity orthopedic problems. *Phys Ther*. 1998;78:19–24.
5. Findley TW, Daum MC. Research in physical medicine and rehabilitation, III: the chart review, or how to use clinical data for exploratory retrospective studies. *Am J Phys Med Rehabil*. 1989;68:150–157.
6. Chevan J, Chevan A. A statistical profile of physical therapists, 1980 and 1990. *Phys Ther*. 1998;78:310–312.
7. Bohannon RW, Cooper J. Total knee arthroplasty: evaluation of an acute care rehabilitation program. *Arch Phys Med Rehabil*. 1993;74:1091–1094.
8. Jette AM, Smith KW, McDermott SM. Quality of Medicare-reimbursed home health care. *Gerontologist*. 1996;36:492–501.
9. Lu-Yao GL, Baron JA, Barrett JA, Fisher ES. Treatment and survival among elderly Americans with hip fractures: a population-based study. *Am J Public Health*. 1994;84:1287–1291.
10. Taylor TK, Domholdt E. Legislative change to permit direct access to physical therapy services: a study of process and content issues. *Phys Ther*. 1991;71:382–389.
11. Polit DF, Hungler BP. *Nursing Research: Principles and Methods*. 5th ed. Philadelphia, Pa: JB Lippincott Co; 1995.
12. McEwen I, ed. *Writing Case Reports: A How-To Manual for Clinicians*. Alexandria, Va: American Physical Therapy Association; 1996.
13. Jones DL, Erhard RE. Diagnosis of trochanteric bursitis versus femoral neck fracture. *Phys Ther*. 1997;77:58–67.
14. Geerdink JJ, Hopkins B, Beek WJ, Heriza CB. The organization of leg movements in preterm and full-term infants after term age. *Dev Psychobiol*. 1996;29:335–351.
15. Plancher KD, Steadman JR, Briggs KK, Hutton KS. Reconstruction of the anterior cruciate ligament in patients who are at least forty years old: a long-term follow-up

and outcome study. *J Bone Joint Surg Am.* 1998;80:184–197.

16. Rosa L, Rosa E, Sarner L, Barrett S. A close look at therapeutic touch. *JAMA.* 1998;279:1005–1010.

17. Mack R, Salmoni A, Viverais-Dressler ZG, Porter E, Garg R. Perceived risks to independent living: the views of older, community-dwelling adults. *Gerontologist.* 1997;37:729–736.

18. Ingram D. Opinions of physical therapy education program directors on essential functions. *Phys Ther.* 1997;77:37–45.

19. Guccione AA, Felson DT, Anderson JJ, et al. The effects of specific medical conditions on the functional limitations of elders in the Framingham Study. *Am J Public Health.* 1994;84:351–358.

20. Powers CM, Boyd LA, Fontaine CA, Perry J. The influence of lower-extremity muscle force on gait characteristics in individuals with below-knee amputations secondary to vascular disease. *Phys Ther.* 1996;76:369–377.

21. van Dijk CN, Lim LSL, Marti RK, Bossuyt PMM. Physical examination is sufficient for the diagnosis of sprained ankles. *J Bone Joint Surg Br.* 1996;78:958–962.

22. Andrews AW, Thomas MW, Bohannon RW. Normative values for isometric muscle force measurements obtained with hand-held dynamometers. *Phys Ther.* 1996;76:248–259.

23. Timm KE. Postsurgical knee rehabilitation: a five year study of four methods and 5,381 patients. *Am J Sports Med.* 1988;16:463–468.

24. Holt P, Winograd CH. Prospective payment and the utilization of physical therapy service in the hospitalized elderly. *Am J Public Health.* 1990;80:1491–1494.

25. Morris JA, MacKenzie EJ, Edelstein SL. The effect of pre-existing conditions on mortality in trauma patients. *JAMA.* 1990;263:1942–1946.

26. Hayden GF, Kramer MS, Horwitz RI. The case-control study: a practical review for the clinician. *JAMA.* 1982;247:326–331.

27. Norton BJ, Strube MJ. Some cautionary comments on the use of retrospective designs to evaluate treatment efficacy. *Phys Ther.* 1988;68:1374–1377.

28. Victor N. The challenge of meta-analysis: discussion: indications and contraindications for meta-analysis. *J Clin Epidemiol.* 1995;48:5–8.

29. Finney DJ. A statistician looks at meta-analysis. *J Clin Epidemiol.* 1995;48:87–103.

30. Pogue J, Yusurf S. Overcoming the limitations of current meta-analysis of randomised controlled trials. *Lancet.* 1998;351:47–52.

31. Glass GV. Primary, secondary and meta-analysis of research. *Educ Res.* 1976;5:3–9.

32. Moreland JD, Thomson MA, Fuoco AR. Electromyographic biofeedback to improve lower extremity function after stroke: a meta-analysis. *Arch Phys Med Rehabil.* 1998;79:134–140.

33. Jansen CWS, Minerbo G. A comparison between early dynamically controlled mobilization and immobilization after flexor tendon repair in zone 2 of the hand: preliminary results. *J Hand Ther.* 1990;3:20–25.

34. Walsh M, Woodhouse LJ, Thomas SG, Finch E. Physical impairments and functional limitations: a comparison of individuals 1 year after total knee arthroplasty with control subjects. *Phys Ther.* 1998;78:248–258.

35. Wiley ME, Damiano DL. Lower-extremity strength profiles in spastic cerebral palsy. *Dev Med Child Neurol.* 1998;40:100–107.

Clinical Case Reports

Contributions of Case Reports to Theory and Practice	Building Problem-Solving Skills
	Testing Theory
Purposes of Case Reports	Persuading and Motivating
Sharing Clinical Experiences	Helping to Develop Practice
Developing Hypotheses for	Guidelines and Pathways
Research	**Format of Case Reports**

Clinical case reports are the means by which clinicians explore the theoretical basis for their practice through thoughtful description and analysis of clinical information from one or more cases. Sometimes dismissed as "not research," as they were in the first edition of this text, several authors consider clinical case reports to be important forms of inquiry in the health sciences. In 1993, Rothstein, in an editor's note in the journal *Physical Therapy*, noted that case reports are "too rare in this journal and in the physical therapy literature in general." [1(p492)] He believes that case reports are useful because they "clarify clinical terminology, concepts, and approaches to problem solving" [1(p495)] through the careful documentation of practice.

Sometimes the terms "case report" and "case study" are used interchangeably as labels for systematic descriptions of practice. However, the term "case study" is also used, particularly by qualitative researchers, to describe a more complex analysis of "the particularity and complexity of a single case" [2(pxi)] within its organizational,

social, or environmental context. For the purpose of this text, the term *case report* will refer to descriptions of clinical practice (covered in this chapter) and *case study* will refer to the more complete descriptions typical of research in the qualitative tradition (see Chapter 13). Case reports, which are nonexperimental descriptions of practice, should also be clearly differentiated from single-system experimental designs, which were discussed in detail in Chapter 10.

Case reports can be developed either retrospectively or prospectively. *Retrospective* case reports are developed when a practitioner realizes that there are valuable lessons to be shared from a case in which the physical therapy episode has been completed. *Prospective* case reports are developed when a practitioner, on initial contact with a patient or sometime early in the course of treatment, recognizes that the case is likely to produce interesting findings that should be shared. When a case report is developed prospectively, there is the potential for excellent control of measurement techniques and complete description of the treatments and responses as they unfold. Unfortunately, the prospective case report suffers from the possibility that the case was managed differently from usual because of the desire to publish the results in the future.

The rest of this chapter examines the ways in which case reports can contribute to theory and practice, cites examples of case reports that fulfill different purposes within the literature, and briefly outlines the format of case reports. Although this chapter focuses on clinical case reports, readers should recognize that case reports can also be used to document educational or administrative practices.

■ CONTRIBUTIONS OF CASE REPORTS TO THEORY AND PRACTICE

The potential value of case reports is illustrated by reviewing the relationships between theory, research, and practice that were originally presented in Chapter 2. Figure 12–1, a modification of Figure 2–9 to include case reports, shows these relationships visually. Clinical observation and logical speculation, which contribute to the development of theory, can be documented or developed in clinical case reports. Theories are put into action in practice, and careful documentation of this practice within case reports can help test the theories. The information presented in case reports may be used directly to change practice, to revise theories, and to suggest areas for future research. This figure suggests, then, that case reports can contribute to the development of knowledge in physical therapy by contributing to theory development, by testing theory, by leading to the revision of theory, and by suggesting areas for further research. This figure also suggests that the information gleaned from case reports can contribute directly or indirectly to changes in practice. This suggestion, however, is not supported by everyone.

Haynes,[3] a physician and epidemiologist, identified several purposes of various forms of

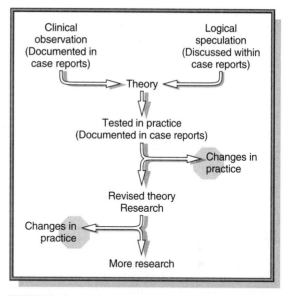

FIGURE 12–1. Modified version of Figure 2–9 showing the contribution of case reporting to the relationship between theory, practice, and research.

scholarly communications and presented a thoughtful analysis of the usefulness of clinical case reports. His analysis is shown in the matrix in Figure 12–2. Research reports of basic science research (sometimes called "bench research") and preliminary reports of clinical research ("field studies") are viewed as communications between scientists because their results are not yet rigorous enough to be applied in routine practice. Research reports of rigorous clinical trials are viewed as communications from scientists to practitioners because the findings within these definitive clinical studies are ready for application to practice. Articles that synthesize the findings of others are seen as communications between practitioners, since they can help clinicians identify and rectify gaps in their knowledge base. Finally, case reports are viewed as communications from practitioners to scientists. This view, which differs from the common perception of case reports as valuable contributions to practice, is supported as follows:

Clinicians who use case reports and case series as guidance for management of their own patients

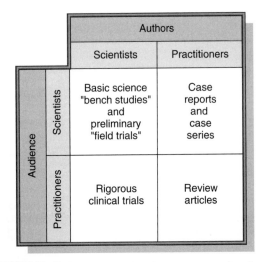

FIGURE 12–2. Matrix showing the purposes of various scholarly communications, delineated by the author and the audience for the communication.
Figure generated from information presented in Haynes RB. Loose connections between peer-reviewed clinical journals and clinical practice. *Ann Intern Med.* 1990; 113:724–728.

are at risk for deceiving themselves and hurting their patients. . . . Some case reports, of course, eventually prove to be important; most do not. Unfortunately, their methods do not permit discrimination of the valid from the interesting but erroneous, and they cannot provide a sound basis for clinical action. Case reports are, however, a fertile source of hypotheses that could lead to systematic observation.[3(pp725–726)]

Thus, Haynes believes that the primary value of case reports is in their contributions to theory and research, rather than their direct contributions to practice. This view of case reports is not presented to discourage practitioners from reading and learning from case reports. Rather, this alternate view is presented to remind practitioners that they need to thoughtfully critique the findings of case reports, just as they would assess the validity of more traditional research reports. In addition, because case reports are presented in the familiar language of practice, rather than the sometimes foreign language of research, clinicians may find that their reading habits gravitate toward case reports. Haynes's ma-

trix of scholarly communications reminds us to broaden our reading habits to include review articles and the reports of rigorous clinical trials.

■ PURPOSES OF CASE REPORTS

Although the general purpose of case reports is to carefully describe practice, the case reports that are presented in the literature show that there are many ways in which this general purpose can be fulfilled. McEwen,[4] in her useful manual on writing case reports, identifies six functions of case reports: sharing clinical experiences, developing hypotheses for research, building problem-solving skills, testing theory, persuading and motivating, and helping to develop practice guidelines and pathways. Recent examples of case reports that fulfill these six functions are presented.

Sharing Clinical Experiences

One clinical experience that is commonly shared through a case report is that of the diagnostic enigma. Jones and Erhard[5] reported on the diagnosis of trochanteric bursitis versus femoral neck stress fracture; Law and Haftel[6] reported on a case in which shoulder, knee, and hip pain were the presenting symptoms of a teenager who was ultimately diagnosed with juvenile ankylosing spondylitis; and Ferraro-Herrera and colleagues[7] reported on a patient for whom autonomic dysfunction was the presenting feature of Guillain-Barré syndrome.

Another common clinical experience that is shared through case reports is the presentation of unusual patients. Manktelow and colleagues[8] presented the case of a patient who experienced a late lateral femoral condyle fracture 2 years after anterior cruciate ligament reconstruction; Simonian and colleagues[9] documented the presentation and treatment of two cases of chronic knee dislocation; and Young[10] documented a successful course of physical therapy for a patient with chronic posterior dislocation of the shoulder.

The clinical experiences documented in case reports do not, however, need to focus on the odd or the unusual in clinical practice. Careful documentation and discussion of commonplace cases can also be instructive. For example, Olson[11] carefully documented the course of treatment for a woman with whiplash-associated chronic headache. Although the diagnosis is not unusual and the treatments were common (motion control exercises and home traction), the case serves as a reminder of how to put a variety of elements together to achieve success with a patient frustrated by previous unsuccessful courses of therapy.

Developing Hypotheses for Research

Although most case reports have the potential to help develop hypotheses for research, some authors include an explicit discussion of the research applications of their work. For example, McCulloch and Kemper[12] presented a case report on the use of vacuum-compression therapy (VCT) for treatment of a nonhealing fasciotomy wound. This technique was initiated after the size of the wound had not changed with 2 weeks of traditional wound care. After describing the successful course of treatment with VCT, the authors made an appropriately tentative conclusion based on this single case: "the case seems to demonstrate the potential benefits of VCT in . . . assisting the healing of wounds . . ." [12(p169)] Based on the case, they recommended that controlled studies with larger number of patients be conducted.

Another case with an explicit connection to future research is the report by Fritz and colleagues[13] of the results of a nonsurgical treatment approach for patients with lumbar spinal stenosis (LSS). They provided readers with a clear indication of the line of research that needs to flow from the case report:

In our view, experimental studies can be performed only after an approach to evaluation, treatment, and outcome assessment has been defined for the population being studied. This case report of two patients with short-term follow-up needs to be followed by reports describing larger series of patients with LSS treated with this approach with longer follow-up periods. If the treatment approach we are recommending produces favorable long-term outcomes in larger series of patients, then a randomized clinical trial would be warranted to compare this approach with the present "standard of care," which consists of the use of medications and nonspecific exercises. Only a randomized clinical trial could produce experimental evidence for the efficacy of the treatment approach we suggest.[13(p971)]

Note that the sequence of events they described corresponds closely to the types of research described in the matrix of communication presented earlier in this chapter. The first research approach that is recommended—a larger descriptive series—is a limited "field trial." If the field trial is promising then a formal randomized clinical trial is recommended to compare this new treatment to existing ones.

Building Problem-Solving Skills

Some clinical case reports contribute to practice by presenting frameworks for problem solving by clinicians. Zimny[14] accomplished this purpose in her case report of the clinical reasoning involved in the evaluation and management of undiagnosed chronic hip pain in a 21-year-old woman. Before describing the case, she reviewed various protocols for examination of the hip and presented several organizational models for reasoning about musculoskeletal pain. The description of the case then showed how these protocols and models could be applied in practice. The results were divided into an "examination" section, in which the results of clinical testing were reported, and an "evaluation" section in which the author's judgments about the meaning of the clinical test results were articulated. This section gave the reader an insider's view of the clinical reasoning that was applied to this case.

Testing Theory

Case reports can provide preliminary tests of various theories about patient management. For example, McClure and Flowers[15] used a case report on treatment of limited shoulder motion to challenge the convex-concave theory of arthrokinematic motion and to present their biomechanical approach to placing tensile stress on appropriate structures.

In another case report, Ford-Smith[16] described the evaluation and treatment of a patient with a 17-year history of benign paroxysmal positional vertigo (BPPV). A prevailing theory about the development of BPPV was presented, and a treatment based on this theory was initiated for the patient described in the report. The success of the treatment provided preliminary support for the theory and the treatment based on the theory.

Persuading and Motivating

Although some are uncomfortable with the idea of immediate application of the results of case reports, others find it appealing that "case reports can help practitioners deal with change, influence administrators, and persuade physicians and insurers of the value of services for particular patients."[4(p11)] One example of a case report with persuasion potential is Schindler and colleagues'[17] report on the functional effect of bilateral tendon transfers on a person with quadriplegia. Rather than reporting on a new technique, this case report extended the findings of almost 20 years of experience with tendon transfers for persons with quadriplegia. The authors of this case indicated that although previous reports had documented improvements in hand function tests and some activities of daily living, none had examined the impact of the surgeries on the amount of assistance needed with various tasks or the amount of equipment needed to accomplish the tasks. For patients who are considering tendon transfer surgery, it is exceedingly important to answer the question of whether the well-documented improvements in hand function lead to any meaningful changes in independence. Although this single case report does not provide a definitive answer to that question, the data in the case report, coupled with the well-documented experiences of the past 20 years, may assist with the decision-making process.

Helping to Develop Practice Guidelines and Pathways

McEwen's final purpose for presenting case reports is that they may help develop practice guidelines and pathways.[4] An excellent example of a case report that accomplishes this purpose is Fritz's[18] report of the application of a classification approach to the treatment of three patients with low back syndrome. This approach to care of patients with low back pain classifies patients according to clusters of signs and symptoms and then provides treatment that "matches" the classification. If adequate testing demonstrates the validity of the classification and the effectiveness of the matched treatments, then classification approaches can be the basis for developing practice guidelines or preferred clinical pathways.

Fritz[18] contributed to these efforts by describing three patients who appeared to have similar pathology, but fell into three different classifications and were successfully treated three different ways with treatments that matched their classifications. This case-based evidence is not sufficient to conclude that this classification approach is valid, but, combined with the positive results of a similar field trial,[19] suggests that this approach may be appropriate to study with rigorous randomized clinical trials.

◼ FORMAT OF CASE REPORTS

Case reports that appear in peer-reviewed journals typically follow the format—or a modified format—of more traditional research reports. First there is an introduction, critical review of the literature, and purpose statement to place the case into the context of what is already known about the phenomenon. Next, the equivalent of the methods section describes the subject, analyzes the presenting problem, presents examination data, outlines the conclusions drawn from the examination data, and describes the intervention. The equivalent of the results section presents the outcomes of care. As is the case with a traditional research report, the results are then placed into context in a discussion and conclusion section in which the authors discuss the meaning and application of the case. Detailed instructions for writing case reports can be found in McEwen's "how-to" manual.[4]

■ SUMMARY

Case reports are systematic descriptions of practice. It is clear that the information in case reports can be used to contribute to the development of theory and the design of research. There are differing opinions about the extent to which the information in case reports should be used directly to change practice. The written format of case reports is analogous to traditional research reports, with introduction, methods, results, and discussion sections.

REFERENCES

1. Rothstein JM. The case for case reports [Editor's Note]. *Phys Ther.* 1993;73:492–493.
2. Stake RE. *The Art of Case Study Research.* Thousand Oaks, Calif: Sage Publications; 1995.
3. Haynes RB. Loose connections between peer-reviewed clinical journals and clinical practice. *Ann Intern Med.* 1990;113:724–728.
4. McEwen I, ed. *Writing Case Reports: A How-To Manual for Clinicians.* Alexandria, Va: American Physical Therapy Association; 1996.
5. Jones DL, Erhard RE. Diagnosis of trochanteric bursitis versus femoral neck stress fracture. *Phys Ther.* 1997;77: 58–67.
6. Law LAF, Haftel HM. Shoulder, knee, and hip pain as initial symptom of juvenile ankylosing spondylitis: a case report. *J Orthop Sports Phys Ther.* 1998;27:167–172.
7. Ferraro-Herrera AS, Kern HB, Nagler W. Autonomic dysfunction as the presenting feature of Guillian-Barré syndrome. *Arch Phys Med Rehabil.* 1997;78:777–779.
8. Manktelow AR, Haddad FS, Goddard NJ. Late lateral femoral condyle fracture after anterior cruciate ligament reconstruction: a case report. *Am J Sports Med.* 1998;26: 587–590.
9. Simonian PT, Wickiewicz TL, Hotchkiss RN, Warren RF. Chronic knee dislocation: reduction, reconstruction, and application of a skeletally fixed knee hinge. *Am J Sports Med.* 1998;26:591–596.
10. Young MS. Electromyographic biofeedback use in the treatment of voluntary posterior dislocation of the shoulder: a case study. *J Orthop Sports Phys Ther.* 1994;20: 171–175.
11. Olson VL. Whiplash-associated chronic headache treated with home cervical traction. *Phys Ther.* 1997;77:417–424.
12. McCulloch JM Jr, Kemper CC. Vacuum-compression therapy for the treatment of an ischemic ulcer. *Phys Ther.* 1993;73:165–169.
13. Fritz JM, Erhard RE, Vignovic M. A nonsurgical treatment approach for patients with lumbar spinal stenosis. *Phys Ther.* 1997;77:962–973.
14. Zimny NJ. Clinical reasoning in the evaluation and management of undiagnosed chronic hip pain in a young adult. *Phys Ther.* 1998;78:62–73.
15. McClure PW, Flowers KR. Treatment of limited shoulder motion: a case study based on biomechanical considerations. *Phys Ther.* 1992;72:929–936.
16. Ford-Smith CD. The individualized treatment of a patient with benign paroxysmal positional vertigo. *Phys Ther.* 1997;77:848–855.
17. Schindler L, Robbins G, Hamlin C. Functional effect of bilateral tendon transfers on a person with C-5 quadriplegia. *Am J Occup Ther.* 1994;48:750–757.
18. Fritz JM. Use of a classification approach to the treatment of 3 patients with low back syndrome. *Phys Ther.* 1998;78:766–777.
19. Delitto A, Cibulka MT, Erhard RE, Bowling RW, Tenhula JA. Evidence for use of an extension-mobilization category in acute low back syndrome: a descriptive validation pilot study. *Phys Ther.* 1993;73:216–228.

13

Qualitative Research

Assumptions of the Qualitative
  Paradigm
Qualitative Designs
  Case Study
  Ethnography
  Phenomenology
  Grounded Theory
Qualitative Methods
  Sampling

Data Collection
  Interview
  Observation
  Artifacts
Data Analysis
  Data Management
  Generating Meaning
  Verification

Research conducted in the tradition of the qualitative paradigm is of growing importance to physical therapy and rehabilitation literature. As health care practitioners begin to conceptualize what they do according to biopsychosocial models of care, rather than focusing solely on a disease-based biomedical model of care, so too must health care researchers embrace research methods that capture the complexity of these new models of care. The qualitative research paradigm, along with the methods that flow from that paradigm, provide a means by which researchers can match their research methods to the complex phenomena they wish to study. This chapter reviews the assumptions of the qualitative research paradigm (originally presented in Chapter 5), introduces the various research designs associated with the qualitative tradition, and discusses a variety of methods and issues related to qualitative research.

■ ASSUMPTIONS OF THE QUALITATIVE PARADIGM

Five central assumptions of the qualitative paradigm were introduced in Chapter 5 and are reviewed here. The first assumption is that the world consists of multiple constructed realities. There are always several versions of reality and the meaning that participants construct from events is an inseparable component of the events themselves. The second assumption is that the investigator and the subject are interdependent and the process of inquiry itself changes both the investigator and the subject. The third assumption is that knowledge is time and context dependent. As a consequence, qualitative research is *idiographic,* meaning that it pertains to a particular case in a particular time and context. The fourth assumption is that it is impossible to distinguish causes from effects. Researchers who adopt the qualitative paradigm believe it is more useful to describe and interpret events than to attempt to control them to establish oversimplified causes and effects. The fifth assumption is that inquiry is value bound. This value-ladenness is exemplified in the type of questions qualitative researchers ask, the way they define and measure constructs, and the way they interpret the results of their research.

■ QUALITATIVE DESIGNS

The qualitative research paradigm encompasses a wide range of designs that flow from the five basic assumptions previously outlined. In fact, the boundaries between different types of qualitative research are far less clear than the boundaries between different quantitative designs. Denzin and Lincoln,[1] in the preface to their *Handbook of Qualitative Research,* articulate this as they describe the process of developing the volume:

> It did not take us long to discover that the "field" of qualitative research is far from a unified set of principles promulgated by networked groups of scholars. In fact, we discovered that the field of qualitative research is defined primarily by a series of essential tensions, contradictions, and hesitations. These tensions work back and forth among competing definitions and conceptions of the field.[1(pix)]

Whereas there is relatively well-standardized terminology for the different classifications of quantitative designs, the terminology for the different types of qualitative research is far less universally accepted. Four sometimes overlapping design strategies are discussed in this section of the chapter. Although it is useful to categorize the design strategies into a manageable number of approaches, readers should recognize that there is disagreement about what defines each approach and that there is considerable overlap between the methods used in the approaches.

To illustrate the similarities and differences between the methods, a single hypothetical research problem is developed in different ways using the four design strategies. Table 13–1 introduces this problem, which focuses on shifts in the supply and demand of physical therapists in the United States.

Case Study

Case study, rather than being a complete design strategy, is one way of structuring a qualitative research project; it is "not a methodological choice, but a choice of object to be studied." [2(p236)] By nature, a case has boundaries that define the limits of the inquiry.[3,4] In the context of the hypothetical problem defined in Table 13–1, the case is identified as one therapist who has been affected by the changing supply and demand for physical therapists by having her position eliminated. The purpose of such a study would be to gain an in-depth perspective on the impact of a layoff on an individual therapist. Having identified the case, the qualitative researcher still has a choice of studying the case through any single or combination of the remaining designs, which are discussed in subsequent sections of this chapter. The researcher who studies a case chooses to emphasize the idiographic nature of qualitative research, and recognizes that the results of the study will be particularly time and context dependent. Another researcher might choose to study the same problem, also guided by the qualitative paradigm, by studying several unrelated therapists whose positions had been eliminated. The purpose of this research would be to understand the phenomenon of therapists being laid off, rather than gaining an in-depth view of the impact of losing a job on an individual therapist.

The previous paragraph identified what was and was not a case study by contrasting the study of an individual therapist with the study of several unrelated therapists. This example leaves open the possibility of two ways of identifying what is and what is not a case: the number of elements and the relationship among the elements.

TABLE 13-1	Hypothetical Research Problems That Match Different Qualitative Design Strategies
Given	During the 1980s and early 1990s the profession of physical therapy in the United States enjoyed unprecedented growth. Opportunities were expanding and salaries were rising. To try to keep up with the demand for practitioners, existing academic programs to prepare physical therapists increased their class sizes and many new programs were developed. The shortage of practitioners meant that both experienced clinicians and new graduates usually had their choice of positions and could work in any setting or geographical region they desired. This situation, with demand far outstripping supply, meant that an entire generation of physical therapists became used to "calling the shots" with respect to where, when, and how they worked.
However	Beginning in the early 1990s, widespread health care cost containment efforts became the norm, thereby reducing demand for physical therapy services. At the same time, the supply of physical therapists was at an all-time high in the United States because of the increased capacity of the educational system to produce new graduates. For the first time in most therapists' careers, new jobs became scarce, moving between jobs became less possible, and finding employment in a desired setting or region was not always feasible. The current situation, with supply outstripping demand, means that the generation of therapists who were used to "calling the shots," or new graduates who expected to "call the shots" have had to make profound changes in how they think and act in relation to their careers.
Therefore	(Case Study) We did an in-depth case study of one physical therapist who entered the job market after the position she had held for 20 years was eliminated.
Therefore	(Ethnography) We used participant-observation to develop an understanding of the phenomenon of unemployment for physical therapists by studying its impact on one physical therapist and her family, friends, and coworkers.
Therefore	(Phenomenology) The purpose of our study was to describe the experience of being laid off and seeking a new job from the point of view of a therapist whose job of 20 years was eliminated.
Therefore	(Grounded Theory) The purpose of our study was to develop a preliminary theory to explain the ways in which therapists deal with the loss of jobs that they have held for more than 10 years.

The relationship among the elements is the key. If a number of therapists who had been laid off from the same facility were studied, the "case study" would be of the impact of therapist layoffs from that particular facility. The researchers would seek information about each therapist's story, but would also find out about how the layoffs were accomplished, the impact on the therapists who remained, and so on. Because of the facility boundary, different things would be learned from this case than would be learned in a qualitative study of several unrelated therapists who were laid off.

There are several good examples of qualitative case studies in rehabilitation. In a multiple case study with very clear boundaries—both in identifying the activity of interest and the people to study—Taylor and colleagues examined the meaning of sea kayaking for three individuals with incomplete quadriplegia.[5] In another example, with boundaries determined by membership in a single academic cohort, Graham studied conceptual learning processes of 10 first-year physical therapy students at one university.[6] Finally, Jensen and colleagues studied dimensions that distinguished master from novice clinicians working in orthopedic settings.[7] In this example, the six cases were selected to represent two ends of a continuum of experience. In addition to studying each case, the researchers examined commonalities among the three master clinicians and among the three novice clinicians, as well as between the master and novice clinicians. These three articles, then, illustrate three different ways of defining the "case" or "cases" of interest.

Ethnography

The purpose of ethnography is to describe a culture. Broadly, *culture* can be defined as the knowledge, beliefs, and behaviors that define a group. The group can be a societal group such as "Americans," "French-Canadians," or "Southeast Asian immigrants." The group can also be a small, specialized unit such as "burn therapists," "members of a wheelchair basketball team," or "physical therapy faculty members at a particular institution." Sometimes the terms *macroethnography* and *microethnography* are used to describe the extent of the group being described.[8(p147)]

The ethnographic approach requires that the researcher, an outsider to the culture, describe the culture from the perspective of an insider. Spradley indicated that "rather than *studying people,* ethnography means *learning from people.*"[9(p3)] The way that one learns from people is often described as *participant-observation.* Participant-observers immerse themselves in a new culture so that they can participate in and experience, in part, what it means to be within this culture. Rather than being complete insiders, however, participant-observers maintain a level of detachment that enables them to analyze, reflect on, and place the happenings within the observed culture into a broader framework. The concept of the researcher as both observer and participant illustrates clearly the qualitative research assumption that the investigator and subject are interdependent. Table 13–1 includes a purpose statement for an ethnographic study consistent with the background information on the changing supply and demand for physical therapists. Whereas the purpose statement for the case study identified only who would be studied, the purpose statement for the ethnographic study also includes information about the methods that will be used as well as the interest in the broader culture surrounding the person being studied.

The nature of ethnography can be illustrated by contrasting quantitative and ethnographic approaches to studying therapists whose positions were eliminated. A quantitative approach to studying such therapists might focus on the financial details of severance packages received by the therapists, the length of time between jobs, the number of résumés sent out in search of a new job, the number of interviews attended before securing a new job, and scores on standardized questionnaires measuring self-esteem and anxiety. The ethnographic approach would require observation and documentation of some of the same activities explored by the quantitative approach but would also focus on the emotions, feelings, and perceptions of one therapist and the people with whom she interacts. To do so, the ethnographer needs to request this information from the participants in the culture being studied. To become a participant-observer, the ethnographer would spend a great deal of time with the therapist being studied, participating in her life for a period of time. For example, the researcher might participate by eating meals with the therapist and her family, sitting with her and her friends on the sidelines of their children's soccer games, and accompanying her to a professional meeting where she hoped to network about jobs with colleagues.

As an observer the researcher might privately note how much spontaneous conversation focused around the job issue, how the heroes and villains of the story were described, or how the tone of such conversation changed over the course of several months. As a participant the researcher would ask direct questions about what had been observed: "A few weeks ago your friends always asked about your job search, but now they seem to wait for you to mention it—do you feel that support for your predicament is fading?" "It is interesting to me that you don't view your previous supervisor as the villain in your being laid off—why is that?" "Your son commented last week that he liked it that you were home more often—has this period of time without a job influenced you to look for a different balance between home and work responsibilities in your next job?" In addition to asking questions of the therapists being studied, the ethnographic researcher would likely question other important members of the "culture": family and friends of the therapist, colleagues within and outside her previous place of employment, and perhaps the therapist's new employer. As a participant, the researcher would recognize that his or her presence changed things in some way—people would say things for the researcher's benefit or would fail to do or say things they might have otherwise done or said if the researcher were not present. In addition, reflecting on and articulating feelings and concerns might change the way that the participants deal with those concerns.

A health-related example of an ethnographic study is Shidler's[10] perspective on life-prolonging treatment decision making in two long-term care centers in Quebec. Methods of study included more than 100 hours of interviews with informants who held many different roles within the long-term care setting, 400 hours of participant-observation, and examination of various documents. The informants included the older adults living in the long-term care centers, their family members, and personnel including physicians, registered and practical nurses, psychosocial workers, clinical administrators, nurse aides, and housekeeping staff. The extensive time spent within each facility and the wide range of informants who were interviewed and observed meant that the researcher was able to generate a complex description of the culture in which life-prolonging treatment decisions were made.

Phenomenology

The purpose of the phenomenological approach to qualitative inquiry is to "focus on the ways

that the life world . . . is produced and experienced by members." [11(p263)] The distinction between the phenomenological and ethnographic approaches, as defined here, can be seen if the ethnographic study of the culture of unemployment in physical therapy is recast as a phenomenological study. The purpose of the ethnography was to describe the culture of unemployment in physical therapy and the methods included participant-observation of the therapist who was laid off as well as members of her social system. As observers as well as participants, ethnographers interpret the many sources of data to provide a unique combination of insider and outsider insights into the situation. Phenomenological research "gives voice" to the person being studied, and requires that the researcher present the subject's view of his or her world. In a phenomenological study of unemployment in physical therapy, the only informants would be those therapists who had become unemployed. For example, what the son of an unemployed therapist thinks of the situation would not be relevant to a phenomenological study. However, the therapist's perception of her son's reaction would be of great importance in describing her experience with being laid off. Table 13–1 lists a sample purpose statement that would be consistent with a phenomenological approach.

The case study described earlier, about the meaning of sea kayaking for individuals with quadriplegia,[5] used a phenomenological approach. The only informants were the individuals with quadriplegia, and the questioning started with an open-ended invitation to relate their views: "Tell me about sea kayaking." In another example, Carpenter[12] studied the experience of spinal cord injury from the perspective of 10 individuals who had sustained traumatic spinal cord injury 3 to 5 years prior to the study. Thus, it can be seen that the scope of the "life world" described within a phenomenological study can vary greatly—from a narrow slice of life about a recreational activity to an all-encompassing view of life after an injury.

Grounded Theory

The grounded-theory approach was developed by Glaser in the 1960s.[13] Grounded theory has been described as a "general methodology for developing theory that is grounded in data systematically gathered and analyzed. Theory evolves during actual research, and it does this through continuous interplay between analysis and data collection." [14(p273)] Because of this interplay between data collection and analysis, grounded theory is often referred to as a constant comparative method. Although initially viewed as a means of generating new theory, contemporary writers also allow that grounded-theory approaches may be used to elaborate and modify existing theories.[15,16] Although the grounded-theory approach shares interview and observational methods with other qualitative approaches, the goal of the research is different. Ethnography and phenomenology are distinguished from grounded-theory research in that the goals of the former are to describe the phenomenon of interest and the goal of the latter is to explain the phenomenon through the analysis of the relationships among concepts. In the hypothetical example of the impact of changing supply and demand for physical therapists, a purpose consistent with a grounded-theory approach would focus on the development of a theory to explain how therapists cope with losing their jobs (Table 13–1).

Jensen and associates' study of novice and experienced clinicians, discussed earlier as a general example of a case study, could be classified as grounded-theory research because one of its purposes was to "develop an initial conceptual framework" [7(p712)] about the work of physical therapists. In this instance, the study was used to elaborate on a previous set of themes distinguishing between novice and experienced physical therapy clinicians.

Another example of the use of the grounded-theory approach, Graham's[6] work on conceptual learning processes of physical therapy students, follows the more classic approach to grounded theory—going in without a theoretical framework and seeing what emerges. She used the constant comparative method to analyze her data and described that process succinctly:

> As I transcribed the first set of interviews, I made notes about potential categories and trends. After the transcriptions were complete, I read each transcribed interview several times. I then coded the data to identify emerging categories and trends. The second set of interviews focused on the trends that emerged from the first set of interviews. The process continued through the final set of interviews. The previously collected data were compared with the newly collected data to identify emerging or changing trends. In this way, existing trends were discarded as new trends developed.[6(pp857–858)]

As noted previously, the boundaries between the qualitative approaches are not clear. Some studies may not fit any of the categories; others may fit more than one of the categories. Labels such as "case study," "grounded theory," "ethnography," and "phenomenology" are important because they provide a way to organize what we know about qualitative research. However, arguments about which definition is the "one true definition" tend to be counterproductive in that they violate one of the basic tenets of qualitative research—the acceptance of multiple realities. Thus, readers should use this classification of qualitative research as one way to organize information and recognize that others may use equally useful alternate classification systems.

■ QUALITATIVE METHODS

The methods of qualitative research are consistent with the assumptions presented earlier in the chapter and often cross the lines between the various research designs associated with qualitative research. This section of the chapter introduces sampling, data collection, and data analysis procedures commonly used by qualitative researchers. More detail about these procedures can be found in several excellent text-books devoted to qualitative research.[17–19]

Sampling

Qualitative researchers use nonprobability sampling methods, originally described in Chapter 8, to identify the individuals who participate within their studies. These individuals are typically referred to as *informants* rather than subjects, reflecting the emphasis on gaining access to their point of view rather than on manipulating them in some way as would be typical in quantitative experimental studies.

In the broadest sense, the sampling method is one of convenience because researchers often study informants they know who meet their study criteria, or facilities or organizations with whom they have connections. Beyond the initial convenient selection of sites or subjects, qualitative researchers often use a combination of purposive sampling and snowball sampling techniques. Recall that purposive sampling involves selecting individuals not for representativeness, but for diversity of views. Researchers studying changes in supply of and demand for physical therapists might believe that it is important to include both male and female therapists as well as therapists who are single without children, those who are primary breadwinners for a family, and those who are secondary sources of income for their families. They might also believe that they should have the perspectives of therapists working in urban and rural settings, as well as therapists in states with different economic climates. Because there is no established sampling frame of therapists whose jobs have been eliminated, researchers would likely use snowball sampling techniques to assemble the purposive sample. To do so, they might identify a few key informants who meet their criteria and ask them to identify others who have gone through similar experiences. In qualitative research, the sampling design often changes as the study progresses. In the first few interviews with therapists

whose jobs had been eliminated, the informants may share the view that it was important for them to have had the choice to accept a lower-level position rather than leaving. If the researchers had not anticipated this as an important dimension of the study, they might now change their purposive sampling procedure to include some therapists who did not have a choice to accept another position within the organization.

If a researcher were planning an ethnographic study, then the informants would include many people other than the therapists who had lost their jobs. At the beginning of the study the researcher would likely anticipate some groups of informants that would be important to the study—family members, friends, and coworkers. However, the researcher would not have enough knowledge of the phenomenon of joblessness in physical therapy to anticipate all of the relevant informants. During contact with initial informants, then, a common question should therefore be, "Who else could provide me with information about xxx?" At a given facility, for example, the evening shift housekeeper may be someone who always seems to know everything about everybody. At the outset, she might not be identified as a potential informant, but some of the initial informants would likely say, "Talk to Bea, she knows everything!" This variation on snowball sampling would help identify additional informants who meet criteria the researcher had anticipated, as well as identify additional classes of informants that had not been anticipated.

Several reports of qualitative research illustrate these sampling principles. Carpenter,[12] in her study of the experiences of individuals after spinal cord injury, used snowball sampling to identify 10 informants. She knew someone who was able to recruit three informants from a peer-support group he facilitated. These three informants then identified others who met the criteria for the study. A variation on snowball sampling was used by Jensen and associates[7] to identify their "master" clinicians. The researchers asked academic coordinators of clinical education in three different regions to identify, or nominate, several therapists who would be considered master clinicians in orthopedic physical therapy. Potential informants who were identified as master clinicians by more than one clinical coordinator were then contacted by one of the researchers to determine their willingness to participate.

Data Collection

Although there are many different design strategies for qualitative research, their implementation rests on a common core of methods. These methods include interviewing, observation, and examination of artifacts.

INTERVIEW. "Asking questions and getting answers is a much harder task than it may seem at first. The spoken or written word has always a residue of ambiguity, no matter how carefully we word the questions." [20(p361)] Interviewing, with all of its ambiguity, is one of the primary ways in which qualitative researchers collect data. Interviews can be classified by the extent of structure, the number of interviewees, and the proximity of the interviewer and interviewee.

With respect to structure, interviews can generally be classified as structured, semistructured, and unstructured. A *structured interview* is essentially an oral administration of a written questionnaire. When a surveyor stops you in the shopping mall to determine whether you have purchased a certain brand of facial tissue within the past 6 weeks, he or she is using a structured interview. The surveyor asks the same questions of everyone and does not deviate from the wording in the question. Structured interviews are most appropriate when relatively factual information is sought. In qualitative research, structured interviews might be used to collect a core of basic information from informants. However, structured interviews are rarely the choice

for capturing the depth and breadth of response that is desired in qualitative research.

Semistructured interviews are based on pre-developed questions, but the format permits the interviewer to clarify questions to help the subject provide more information for the study. Semistructured interviews are appropriate when information of a somewhat abstract nature is sought. Qualitative researchers who are testing theory (rather than developing it) or verifying information (rather than collecting it for the first time) may use semistructured interviews for these components of their data collection efforts. Triggs Nemshick and Shepard[21] used semistructured interviews to study the 2:1 student-instructor clinical education model and to extend and modify the conceptual framework they developed in advance of the study. Although they asked the same eight questions of all respondents, the unstructured format left them free to elaborate on questions as requested by the informants or to follow up on information volunteered by the informants.

Unstructured interviewing is the general method used by qualitative researchers to come to an understanding of the opinions and beliefs of informants. In an unstructured interview, researchers have a general idea of the topics that they hope to cover during the interview. However, the order and way in which the topics are covered are left to the interviewer as he or she interacts with subjects. The interviewer is free to follow up on unexpected responses that lead in a direction that was unanticipated by the researcher. In addition, unstructured interviews can change from interviewee to interviewee as the researcher gains more insight into the situation being studied. Suppose that Informant A volunteers his belief that the whole reorganization process that led to the elimination of jobs was just a way to eliminate a particularly problematic supervisor in the department. The researcher, who may not have anticipated a need to determine beliefs about the motives behind the reorganization effort, might follow this thread in subsequent interviews to determine whether others share Informant A's belief. Graham[6] used unstructured interviewing to collect data from the students in her study of conceptual learning processes of physical therapy students. Because she went into the study without a preconceived theory about conceptual learning processes of physical therapy students, it was appropriate that she go into the interviews in a consistent manner—without a preconceived set of questions.

With respect to the number of interviewees, researchers must determine whether they wish to interview informants singly or in groups. Individual interviews may elicit more confidential information about the informant or more frank information about other individuals within the setting. Group interviews may make the interviewer seem less intimidating and the responses of some group members may prompt other members to remember or share additional information. In any given study, it may be appropriate to conduct individual interviews, group interviews, or both.

With respect to the proximity of the interviewer and interviewee, the options are expanding because of the availability of new communication technologies. In-person interviews allow for the best opportunity to establish rapport and observe nonverbal cues of the interviewee. Telephone interviews do not permit observation of nonverbal behaviors, but may give the interviewer access to informants who are unavailable in person. Interactive two-way video hookups provide an opportunity to see the informants being interviewed at a distance. Electronic mail provides an opportunity to communicate with others in an informal, conversational way and various forms of electronic conferencing offer an electronic equivalent of the group interview situation.

Whichever style of interviewing is used, the researcher must consider several common concerns. First, the interviewer's vocabulary must match that of the individuals being interviewed. Second, interviewers must be sensitive to the meaning of specific words that they use. For ex-

ample, when interviewing individuals who are members of racial or ethnic groups, the interviewers should determine subjects' preferences for identifying terms such as *black* versus *African American, American Indian* versus *Native American,* and *Latino* versus *Hispanic.*

Third, interviewers must do what they can to establish rapport and make the interviewee comfortable. Friendly chit-chat and social conventions such as talking about the weather, taking coats, offering coffee or soft drinks, and the like can all be used to place the subject at ease in the research situation. The interviewees' comfort may be enhanced if the interview takes place on their turf—their office, their home, or a public place of their choosing.

Fourth, interviewers must ensure that subjects give their informed consent to participate in the interview. The interviewer should specify the purposes of the study, emphasize the provisions for confidentiality of responses, and make it clear that the subject can terminate the interview at any time. If the researcher is going to audiotape or videotape the interview, the subject needs additional assurances about the provisions for confidentiality of the recorded information. In research conducted using interviews, the primary risk to the subject is often the breach of confidentiality; informed consent is therefore often accomplished verbally rather than in writing so there is no written record of the names of those who participated in the study.

OBSERVATION. Qualitative researchers frequently use observation as an adjunct to interviews. The observational role has been described as a continuum between complete observation and complete participation. Along this continuum, four points have been defined: complete participant, participant-as-observer, observer-as-participant, and complete observer. These terms, originated by Gold in the 1950s, have been reconceptualized by contemporary qualitative researchers.[22]

When the researcher is a complete participant this means that he or she is a full, legitimate member of the setting being studied. This usually involves "opportunistic research" wherein a researcher recognizes a good research opportunity within an organization to which he or she already belongs.

In the participant-as-observer model the researcher assumes limited membership roles within a community for the purpose of conducting the research. This role has generated controversy in past research, mostly in sociological studies of illegal or socially unacceptable behavior, when researchers have inserted themselves into a community without disclosing their role as a researcher. This model of observation can, however, be accomplished with the knowledge and consent of the members of the community. If, for example, a researcher wished to gain an insider perspective to a physical therapy department as it is reorganized, the researcher might work as a therapist within the department for several hours a day, and assume a visible role as researcher for the rest of each day.

In the observer-as-participant model the researcher does not assume membership roles within the community. Rather, the researcher is available for relatively brief periods during which interviews and observations take place. Despite the relatively brief contact, the researcher recognizes that the very process of implementing the study changes the environment. The concept of the participant-observer, discussed earlier in the chapter, is generally broad enough to include both the observer-as-participant and participant-as-observer levels along this continuum.

In the complete observer model the researcher assumes the role of the "objective observer" who does not change the situation being observed. Qualitative researchers generally believe that this end of the continuum is not possible to achieve, because the mere presence of the investigator changes the dynamics of the situation.

The kinds of observations that one makes are dependent on the purpose of the research. In general, observations relate to the nonverbal behaviors of individual informants, interpersonal exchanges among informants, and the physical setting associated with the problem. In the study of therapists whose positions were eliminated, the researcher might note posture, hand gestures, and the tone of voice of individual informants; might note that Informants A, E, and G not only share similar views of the situation but also tend to sit together at staff meetings; and might observe that the bulletin board in the staff office still has postings of memos from the therapist whose job was eliminated. Some of these observations may confirm information gained in the interviews and other observations may require follow-up in interviews. For example, a researcher might ask the following: "I notice that memos from Therapist A are still up on the board; is this a deliberate attempt to keep her influence alive in the department, or doesn't anyone ever look at the bulletin board?"

There are several ethical issues involved with observation in qualitative research. When one interviews informants, there is a formal opportunity to discuss the study and gain the informed consent of the informant. Observation, however, may result in the inclusion of information about the behavior of members of the community who did not specifically agree to participate in the research. Even if observation occurs in public places, people who are observed may feel that their privacy has been violated. If descriptions of observations are sufficiently detailed, readers of the research results may be able to identify the participants, even if an attempt has been made to disguise the identity of the setting or of the particular informants. As discussed earlier, researchers who assume increasingly legitimate membership roles within the communities they study will likely interact with many people who are unaware of their research role—even if key members of the community have given informed consent to the project.

ARTIFACTS. Artifacts are sometimes known as the "material traces" associated with the research, or as the "material culture" of the setting.[23] Artifacts include any physical evidence that contributes to the understanding of the problem at hand. Some artifacts will be readily available and observable to the researcher; others will require that the researcher inquire about their existence or look in archives or public document depositories to locate them. Artifacts can be broadly divided into written documents, written records, objects, and the environment.

Although the terms "documents" and "records" are often used interchangeably, Hodder believes that it is useful to distinguish between them.[23] He defines *written documents* as unofficial or personal writings. For our hypothetical study of therapists whose jobs have been eliminated, one set of relevant documents might include informal correspondence on the job—perhaps a trail of electronic mail messages between a therapist and her immediate supervisor about the possible reorganization of the department or working papers of a reorganization committee. Personal writings might include a journal that the therapist keeps, letters between the therapist and an out-of-town friend, and the updated résumé and cover letter she prepared when beginning her job search.

Records are then defined as official documents. In our hypothetical study records that are relevant might include licenses of the practitioners involved, annual performance reviews, official salary schedules, and the formal letters notifying therapists of the elimination of their positions. Some records, such as birth, death, marriage, and professional licensure, are public and can be obtained by the researcher—or anyone else. Other records, including medical records, are private and require the cooperation and permission of those who have access to the private records.

Objects can send powerful qualitative messages. Think about the gift that might be given by coworkers to the therapist whose job was eliminated. A memory book of photos and letters from coworkers says one thing; a gift basket with cheeses and jams says another; and a box of straight pins and a doll that superficially resembles the new supervisor says another! Clearly,

the researcher would not conclude that the relationship between the departing therapist and her coworkers was close, distant, or diabolical based on the gift alone—but the gift would be a part of the pattern of evidence that would describe this relationship. Other common objects to be studied include photographs and personal effects in the offices or homes of informants.

The environment offers other artifactual evidence that may be important to the research. For example, in my own back yard, the pattern of beaten down grass provides clear evidence of the movement patterns of the dogs during the day and the pattern of brown foliage on the lower branches of isolated shrubs indicates their status as "watering" points! In a more relevant example, the retention of memos on the bulletin board, described earlier as an observation, might also be considered an artifact. Whether one considers them to be artifacts or observations, they can provide evidence that supplements the data gathered directly from informants.

Artifacts, then, provide material evidence that contributes to the breadth and depth of information collected by the qualitative researcher. Unlike archaeologists or criminal forensic investigators, qualitative researchers rarely base their conclusions on the analysis of artifacts alone. Rather, they use artifacts to supplement the data they collect through interview and observation.

Data Analysis

Data analysis in qualitative research is a process that differs greatly from data analysis in quantitative research. Whereas quantitative researchers typically describe their conclusions in statistical, probabilistic terms, qualitative researchers typically describe their conclusions in interpretive narratives that provide "thick description" of the phenomenon being studied. Generating this narrative rests on three general steps in the data analysis process—data management, generating meaning, and verification.

DATA MANAGEMENT

Data management relates to the collection, storage, and retrieval of information collected within the study. One of the consequences of seeking depth and breadth of information from multiple sources is that the amount of data becomes voluminous. A 30-minute interview with one informant might yield 20 pages of verbatim transcript based on an audiotape of the interview, 12 marginal notes on the transcript to remind the researcher of things to follow up on with future informants, and 2 pages of handwritten observations. If one does three interviews with each of 10 informants, this could easily result in more than 600 pages of data! Clearly, the qualitative researcher needs to develop a system for organizing and storing the information collected throughout the study.

One of the keys to the organization of data is the identification of the source of the data. Researchers come up with an identification code that enables them to determine where a piece of data came from originally. For example, a code of JP/I/02/07 might refer to the 7th page of the transcript of the 2nd interview conducted with an informant with the code initials JP. A code of MM/R/12/02 might refer to the 2nd page of the 12th record that was authored by an informant with the code initials MM.

A second key to the organization and reduction of data is a code-and-retrieve system. The coding system is the means by which the researcher labels the themes that emerge as the data are amassed. Box 13–1 shows a coded portion of Stikeleather's study of injured workers' perceptions of the workers' compensation process.[24] The nine text fragments included in Box 13–1 are only a small proportion of the hundreds of fragments that were coded for this participant. Although this code-and-retrieve process is, in part, a data management project, deciding how to code the data becomes a highly analytical process. This process involves several levels of coding as basic concepts are consolidated into larger groupings of ideas. Thus, the process of managing and analyzing the data generally occurs simultaneously.

From a technical standpoint, qualitative researchers used to generate hundreds, sometimes thousands, of index cards in the course of a study. Each card would include a coded snippet of interview, observation, or reflection, cross-referenced to the original source of the data. The researchers would sort and resort the cards, seeking to understand the relationships among the various themes that emerge. Today, many qualitative researchers use word-processing or relational database programs with search and sort properties to manage this process. In addition, several commercial software products have been designed to help qualitative researchers with the code-and-retrieve process, as well as the process of identifying relationships among concepts.[19(p316)]

GENERATING MEANING

After the data are coded, the researcher's job is to generate meaning from the data by noting themes, patterns, and clusters within the data, as well as identifying relationships among the themes and clusters. This is a reflective process that requires that the researcher "try on" ideas based on a portion of the data, test them against other portions of the data, and modify them as needed. In Stikeleather's study of the workers' compensation process, she began to group codes together under larger themes.[24] For example, the codes "health over work," "report injury quickly," "learned to protect against injury," and "educate" were all grouped into an "educate/protect self" theme. Other codes were grouped to generate the themes of "continued health problems," "physician caring," "work environment," and so forth. Finally, the relationships among the various themes were examined. For each of the participants in her qualitative study, Stikeleather generated a diagram showing the relationships among the themes for that participant. The diagram and a narrative story line expounding on the meaning of each theme and the relationship among the themes constituted the "within-case" portion of her study. In addition, when there is more than one case, re-

BOX 13-1

Excerpt of Coded Data

Jill Stikeleather, a physical therapist interested in work-related injury, conducted an exploratory qualitative study of injured workers' perspectives of the workers' compensation process.[24] Stikeleather used HyperRESEARCH, a coding and theory building program,[19(p316)] to assist in managing the coding process. The excerpt reported here has been sorted by codes and is not the continuous narrative of the interview. Each piece of text is linked to this particular interview by the letter-and-number identifier generated by the researcher, by the conceptual code words she assigned to the text, and by whether the statements are by the participant (P) or the interviewer (I).

DMV00339, financial security
P: Be able to stay around to retire. That is my biggest concern. You know, I look at it this way . . . I've worked too long at this job not to get nothing out of it.

DMV00339, health over work
P: I'm going back with a whole different attitude. I am taking a lunch hour every day. I am taking one hour. I am not running any longer, because all that does is get you hurt. I'm gonna do the job by the book.

DMV00339, learned to protect against injury
P: I've learned an awful lot being in therapy. How to keep yourself from getting hurt, you know. And I'm learning finally after all these years to slow down and think about what I'm doing before I try to do it.

DMV00339, learned to protect against injury
P: Well, I'm getting so that any injury on the job, I report, regardless of how small it is. Because now I know it can escalate into something worse. I: So you sort of learned your lesson with the knee?
P: Yes. And the best thing I ever did was report my shoulder the day it happened, too.

DMV00339, learned to protect against injury
P: So you know, if you do it the wrong way, and that's why when I'm out on the job, or even at home, but I don't lift heavy things at home, if I can get out of it.

DMV00339, legitimacy questioned
P: I mean, I was shocked, because any doctor that the clinic has ever referred me to has either told me that "my backache was due to my period," "my ankle was all right even though I didn't look at the x-rays," or "you have arthritis." You know, it was like, "Go on, out of here, goodbye."

DMV00339, legitimacy questioned
P: The first time they put it in a cast for 6 weeks. Then the second time, "Well, there's nothing wrong with you, go back to work." That's basically what it was.

DMV00339, legitimacy questioned
P: But on like ankle and sometimes back, they tend to talk among themselves and say "Oh, she's faking." But now they've got a younger girl to pick on, so . . . and she is faking half the time!

DMV00339, pushing self/no choice
P: And it's like, I retire in 3.5 years, you know, and it's like I'm just going to have to grin and bear it. I can't quit my job.

searchers typically do a "cross-case" comparison to search for similarities and differences among the cases. Stikeleather, for example, noted that one of her participants found the workers' compensation system to be more supportive than the other participants and explored reasons why the one worker's experience was so different from the rest.

Generating meaning from qualitative data, then, involves an interpretive process in which data are reduced into small components (coding), reorganized into larger components (themes), and then displayed in ways that illustrate the relationships among components. This process is an iterative one, meaning that the researcher goes back and forth among the steps several times, making modifications along the way until the final analysis of relationships among themes fits with the data. This sequence of steps is illustrated nicely in a diagram of the 2:1 clinical education experience, based on the research of Triggs Nemshick and Shepard.[21] Reproduced here as Figure 13–1, the bullets represent the codes, the boxes represent the themes, and the placement of the boxes and the arrows connecting the boxes represent the relationships among the themes. Several texts provide detailed guidance on the process of generating meaning from qualitative data.[17,19,25]

VERIFICATION

A final step in data analysis is the process of verifying the conclusions that have been drawn.[19] Without some verification process, qualitative research results remain open to the criticism that the researcher found what he or she was hoping to find. One form of verification is the triangulation of results. This is done by comparing multiple sources of information to determine whether they all point to similar conclusions.

A second form of verification is the use of multiple researchers to code data independently. Typically, two or more researchers will independently code a small amount of data at the beginning of the study, compare their results, discuss discrepancies, and code another small set of data until they are satisfied that they have a common understanding of what the codes mean. If they then divide up the data so that each codes just a portion of the data, they may complete periodic reliability checks to ensure that they remain consistent throughout the course of the study.

A third form of verification is called member checking. In this process, informants review the interpretive "story" that the researcher has generated and have the opportunity to correct technical errors or take issue with ways in which the researcher has interpreted their situation. The researcher uses this information to revise the story, or at least to indicate points of departure between his or her views and the views of the informants.

A final way of verifying the data analysis process is to have an outside researcher audit the analysis. Through this process the outsider does a detailed "walk through" of the data analysis to determine whether the steps the researcher took and the conclusions that were drawn at each step make logical sense and appear to fit the data. Comments from the auditor are carefully considered and, as is the case with member checks, used to either revise the results or indicate points of departure between the researcher and the auditor.

The various pieces of qualitative research that have been cited throughout this chapter illustrate, in the aggregate, all four classes of verification techniques. Graham[6] and Jensen and colleagues[7] used multiple sources of data to triangulate results. Triggs Nemshick and Shepard both coded one third of their data and documented a high level of agreement between their independent coding schemes.[21] Graham[6] and Taylor and colleagues[5] used member checks to solicit feedback from their participants. Finally, Graham[6] and Carpenter[12] asked colleagues to audit their data analysis process. By implementing these verification steps, qualitative researchers help to establish the credibility of qualitative findings by subjecting themselves to

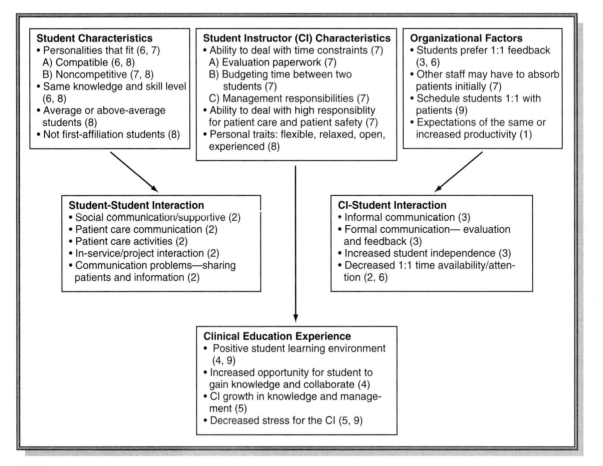

FIGURE 13-1. Conceptual model representing factors influencing the 2 : 1 clinical education experience. The numbers of the questions asked by the researcher are shown in parentheses. The bulleted items correspond to codes, the boxes to themes, and the arrangement of boxes and arrows to the relationship among themes.
From Triggs Nemshick M, Shepard KF. Physical therapy clinical education in a 2 : 1 student-instructor education model. *Phys Ther*. 1996;76:979. Used with permission of the American Physical Therapy Association.

external review and demonstrating to skeptics that "qualitative" is not synonymous with "arbitrary."

SUMMARY

Qualitative research includes a broad group of designs that generally follow five assumptions: that reality is constructed by participants, that researchers and subjects are interdependent, that research results are time and context dependent, that differentiating between causes and effects is not generally possible, and that research is a value-laden process. Although many different terms are used to describe qualitative design strategies, major approaches include case studies, ethnography, phenomenology, and grounded theory. Sampling in qualitative research generally includes convenience sampling, often selecting informants purposively through snowball sampling procedures. Common data collection methods include interviews, observation, and collection and review of artifacts. The data analysis process includes methods for managing large volumes of data from different sources; ways of generating meaning from codes, themes, and relationships among themes; and techniques to verify the conclusions.

REFERENCES

1. Denzin NK, Lincoln YS. Preface. In: Denzin NK, Lincoln YS, eds. *Handbook of Qualitative Research*. Thousand Oaks, Calif: Sage Publications; 1994.

2. Stake RE. Case studies. In: Denzin NK, Lincoln YS, eds. *Handbook of Qualitative Research*. Thousand Oaks, Calif: Sage Publications; 1994.

3. Stake RE. *The Art of Case Study Research*. Thousand Oaks, Calif: Sage Publications; 1995:2.

4. Yin RK. *Applications of Case Study Research*. Thousand Oaks, Calif: Sage Publications; 1993.

5. Taylor LPS, McGruder JE. The meaning of sea kayaking for persons with spinal cord injuries. *Am J Occup Ther*. 1996;50:39–46.

6. Graham CL. Conceptual learning processes in physical therapy students. *Phys Ther*. 1996;76:856–865.

7. Jensen GM, Shepard KF, Gwyer J, Hack LM. Attribute dimensions that distinguish master and novice physical therapy clinicians in orthopedic settings. *Phys Ther*. 1992;72:711–722.

8. Germain C. Ethnography: the method. In: Munhall PL, Oiler CJ, eds. *Nursing Research: A Qualitative Perspective*. Norwalk, Conn: Appleton-Century-Crofts; 1993.

9. Spradley JP. *The Ethnographic Interview*. Fort Worth, Tex: Holt, Rinehart & Winston; 1979.

10. Shidler S. A systemic perspective of life-prolonging treatment decision making. *Qual Health Res*. 1998;8:254–269.

11. Holstein JA, Gubrium JF. Phenomenology, ethnomethodology, and interpretive practice. In: Denzin NK, Lincoln YS, eds. *Handbook of Qualitative Research*. Thousand Oaks, Calif: Sage Publications; 1994.

12. Carpenter C. The experience of spinal cord injury: the individual's perspective—implication for rehabilitation practice. *Phys Ther*. 1994;74:614–629.

13. Glaser BG, Strauss AL. *The Discovery of Grounded Theory: Strategies for Qualitative Research*. Chicago, Ill: Aldine Publishing Co; 1967.

14. Strauss A, Corbin J. Grounded theory methodology. In: Denzin NK, Lincoln YS, eds. *Handbook of Qualitative Research*. Thousand Oaks, Calif: Sage Publications; 1994.

15. Strauss A. *Qualitative Analysis for Social Scientists*. Cambridge, England: Cambridge University Press; 1987.

16. Vaughan D. Theory elaboration: the heuristics of case analysis. In: Becker H, Ragin C, eds. *What Is a Case?* Cambridge, England: Cambridge University Press; 1992.

17. Denzin NK, Lincoln YS, eds. *Handbook of Qualitative Research*. Thousand Oaks, Calif: Sage Publications; 1994.

18. Morse JM, Field PA. *Qualitative Research Methods for Health Professionals*. 2nd ed. Thousand Oaks, Calif: Sage Publications; 1995.

19. Miles MB, Huberman AM. *Qualitative Data Analysis: An Expanded Sourcebook*. 2nd ed. Thousand Oaks, Calif: Sage Publications; 1994.

20. Fontana A, Frey JH. Interviewing: the art of science. In: Denzin NK, Lincoln YS, eds. *Handbook of Qualitative Research*. Thousand Oaks, Calif: Sage Publications; 1994.

21. Triggs Nemshick M, Shepard KF. Physical therapy clinical education in a 2:1 student-instructor education model. *Phys Ther*. 1996;76:968–981.

22. Adler PA, Adler P. Observational techniques. In: Denzin NK, Lincoln YS, eds. *Handbook of Qualitative Research*. Thousand Oaks, Calif: Sage Publications; 1994.

23. Hodder I. The interpretation of documents and material culture. In: Denzin NK, Lincoln YS, eds. *Handbook of Qualitative Research*. Thousand Oaks, Calif: Sage Publications; 1994.

24. Stikeleather SJ. *Injured Workers' Perspective on Claiming Compensation for Work-Related Injuries*. Doctoral dissertation in progress. West Lafayette, Ind: Purdue University; 1998.

25. Coffey A, Atkinson P. *Making Sense of Qualitative Data: Complementary Research Strategies*. Thousand Oaks, Calif: Sage Publications; 1996.

14

Epidemiology

Ratios, Proportions, and Rates	**Screening and Diagnosis**
Ratios	Sensitivity and Specificity
Proportions	*Receiver-Operator Curves*
Rates	*Likelihood Ratios*
Prevalence	Predictive Value
Incidence	**Nonexperimental Epidemiological Designs**
Relationship Between Incidence and Prevalence	Cross-Sectional Studies
Crude, Specific, and Adjusted Rates	Case-Control Studies
Relative Risk: Risk Ratios and Odds Ratios	Cohort Studies

Epidemiology has been defined as the "study of the distribution and determinants of states of health and illness in human populations." [1(p4)] This definition articulates a descriptive role for epidemiological research (studying distributions of health and illness), as well as an analytical role (studying determinants of health and illness). The other critical component of this definition is the emphasis on populations—epidemiological research tends to focus on large groups of people. As such, it has important applications in public and community health. This public health function is illustrated in Box 14–1, which relates a classic story of an early epidemiological project that helped to establish the transmission of cholera via contaminated water.

With its emphasis on the study of large groups, epidemiological research tends to focus on describing the characteristics of existing groups of people or analyzing the relationships among various health and demographic factors as they unfold within certain subgroups or across time. Both of these foci are nonexperimental in nature because they document existing health and illness states rather than attempting to change these states by introducing a controlled treatment. Despite this predominantly nonexperimental focus, some epidemiological research may be experimental in nature and follows the principles outlined in Chapter 9.

This chapter is organized around three major sections. The first section examines the use of ratios, proportions, and rates to describe various

BOX 14-1

Dumping in and Pumping from the Thames: An Epidemiological Study of Cholera in 19th-Century London

Routine collection of population data allowed British physician John Snow to investigate the epidemic of cholera that took place from 1848 to 1854. He noticed that deaths from cholera were particularly high in those areas of London that were supplied by two water companies, the Lambeth Company and the Southwark and Vauxhall Company. The two companies served about two thirds of London's residents, and their water mains were often interwoven in such a manner that houses on the same street or even next door to each other were receiving water from different sources. Both companies obtained water from an area of the Thames River heavily polluted with sewage. However, at some time between 1849 and 1854, the Lambeth Company changed its source of water to a part of the Thames River that was less contaminated. The rates of cholera declined in those areas that were supplied by the Lambeth Company, but rates of cholera remained the same in those areas supplied by the Southwark and Vauxhall Company. Snow recognized the opportunity to test his hypothesis that contaminated water was related to cholera by making use of the natural experiment that existed. He actually walked house to house in the area served by the two water companies and was able to determine the source of water for every dwelling. He noted that no experiment could have been devised that would test the relationship between cholera and the water supply more thoroughly. More than 300,000 people of each sex and every age, occupation, and socioeconomic group were divided into two groups without their choice and, often, without their knowledge. One group received water contaminated with the sewage of London, and the other group did not. The results in 1853–1854 were dramatic:

Water Company	Number of Houses	Deaths from Cholera	Deaths per 10,000 Houses
Southwark and Vauxhall	40,046	1263	315
Lambeth	26,107	98	37
Rest of London	256,423	1422	59

However, Snow also was aware that many other factors could account for the differences in cholera rates, and he investigated variations in the data as possible clues to further understanding of the epidemic. Snow's achievements were remarkable for the times. As one of the first epidemiologists, he outlined the frequency and distribution of cholera and found evidence of a cause or determinant of the outbreak. Snow logically organized data, recognized and analyzed a natural experiment, and did so prior to the era of bacteriology.

Excerpted from Harkness GA. *Epidemiology in Nursing Practice*. St. Louis, Mo: Mosby–Year Book, Inc.; 1995:6–9. Used with permission. The data within the excerpt are originally from Snow J. *On the Mode of Communication of Cholera*. 2nd ed. London: Churchill; 1855

health and illness phenomena. The second section presents a variety of concepts that are important to the understanding of screening and diagnostic processes. The final section presents nonexperimental epidemiological designs that compare health and illness in different naturally occurring groups.

■ RATIOS, PROPORTIONS, AND RATES

Researchers and practitioners are often interested in documenting "how many" cases of particular diseases or injuries occur in different groups, regions, or time frames. However, raw frequency counts of cases are rarely valuable because they are not directly comparable across groups of different sizes or across varied time frames. In Box 14–1, for example, the number of deaths from cholera in households supplied by the different water companies was not meaningful until it was expressed as the number of deaths per 10,000 houses supplied by each company. Changing frequencies into meaningful epidemiological data depends on the calculation of various ratios, proportions, and rates. The discussion of these concepts is accompanied by a hypothetical example related to ankle sprains on a college campus (Table 14–1).

Ratios

A *ratio* expresses the relationship between two numbers by dividing the numerator by the denominator. The numerator of a ratio is not necessarily a subset of the denominator. The simple formula for a ratio is therefore:

$$\text{Ratio} = a/b \qquad \text{(Formula 14–1)}$$

An example is the ratio of inversion to eversion

TABLE 14–1	Hypothetical Data on Ankle Sprains, University A, 1999–2000
Number at risk during the year	12,237
Athletes	1,216
Nonathletes	11,021
Number surveyed at beginning of year	9,857
Number of ankle sprains at beginning of year	61
Total new ankle sprains during year	436
Distribution by type of sprains	
Inversion sprains	401
Eversion sprains	35
Distribution by activity level of individual	
Athletes	170
Nonathletes	266

ankle sprains. Our hypothetical data, shown in Table 14–1, shows that of a total of 436 new ankle sprains documented during the 1999–2000 academic year, 401 were inversion sprains (*a* in Formula 14–1) and 35 were eversion sprains (*b* in Formula 14–1). This divides out to a ratio of 11.46 to 1 ($401 \div 35 = 11.46$). The notation for ratios is that a colon (:) is used for the "to" so that the ratio of inversion to eversion ankle sprains would be expressed as 11.46:1. The interpretation of this ratio is that there were almost $11\frac{1}{2}$ inversion ankle sprains for every eversion ankle sprain reported on the campus of University A during the 1999–2000 academic year.

Proportions

A *proportion* is a fraction in which the numerator is a subset of the denominator. The formula for a proportion is:

$$\text{Proportion} = a/a + b \qquad \text{(Formula 14–2)}$$

If we wish to know what proportion of ankle sprains are inversion sprains, then we must divide the number of inversion sprains (a) by the total number of ankle sprains, or the sum of the inversion sprains (a) and the eversion sprains (b). Thus, the proportion of inversion sprains is $401/(401 + 35) = .9197$. Proportions are often converted to percentages by multiplying by 100. Thus, we find that 91.97% of ankle sprains at University A are inversion sprains. Sometimes very small proportions are multiplied by constants larger than 100 in order to express them as whole numbers rather than decimals.

Rates

A *rate* is a proportion expressed over a particular unit of time. In epidemiology, rates are used to express the change in a health variable in the population at risk over a period of time. Because rates often describe fairly rare events in large populations, the number that is calculated is often a decimal beginning with one or more zeros. At University A, the rates of new inversion and eversion ankle sprains in a year are as follows:

Rate of new inversion sprains per year = 401/12,237 = .03277

Rate of new eversion sprains per year = 35/12,237 = .00286

Because it is difficult to conceptualize these small decimal values, rates are multiplied by a constant to obtain values that are whole numbers. To use the same constant to express both inversion and eversion ankle sprain rates as whole numbers, we need to multiply each rate by 1000, as follows:

Rate of new inversion sprains = [401/12,237] × 1000 = 32.77 per 1000 people per year

Rate of new eversion sprains = [35/12,237] × 1000 = 2.86 per 1000 people per year

When rates are multiplied by a constant, it is important to include the constant when listing the rate so that readers know whether the rate is, for example, for 1000 people or 1 million people.

Epidemiologists use ratios, percentages, and rates to express many important concepts. Two of the most common are prevalence and incidence. Each of these can be expressed in crude, specific, and adjusted forms.

Prevalence

Prevalence expresses the proportion of a population who exhibit a certain condition at a given point in time.

Prevalence = Existing cases/Population examined at a given point in time (Formula 14–3)

Because the proportion is often small, it is usually multiplied by an appropriate constant. Because prevalence is a value at a given time, rather than a value calculated over a given pe-

riod of time, it is a proportion rather than a rate. To determine prevalence, one must consider what individuals will be counted in the numerator and denominator of Formula 14–3.

The numerator will contain all of the cases of the desired condition at the time of measurement. Consider the example of multiple sclerosis. Because the symptoms of multiple sclerosis come and go and may resemble other disorders, at any one point in time, there are many individuals who have the disease but have not been diagnosed. Once diagnosed, however, the condition is presumed to exist for a lifetime. Therefore, the difficulty in defining cases of multiple sclerosis is in knowing when the disease begins, not when it ends.

Contrast this with the case of acute conditions that have more distinct beginnings, but less clear endpoints. An ankle sprain might be defined as posttraumatic pain, swelling, bruising, or instability that results in an inability to participate fully in desired activities. With this definition one would count all of the following as cases: an individual who sprained her ankle 2 days ago and is still walking gingerly, an intercollegiate athlete who sprained his ankle 3 weeks ago and is now practicing with the team but not yet back on the game roster, and a recreational athlete who sprained her ankle 3 years ago and gave up racquetball because of chronic instability. One would not count an individual who "twisted" his ankle but did not experience swelling, bruising, or functional difficulties, nor would one count an individual who sustained a sprain in the past but has no residual swelling or instability and has returned to full function.

The denominator will contain all of the people "examined" to determine whether they have the condition. Sometimes this number represents an actual examination of the individuals in the population; other times the number is determined from responses to a survey or numbers of cases within a large health care system or health insurer database.

To determine the prevalence of ankle sprains at University A, researchers would need to pick a reporting date and a mechanism to obtain the information. Knowing that all members of the community need to renew parking permits during the first week of September, the researchers might set up shop at the parking permit window and administer a brief survey to all members of the campus who were willing to participate. If they administered 9857 questionnaires and identified 61 cases of ankle sprain, then prevalence would be calculated as follows:

Prevalence of ankle sprains at the beginning of the academic year = [61/9857] × 1000 = 6.19

When reporting the prevalence it is important to include the constant and the point in time that the data were collected. In a report about ankle sprains at University A, the researchers might, after presenting their definition of what constituted an ankle sprain, write that "the prevalence of ankle sprains in the academic community at the beginning of the academic year was 6.19 sprains per 1000 people."

Incidence

Incidence is the rate of new cases of a condition that develop during a specified period of time. The numerator represents the number of new cases and the denominator represents the number in the population at risk:

Incidence = New cases during time period/Population at risk during time period
(Formula 14–4)

As with other values, the incidence is often multiplied by a constant so that it can be expressed as a whole number rather than as a decimal.

To determine the incidence of ankle sprains at University A, researchers would need to set up a monitoring system to ensure good reporting of ankle sprains among members of the university community. For the purposes of this example, we will make the following (unrealistic) assumptions: (1) all members of the community will seek care for sprained ankles, (2) all will seek care at the campus health center or the athletic training center, and (3) all the professionals providing the care will use the same operational definition of ankle sprain and will report the number of new cases accurately. In the real world, determining incidence is complicated because people do not always seek medical care for new conditions, the care they receive occurs in many different places, and the providers they see define conditions differently and report them inconsistently. In our ideal world, we have already established the number of new cases of ankle sprain at University A to be 436 during the 1999–2000 academic year (Table 14–1). Thus, 436 is the numerator of the incidence formula.

The denominator for incidence is the population at risk during the time period being measured. Determining this number is harder than it seems! First, one must determine the number in the "population." However, the number of individuals in a population usually varies over the course of the time period being studied. One common way to handle this is to use the number in the population at the midpoint of the period of study. For our ankle sprain example the 1999–2000 academic year could be defined as September 1, 1999 to August 31, 2000, with a midpoint at March 1, 2000. This is probably a good date in the academic calendar because it avoids the peak enrollment time of early September, as well as the valley of summer enrollments. Incidence studies frequently use the calendar year as the reporting period with July 1 as the midpoint for determining the denominator.

The second difficulty in determining the denominator for an incidence calculation is in determining who is "at risk." If some conditions affect only one sex, or are virtually unheard of in certain age groups, then the population at risk should include only those of the appropriate sex or age. If having the condition means that one is no longer at risk of developing a new case of the disease (e.g., multiple sclerosis), then individuals with the condition at the start of the reporting period should be excluded from the denominator. In contrast, if the condition of interest can occur multiple times in the same individuals, then even those with the condition at the start of the reporting period remain at risk for new events. In the example of ankle sprains, the 61 people with ankle sprains during the first week of September 1999 remain at risk for a new ankle sprain during the academic year and are not excluded from the denominator. Therefore, the incidence of ankle sprains at University A would be calculated as follows:

Incidence of ankle sprains during 1999–2000 = [436/12,237] × 1000 = 35.63

Note that the constant of 1000 was used, even though we could have multiplied by a constant of 100 to get a value that was a whole number. Because incidence and prevalence are often reported together, it is helpful to express them in terms of the same multiple of the population. Since the constant of 1000 was used to express the prevalence, this was used to express the incidence as well. When reporting incidence rates, it is important to include the time period studied and the population multiplier. In a report about ankle sprains at University A, researchers would indicate that the "incidence of ankle sprains during the 1999–2000 academic year was 35.63 per 1000 people in the academic community."

Relationship Between Incidence and Prevalence

The relationship between incidence rates and prevalence depends on the nature of the condition being examined. For diseases or injuries that are of short duration (either rapidly resolving or quickly fatal), the incidence is often greater than the prevalence. Consider the common cold— during the course of a year, most people get a new cold at some point (high incidence), but far fewer have colds at the same time (lower prevalence). Of course, this general statement is complicated by the seasonal nature of colds—it sometimes seems like everyone has them at once! The hypothetical ankle sprain example in this chapter exhibits this relationship between incidence and prevalence: the incidence is high (35.63 per 1000 people during the 1999–2000 academic year) compared to the prevalence (6.19 sprains per 1000 people at the beginning of September 1999).

For conditions that are of long duration, incidence is often lower than prevalence. Consider the case of Parkinson's disease. Reports of crude prevalence range from approximately 65 to 187 cases per 100,000 population, depending on geographical region.[2] The annual incidence is much lower, ranging from approximately 4 to 20 new cases per 100,000 population across the same regions.[2] Similar patterns can be expected with conditions such as multiple sclerosis, spinal cord injury, cerebral palsy, and diabetes.

Readers of the literature should be aware that even though "incidence" and "prevalence" have the specific meanings outlined here, sometimes the terms are used inaccurately as general measures of frequency. While preparing this chapter, I was talking to a colleague who indicated that she knew that incidence and prevalence had specific, different meanings, but that she could never remember which was which. The following mnemonic device, based on the first three letters of each word, is offered to help readers remember which is which:

Incidence = **N**ew **C**ases (**INC**idence)

PRevalence = **E**xisting cases (**PRE**valence)

Crude, Specific, and Adjusted Rates

Although rates are sometimes calculated for purely descriptive purposes, researchers often wish to compare the rates with one another. They may wish to compare their sample with established population norms; they may wish to determine whether the rate within their population has changed over time; or they may wish to see whether their rates are approaching some desirable target rate. Making valid comparisons, however, depends on comparing the rates for similar populations. To generate the data appropriate for these "apple-to-apple" comparisons, researchers often modify their rates in several different ways.

Crude rates are rates calculated using the entire population at risk. Generating a crude rate is usually the starting point for the researcher's calculations. The incidence rate of 35.63 ankle sprains per 1000 people during the 1999–2000 academic year is a crude rate. In certain circumstances crude rates are systematically modified to become specific and adjusted rates.

Specific rates are rates for specified subgroups of the population. In our ankle sprain example we might wonder whether athletes and nonathletes had different rates of ankle sprains. To determine this, we would first need an operational definition of athlete (perhaps someone who participates in recreational or intercollegiate team sports or individual physical activities an average of two times per week). Next, we would need to determine the number of athletes and nonathletes for the denominators of our specific rates. Finally, we would need to know how many of our 436 new cases occurred in athletes versus nonathletes. Figure 14–1, which presents a 2 × 2 matrix containing this hypothetical information, shows that the specific incidence for athletes appears to be much higher (139.80 per 1000 athletes) than it is for the nonathletes (24.14 per 1000 nonathletes).

If we wished, we could get even more specific. Among athletes, we might generate sport-specific incidence rates to determine whether there is a higher incidence among basketball, volleyball, and soccer players than among swimmers, golfers, and baseball/softball players. We also might determine competition-specific rates to look at incidence in recreational versus intercollegiate athletes. In addition, we might suspect that there are age or gender differences in ankle sprain incidence and calculate age- and sex-specific rates as well.

Adjusted rates are used when one wishes to compare rates across populations with different proportions of various subgroups. Let's assume that we got our hands on the injury statistics for

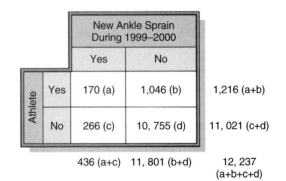

FIGURE 14–1. Crude and specific incidence rates of ankle sprain at University A during the 1999–2000 academic year.

Crude incidence rate: [(a + c)/(a + b + c + d)] × constant = [436/12,237] × 1000 = 35.63 per 1000 people.

Specific incidence rate for athletes: [a/(a + b)] × constant = [170/1216] × 1000 = 139.80 per 1000 athletes.

Specific incidence rate for nonathletes: [c/(c + d)] × constant = [266/11,021] × 1000 = 24.14 per 1000 nonathletes.

University B and note that their ankle sprain incidence for the year was only 100.8 sprains per 1000 athletes. Initially concerned because University A's incidence for athletes seems so much higher, you realize that the rates must be adjusted before you can make a valid comparison. Table 14–2 shows the specific, unadjusted rates for each university. A much higher proportion of athletes at University A are soccer players than at University B. Furthermore, you can see that soccer players at both universities have a high incidence of ankle sprains. To compare "apples to apples" you need to mathematically adjust the proportion of athletes in each sport at one university so that it matches the proportion at the other university, and then adjust the presumed number of injuries and the incidence rates in light of the new proportions. Table 14–3 shows how this is done, by adjusting the University A data to match the proportions at University B. For example, at University B, only 1.6% of their athletes are soccer players. If University A, with

TABLE 14-2 Hypothetical Sport-Specific Incidence Rates at Universities A and B

	University A			University B		
Category	No. of Sprains	No. (%) in Group	Incidence of Sprains (per 1000)	No. of Sprains	No. (%) in Group	Incidence of Sprains (per 1000)
Recreational	109	968 (79.6)	112.6	81	821 (84.5)	98.7
Intercollegiate						
Soccer	49	92 (7.6)	532.6	9	16 (1.6)	562.5
Baseball/Softball	8	74 (6.1)	108.1	5	68 (7.0)	73.5
Swimming	4	82 (6.7)	48.7	3	67 (6.9)	44.8
Total	170	1216 (100.0)	139.80	98	972 (100.0)	100.82

1216 athletes overall, had only 1.6% soccer players, then they would have 19 soccer players (1216 × .016 = 19.456). If these 19.46 players sustained ankle injuries at the same rate that the original 92 players did (532.6 per 1000 players), you would expect them to have sustained roughly 10.36 injuries during the year (19.46 × 0.5326 = 10.36). First, the University B subgroup proportions are used to adjust the proportions in the University A population. Then, the University A incidence rates are applied to the new proportions to calculate the adjusted injury numbers.

This adjustment is done for each subgroup within the population, as shown in Table 14–3. If University A had the same distribution of athletes as University B, then you would expect University A to have 139.35 ankle sprains among athletes for an adjusted incidence of 114.60 sprains per 1000 athletes. This process shows that the adjusted incidence rates are more similar to University B (114.60 compared to 100.82) than the original unadjusted rates (139.80 compared to 100.82).

Relative Risk: Risk Ratios and Odds Ratios

Epidemiologists often wish to move beyond describing groups to compare the probability that different groups with different characteristics will

TABLE 14-3 Adjusted Hypothetical Sport-Specific Incidence Rates at University A

	University A			University A—Adjusted		
Category	No. of Sprains	No. (%) in Group	Incidence of Sprains (per 1000)	No. of Sprains	No. (%) in Group	Incidence of Sprains (per 1000)
Recreational	109	968 (79.6)	112.6	115.70	1027.52 (84.5)	112.6
Intercollegiate						
Soccer	49	92 (7.6)	532.6	10.36	19.46 (1.6)	532.6
Baseball/Softball	8	74 (6.1)	108.1	9.20	85.12 (7.0)	108.1
Swimming	4	82 (6.7)	48.7	4.09	83.90 (6.9)	48.7
Total	170	1216 (100.0)	139.80	139.35	1216 (100.0)	114.60

be affected by disease or injury in some way. That is, they seek to determine the relative risk of disease or injury of two different groups. There are two important ways in which relative risk is calculated—using risk ratios and using odds ratios. The distinction between the two is important and warrants careful consideration of the examples that follow.

The risk ratio is calculated by creating a ratio of the incidence rate for one subgroup and the incidence rate for another subgroup. In our example of ankle sprain, we saw that athletes sustained ankle sprains at a rate of 139.80 per 1000 people and that nonathletes sustained ankle sprains at a rate of 24.14 per 1000 people (see Fig. 14–1). If we create a ratio out of these two numbers (139.80/24.14), we find that the athletes are 5.79 times as likely to sustain ankle sprains as nonathletes. Earlier we used a 2 × 2 matrix to organize our data. The formula for determining the risk ratio is often given with a standard form of this table in mind (Fig. 14–2). The risk ratio is defined as:

$$\text{Risk ratio} = [a/(a + b)]/[c/(c + d)]$$
$$\text{(Formula 14–5)}$$

Note that this is calculated by "working" the table horizontally—determining the incidence of ankle sprains for the row that represents athletes and then determining the incidence for the row that represents nonathletes. We can compute relative risks this way because we have measured the entire population of interest and the totals for each row [(a + b) and (c + d)] give us meaningful information about the number of athletes and nonathletes in the population.

Many epidemiological researchers, however, do not have access to an entire population of interest. Instead of measuring the entire population of interest, the researcher identifies a number of individuals who have the condition or risk factor of interest. The researchers then seek out matched controls without the condition or risk factor in order to create a comparison group. Figure 14–3A and B show two new sets of hypothetical data used to determine the relative risk of ankle sprains in athletes and nonathletes. In Figure 14–3A the researchers identified one control for each case; in Figure 14–3B they identified three controls for each case. In both parts of Figure 14–3 the numbers for those with ankle sprains remains constant. In addition, the distribution of athletes and nonathletes without ankle sprains remains the same even though the absolute numbers change from Part A to Part B. Watch what happens mathematically if we apply the risk ratio formula to these tables. Figure 14–3 shows that the risk ratio is different for the two parts of the figure. This is because the totals in the margin change as the number of control subjects changes. Because the totals in the margins reflect the sampling design, and not the actual totals in the population, it is not valid to use the risk ratio in this situation.

When computing risk ratios is not valid, then a value known as the odds ratio is used to estimate relative risk. To understand the difference between these two ratios, the difference between proportions and odds must be clarified. To use a common example,[3(p91)] consider a baseball player who has one hit (and three misses) in four times at bat in a game. A hit is represented by *a* and a miss is represented by *b*. The formula for a proportion is a/(a + b), which in this case means that the proportion of hits is 1/4, or 0.250. The proportion divides the "part" by the "whole." In contrast, odds are determined by creating a ratio between hit and misses, or a/b. The odds divides one "part" by the other

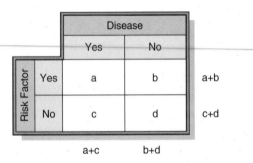

FIGURE 14–2. Standard table for determining relative risk.

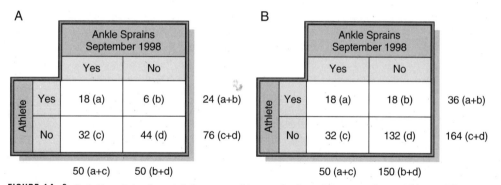

FIGURE 14–3. Relative risk of sustaining an ankle sprain for athletes and nonathletes. The two parts of the figure demonstrate the problem of calculating risk ratios when the total population of interest has not been studied. Because the totals in the row margins reflect the sampling design rather than the proportion of injury in the population, the risk ratio changes from **A** to **B**. The odds ratio, which does not depend on the totals in the margins, remains the same.

A. Hypothetical study in which one control subject is identified for each case.

Proportion of athletes with ankle sprains = a/(a + b) = 18/24 = 0.75
Proportion of nonathletes with ankle sprains = c/(c + d) = 32/76 = 0.42
Risk ratio = [a/(a + b)]/[c/(c + d)] = 0.75/0.42 = 1.79

Odds of someone with an ankle sprain being an athlete = a/c = 18/32 = 0.5625
Odds of someone without an ankle sprain being an athlete = b/d = 6/44 = 0.1364
Odds ratio = (a/c)/(b/d) = 0.5625/0.1364 = 4.124

B. Hypothetical study in which three controls are identified for each case.

Proportion of athletes with ankle sprains = a/(a + b) = 18/36 = 0.500
Proportion of nonathletes with ankle sprains = c/(c + d) = 32/164 = 0.195
Risk ratio = [a/(a + b)]/[c/(c + d)] = 0.500/0.195 = 2.56

Odds of someone with an ankle sprain being an athlete = a/c = 18/32 = 0.5625
Odds of someone without an ankle sprain being an athlete = b/d = 18/132 = 0.1364
Odds ratio = (a/c)/(b/d) = 0.5625/0.1364 = 4.124

"part." In this baseball example, the odds of getting a hit is 1 : 3 or 0.333.

Returning to the ankle sprain example, the totals in the margins of the rows in Figure 14–3 are not meaningful because they do not represent the "whole" population of interest; instead they reflect the sampling design of the researchers. When this is the case, researchers use an odds ratio, rather than a risk ratio based on proportions, to estimate relative risk among subgroups.

The odds ratio uses only the numbers found within the table (not those in the margin) and

works the table "vertically." In Figure 14–3A the odds of a person with an ankle sprain being an athlete is (18/32) or 0.5625. The odds of a person without an ankle sprain being an athlete is (6/44) or 0.1364. The odds ratio is simply the ratio of these two odds. The conceptual formula for the odds ratio is given below, along with a common algebraic simplification:

$$\text{Odds ratio} = (a/c)/(b/d) = ad/bc$$

(Formula 14–6)

In contrast to the changing value of the risk ratio between Figures 14–3A and 14–3B, the odds ratio remains the same whether the researcher selects one or three controls for each case.

Epidemiologists use measures such as incidence, prevalence, risk ratios, and odds ratios to describe the distribution of disease and injury within populations and population subgroups. Reports of epidemiological studies frequently report these measures, or variations on these measures. Readers who encounter a rate, proportion, or ratio with which they are unfamiliar should be able to apply the general principles in this section to gain a general understanding of the unfamiliar measure.

■ SCREENING AND DIAGNOSIS

A common function of epidemiological research is to evaluate the usefulness of various screening and diagnostic tests. Four key proportions are used to compare the usefulness of the test being evaluated to a criterion test that is considered the "gold standard." These four proportions are the sensitivity, specificity, positive predictive value, and negative predictive value. They are generally represented by a standard 2 × 2 table, as shown in Figure 14–4.

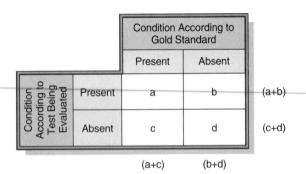

FIGURE 14–4. Illustration of traditional epidemiological concepts. Sensitivity = a/(a + c). Specificity = d/(b + d). Positive predictive value = a/(a + b). Negative predictive value = d/(c + d).

Sensitivity and Specificity

Sensitivity and specificity compare the conclusions of the new test with the results on the criterion test. They are determined by "working" the 2 × 2 table vertically. The *sensitivity* of a test is the proportion or percentage of individuals with a particular diagnosis who are correctly identified as positive by the test. The *specificity* is the proportion or percentage of individuals without a particular diagnosis who are correctly identified as negative by the test.

Sensitivity = a/(a + c)   (Formula 14–7)

Specificity = d/(b + d)   (Formula 14–8)

These two epidemiological concepts are illustrated in Figure 14–5, which uses data from Clark and associates'[4] study of ankle joint effusion and occult ankle fractures. A series of patients with severe ankle sprains, but without apparent fractures on plain radiographs, was studied with plain radiographs and computed tomography (CT). The "gold standard" for identifying ankle fractures was CT of the ankle. The new test involved measuring the extent of ankle joint effusion on the plain radiographs. They found that an ankle effusion of 15 mm or more on plain radiography had a sensitivity of 83.3% for detecting occult ankle fractures. This means that 83.3% of patients with fractures also had an effusion of 15 mm or more. When testing patients without occult fractures, they found that an effusion of less than 15 mm had a specificity of 85.7%. This means that 85.7% of the patients without occult fractures had effusions of less than 15 mm.

When test results can take more than two values, as in this study, then the researchers need to determine the "cutoff" score for differentiating between positive and negative results. Figure 14–6 shows an approximate reconstruction of the results of the two tests for all 26 patients in the series. If the criteria for a positive result is set at 12 or more mm of effusion, then the sensitivity of the test would be 100%, since all 12

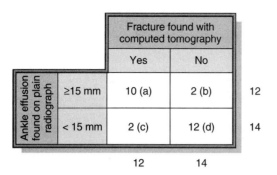

		Fracture found with computed tomography		
		Yes	No	
Ankle effusion found on plain radiograph	≥15 mm	10 (a)	2 (b)	12
	< 15 mm	2 (c)	12 (d)	14
		12	14	

FIGURE 14–5. Calculation of sensitivity, specificity, positive predictive value, and negative predictive value.
From data presented in Clark TWI, Janzen DL, Logan PM, Connell DG. Improving the detection of radiographically occult ankle fractures: positive predictive value of an ankle joint effusion. *Clin Radiol.* 1996;51: 632–636.

Sensitivity = a/(a + c) = 10/12 = 0.833 = 83.3%
Specificity = d/(b + d) = 12/14 = 0.857 = 85.7%
Positive predictive value = a/(a + b) = 10/12 = 0.833 = 83.3%
Negative predictive value = d/(c + d) = 12/14 = 0.857 = 85.7%

Observant readers will note that in this example the sensitivity and the positive predictive value are the same, and the specificity and negative predictive value are the same. This is because the number of false positives and false negatives happens to be the same in this example. In most examples, this will not be the case and all four of the proportions will take different values.

patients with fractures visualized by CT had an effusion of 12 mm or more. However, the specificity would be only 64.3%, since this permissive criterion would result in many false positives. If the criteria for a positive result is set at 18 or more mm of effusion, then the specificity of the test would be 100%, since all 14 patients without fractures had effusions of less than 18 mm. However, the sensitivity would be only 58.3% since this stringent criterion would result in many false negatives. Test developers work to determine an intermediate cutoff score that results in a desirable balance between the sensitivity and specificity of the test.

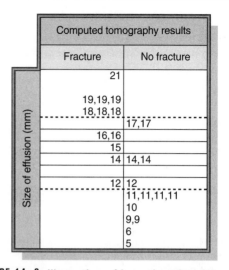

FIGURE 14–6. Illustration of how changing the cutoff score influences sensitivity and specificity. If the cutoff is between 11 and 12 mm, sensitivity is maximized. If the cutoff is between 17 and 18 mm, specificity is maximized.

Sensitivity if cutoff set at 12 or more mm: (12/12) × 100 = 100.0%
Specificity if cutoff set at 12 or more mm: (9/14) × 100 = 64.3%

Sensitivity if cutoff set at 18 or more mm: (7/12) × 100 = 58.3%
Specificity if cutoff set at 18 or more mm: (14/14) × 100 = 100.0%

Data reconstructed from Clark TWI, Janzen DL, Logan PM, Connell DG. Improving the detection of radiographically occult ankle fractures: positive predictive value of an ankle joint effusion. *Clin Radiol.* 1996; 51:632–636.

RECEIVER-OPERATOR CURVES. One way that this process is visualized is through development of a receiver-operator curve (ROC). Clark and colleagues[4] created such a curve with their data, as shown in Figure 14–7. The heavy line with the triangles for points represents a test with an ideal cutoff point—at 100% sensitivity and 100% specificity (the upper left-hand corner of the graph). In practice, tests generally deviate from this ideal, as is the case with the use of the extent of ankle effusion to predict occult ankle

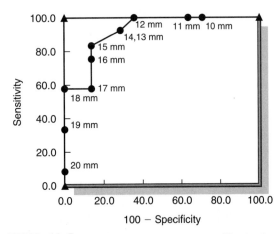

FIGURE 14–7. Receiver-operator curve illustrating how changing the cutoff score influences the sensitivity and specificity of a test. In general, the ideal cutoff score is the one closest to the upper left-hand corner of the graph.

fractures (the circular points on the graph). These points demonstrate visually that cutoff scores of 20, 19, and 18 mm result in perfect specificity but low sensitivity; and the cutoff scores of 12, 11, and 10 mm result in perfect sensitivity but low specificity. The cutoff score of 15 mm results in the best balance between sensitivity and specificity—it is the point closest to the ideal point in the upper left-hand corner. When two points are approximately equidistant from this ideal point, then researchers consider the impact of false positives (needlessly worrying the healthy) or false negatives (falsely reassuring the ill) in determining which cutoff score to select. If the disease being screened for is serious, but treatable in early stages, then the researchers would probably choose the cutoff score with somewhat lower specificity and higher sensitivity so that the probability of false negatives would be lower. If the disease being screened for is less serious and can be effectively treated even at later stages of the disease, then the researchers would probably choose a cutoff score with lower sensitivity and higher specificity so that the probability of false positives would be lower.

LIKELIHOOD RATIOS. An important way that sensitivity and specificity are used is in the calculation of likelihood ratios:

Likelihood ratio of a positive test =
Sensitivity %/(100 − Specificity %)

(Formula 14–9)

Likelihood ratio of a negative test =
(100 − Sensitivity %)/Specificity %

(Formula 14–10)

A likelihood ratio of a positive test of 1.0 does not help to rule in disease because the false positives (100 − specificity) are as likely as true positives (sensitivity). The higher the likelihood ratio of a positive test, the more information the test gives for ruling in a disease or injury.

A likelihood ratio of a negative test of 1.0 does not help to rule out disease because the false negatives (100 − sensitivity) are as likely as the true negatives (specificity). The lower the likelihood of a negative test, the more information the test gives for ruling out a disease or injury.[5(pp178–179)] Likelihood ratios are also a good way to determine the information provided by tests that have multiple levels of cutoff points.[3(p92)]

One important characteristic of sensitivity and specificity is that they are unaffected by the proportion of individuals with the disease or injury of interest. Because they are each calculated from one column of the 2 × 2 table, the number of individuals in the other column does not affect their value. Thus, ankle effusion measurement should yield similar sensitivity and specificity whether it is applied to a group with minor ankle sprains with few fractures or to a group with severe sprains and many fractures.

Predictive Value

Although sensitivity and specificity are useful concepts, they only tell half the story about diagnostic and screening tests. The other half of the story is told by the positive and negative predictive values. The *positive predictive value* is the percentage of individuals identified by the test as positive who actually have the diagnosis. The *negative predictive value* is the percentage of those identified by the test as negative who actually do not have the diagnosis. These values are found by "working" the table horizontally:

Positive predictive value = a/(a + b)

(Formula 14–11)

Negative predictive value = c/(c + d)

(Formula 14–12)

Because the table is worked horizontally, the predictive values vary greatly depending on the proportion of individuals with and without the disease or injury. This is illustrated in Figure 14–8A and B, which maintain the sensitivity and specificity values of the original study. What is varied, though, is the proportion of total cases with and without an ankle fracture. In the original study 46% of the cases had an ankle fracture identified through CT. In Figure 14–8A, only 4% of the cases have an ankle fracture; and in Figure 14–8B 94% of cases have an ankle fracture. When dealing with a population with only a 4% probability of having a fracture, the predictive value of a positive test is only 20%—this means that 80% of positive test results would be false positives. Although this sounds bad, the upside is that the predictive value of a negative test is 99%—there would be very few false-negative results. Conversely, when dealing with a population with a 94% probability of having a fracture, the predictive value of a positive test is 99% and the predictive value of a negative test is only 23%. Because the positive and negative predictive values are dependent on the proportion of diseased or injured individuals within the population studied, this proportion should always be specified when the predictive values are reported.

This characteristic of the predictive values has a great deal of impact for clinicians who are performing diagnostic or screening tests. To know how to interpret the predictive value of a

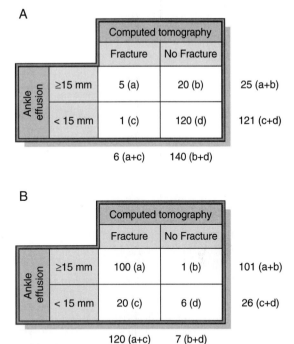

FIGURE 14–8. Changing the prevalence of fractures influences the predictive values, but not the sensitivity and specificity.

A. Illustration with prevalence of 4%.

Sensitivity = a/(a + c) = 5/6 = 83%
Specificity = d/(b + d) = 120/140 = 86%
Positive predictive value = a/(a + b) = 5/25 = 20%
Negative predictive value = d/(c + d) = 120/121 = 99%

B. Illustration with prevalence of 94%

Sensitivity = a/(a + c) = 100/120 = 83%
Specificity = d/(b + d) = 6/7 = 86%
Positive predictive value = a/(a + b) = 100/101 = 99%
Negative predictive value = d/(c + d) = 6/26 = 23%

test, the clinician should estimate the "pretest" probability of the patient having the condition. If an asymptomatic individual is being screened, then the probability of having the condition is low. In this instance the predictive value of a positive test is likely to be low, but the predictive value of a negative test is apt to be high. If an individual with a history and physical examination that is highly suggestive of the condition is tested, then the predictive value of a positive test is likely to be high and the predictive value of a negative test is likely to be low. Applying this information to the example of ankle effusion, a clinician who notes a 15-mm ankle effusion on the plain radiograph of a patient experiencing an uncomplicated recovery from ankle sprain would likely not order a CT to look for an occult fracture. The assumption would be that the patient belongs to a population similar to the one in Figure 14–8A, and the positive ankle effusion has a high probability of being a false positive. In contrast, if a clinician notes a 15-mm ankle effusion on the radiograph of a patient with a great deal of swelling and discoloration, malleolar tenderness, and inability to bear weight 72 hours postinjury, a follow-up CT would likely be ordered to look for an occult fracture. The assumption would be that the patient belongs to a population similar to the one in Figure 14–8B and the positive ankle effusion has a high probability of being a true indication of an occult fracture.

This section of the chapter has only introduced the complex interrelationships among sensitivity, specificity, likelihood ratios, prevalence, and predictive values. Several excellent texts present a fuller description of these topics.[5–8]

■ NONEXPERIMENTAL EPIDEMIOLOGICAL DESIGNS

Three common nonexperimental designs are used to implement epidemiological research: cross-sectional, case-control, and cohort designs. Figure 14–9 shows how each design is related to the timing of various elements of the design. Cross-sectional studies are used to document the status of a group at a particular point in time. With case-control studies, researchers identify individuals with the condition of interest (the

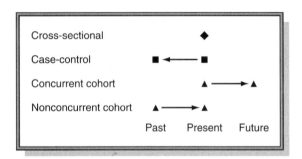

FIGURE 14–9. The epidemiological designs can be characterized by the timing of measurements, as well as the direction in which the logic of the design proceeds. Data are collected at one point in time for cross-sectional studies, researchers work from effects to causes in case-control designs, and they work from causes to effects in two variations on cohort designs.

cases) and controls without the condition of interest (the controls). They then look into the past for the presence or absence of risk factors that might explain the presence or absence of the condition. In effect, in case-control studies the researchers start with an effect and go looking for a cause. With cohort studies (termed also "concurrent cohort studies") researchers identify individuals with various risk factors and look into the future to see if the condition of interest develops. In a variation on cohort studies, sometimes termed "historical cohort studies" or "nonconcurrent cohort studies," the researchers identify a group of interest, identify risk factors from the past, and then determine whether a condition of interest is present or absent. In both variations of cohort studies the researchers start with the cause and look for the effect.

In the research design overview presented in Chapter 6, the terms prospective and retrospective were defined in terms of the timing of data collection in relation to the development of the research problem. It was also noted that alternate definitions of these two terms are sometimes used to describe the "direction" in which the research proceeds. According to these alternate definitions, a *prospective study* proceeds from cause to effect, as do the cohort designs.

A *retrospective study* proceeds from effect to cause, as do the case-control designs. In this text, the terms will refer to the timing of data collection, as recommended by Friedman.[8] When referring to the direction in which the research proceeds, the terms cohort and case-control will be used.

Cross-Sectional Studies

Cross-sectional studies are used to document health status at a single point in time for each subject within the study. In some instances the point in time may be a range of calendar dates (e.g., a study in which fitness levels of top executives in a particular company were collected between January and March of one year); in other instances the point in time may be a particular event (e.g., a study of fitness levels of top executives as they turn 60 years old). In studies that document health status, the point in time is often the point of entry into a health system. This was the case for Fallat and associates' study of sprained ankle syndrome.[9] Over a 33-month period they conducted a standardized examination of all patients presenting to a hospital emergency room with acute "twisted" ankles. Even though the study was conducted over an almost 3-year period, each of the over 600 patients within the study was assessed only once. The "point in time" that makes this a cross-sectional study was the "event" of presenting to an emergency room with a complaint of a twisted ankle.

Many reports of case-control and cohort research include a cross-sectional component that describes the patient groups at a single point in time. For example, Prencipe and colleagues[10] conducted a study of stroke, disability, and dementia among elders in rural Italy. Although their main purpose was to document the relationship between stroke and dementia (done through a nonconcurrent cohort design, to be described later), their results also included age- and sex-specific prevalence rates for stroke in the population they surveyed.

Case-Control Studies

The defining characteristic of a case-control study is that the researchers start with "effects" and look for "causes." First, the researchers identify individuals with the effect of interest (the cases). Second, they identify appropriately matched individuals without the effect of interest (the controls). Third, they evaluate all the subjects (cases and controls alike) to determine the presence or absence of various factors hypothesized to cause the effect of interest. This evaluation may involve review of records to determine previous health status, may involve collection of new information that asks subjects to recall past behaviors or events, or may involve observation of characteristics that were presumed to have existed before the effect of interest occurred. Finally, they conduct statistical analyses to determine whether individuals with the presumed causes have a higher relative risk of being a case than a control.

Morris and colleagues[11] used case-control methods to determine the effect of preexisting conditions on mortality in trauma patients. A computerized database with information on all discharges from California acute care hospitals assured a large, representative sample. The effect of interest was death from trauma, and the cases were 3074 of almost 200,000 trauma patients in the database who died from their injuries. The researchers matched each case with up to four trauma survivors discharged from the same hospital, within the same age grouping, and with a similar severity of injury. They then collected information about 11 preexisting health conditions. Finally, they determined the relative risk of dying (the risk of having the "effect" of interest) for patients with the various preexisting conditions (the presumed "causes"). Using odds ratios, they determined that individuals with cirrhosis were 4.7 times more likely to die from trauma than individuals without cirrhosis, and that individuals with chronic obstructive pulmonary disease were 1.8 times more likely to die from trauma.

Another case-control study with a closer tie

to rehabilitation is Clemson and associates' study of hazards in the home and risk of falls and hip fractures.[12] Their method of identifying cases and controls yielded, in effect, two studies within a single report. For one study the cases were 43 patients with recurrent falls (two or more falls in the past year) and the controls were 157 nonfallers; for the other study the cases were 52 patients with hip fractures compared with 195 patients without hip fractures. Thus, the effects of interest were falls and fractures. The presumed causes were hazards in the home, as assessed by occupational therapists. Using odds ratios, the researchers found, among other things, that individuals in homes with hazardous toilet railings had more than 11 times the risk of falls or hip fractures as those with safe railings.

These two studies illustrate some of the positive and negative features of case-control methods. In the study of the association between preexisting conditions and death from trauma, the case-control methods enabled the researchers to study a large number of trauma cases in a cost-effective manner. If the researchers had tried to implement this study with a cohort design, they would have had to enroll tens of thousands of patients and follow them for years until enough of the subjects sustained trauma for which they were hospitalized—and until they had a large enough subgroup of patients who died from the trauma. This illustrates one of the chief advantages of the case-control design over other designs—the ability to study a reasonable number of individuals with relatively rare conditions without needing to observe the entire population at risk for long periods of time.

A second advantage of the case-control design is that it enables researchers to study things that might not otherwise be ethical to study. In the study of home hazards, one would clearly not be able to study this experimentally by randomly placing patients into hazardous and nonhazardous home environments! One would not even be able to study this ethically with a nonexperimental cohort design. To do so would involve identifying a group of older persons to study, evaluating their homes for hazards, and

then doing nothing about those hazards until you saw who did and who did not fall or fracture their hips. Ethical practice would demand that subjects at least be given advice about how to remedy the hazards that were identified—and if enough patients took that advice the level of hazards across the homes would become much more uniform, and one of the variables of interest would be nearly eliminated. Therefore, the case-control method, in which hazards that were presumed to exist prior to the fall or fracture are identified after the return home, provides an ethical way to study this potential relationship.

One of the chief concerns about case-control designs is the manner in which the presumed causes are documented or identified. In the study of death after trauma, the preexisting conditions were pulled from abstracts of the discharge summaries of the patients. Because of the emergent nature of the trauma care, many of the patients in the study may have had an incomplete list of preexisting conditions. In particular, it seems reasonable to assume that patients who survive trauma are cared for long enough to fill in the aspects of their medical histories that may have been neglected in the press of emergency care following the trauma. A complete medical history may never be taken on those patients who die very soon after trauma, and, therefore, preexisting conditions may be selectively underreported in the cases compared with the controls.

In the study of hazards in the home, the hazards were evaluated after the fall or fracture and after the patient had returned home. The assumption was made that the home environment was similar at discharge as it was prior to the fall. If a sufficient number of concerned children or neighbors have taken up throw rugs, installed toilet safety rails, replaced burned out light bulbs, and tightened rickety stair railings during the hospitalization of the person who fell or fractured the hip, then this assumption would not be valid. In addition, if this effort to reduce hazards is done more often for those who fall or fracture a hip, and less often for those who have not fallen, then this selective reduction in hazards for certain groups of subjects would be of particular concern to the validity of the project.

Cohort Studies

Cohort designs are characterized by their progression from cause to effect. In a cohort study individuals are selected because they do not have the disease or injury of interest, and can be classified as to their status on a risk factor or factors of interest. The "healthy" individuals (at least with respect to the disease or injury of interest) in the different risk categories are followed for a period of time to compare their relative risks of developing the disease or injury of interest.

There are two variants of the cohort design. In the first, the subjects are identified in the present and followed into the future to see who does and does not develop the outcome of interest. This variant is either known simply as a cohort design or as a *concurrent cohort design*. In the second variant, the subjects are placed into risk factor groupings based on data collected in the past. Then, they are measured in the present or future to determine who develops the outcome of interest. This variant is either known as a *historical cohort design* or a *nonconcurrent cohort design*. In both variants, the researcher establishes the presence or absence of the risk factor first, and then determines the presence or absence of the outcome of interest. This is the reverse of the case-control design, in which the outcome is established before the risk factors are identified.

A concurrent cohort design was used by Rothweiler and colleagues[13] to study the effect of age at the time of injury on psychosocial outcomes in traumatic brain injury. Over 400 patients with brain injury were studied at 1 month and 1 year postinjury to determine their psychosocial functioning. The independent variable was age, with five levels: 18 to 29 years, 30 to 39 years, 40 to 49 years, 50 to 59 years, and 60 years and older. The dependent variable was psychosocial functioning as measured by the Glasgow Outcome Scale, postinjury living situation,

and postinjury employment status. They found that, in general, older individuals who sustain traumatic brain injury experience more psychosocial dysfunction than younger individuals.

The study of stroke, disability, and dementia, mentioned earlier when describing cross-sectional studies, used a nonconcurrent cohort design to answer the main question of interest of whether patients with stroke have a higher risk of dementia than individuals without stroke.[10] The grouping of patients into stroke and stroke-free categories was based on a door-to-door survey done by a lay researcher, with confirmation of dementia and stroke status by a neurologist. The strokes that were identified had to have occurred prior to the "prevalence day" established by the researchers. This ensured that the "direction" of the study was from possible cause (a stroke, in the past) to effect (dementia, in the present). Odds ratios, adjusted for age and sex differences between the stroke and stroke-free groups, showed that the individuals with stroke had 5.8 times the risk of dementia than those without stroke.

■ SUMMARY

Epidemiology is the study of the distribution and determinants of disease and injury in populations. Common measures used in epidemiology include ratios, proportions, and rates. Prevalence is the proportion of existing cases of a disease or injury in a population at a particular point of time. Incidence is the rate of development of new cases of a disease or injury in a population at risk. Relative risk of disease or injury in different groups is expressed with risk ratios and odds ratios. Screening and diagnostic tests are evaluated by measures of sensitivity (the proportion of patients with the condition who test positive), specificity (the proportion of patients without the condition who test negative), and the likelihood ratios (usefulness for ruling in and ruling out diagnoses). In addition, predictive values for positive and negative tests can be calculated for populations with different proportions of individuals with disease or injury. Common epidemiological research designs include cross-sectional studies (subjects measured at one point in time), case-control studies (researchers work backward from effect to cause), and cohort studies (researchers work forward from cause to effect).

REFERENCES

1. Harkness GA. *Epidemiology in Nursing Practice*. St. Louis, Mo: Mosby–Year Book; 1995.
2. Tanner CM, Goldman SM. Epidemiology of Parkinson's disease. *Neurol Clin*. 1996;14:317–335.
3. Jekel JF, Elmore JG, Katz DL. *Epidemiology, Biostatistics, and Preventive Medicine*. Philadelphia, Pa: WB Saunders Co; 1996.
4. Clark TWI, Janzen DL, Logan PM, Connell DG. Improving the detection of radiographically occult ankle fractures: positive predictive value of an ankle joint effusion. *Clin Radiol*. 1996;51:632–636.
5. Riegelman RK, Hirsch RP. *Studying a Study and Testing a Test: How to Read the Health Science Literature*. 3rd ed. Boston, Mass: Little, Brown & Co; 1996.
6. Sackett DL, Haynes RB, Guyatt GH, Tugwell P. *Clinical Epidemiology: A Basic Science for Clinical Medicine*. 2nd ed. Philadelphia, Pa: Lippincott-Raven Publishers; 1991.
7. Gerstman BB. *Epidemiology Kept Simple: An Introduction to Classic and Modern Epidemiology*. New York, NY: Wiley-Liss; 1998.
8. Friedman GD. *Primer of Epidemiology*. 4th ed. New York, NY: McGraw-Hill; 1994.
9. Fallat L, Grimm DJ, Saracco JA. Sprained ankle syndrome: prevalence and analysis of 639 acute injuries. *J Foot Ankle Surg*. 1998;37:280–285.
10. Prencipe M, Ferretti C, Casini AR, Santini M, Giubilei F, Culasso F. Stroke, disability, and dementia. *Stroke*. 1997; 28:531–536.
11. Morris JA, Mackenzie EJ, Edelstein SL. The effect of pre-existing conditions on mortality in trauma patients. *JAMA*. 1990;263:1942–1946.
12. Clemson L, Cumming RG, Roland MA. Case-control study of hazards in the home and risk of falls and hip fractures. *Age Ageing*. 1996;25:97–101.
13. Rothweiler B, Temkin NR, Dikmen SS. Aging effect on psychosocial outcome in traumatic brain injury. *Arch Phys Med Rehabil*. 1998;79:881–887.

Outcomes Research

Purpose of Outcomes Research
  Efficacy
  Effectiveness

Frameworks for Outcomes Research
  International Classification of Impairments, Disabilities, and Handicaps
  Nagi Formulation
  Issues and Refinements

Measurement Tools for Outcomes Research
  Quality of Life
  Health-Related Quality of Life
  SF-36 and SF-12
  Sickness Impact Profile
  Functional Status Questionnaire
  Condition-Specific Tools
  Oswestry Low Back Pain Disability Index
  Lysholm Knee Rating Scale
  Satisfaction

Design Issues for Outcomes Research
  Database Research
  Review of Existing Medical Records
  Abstracts of Medical Records
  Insurance Claims Databases
  In-House Database Development
  Participation in National Outcomes Databases
  Analysis Issues
  Case Mix Adjustments
  Techniques for Dealing with Missing Data
  Survival Analysis
  Comparisons Across Scales
  Multivariate Statistics

The outcomes movement in health care policy, practice, and research has received widespread recognition during the 1990s. Most writers attribute the emergence of the outcomes movement to (1) the need for cost containment in the health care sector,[1-3] (2) the need to examine outcomes other than mortality when dealing with the increasingly prevalent chronic diseases of an aging society,[3,4] and (3) the need to determine "best practices" and thereby reduce the great variations in medical care that occur for reasons apparently unrelated to the characteristics of the group receiving the care.[1-5] Contemporary authors[4,6] credit the conceptual basis for outcomes assessment to Donabedian, whose "structure, process, outcomes" framework influenced the design of the *Medical Outcomes Study* (MOS), an important outcomes project initiated in the late 1980s.[7]

As with many emerging movements, there is

neither widespread agreement about the definitions of various components related to health care outcomes nor agreement as to the boundaries of the outcomes movement. Consequently, the terms "outcomes" and "outcomes research" are used in different ways by the many participants in and observers of the health care system. One area of commonality, however, appears to be a shift in emphasis from looking for narrow biological effects of treatments delivered under highly controlled conditions to assessing the broad biopsychosocial impact of treatments implemented in typical clinical settings.[2-4,8] This shift, from what is often termed "efficacy" to what is characterized as "effectiveness" has profound implications for the conduct of outcomes research. These implications extend from the nature of the overall research design to the selection of the dependent measures of interest. A general text that addresses many of these issues is Kane's *Understanding Health Care Outcomes Research.*[9]

The purpose of this chapter is to present an overview of the emergence of outcome measures in rehabilitation research. First, the purpose of outcomes research is explored by contrasting the concepts of efficacy and effectiveness. Second, broad frameworks for outcomes research are presented. Third, a variety of measurement tools consistent with these frameworks are described. Finally, design and implementation issues related to outcomes research are addressed.

■ PURPOSE OF OUTCOMES RESEARCH

One thing that has fairly consistently been used to discuss the outcomes movement is the differentiation between "efficacy" and "effectiveness." Although he does not use these words, Kane[10] identified the tension between these two concepts and between the research models that support each concept:

> If the practice of medicine (including rehabilitation) is to become more empiric, it will have to rely on epidemiological methods. Although some may urge the primacy of randomized clinical trials as the only path to true enlightenment, such a position is untenable for several reasons. First, the exclusivity of most trials is so great that the results are difficult to extrapolate to practice. Such trials may be the source of clinically important truths, but these findings will have to be bent and shaped to fit most clinical situations. Second, researchers do not have the time or resources to conduct enough trials to guide all practice. Instead, we need a more balanced strategy that combines targeted trials with well-organized analysis of carefully recorded clinical practice.[10(pJS22)]

This observation emphasizes the importance of studying health care under ideal conditions through highly controlled experimental studies (randomized clinical trials) as well as through well-organized analysis of clinical practice as it actually occurs (outcomes research). These contrasting approaches are often thought of as assessing "efficacy" versus "effectiveness."

Efficacy

Efficacy is usually defined as the biological effect of treatment delivered under carefully controlled conditions. The research method that is best suited to determining efficacy is the randomized controlled trial, in which researchers control for a variety of factors that would interfere with an understanding of the impact of the treatment of interest. Thus, subjects are selected to be relatively homogeneous, treatments are implemented in uniform ways, and dependent variables are selected because they are objective and relate directly to the expected biological effect of the treatment. Research to determine efficacy focuses on the "does it work?" and "is it safe?" questions, and does not often examine issues of cost, feasibility, and acceptability to practitioners and patients.

Effectiveness

In contrast, effectiveness is defined as the usefulness of a particular treatment to the individuals receiving it under typical clinical conditions. Nonexperimental research methods are generally seen as best suited to determining effectiveness. Rather than manipulating the treatment patients receive, as well as the conditions under which they receive it, researchers implementing nonexperimental designs examine the effectiveness of actual treatment that has already occurred or observe actual treatment as it is delivered. This is a messy process that usually results in heterogeneous groups of subjects, treatments that are implemented in various ways by different clinicians and patients, and dependent variables that focus on broader outcomes of interest to patients, payers, and practitioners.

FRAMEWORKS FOR OUTCOMES RESEARCH

The shift from looking at narrow efficacy to broader effectiveness has required that practitioners develop broad-based frameworks to guide the way that they think about disease and injury, as well as the consequences of disease and injury. Two frameworks that have received widespread discussion within the rehabilitation literature include the Nagi formulation[11] and the World Health Organization's *International Classification of Impairments, Disabilities, and Handicaps* (ICIDH).[12] The similarities and differences between these two frameworks have been discussed in detail by Verbrugge and Jette.[13–15] Each of the two frameworks are presented here, followed by a summary of issues and refinements that have been articulated by others.

International Classification of Impairments, Disabilities, and Handicaps

The World Health Organization (WHO) published its ICIDH in 1980.[12] This classification is a supplement to the *International Classification of Diseases, Ninth Revision* (ICD-9), needed because of the inadequacies of the ICD-9 in addressing the long-term impact of chronic diseases. The ICIDH, as can be inferred from its name, conceptualizes the long-term sequelae of disease as impairments, disabilities, and handicaps, as described in the top row of Figure 15–1. For example, a man with osteoarthritis experiences inflammation (the disease, manifested at the cellular level) that leads to muscle weakness and valgus deformity at the knees (the impairments, at the tissue, organ, or system level). The person has difficulty walking long distances or climbing stairs (the disability, at the level of the person) and he changes from a field position as a police officer to a desk job because the demands of and architectural barriers in the field involve more walking and stair climbing than is tolerable (the handicap, at the level of society and the environment). A revision of the ICIDH is expected to be published in 1999.[16]

Nagi Formulation

Saad Nagi, a sociologist, first presented his formulation in 1965.[17] He revisited his original formulation as an appendix to a report of the Committee on a National Agenda for the Prevention of Disabilities,[11] a group appointed jointly by the Centers for Disease Control and Prevention and the National Council on Disabilities. His scheme describes active pathology, impairment, functional limitation, and disability, as shown in the middle row of Figure 15–1. Using the same example of a person with arthritis, we can see how the Nagi scheme differs from the ICIDH framework. A man with osteoarthritis experiences inflammation (the active pathology, manifested at the cellular level) viewed as a component of muscle weakness and valgus deformity at the knees (the impairments, at the tissue, organ, or system level). He has difficulty walking long distances or climbing stairs (the functional impairment, at the level of the person) and he gives up his position as a field-based police officer because it involves more walking and stair climbing than is tolerable (the disability, at the level of social functioning).

International Classification of Impairments, Disabilities, and Handicaps[12]

Disease	Impairment	Disability	Handicap
The intrinsic pathology or disorder	Loss or abnormality of psychological, physiological, or anatomical structure or function at organ level	Restriction or lack of ability to perform an activity in a normal manner	Disadvantage due to impairment or disability that limits or prevents fulfillment of a normal role (depends on age, sex, sociocultural factors for the person)

Nagi Model[11]

Active Pathology	Impairment	Functional Limitation	Disability
Interruption or interference with normal processes, and efforts of the organism to regain normal state	Anatomical, physiological, mental, or emotional abnormalities or loss	Limitation in performance at the level of the whole organism or person	Limitation in performance of socially defined roles and tasks within a sociocultural and physical environment

Comments

These two categories are similar within both models, focusing on abnormalities at the cellular, tissue, organ, or system level—but not at the level of the organism or person.	The differences between the two models are in these three categories. The categories focus on person-level issues, although they draw the lines between these issues in different ways. The differentiation is related to tasks or attributes (characteristics of the person by himself or herself), roles (the person in relation to others), and the person in the context of the broader society and environment. "Disability" in the ICIDH model seems to cover both "functional limitation" and part of "disability" in the Nagi model. "Disability" in the Nagi model seems to cover part of "disability" and part of "handicap" in the ICIDH model.

FIGURE 15–1. Comparison of the International Classification of Impairments, Disabilities, and Handicaps (ICIDH) with the Nagi model.
The verbal descriptions of the models are from Jette AM. Physical disablement concepts for physical therapy research and practice, *Phys Ther.* 1994;74:380–386. Their presentation has been modified to show how the categories are related across the models, as described in the comment portion of the

Issues and Refinements

A variety of individuals and groups have identified concerns with either or both frameworks or have suggested refinements to either scheme. Although a comprehensive critical discussion of the frameworks is beyond the scope of this chapter, a few of the major discussion points are provided here. Jette[15] finds the differences between the schemes to be more than just semantic, and identifies a critical issue as one of differentiating between "attributes" and "relational concepts." In his opinion, the Nagi scheme wisely provides for clear differentiation between a functional limitation and a disability. The former is an attribute of the person and the latter extends to the point at which it affects social functioning, a relational concept. In contrast, he notes that the ICIDH scheme includes both attribute and relational concepts within the "disability" category, and the "handicap" category does not classify the individual, but rather classifies the social and environmental circumstances that place an individual with a disability at a disadvantage. One group, the National Center for Medical Rehabilitation Research,[14] has retained Nagi's differentiation between functional limitation and disability, and has added "societal limitation," a concept that closely parallels the ICIDH concept of "handicap."

Pope and Tarlov[18] have added quality of life as a global concept influenced by the full spectrum of problems from disease to disability. In addition, they introduced the idea that risk factors and modifiers feed into the development of disability at different points, creating a multidimensional disabling process. Verbrugge and Jette[13] have also extended the schemes to look at the process of disablement, which they believe is influenced by the presence of risk factors, buffers, and exacerbators. Duncan has pointed out that the disablement process is not always unidirectional.[19] Using the example of health status after stroke, she notes that secondary impairments such as weakness and loss of range of motion may develop from inactivity related to functional limitations in mobility.

Some authors have identified measurement issues related to the various disablement concepts. Verbrugge and Jette[13] identify the importance of distinguishing between intrinsic disability (difficulty experienced when external assistance, either equipment or personnel, is not available) and actual disability (difficulty experienced when external assistance is available). In a different way of looking at function, Liang[20] identified three domains that enter into function: capacity (the level of impairment), will (psychological factors such as motivation and

self-confidence), and need (the social and environmental context). For example, a woman with osteoarthritis affecting the knees may use an elevator rather than stairs at work but she may enjoy hiking on trails with steps on the weekends. Her capacity for stair climbing is present 7 days a week, the need to climb stairs during the week is obviated by the presence of the elevator, and her will to continue to participate in an enjoyable recreational activity dominates on the weekend. Measurement of this person's (or any person's) functional level, then, is difficult, because of the complex interplay between these domains.

Despite the differences between the frameworks, the complexity of the disablement process, and the difficulties with measurement within either framework, these frameworks convey a central message that has shaped outcomes research in rehabilitation. The message is that impairment-level measures are insufficient for the study of person-level concepts such as functional limitation and disability. Medical and rehabilitation professionals have received this message and have changed the ways in which they measure outcomes in both clinical and research settings. The next section of this chapter highlights measures that reflect the person-level outcomes represented by the functional limitation, disability, and handicap categories within the disablement models.

■ MEASUREMENT TOOLS FOR OUTCOMES RESEARCH

Clinicians and researchers have long used measures of pathology (e.g., laboratory values and imaging techniques) and measures of impairment (e.g., range of motion, muscle performance) to guide their practice and to serve as dependent measures in research studies. Outcomes research, or an outcomes focus to practice, generally means that researchers and practitioners supplement these measures of pathology and impairment with person-level measures of functional limitation, disability, or handicap. This section of the chapter is designed to provide an overview of these person-level measures. A few representative measures are listed here; additional measures are presented in Chapter 19, which reviews measurement tools of all types.

Quality of Life

Quality of life is a global concept that can include elements as diverse as perceptions of health, satisfaction with the work environment, quality of family and social relationships, satisfaction with schools and neighborhoods, productive use of leisure time, connections with one's spiritual nature, and financial well-being. Although problems in many of these areas can lead to health-related problems associated with stress, poor eating habits, sedentary lifestyles, and tobacco, alcohol, and drug use, global measures of quality of life are so broad as to have limited use in health care research and practice settings.

Health-Related Quality of Life

Because quality of life, as a global concept, is limited in its usefulness in health care research, a variety of measures of health-related quality of life (HRQL) have been developed. These measures have also been termed "health status" and "outcomes" measures. They may also be referred to as "generic" tools because they are designed for use with individuals with health conditions of all types. There is general agreement that measures of HRQL should include elements related to physical, psychological, and social functioning. Because many of these measures have been well-described by others,[21–24] only a few will be described here.

SF-36 AND SF-12. The Medical Outcomes Study (MOS), begun in the late 1980s, was designed to develop patient outcome tools and to monitor variations in outcome on the basis of differences

in health care systems, clinician styles, and clinician specialties.[7] One of the major tools to come out of this study is the Short Form-36, commonly known as the SF-36. The self-report includes 36 items covering the eight domains of physical functioning, role limitation due to physical problems, role limitation due to emotional problems, social functioning, mental health, pain, energy/fatigue, and general health perceptions. The SF-36 is scored to produce a profile of the eight domains, each with scores ranging from 0 to 100, with higher scores representing better health. Although this tool takes only about 10 minutes to complete, the desire for an even briefer tool has led to its modification into a shorter tool known as the SF-12. This 12-item tool includes one or two items from each of the eight components of the SF-36.[25]

The SF-36 has been used as one of the major health status measures collected for the Focus on Therapeutic Outcomes (FOTO) database. In reports of outcomes of physical therapy episodes for patients with knee and spinal impairments, scores on the eight subscales were standardized so that they could be compared with general population scores.[26,27] At the initiation of treatment the patients had scores below the population norms in most areas, most notably bodily pain, physical functioning, and role limitations due to physical problems. The data from the conclusion of treatment showed significant improvements in many areas, most notably in physical functioning and bodily pain.

SICKNESS IMPACT PROFILE. The Sickness Impact Profile (SIP) is a 136-item self-report that takes about 30 minutes to complete.[28] It is used to evaluate the physical dimensions of ambulation, mobility, and body care; the psychosocial dimensions of social interaction, communication, alertness, and emotional behavior; and other dimensions related to sleep/rest, eating, work, home management, and recreational pastimes. The instrument is scored on a percentage basis, with higher scores representing greater levels of disability. The SIP was used to document health status of patients with transmetatarsal amputation and diabetes, compared with age- and sex-matched individuals without either condition.[29]

FUNCTIONAL STATUS QUESTIONNAIRE. The Functional Status Questionnaire (FSQ) is a 34-item self-report that, like the SF-36, takes about 10 minutes to complete.[22,24] It measures physical function (basic and intermediate activities of daily living), emotional function (anxiety and depression and quality of social interaction), social performance (occupational function and social activities), and a group of other functions (sexual function, global disability, global health satisfaction, and social contacts). The FSQ was used by Boström and colleagues to study predictors of disability in patients with rheumatoid arthritis.[30]

Condition-Specific Tools

In addition to generic health status instruments, a variety of condition-specific tools have been developed. Two book references provide additional insight into condition-specific tools. Atherly provides an overview of differences between condition-specific and generic measures[31] and Pynsent and associates provide information about a variety of condition-specific or region-specific outcome tools in orthopedics.[32] For the purposes of this chapter, two of the many condition-specific tools in use are highlighted, namely, the Oswestry Low Back Pain Disability Index[33] and the Lysholm Knee Rating Scale.[34] References for additional condition-specific tools are provided in Chapter 19.

OSWESTRY LOW BACK PAIN DISABILITY INDEX. The Oswestry tool is a self-report of perceived disability related to low back pain.[33] It measures 10 areas, including pain intensity, changing pain status, personal hygiene, lifting, walking, sitting, standing, sleeping, social activity, and traveling. Unlike the generic tools, which measure physical, psychological, and social functioning, this tool focuses mostly on physical dimensions, with some social dimensions. The scoring is from 0 to 100 points, with higher scores representing

higher percentages of disability. Jette and Jette's study of spine impairments, described earlier in the SF-36 section,[26] used the Oswestry questionnaire as a condition-specific adjunct to the use of the SF-36 to document health status. Perhaps because of its specific focus on low back disability, some of the most impressive improvements documented in the study were in the Oswestry scores.

LYSHOLM KNEE RATING SCALE. The Lysholm Knee Rating Scale assesses eight areas of knee dysfunction: limp, support, locking, instability, pain, swelling, ability to squat, and ability to negotiate stairs.[34] The highest score possible is 100, with higher scores representing better function. Unlike the generic health status instruments or the Oswestry questionnaire, the Lysholm scale does not measure psychological or social aspects of knee dysfunction. Instead, it focuses on impairments (limp, support, locking, instability, pain, swelling) and functional limitations (ability to squat and to negotiate stairs). Jette and Jette's study of knee impairments, described earlier in the SF-36 section,[27] used the Lysholm scale as an adjunct measure of outcome after physical therapy. As was the case with the study of spinal impairments, the greatest improvement seen after treatment was in the condition-specific Lysholm score rather than in the overall measures of health-related quality of life.

Satisfaction

Satisfaction is seen as an important outcome of treatment, as well as an indicator of the effectiveness of various structures and processes within the health care system. The health status measures described in the previous section may demonstrate changes in status over the course of treatment yet still fail to indicate whether the extent of change met the expectation of the patient. Measurements of patient satisfaction provide this important perspective. In addition to satisfaction with the outcomes of care, patients' opinions are often sought on other structural and process dimensions of the health care system: accessibility and convenience of care, availability of resources, continuity of care, efficacy/outcomes of care, finances, humaneness, information gathering, information giving, pleasantness of surroundings, and quality/competence of caregiver.[34] Input into the structure and process of health care is seen as important because this input can help health care entities organize themselves more effectively. In addition, satisfaction may be indirectly related to clinical outcomes if it affects appointment-keeping and adherence to treatment recommendations. In a review article about satisfaction research, Di Palo discussed several national efforts to collect satisfaction data.[35] As is the case with health status tools, both global and condition-specific satisfaction tools have been developed. In addition, many tools are developed by individual facilities for their own use each year. In contrast to the health status tools, a few of which enjoy widespread popularity for clinical and research use, there seems to be, as yet, no clear "winners" in the satisfaction instrument sweepstakes. Maciejewski and associates provide an overview of many of the issues related to measurement of satisfaction in health care settings.[36]

■ DESIGN ISSUES FOR OUTCOMES RESEARCH

Although research of any type can have person-level outcomes as dependent measures, outcomes research, as defined by the focus on effectiveness, is more than concerned with changing the dependent measures of interest. It also involves a commitment to studying care as it actually occurs, rather than under the ideal, controlled conditions of experimental research. Therefore, for the purpose of this chapter, outcomes research is also assumed to imply a set of methods related to the assessment of care as it occurs in the real world. The design elements that characterize outcomes research, as they are presented here, include nonexperimental design

and the analysis of information contained in various health care databases.

Database Research

The databases used in outcomes research can be medical records themselves, computerized abstracts of medical records, health care insurance claims databases, databases generated within one's own clinic or within a network of clinics associated with a large medical conglomerate, or participation in commercial databases that combine data from clinical entities from many regions.

REVIEW OF EXISTING MEDICAL RECORDS. Medical records themselves may be used as sources of data in outcomes projects. The biggest advantage to using medical records is that they contain a great deal of information that can be evaluated in context. However, this advantage is balanced by at least two disadvantages. First, reviewing records is a time-consuming process that requires the personnel extracting the data to make judgment calls about which of the many pieces of information is relevant to the questions at hand. Second, the information in medical records is often inconsistent and incomplete. Both of these disadvantages have the impact of reducing the available sample size that can be generated for a given project.

ABSTRACTS OF MEDICAL RECORDS. The various reporting mechanisms required for billing, reporting, and accreditation processes mean that records of hospitalization are routinely abstracted, summarized on a "facesheet," and computerized at discharge. Use of this computerized information is time efficient for the researcher and generally ensures that there is a common data set on all patients of interest. One problem with the abstracted information is that there may be errors in coding the information, including diagnoses, comorbidities, and complications (either by physicians, clinic clerks, or medical records personnel). A study that compared facesheet information with information in the medical chart of patients with hip fracture found that there was an error rate of 12% related to diagnoses, 17% related to complications, and 16% related to surgical procedures.[37]

In addition to this concern about the accuracy of the data, the information in the abstract is often less specific than desired by the researcher, so "proxy" measures are used instead of the real measures of interest. For example, researchers who wish to eliminate chronically depressed patients from their sample might screen out patients taking antidepressant medication. If antidepressant medications are used for conditions other than chronic depression, or if many patients receive antidepressants for a short period of time after an acute health care event, then many relevant patients may be excluded from the study. Conversely, if depression is prevalent but often untreated, then many depressed patients may not be screened from the analysis.

INSURANCE CLAIMS DATABASES. Insurance claims databases, which often share a great deal of information with administrative facesheets, are frequently used for outcomes studies. Examples relevant to physical therapy include research on hip fracture outcomes using Medicare claims data,[38] and use of Blue Cross–Blue Shield claims to assess the number of visits and costs of care when patients were seen for physical therapy with and without physician referrals.[39]

In a review of the use of claims databases for outcomes research, Motheral and Fairman[40] identify several challenges to the effective use of this data source. One central advantage to claims databases is that, because of their link to reimbursement for services, they tend to be complete. In addition, they offer access to large numbers of patients at relatively low cost, without ethical concerns related to how treatment is delivered. However, claims databases suffer from limitations on the number of diagnoses, comorbidities, and procedures that are listed, making it difficult to adjust for differences in severity of illness among groups of patients that the re-

searcher hopes to compare. Another potential disadvantage is that when reimbursement policies change, concomitant changes in coding strategies may reflect the policy change rather than a change in practice. In addition, person-level outcomes, such as health-related quality of life, that are so important to determining effectiveness are generally not available through insurance claims databases. Outcomes such as mortality, discharge location, or readmission dates may provide the only insights into the impact of the treatment episodes for the people being treated. Finally, insurance claims data are only available on individuals who are insured, making it difficult to generalize results to groups that are uninsured.

IN-HOUSE DATABASE DEVELOPMENT. To solve many of the problems with the use of medical records, abstracts of medical records, and insurance claims databases, facilities may choose to develop and manage their own outcomes databases. Experience in developing such a database was described by Shields and colleagues[41] and suggestions for those planning to "go it alone" in database development were summarized in a recent article in the popular literature of physical therapy.[42]

Developing one's own database is a time-consuming, expensive venture. In the project described by Shields and colleagues,[41] staff at the University of Iowa Hospitals and Clinics began the development process in 1986, began collecting data in 1991, and began retrieving data in 1993. This long-term commitment was feasible for a teaching hospital with a research mission and access to university resources in instrument development, computer systems, and research design and analysis. Hospitals in large systems, extended care and rehabilitation facilities that are parts of nationwide systems, or outpatient clinics that are affiliated with national corporations may also have the resources to pursue this type of a database and may find competitive business reasons to collect this information even if they do not have primary research missions.

Despite the time and money involved in creating an in-house database, there are many benefits to doing so. In-house outcomes systems may have high levels of utilization by staff members who participate in the development process, have local control of the training process for staff members who contribute information to the database, and have staff who are able to design data collection tools to answer specific questions of interest within the setting.

PARTICIPATION IN NATIONAL OUTCOMES DATABASES. Clinical leaders who wish to involve their facilities in outcomes research may not believe that developing an in-house database is the best solution. They may not have the resources to develop and maintain a system, and they may wish to be able to compare the care at their facilities with that delivered in other centers. Participating in a national outcomes database gives clinics access to the needed resources and allows them to "benchmark" their practices against other similar clinics in the database. In addition, in comparison to in-house databases, the pooling of data from many clinics may increase sample size, enhance statistical power, and improve the generalizability of research results generated from the database. A recent article in the popular literature of physical therapy described the various national, commercial databases to which physical therapy practices can belong.[43]

Although participation in a national outcomes database has the advantages of access to resources and benchmarking information, there may be considerable reluctance on the part of therapists to participate in the process. Russek and colleagues[44] conducted a study to determine therapist attitudes toward standardized data collection. Disappointed by the level of therapist participation in data collection for a database for a multisite corporation with 71 clinics nationwide, they surveyed therapists who should have been able to participate in the data collection effort. This study identified five major factors concerning attitudes about standardized data collection: inconvenience of the data collection tool, acceptance of the operational definitions used for the data collection effort, lack of automation

of the process, the paperwork load within the clinic in general, and training issues. They also found that clinics with a staff member responsible for the organization and management of the data collection effort tended to have higher levels of participation. Together, these factors seem to indicate that clinics who wish to participate in national outcomes databases should attend to the convenience of doing so for individual staff members, and should also work to enhance "buy-in" by providing local support to the effort and improving the training of therapists for the data collection effort.

Analysis Issues

The design of outcomes research studies has a major impact on the way in which the data are analyzed. Because the foundation needed to understand statistical analysis issues has not yet been laid (see Section 6, Chapters 20 through 24), these statistical issues are introduced briefly here and followed up in more detail in Section 6.

CASE MIX ADJUSTMENTS. Because outcomes research studies tend to be nonexperimental in nature, the researcher has little or no control over which patients are placed into which groups within the study. Thus, there are often important differences among study groups, some of which occur because there are systematic biases in the way that clinical decisions are made. For example, older adults with more active lifestyles may seek total knee replacement as a treatment for osteoarthritis, whereas less active patients may choose more conservative care. Differences in outcomes between these two groups, then, might be the result of preoperative lifestyles rather than the treatment of interest. In addition, if the outcomes reported are to be compared with outcomes in other facilities or regions, then researchers need to assure that they are "benchmarking" themselves against comparable groups.[45,46]

There are two general ways to deal with case mix problems in outcomes research. The first is to stratify the groups and compare only those subgroups that have, for example, similar ages, comorbidities, or disease severity. The second way of managing case mix problems is to mathematically adjust the data so that two groups with, for example, different average ages are equalized in some way. Sometimes this is done by "weighting" subgroups within the analysis, much as epidemiological rates are adjusted for valid comparisons between groups (see Chapter 14). Smith,[47] Nitz,[48] and Derose[49] provide guidance about risk adjustment for severity, comorbidity, and demographic and psychosocial factors, respectively.

TECHNIQUES FOR DEALING WITH MISSING DATA. Because the databases used for outcomes research are often developed for other purposes, missing data is a frequent problem. One solution is to simply delete variables or patients for which there is incomplete data. The other general solution is to use a variety of statistical methods to estimate, or "impute" what the missing score might have been. If the researcher has good ways of imputing missing data, this is often preferred to deleting cases, as it maintains larger sample sizes.[50]

SURVIVAL ANALYSIS. Because the data in existing databases often include events such as death, readmission, and discharge, outcomes research reports often use a technique called survival analysis to analyze the timing of these events. In general, survival analysis involves creating a graph that indicates the cumulative proportion of individuals for whom an event has or has not occurred (y axis) against time (x axis). There are several different ways of creating survival analysis graphs, some of which result in smooth curves and some of which result in stair-step graphs (Kaplan-Meier method).[50] Survival analysis can be used to show the pattern of achievement of the milestone for a single group, or it can be used to compare patterns across groups. Figure 15–2 shows the survival curves generated

in Hoenig and colleagues'[51] study of the timing of surgery and rehabilitation care after hip fracture. In this study, most of the surviving patients regained ambulation ability after hip fracture. Therefore, the outcome of "ambulation," per se, was not a good indicator of differences between treatment regimens. However, the time it took until ambulation occurred turned out to be a useful measure. The survival curves, for example, show that those receiving high-frequency physical therapy (PT) and/or occupational therapy (OT) (more than five visits per week) ambulated earlier than those who received low-frequency PT or OT, regardless of whether the surgical repair was done early (within 2 days of hospitalization) or late.

COMPARISONS ACROSS SCALES. Outcome studies often involve several different dependent variables, and some of these dependent variables contain multiple subscales. Often, the different tools are scored differently and have different scales of measurement. In addition, the groups being studied may show more or less variability on the different measures, which also influences the interpretation of changes in scores. If a researcher wishes to know which of the many different variables changed the most, then the changes need to be expressed on a common scale that captures both the size of the change as well as the variability within the group. The usual scale that is used is a measure of *effect size,* which expresses the difference between two means in terms of the amount of variability within the data. An effect size of 1.0 indicates that the difference between the means of two groups is the same size as the standard deviation, a measure of variability within each group. Effect sizes less than 1.0 mean that the difference between the means is smaller than the standard deviation, and effect sizes larger than 1.0 mean that the difference is greater than the standard deviation. The conceptual basis for effect size will be clearer after a review of Chapters 20 and 22, which lay the statistical foundation needed for a full understanding of effect sizes. For now, it is enough to know that the use of effect sizes en-

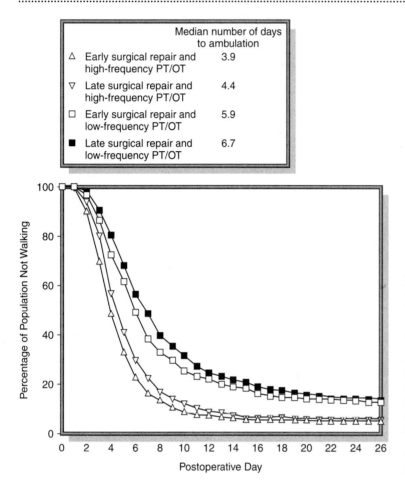

FIGURE 15–2. Illustration of the use of survival curves. The curves show the probability and timing of ambulation according to timing of surgical repair and the frequency of physical and occupational therapy (PT/OT).
From Hoenig H, Rubenstein LV, Sloane R, et al. What is the role of timing in the surgical and rehabilitative care of community-dwelling older persons with acute hip fracture? *Arch Intern Med.* 1997;157:513–520. Used with permission of the American Medical Association.

ables the researcher to compare the magnitude of change across many different variables. Jette and Jette used effect sizes to evaluate changes in SF-36 scores and Lysholm Knee Rating Scale scores over an episode of physical therapy for patients with knee impairments.[27] Figure 15–3 shows a radar graph of their results. In a radar graph, each dependent variable is displayed as a "spoke" coming from a common center. The scale on each spoke is the same, and in this example represents effect size, marked in $\frac{1}{10}$ of a standard deviation increment. It is readily apparent from this graph that the biggest changes were seen in Lysholm scores and in the bodily pain and physical function subscales of the SF-36.

MULTIVARIATE STATISTICS. The final analysis issue covered here also stems from the multiple dependent variables that are often measured in outcomes studies. Because of these many variables, researchers often use statistical tools that enable them to analyze many dependent variables simultaneously. The general term for these types of statistical tools is *multivariate*. Although the descriptions of multivariate results often appear intimidating, they rest on many of the same statistical foundations as do the simpler univariate statistics that handle one dependent variable at a time. Chapters 20 through 24 cover the statistical information needed to become comfortable reading and interpreting the results of both univariate and multivariate analyses.

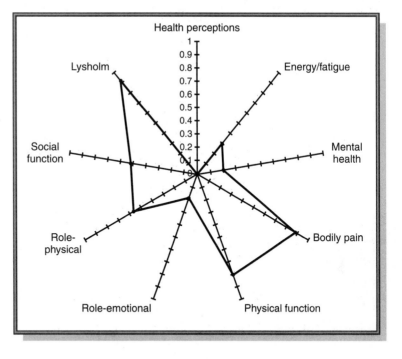

FIGURE 15–3. Use of effect sizes in a radar graph format to display changes in SF-36 and Lysholm scores over a physical therapy episode for patients with knee impairments. Changes are presented as effect sizes for each outcome and are represented by a point on an arm of the radar graph. The center of the graph is no change. Each hatch mark represents a change of $\frac{1}{10}$ of a standard deviation. From Jette DU, Jette AM. Physical therapy and health outcomes in patients with knee impairments. *Phys Ther.* 1996;76:1178–1187. Used with permission of the American Physical Therapy Association.

■ SUMMARY

Outcomes research refers to a broad group of research designs that evaluate the overall effectiveness of clinical care as it is delivered in actual practice, rather than the physiological efficacy of treatments given under tightly controlled circumstances to narrowly defined groups of subjects. Evaluating effectiveness often includes measurements of functional limitation, disability, and handicap, as defined by the Nagi model or the World Health Organization's International Classification of Impairment, Disabilities, and Handicaps, in addition to the more traditional measures of pathology and impairment. This broader conceptualization of health status is often referred to as "health-related quality of life" and can be measured by a number of generic, condition-specific, or satisfaction tools. Outcomes research studies generally rely on databases that are generated by review of medical records, computerized abstracts of medical records, insurance claims data, in-house data

collection efforts, or commercial concerns that provide standardized data collection forms and analysis services. Statistical analysis of outcomes research is often complex and must address issues of case mix, missing data, survival analysis, comparisons across different scales, and analysis of many dependent variables simultaneously.

REFERENCES

1. Epstein AM. Sounding board: the outcomes movement—will it get us where we want to go? *N Engl J Med.* 1990;323:266–270.
2. Keller RB, Rudicel SAZ, Liang MH. Outcomes research in orthopaedics. *J Bone Joint Surg Am.* 1993;75:1562–1574.
3. Nyiendo J, Haas M, Hondras MA. Outcomes research in chiropractics: the state of the art and recommendations for the chiropractic research agenda. *J Manipulative Physiol Ther.* 1997;20:185–197.
4. Bradham DD. Outcomes research in orthopedics: history, perspectives, concepts, and future. *Arthroscopy.* 1994; 10:493–501.
5. Birkmeyer JD. Outcomes research and surgeons. *Surgery.* 1998;124:477–483.
6. Jette AM. Outcomes research: shifting the dominant research paradigm in physical therapy. *Phys Ther.* 1995; 75:965–970.
7. Tarlov AR, Ware JE, Greenfield S, Nelson EC, Perrin E,

Zubkoff M. The Medical Outcomes Study: an application of methods for monitoring the results of medical care. *JAMA*. 1989;262:925–930.

8. Faust HB, Mirowski GW, Chuang T-Y, et al. Outcomes research: an overview. *J Am Acad Dermatol*. 1997;36: 999–1006.

9. Kane RL. *Understanding Health Care Outcomes Research*. Gaithersburg, Md: Aspen Publishers; 1997.

10. Kane RL. Improving outcomes in rehabilitation: a call to arms (and legs). *Med Care*. 1997;35(suppl):JS21–JS27.

11. Nagi SZ. Disability concepts revisited: implications for prevention. In: Pope AM, Tarlov AR, eds. *Disability in America: Toward a National Agenda for Prevention*. Washington, DC: National Academy Press; 1991:309–327.

12. *International Classification of Impairments, Disabilities, and Handicaps*. Geneva, Switzerland: World Health Organization; 1980.

13. Verbrugge LM, Jette AM. The disablement process. *Soc Sci Med*. 1994;38:1–14.

14. Jette AM. Physical disablement concepts for physical therapy research and practice. *Phys Ther*. 1994;74: 380–386.

15. Jette AM. Disablement outcomes in geriatric rehabilitation. *Med Care*. 1997;35(suppl):JS28–JS37.

16. Hamilton BB. Comments on: Jette AM. Disablement outcomes in geriatric rehabilitation. *Med Care*. 1997; 35(suppl):JS28–JS37.

17. Nagi S. Some conceptual issues in disability and rehabilitation. In: Sussman M, ed. *Sociology and Rehabilitation*. Washington, DC: American Sociological Association; 1965:100–113.

18. Pope AM, Tarlov AR, eds. *Disability in America: Toward a National Agenda for Prevention*. Washington, DC: National Academy Press; 1991.

19. Duncan PW. Stroke disability. *Phys Ther*. 1994;74: 399–407.

20. Liang MH. Comments on: Jette AM. Disablement outcomes in geriatric rehabilitation. *Med Care*. 1997;35 (suppl):JS28–JS37.

21. Jette DU. *Orthopaedic Physical Therapy: Home Study Course 96-2: Topics in Orthopaedic Physical Therapy Assessment*. Alexandria, Va: Orthopaedic Section of American Physical Therapy Association; 1996.

22. McHorney CA, Tarlov AR. Individual-patient monitoring in clinical practice: are available health status surveys adequate? *Quality Life Res*. 1995;4:293–307.

23. Maciejewski M. Generic measures. In: Kane RL, ed. *Understanding Health Care Outcomes Research*. Gaithersburg, Md: Aspen Publishers; 1997:19–52.

24. Jette AM. Using health-related quality of life measures in physical therapy outcomes research. *Phys Ther*. 1993;73: 528–537.

25. Ware JE, Kosinski M, Keller SD. A 12-item short-form health survey: construction of scales and preliminary tests of reliability and validity. *Med Care*. 1996;34: 220–223.

26. Jette DU, Jette AM. Physical therapy and health outcomes in patients with spinal impairments. *Phys Ther*. 1996;76: 930–945.

27. Jette DU, Jette AM. Physical therapy and health outcomes in patients with knee impairments. *Phys Ther*. 1996;76: 1178–1187.

28. Bergner M, Bobbitt RA, Carter WB, Gilson BS. The Sickness Impact Profile: development and final revision of a health status measure. *Med Care*. 1981;19:787–805.

29. Mueller MJ, Salsich GB, Strube MJ. Functional limitations in patients with diabetes and transmetatarsal amputations. *Phys Ther*. 1997;77:937–943.

30. Boström C, Harms-Ringdahl K, Nordemar R. Shoulder, elbow and wrist movement impairment—predictors of disability in female patients with rheumatoid arthritis. *Scand J Rehabil Med*. 1997;29:223–232.

31. Atherly A. Condition-specific measures. In: Kane RL, ed. *Understanding Health Care Outcomes Research*. Gaithersburg, Md: Aspen Publishers; 1997:53–66.

32. Pynsent P, Fairbank J, Carr A. *Outcome Measures in Orthopaedics*. Oxford, England: Butterworth-Heinemann; 1993.

33. Fairbank J, Couper J, Davies J, O'Brien J. Oswestry Low Back Pain Disability Index. *Physiotherapy*. 1980;66: 271–273.

34. Tegner Y, Lysholm J. Rating systems in the evaluation of knee ligament injuries. *Clin Orthop*. 1985;190:43–49.

35. Di Palo MT. Rating satisfaction research: is it poor, fair, good, very good, or excellent? *Arthritis Care Res*. 1997;10:422–430.

36. Maciejewski J, Kawiecki J, Rockwood T. Satisfaction. In: Kane RL, ed. *Understanding Health Care Outcomes Research*. Gaithersburg, Md: Aspen Publishers; 1997: 67–89.

37. Fox KM, Reuland M, Hawkes WG, et al. Accuracy of medical records in hip fracture. *J Am Geriatr Soc*. 1998;46:745–750.

38. Lu-Yao GL, Baron JA, Barrett JA, Fisher ES. Treatment and survival among elderly Americans with hip fractures: a population-based study. *Am J Public Health*. 1994; 84:1287–1291.

39. Mitchell JM, de Lissovoy G. A comparison of resource use and cost in direct access versus physician referral episodes of physical therapy. *Phys Ther*. 1997;77:10–18.

40. Motheral BR, Fairman KA. The use of claims databases for outcomes research: rationale, challenges, and strategies. *Clin Ther*. 1997;19:346–366.

41. Shields RK, Leo KC, Miller B, Dostal WF, Barr R. An acute care physical therapy clinical practice database for outcomes research. *Phys Ther*. 1994;74:463–470.

42. Reynolds JP. Database dreams. *PT—Magazine of Physical Therapy*. 1997;5(3):50–58.

43. Reynolds JP. Are you ready to join an outcomes database? *PT—Magazine of Physical Therapy*. 1998;6(10): 36–67.

44. Russek L, Wooden M, Ekedahl S, Bush A. Attitudes toward standardized data collection. *Phys Ther*. 1997;77: 714–729.

45. Pryor DB, Lee KL. Methods for the analysis and assessment of clinical databases: the clinician's perspective. *Stat Med*. 1991;10:617–628.

46. La Valley MP, Anderson JJ. Statistical and study design issues in assessing the quality and outcomes of care in rheumatic diseases. *Arthritis Care Res*. 1997;10: 431–440.

47. Smith M. Severity. In: Kane RL, ed. *Understanding Health Care Outcomes Research*. Gaithersburg, Md: Aspen Publishers; 1997:129–152.

48. Nitz NM. Comorbidity. In: Kane RL, ed. *Understanding Health Care Outcomes Research*. Gaithersburg, Md: Aspen Publishers; 1997:153–174.

49. Derose S. Demographic and psychosocial factors. In: Kane RL, ed. *Understanding Health Care Outcomes Research*. Gaithersburg, Md: Aspen Publishers; 1997; 175–209.

50. Jekel JF, Elmore JG, Katz DL. *Epidemiology, Biostatistics, and Preventative Medicine*. Philadelphia, Pa: WB Saunders Co; 1996:154–158.

51. Hoenig H, Rubenstein LV, Sloane R, Horner R, Kahn K. What is the role of timing in the surgical and rehabilitative care of community-dwelling older persons with acute hip fracture? *Arch Intern Med.* 1997;157:513–520.

Survey Research

Scope of Survey Research

Types of Information

Types of Items
   Open-Format Items
   Closed-Format Items
   Multiple Choice
   Likert-Type
   Semantic Differential
   Q-Sort

Implementation Overview

Mailed Questionnaires
   Access to a Sampling Frame
   Researcher-Developed Versus
      Existing Instruments

Questionnaire Development
   Drafting
   Expert Review
   First Revision
   Pilot Test
   Final Revision
   Motivating Prospects to Respond
   Implementation Details

Interviews
   Access to Prospective Subjects
   Development of Interview
      Schedules
   Motivating Prospects to Participate
   Implementation Details

Survey research is a form of inquiry that rests on the assumption that meaningful information can be obtained by asking the parties of interest what they know, what they believe, and how they behave. This chapter defines the scope of survey research, identifies the type of information that can be gleaned from survey research, presents a variety of types of items that are used within questionnaires, and addresses a variety of implementation details for mailed surveys and in-person or telephone interviews.

■ SCOPE OF SURVEY RESEARCH

Surveys have been defined as "systems for collecting information to describe, compare, and predict attitudes, opinions, values, knowledge, and behavior."[1(p21)] More specifically, survey research relies on self-reported information from participants, rather than on observations or measurements taken by the researcher. For example, consider ways of studying the extent to which patients adhere to a prescribed exercise regimen. One way to study this topic would be to ask patients how often they participate in the exercises or to ask more pointed questions to determine their recall of important details about the exercise program. This self-report information could be collected with survey methods in a face-to-face interview, by administering a questionnaire over the telephone, or with a mailed questionnaire. An assumption of the survey approach is that patients would provide accurate information about their participation level.

In contrast, this topic could also be studied by having researchers score patients in some way as they observe them demonstrating the prescribed exercise routine. An assumption of the observational approach is that patients who were adherent to the prescribed regimen would demonstrate the program correctly without prompting and those who were not adherent would perform the regimen incorrectly or would require prompting from the researcher. Neither the survey approach nor the observational approach is inherently superior for studying this topic. Each rests on assumptions that will not be met in all cases—some patients will exaggerate their exercise participation if surveyed and some patients who faithfully perform their exercises may become flustered in front of the researcher and require prompting to demonstrate the regimen. Researchers need to consider which of the potential problems to avoid when they make decisions among the approaches that could be taken with a given topic.

To place survey research into the context of other forms of research, recall the six-celled matrix of research types presented earlier in Chapter 6 (Fig. 6–4) and repeated in Chapter 11 (Fig. 11–1). One dimension of the matrix is the purpose of the research. Survey techniques can be used for all three purposes: describing phenomena, analyzing relationships among variables, and analyzing differences among groups or across time.

The second dimension of the matrix is the timing of data collection. Clearly, surveys can be prospective, with self-reported information collected to answer specific research questions developed by the researchers. It is equally clear that self-reported information may be used retrospectively—that is, data collected for one purpose might be extracted and reanalyzed to meet another research need. For example, Chevan and Chevan used US Bureau of the Census data to develop a profile of physical therapists.[2] However, most would not label this study "survey research." Instead, they would refer to it as a secondary analysis. The term *survey research* is generally used to describe original, prospective collection of self-reported data.

The third dimension of the matrix is whether the research is experimental or nonexperimental in nature. Clearly, survey research can be nonexperimental, with no controlled manipulation of independent variables. It is equally clear that self-reported information can be used in experimental research—as was the case when Balogun and associates studied the impact of educational programs on physical therapist and occupational therapist student attitudes toward working with individuals with acquired immunodeficiency syndrome (AIDS).[3] This project was experimental in nature because there was controlled manipulation of the type of education received. Researchers surveyed participants to determine self-reported attitudes across time (preeducation, mideducation, and posteducation). However, most would not label this study as "survey" research; they might label it as an experimental, educational research project. Thus, although survey research can be experimental in nature, the term is generally reserved for nonexperimental studies using self-reported information.

In summary, survey research can be used to meet the purposes of description, analysis of relationships, or analysis of differences. The term "survey research" is generally reserved for nonexperimental research with prospective collection of self-reported data. It is important to recognize that although all survey research projects use self-reported information, not all research projects that use self-reported information are considered survey research. Studies that use self-reported information retrospectively or in the context of experimental research are generally not referred to as survey research.

TYPES OF INFORMATION

The scope of information that can be obtained through self-report instruments is vast. Concrete facts, knowledge, and behavior can be documented, as can abstract opinions and personal characteristics. The physical therapy literature contains many examples of each of the five types of survey information just mentioned; one example of each follows. Rozier and colleagues collected factual information about salaries of male and female physical therapist managers.[4] Clark and colleagues used survey methods to study physical therapists' knowledge regarding battered women.[5] Bashi and Domholdt studied the behaviors of physical therapists in Indiana with respect to their use of on-the-job trained support personnel.[6] Rozier and colleagues explored the opinions of therapists about factors they considered important to success in their careers as physical therapists.[7] As a part of this career success study, Rozier and colleagues also used self-reported information to determine a personal characteristic of respondents—their self-esteem as measured by the Rosenberg Self-Esteem Scale.[7]

TYPES OF ITEMS

Although the format of interview and questionnaire items is limited only by the creativity of the researcher, several standard item formats exist. The broadest distinction among item types is open- versus closed-format items. The closed-format items presented in this chapter are divided further into multiple-choice, Likert-type, semantic differential, and Q-sort items.

Open-Format Items

Open-format items permit a flexible response. Interviews frequently include open-format items,

and it is these open-format items that allow for the greater breadth of response that is a major advantage of using the interview in survey research. Suppose that a researcher is interested in identifying the sources of job satisfaction and dissatisfaction for hospital-based physical therapists. An open-format interview question might be, "What about your job is satisfying to you?" Respondents would be free to structure their responses as desired. Some might emphasize aspects of patient care, others might focus on working with a respected leader within the department, others might discuss the quality of interactions among coworkers, and others might list several different satisfying aspects of their work.

Questionnaires may also include open-format items, although the depth of response depends on the respondents' ability to communicate in writing and their willingness to provide an indepth answer in the absence of an interviewer who can prompt them and provide encouragement during the course of their response.

The major difficulty with open-format items is their analysis. The researcher must sift and categorize the responses into a relatively small number of manageable categories. The literature on the qualitative research paradigm provides guidelines for the classification of responses from open-format items, as discussed in Chapter 13. The categorization of responses from open-format items is sometimes used to generate the fixed alternatives needed for closed-format items.

Closed-Format Items

Closed-format items restrict the range of possible responses. Mailed questionnaires often include a high proportion of closed-format responses. In addition, highly structured interviews may use closed-format responses. In such a case, the interview becomes an orally administered questionnaire and the breadth of response characteristic of the interview format is lost. Four types of closed-format items are discussed below:

multiple-choice, Likert-type, semantic differential, and Q-sort items.

MULTIPLE-CHOICE. Multiple-choice items can be used to measure knowledge, behavior, opinions, or personal characteristics. Some researchers design closed-format items that allow some flexibility of response by including "other" as a possible response category and permitting respondents to write in a response of their choice.

In a variation of the multiple-choice item, a vignette may be used as the stem of the item. A vignette is a short story or scenario that sets a scene. Kvitek and associates used vignettes to determine the goals that physical therapists would set for two different patients with amputations.[8] Each patient's age, level of amputation, occupation, and marital status were described in the vignettes. Vignettes permit researchers to evaluate responses to a complex circumstance that may better approximate clinical settings than traditional multiple-choice items.

LIKERT-TYPE. Likert-type items, named for their originator, are used to assess the strength of response to a declarative statement. The most typical set of responses includes "strongly agree," "agree," "undecided," "disagree," and "strongly disagree." Many others are available, a few of which are "very important" to "very unimportant," "strongly encourage" to "strongly discourage," and "definitely yes" to "definitely no."[9] Likert-type items (with ratings from "negative effect" to "positive effect") were used by Rozier and colleagues to determine the perceived impact of various factors (i.e., age, family responsibilities) on the career success of physical therapists.[7]

SEMANTIC DIFFERENTIAL. Semantic differential items are based on the work of Osgood and colleagues in the 1950s.[10] Semantic differential items consist of adjective pairs that represent different ends of a continuum. The respondent indicates the place on the continuum that best represents the item or person being described. If semantic differential items were used to study physical therapists' opinions about their de-

partment, word pairs such as "cohesive–fragmented," "invigorating–dull," and "organized–disorganized" might be used to elicit their opinions. Semantic differential items were used by Streed and Stoecker to assess the levels of stereotyping in physical therapy and occupational therapy students.[11]

Q-SORT. A Q-sort is a method of forced-choice ranking of many alternatives.[12] It could be used to study job satisfaction of physical therapists. To do so, the researcher would generate a set of, say, 50 items about the job that might be important to physical therapists. Example items might be "chance to rotate among services," "weekends off," and "availability of physical therapist assistants." Each item would be written on a single card. Each therapist in the study would be asked to sort the cards into categories based on a preset distribution. For example, for our 50-card sort there might be five categories with the following forced distribution: exceedingly important (4 cards), very important (10 cards), moderately important (22 cards), minimally important (10 cards), and of negligible importance (4 cards). This distribution would force therapists to differentiate among a set of job satisfaction items by identifying the very few that are most important as well as the very few that are least important. Responses could be quantified by assigning numerals to each category (exceedingly important = 5; of negligible importance = 1) and adding the scores for each item across therapists. Items with the highest scores would be those that were consistently placed in the more important categories. Kovach and Krejci used Q-sort methodology to determine the factors that staff members in long-term care facilities perceived were most important in improving care for residents with dementia.[13]

IMPLEMENTATION OVERVIEW

There are three classic methods of collecting survey data: personal interviews, telephone interviews, and written questionnaires. Although written questionnaires can be administered in person, the most common method is to administer them through the mail. Each of the three methods has its advantages and disadvantages, as indicated in Table 16–1.

Survey research is sometimes viewed as an "easy" approach to research—write a few questions, interview subjects or mail out questionnaires, and wait for the information to come pouring in. Unfortunately, this view sometimes leads to surveys that are conducted casually and lead to a superficial or distorted understanding of a topic based on the responses of a few. In contrast, well-designed and well-implemented survey research involves meticulous attention to the details of sampling, interview, or questionnaire design; interview implementation or questionnaire distribution; and follow-up. Dillman's classic text on the "total design method" of implementing surveys[14] and the more recent *Survey Kit*[15] (a set of nine slim volumes covering different aspects of survey research) provide prospective researchers with the information needed to implement survey research in rigorous

ways to produce valid and reliable information. Procedural guidelines for conducting mailed surveys and interviews are offered in the next two sections of this chapter.

■ MAILED QUESTIONNAIRES

Compared with interviews, mailed surveys cost less and permit a broader sampling frame and larger numbers of subjects. Despite these advantages, mailed surveys may also have the disadvantages of unavailability of appropriate mailing lists of subjects, low response rates, inability to gain information from individuals who cannot read, and lack of control over who actually responds to the questionnaire. Borque and Fielder[16] present the details of conducting mailed surveys in one volume of the *Survey Kit*. The next section of this chapter presents an overview of details related to access to a sampling frame, deciding between researcher-developed and existing self-report instruments, questionnaire development, motivating prospects to respond, and implementation details.

TABLE 16–1 Advantages and Disadvantages of Interviews and Questionnaires

	Method		
Characteristic	*Personal Interview*	*Telephone Interview*	*Mailed Questionnaire*
Time	Very time-consuming	Time-consuming	Efficient
Cost	Personnel to do interviews, travel	Personnel to do interviews, long-distance telephone	Clerical personnel, printing and mailing
Geographical distribution of respondents	Greatly limited unless well-funded	Somewhat limited unless well-funded	Least limited because mailing is less expensive than travel
Depth of response	Can be extensive	Somewhat limited	Limited
Anonymity	Difficult to achieve	Difficult to achieve	Easily achieved
Literacy of respondents	Can sample those unable to read/write	Can sample those unable to read/write	Respondents must be able to read and write
Ability to clarify questions	Possible	Possible	Impossible
Scheduling	Must coordinate researcher's and respondents' schedules	Must coordinate researcher's and respondents' schedules	Completed at respondents' convenience

Access to a Sampling Frame

When survey data are collected through a mailed questionnaire, potential subjects can often be identified from the mailing lists of various groups. Mailing labels of member addresses are available from sources such as professional associations. For example, if a researcher is interested in physical therapists' opinions on a certain topic, then purchasing mailing labels from the American Physical Therapy Association or state physical therapist licensing agencies may be indicated. A researcher interested in surveying rehabilitation directors at acute care hospitals across the United States might purchase American Hospital Association labels as probably the best route to the appropriate people. When labels are ordered, the researcher can often specify several inclusion and exclusion criteria, as well as ask for a random sampling of labels meeting those criteria. In one step, then, the researcher can define the population, sample from that population, and obtain the labels needed to do the mailing. More details about sampling procedures are provided in Chapter 8.

Researcher-Developed Versus Existing Instruments

Researchers who wish to collect data through survey methods are faced with the question of whether to develop their own questionnaire or use an existing self-report instrument. A literature review should be done to determine what instruments have been used in related studies. Existing instruments that are commercially available and frequently cited in the literature can be identified from references such as the *Mental Measurements Yearbook* and *Tests in Print*.[17,18] The text *Instruments for Clinical Health Care Research* includes descriptions of existing measures for constructs such as quality of life, coping, hope, self-care, and body image.[19] An instrument that was developed for a single study can often be obtained by writing the researcher. Even if an instrument has been used only once

before, there is a base of information about the tool on which subsequent research can build. Researchers are encouraged to use or adapt existing self-report tools that meet their needs before they develop their own.

Questionnaire Development

When researchers determine that they require unique information for their study, they must develop their own questionnaire. There are five basic steps to questionnaire development: drafting, expert review, first revision, pilot test, and final revision.

DRAFTING. The first step in developing a questionnaire is to draft items for consideration for inclusion in the questionnaire. Before writing any items, the researcher needs to reexamine the purposes of the study and outline the major sections the questionnaire needs to include to answer the questions under study. Researchers seem to have an almost irresistible urge to ask questions because they seem interesting, without knowing how the answers will be used. This lengthens the questionnaire and may decrease the number of subjects who respond. Several authors have provided specific suggestions for questionnaire design and format.[9,14,15,20]

Even for the first draft, the researcher must begin to consider issues of format and comprehensibility. The items in a questionnaire are often divided into topical groups to break the questionnaire into more easily digestible parts. In addition, because different topics may require items with different formats, the section headings provide for a transition between different types of items. Some recommend that easier items be placed first on the questionnaire, with more difficult items presented later. The thought behind this is that the easy initial questions will get respondents interested in the questionnaire so that they will follow through with the more difficult questions that come later. For similar reasons, some recommend that demographic questions come last. It is thought that completing the demographic questions first will either bore respondents or offend them with questions about sensitive areas such as salary.

The readability of the type used in the questionnaire is important. The smallest readable type is generally considered to be 10-point type. Twelve-point type is more readable and is probably preferable for most questionnaires. If the population is expected to have difficulty with vision or if reading skills are likely to be low, 14-point type may be useful. The drawback of larger type is that the questionnaire physically becomes longer.

The type font is also important; researchers should not use atypical fonts that may be difficult to read. With the widespread availability of personal computers and low-cost desktop publishing services, any researcher should be able to produce an attractive, inviting questionnaire at a reasonable cost.

A second aspect of readability is the reading level required to understand the questionnaire. College-educated researchers are so accustomed to reading and writing that they forget that their writing is likely to be at an academic level that many will not be able to comprehend. To increase readability, researchers should write clearly and avoid jargon.

The instructions on how to complete the survey also must be extremely clear and specific (e.g., "Check one box," "Circle as many items as apply," and "Write in your age in years at your last birthday"). If the same format of questions is used throughout a questionnaire, the instructions need to be given only once. If the format of questions changes from item to item, instructions should be provided for each item.

Researchers designing questionnaires must decide whether to include space for data coding on the questionnaire itself. Data coding is used to turn answers to questions into numbers suitable for analysis. Figure 16–1 shows an example of a questionnaire page with a data coding column completed, based on the work of Bashi and Domholdt.[6] Some researchers do not like to include a data-coding column on questionnaires because they believe it is distracting to the respondent and takes up unnecessary space.

The researcher must also consider format and printing decisions such as the color of paper, the size and arrangement of pages, and the amount of white space on the questionnaire. The color of paper should be fairly light to ensure good readability. Good-quality paper should be used because it is the first means by which the potential respondent determines whether the questionnaire is worth responding to. One format that has been recommended is a booklet.[14] A four-page questionnaire could be made by printing on both sides of a single sheet of 11″ × 17″ paper and folding it in half to make an 8 1/2″ × 11″ booklet. One benefit of such a booklet is that because multiple sheets of paper are not needed, none will inadvertently get separated from one another. Another benefit is that the familiar booklet form should lead to fewer skipped questions; if single pages are printed front and back and stapled together, the reverse side of one sheet may be omitted by some respondents. The booklet may also have the appearance of being more professional, thereby increasing the return rate for the study.

EXPERT REVIEW. Once the draft is written the researcher needs to undertake the second step in questionnaire development: subjecting the questionnaire to review by a colleague knowledgeable about the topic under study. This is essentially a check for content validity. Did the colleague think that all the important elements of the constructs under study were addressed? Were questions understandable? Were terms defined satisfactorily? In addition to providing feedback on the content of the questionnaire, a colleague can also assess the format of the questionnaire.

FIRST REVISION. After the expert review, the researcher makes revisions in the questionnaire based on the expert's feedback. If the selected colleague makes no recommendations for change, the researcher probably needs to find another more critical colleague to review the work.

27. At some point during my professional career,
     utilization of aides for patient treatment has presented
     me with ethical dilemmas. (Circle appropriate letter)

     a. Strongly agree
     b. Agree
     c. Disagree   1. _4_
     d. Strongly disagree
     e. Unable to decide

28. I am comfortable with aide involvement in patient   2. _2_
     treatment at my current job. (Circle appropriate
     letter)

     a. Strongly agree
     b. Agree
     c. Disagree
     d. Strongly disagree
     e. Unable to decide

                                                             3. _5_

29. I am satisfied with the Indiana Physical Therapy
     Practice Act's guidelines regarding utilization of aides
     in patient treatment. (Circle appropriate letter)

     a. Strongly agree
     b. Agree
     c. Disagree
     d. Strongly disagree
     e. Unable to decide

FIGURE 16–1. Questionnaire excerpt, with coding column. The circled letters are
converted to numbers before data entry.

PILOT TEST. The next step is to pilot test the instrument on the types of subjects who will complete the questionnaire. When pilot testing, it is useful to have subjects indicate the time it took them to complete the questionnaire. The final item on the pilot questionnaire should be a request for the subjects to review the questionnaire and write any comments they might have about the nature and format of the items.

When the pilot surveys are returned, the researcher should determine the return rate of the questionnaires and look for troublesome response patterns. For example, if only 40% of the pilot subjects return questionnaires, then the researcher should not expect a better return rate from actual subjects. The researcher should attempt to determine the reasons for nonresponse to the pilot survey so that corrective measures can be taken on the final questionnaire.

Patterns to be looked for among responses to the pilot testing are missing responses, lack of range in responses, many responses in the "other" category, and extraneous comments. For example, if one used several Likert-scale items and all the respondents answered "strongly agree," this may mean the item was worded so positively that no reasonable person would ever disagree with the statement. Rewording should create an item that is more likely to elicit a range of responses. Assume that the purpose of a survey is to determine physical therapists' attitudes toward long-term care of the elderly. An item worded "Quality long-term care for the elderly is an important component of the health care system in the United States" would be difficult to disagree with. Rewording the item to read "Funding for long-term care of the elderly should take priority over funding for public education" requires the respondent to make choices between funding priorities and would likely elicit a greater range of responses.

An item repeatedly left unanswered may indicate that placement of the item on the page is a problem, the item is so sensitive that people do not wish to answer it, or the item is so complicated that it takes too much energy to answer it. A multiple-choice item frequently answered with the response category of "other" may indicate that the choices given were too limited.

FINAL REVISION. Rewording of items, elimination of items, addition of items, or revision of the questionnaire format may all be indicated by the results of the pilot study. If a great many problems were identified in the pilot study, the researcher may wish to retest the questionnaire on a small group of subjects before investing the money and time in the final questionnaire.

Motivating Prospects to Respond

Once the individuals to whom a questionnaire will be sent are identified, it is the researcher's job to sell them on the idea of completing the questionnaire. The cover letter that accompanies the survey is the major sales tool. It must be attractive, be brief but complete, and provide potential respondents with a good reason to complete the study. Figures 16–2 and 16–3 provide two examples of cover letters annotated with comments on their good and bad points. Other methods of motivating subjects are the inclusion of incentives in the initial mailing (inexpensive, lightweight items like a packet of instant cocoa

or a dollar bill), entry into a random drawing for a more valuable incentive when the completed questionnaire is returned, or offering the results of the study when the analysis is complete.

Implementation Details

There are a number of implementation details that need to be planned when sending mailed surveys: addressing options, envelopes, postage, and follow-up. If the researcher has a choice between printing the address directly on the outer envelope versus using mailing labels, the former has the advantage of appearing to be more individualized. If the questionnaire packet that goes to prospective participants fits in a business-sized envelope, the researcher can choose between enclosing a folded business-sized return envelope or using a slightly smaller return envelope designed to fit flat within a business envelope. The latter option provides for a flatter packet and a more professional look. The budget may dictate whether bulk or first class mailing rates are used to send the questionnaires. Whenever possible, first class mailing should be done, since bulk mail receives lower priority and may not be delivered in a timely fashion. The researcher will need to decide whether to use first class or business-reply postage for return envelopes. First class postage must be affixed to each return envelope with the knowledge that a proportion of the investment in return postage will be lost to nonrespondents. Business-reply postage costs more per envelope than first class postage, but this higher cost is charged only on the returned envelopes. The researcher will need to compare costs between these postage options, assuming various return rates, to make a good decision about which option will be more cost-effective.

Plans for follow-up mailings, if needed to achieve the desired return rate, need to be made in advance of the first mailing. To provide for the possibility of following up nonrespondents, the researcher numbers the master list of subjects

October 8, 1999

(A)   Dear Program Director:

(B)   We are students in the master's degree program in physical

therapy at the University of Anytown. For our research

project we are studying the content of physical therapy

(C)   curriculums in geriatrics to determine whether enough

attention is paid to geriatrics education for physical

therapists. Please complete this survey and return it to us

(D)   at the following address by October 15, 1999:

University of Anytown

(E)   1256 Holt Road

Anytown, IN   46234

(F)   Thank you for your participation. If you would like a

summary of the results, please write your name and address

on the last page of the survey.

Sincerely,

(G)

(H)   Jodi Beeker   Jonathon Mills

Physical Therapy Student   Physical Therapy Student

FIGURE 16–2. Example of a poor cover letter for a questionnaire. (A) There is no personalization of greeting to potential respondents. (B) When the first sentence indicates that the researchers are students, potential respondents may assume that the research is being done only because it is required. (C) The second sentence indicates a bias on the part of the researchers. (D) Because of the early return date, the potential respondents might not receive the questionnaire until 1 or 2 days before the deadline. (E) The researchers have obviously not included a self-addressed, stamped return envelope and are asking potential respondents to bear part of the cost of the study. (F) The mechanism for respondents to indicate their interest in the study results destroys the anonymity of the questionnaire. (G) Lack of signatures (or photocopied signatures) indicates an impersonal approach to potential respondents. (H) There is no way, other than through the mail, to contact the student researchers if the potential respondent has questions about the study.

University of Anytown
1256 Holt Road
Department of Physical Therapy

Anytown, Indiana 46234
(317) 555-4300

(A)

October 8, 1999

Elizabeth Domholdt, PT, EdD
Dean, Krannert School of Physical Therapy
University of Indianapolis
1400 E. Hanna Avenue
Indianapolis, IN 46227

(B) Dear Dr. Domholdt:

(C) We are requesting your participation in a survey of physical therapy programs in the United States to determine the characteristics of geriatric education within physical therapy curriculums. We know that directors of physical therapy education programs are faced with dilemmas about the breadth and depth of content that should be included in today's overcrowded physical therapy curriculums. We believe that a compilation of information about geriatrics curriculum content will be helpful to physical therapy

(D) educators as they determine the amount of emphasis they wish to place on geriatric education within their own curriculums.

(E) In pilot testing, the enclosed questionnaire took an average of less than 10 minutes to complete. We would greatly appreciate your time in completing the questionnaire and

(F) returning it in the enclosed envelope by **November 8, 1999**. If you would like a copy of the results, please complete the enclosed postcard and return it separately from the

(G) questionnaire.

Thank you in advance for your consideration. If you have any questions or concerns about the study, please feel free to contact any of us at the address or telephone numbers listed.

Sincerely,

(H) *Jodi Beeker*   *Jon Mills*   *Jan Woolery*

Jodi Beeker   Jon Mills   Jan Woolery, PT, PhD
PT Student   PT Student   Associate Professor

(I) (317) 555-4321   (317) 555-6789   (317) 555-4378

FIGURE 16–3. Example of a good cover letter for a questionnaire. (A) Letterhead paper is used to indicate affiliation of the researchers. (B) The greeting is personalized. (C) Introductory paragraph is neutral on the subject matter. (D) The last sentence of the introductory paragraph indicates the usefulness of findings; this provides a reason for completing the questionnaire. (E) The time required of respondents is indicated. (F) The return date gives respondents a few weeks to reply. (G) The mechanism for obtaining survey results does not violate the anonymity of responses. (H) Signing each cover letter individually provides a personal touch. (I) Telephone numbers for students and the name and telephone number of a responsible faculty member provide a mechanism by which potential respondents can contact them about the survey.

and in the envelope going to each subject places a return envelope or postcard with that subject's number on it. When the questionnaire is returned, the number is marked on the master list as returned, and the return envelope is discarded, maintaining the confidentiality of the subject responses to the questionnaire.

A postcard system for follow-up maintains even greater anonymity. A numbered postcard is included with the questionnaire packet, and the subject is instructed to mail the postcard and questionnaire back separately so that the questionnaire and subject number will never be directly linked as they are if the return envelope is coded. The disadvantages of the postcard system are that it increases mailing and printing costs and subjects may forget to mail the postcard.

If the return rate is lower than desired by a week to 10 days after the first responses were due, a second mailing to nonrespondents should be done. This follow-up packet should contain a new cover letter and a duplicate copy of the questionnaire. It is often appropriate to differentiate between first and second returns so that one can check to see whether there is a difference of opinions between those who initially responded and those who required a second prodding. This can be done by using a different-colored questionnaire for the follow-up mailing or by making an inconspicuous mark on all the questionnaires sent with the second mailing. If the first respondents were positive and the second respondents somewhat more negative on the issues studied, this is an indication that overall opinion may not be as positive as that of the initial respondents.

One specialized questionnaire approach, the *Delphi technique,* assumes that several mailings will go to all participants. This technique uses several rounds of questionnaires that compensate for some of the limitations of administration of a single questionnaire. The Delphi technique was designed as a consensus-generating technique that eliminates the interpersonal factors that influence group decisions made in tradi-

tional meetings. These factors include the undue influence of a dominant personality and the willingness of less vocal members to acquiesce for the sake of achieving consensus.[21]

In a Delphi study, respondents complete and return a first-round questionnaire. A group of experts evaluates the first-round responses and compiles results; the results are returned to the respondents for review and comment (the second round). The experts review the second-round responses and compile results; again, the results are sent back to the respondents for a third round. This iterative sequence is repeated until the responses from a round are consistent with the responses of the previous round. Ingram used a Delphi approach to determine physical therapist educational program directors' opinions about essential functions for physical therapy students.[22]

■ INTERVIEWS

Compared with mailed surveys, interviews can achieve greater depth of response, maintain control over who actually responds, determine the opinions of those who cannot read, and have higher response rates. Despite these advantages, interviews may also have the disadvantages of difficulty coordinating researcher and subject schedules; lack of anonymity of responses; and high personnel, travel, or telephone costs. Frey and Oishi[23] present the details of implementing telephone and in-person interviews in one volume of the *Survey Kit.* The following sections of this chapter present an overview of details related to access to prospective subjects, development of the interview schedule, motivating prospects to participate, and implementation.

Access to Prospective Subjects

Because of the high cost of interviews, their use is often confined to studies that require fewer subjects in well-defined groups. Examples include studies of patient satisfaction with care delivered at a single location, and opinions and attitudes of students who have participated in a particular education program. Because of the focused nature of many interview studies, the need to purchase extensive lists of names, addresses, and telephone numbers is not needed, as the researcher already has access to the prospective participants. When polling of the general population is done by telephone, a variety of techniques for random digit dialing are used. As was the case with mailed questionnaires, it may be appropriate to sample from a larger population of eligible participants, according to the various procedures outlined earlier in Chapter 8.

Development of Interview Schedules

Physical therapists who use interviews to collect data generally ask questions that they have developed themselves. The researcher must decide whether structured, semistructured, or unstructured interviews are appropriate based on the nature of information desired. Details about interview styles can be found in Chapter 13.

When conducting a survey with interviews, the "interview schedule" is the corollary to the mailed questionnaire in mail surveys. The basic steps of drafting, reviewing, revising, and pilot testing are completed as they would be when developing a mailed questionnaire. The interview schedule needs to be formatted so that the sequence of items, along with instructions and explanatory text, is clear. If the interviews are highly structured, the instructions are usually expanded into scripts with a conversational tone. If the data are to be collected through telephone interviews, each question must be relatively simple so that respondents can comprehend all their response choices without a visual cue. In-person interviews can include more complex questions if visual aids are provided for respondents.

Motivating Prospects to Participate

When implementing mailed surveys, the cover letter to the survey serves as the main tool for motivating subjects to participate. In interview surveys this same function can be served by advance letters, precalls, or introductory scripts. An advance letter outlines the purposes of the study, the requirements for participation, and notifies prospective participants how they will be contacted to determine their willingness to participate. The same general guidelines for effective cover letters for mailed surveys apply to advance letters for interview surveys. Sometimes a precall (either by telephone or in person) is used instead of a letter. This allows the interviewer to answer any questions the prospective participant may have, to secure the participant's consent, and to schedule a time for the interview. In large-scale telephone surveys the first few sentences uttered by the interviewer may be the only "advance" notice that participants have of the study. Because many people routinely refuse to interact with telephone solicitors, researchers must develop an introductory script that clearly and quickly differentiates the study call from the many sales calls received by prospective participants.

Once a subject has agreed to participate in the study, the interviewer's role becomes one of keeping subjects at ease to maximize their responses to questions and to motivate and engage them to provide thoughtful, accurate responses.

Implementation Details

Implementation details of concern to researchers conducting interview surveys include securing a location for calling or interviewing in person, providing for the comfort of in-person participants, maintaining appropriate supplies, training interviewers, and tracking contacts with prospective participants.

The location for telephone interviews needs

to include a quiet environment so that the interviewer can hear participants and give them their full attention. If many interviewers are being used, a centralized calling area that enables the researcher to monitor the quality of the calls and answer questions as they arise is helpful. If in-person interviews take place on the subjects' turf, the interviewer needs to be prompt. If the interviews are being conducted at, for example, the interviewer's office, then a receptionist should be available to greet arriving subjects or take calls from subjects who will be late or unable to keep their appointment. The comfort of participants should be taken into account by providing a comfortable seating area, an appropriate arrangement of interviewer and participant, and making water or soft drinks available during the interview.

The interviewer needs to be prepared with an adequate supply of paper and working pens or pencils. If the interviews are to be recorded, the interviewer needs to be familiar with the recording equipment and ensure that the supply of tapes and batteries is adequate to meet the needs of the day.

When several interviewers are used within a study, the primary researcher needs to provide for their training. An interviewer manual should be developed and ought to include information on interviewing techniques and guidelines, the responsibilities of the interviewers, the rationale for interview questions, and a complete set of forms and procedures. The training process should include demonstration of good interview techniques, practice interviews, and observation and feedback to new interviewers.

■ SUMMARY

Surveys are systems for collecting self-reported information from participants. In general, the term "survey research" is applied to nonexperimental research with prospective data collection. Self-report instruments can be used to collect facts, determine knowledge, describe behavior, determine opinion, or document personal characteristics. Self-report instruments can include open- and closed-format items. Closed-format items include multiple-choice items, Likert-type scales, semantic differentials, and Q-sorts. Sound survey design requires meticulous attention to the details of sampling, interview, or questionnaire design; interview implementation or questionnaire distribution; and follow-up.

REFERENCES

1. Fink A. *The Survey Kit, Volume 5: How to Design Surveys.* Thousand Oaks, Calif: Sage Publications; 1995.
2. Chevan J, Chevan A. A statistical profile of physical therapists, 1980 and 1990. *Phys Ther.* 1998;78:301–312.
3. Balogun JA, Kaplan MT, Miller TM. The effect of professional education on the knowledge and attitudes of physical therapist and occupational therapist students about acquired immunodeficiency syndrome. *Phys Ther.* 1998;78:1073–1082.
4. Rozier CK, Hamilton BL, Hersh-Cochran MS. Gender-based income differences for physical therapist managers. *Phys Ther.* 1998;78:43–51.
5. Clark TJ, McKenna LS, Jewell MJ. Physical therapists' recognition of battered women in clinical settings. *Phys Ther.* 1996;76:12–18.
6. Bashi HK, Domholdt E. Use of support personnel for physical therapy treatment. *Phys Ther.* 1993;73:429–436.
7. Rozier CK, Raymond MJ, Goldstein MS, Hamilton BL. Gender and physical therapy career success factors. *Phys Ther.* 1998;78:690–704.
8. Kvitek SDB, Shaver BJ, Shepard KF. Age bias: physical therapists and older patients. *J Gerontol.* 1986;41:706–709.
9. Fink A. *The Survey Kit, Volume 2: How to Ask Survey Questions.* Thousand Oaks, Calif: Sage Publications; 1995.
10. Osgood CE, Suci GJ, Tannenbaum PH. *The Measurement of Meaning.* Urbana, Ill: University of Illinois Press; 1957.
11. Streed CP, Stoecker JL. Stereotyping between physical therapy students and occupational therapy students. *Phys Ther.* 1991;71:16–24.
12. Stephenson W. *The Study of Behavior: Q Technique and Its Methodology.* Chicago, Ill: University of Chicago Press; 1975.
13. Kovach CR, Krejci JW. Facilitating change in dementia care: staff perceptions. *J Nurs Adm.* 1998;28(5):17–27.
14. Dillman DA. *Mail and Telephone Surveys: The Total Design Method.* New York, NY: John Wiley & Sons; 1978.
15. Fink A, ed. *The Survey Kit.* Thousand Oaks, Calif: Sage Publications; 1995.
16. Borque LB, Fielder EP. *The Survey Kit, Volume 3: How to Conduct Self-Administered and Mail Surveys.* Thousand Oaks, Calif: Sage Publications; 1995.
17. Impara JC, Plake BS, eds. *The Thirteenth Mental Measurements Yearbook.* Lincoln, Neb: Buros Institute of Mental Measurements of the University of Nebraska–Lincoln; 1998.

18. Murphy LL, Conoley JC, Impara JC, eds. *Tests in Print IV.* Lincoln, Neb: Buros Institute of Mental Measurements of the University of Nebraska–Lincoln; 1994.

19. Frank-Stromborg M, Olsen SJ. *Instruments for Clinical Health Care Research.* 2nd ed. Sudbury, Mass: Jones and Bartlett Publishers; 1997.

20. Sudman S. *Asking Questions.* San Francisco, Calif: Jossey-Bass Publishers; 1982.

21. Goodman CM. The Delphi technique: a critique. *J Adv Nurs.* 1987;12:729–734.

22. Ingram D. Opinions of physical therapy education program directors on essential functions. *Phys Ther.* 1997;77:37–45.

23. Frey JH, Oishi SM. *The Survey Kit, Volume 4: How to Conduct Interviews by Telephone and In Person.* Thousand Oaks, Calif: Sage Publications; 1995.

Measurement

Measurement Theory

Definitions of Measurement

Scales of Measurement
Nominal Scales
Ordinal Scales
Interval Scales
Ratio Scales
Determining the Scale of a
Measurement

Types of Variables

**Statistical Foundations of
Measurement Theory**
Frequency Distribution
Mean
Variance
Standard Deviation
Normal Curve
Correlation Coefficient

Standard Error of Measurement

Measurement Frameworks

Measurement Reliability
Two Theories of Reliability
Components of Reliability
Instrument Reliability
Intrarater Reliability
Interrater Reliability
Intrasubject Reliability
Quantification of Reliability
Relative Reliability
Absolute Reliability

Measurement Validity
Construct Validity
Content Validity
Criterion Validity

Physical therapists use measurements to help them decide what is wrong with a patient, how to treat a patient, and when to discontinue treatment. Health care insurers rely on these measurements when they make decisions about whether to reimburse the patient or physical therapist for treatment. Researchers use measurements to quantify the characteristics they study. In fact, some investigators focus the majority of their research on the evaluation of physical therapy measures. However, knowledge about the usefulness of measurements is not reserved for these research specialists—clinicians also need to understand the meaning and usefulness of the measures they use. The editorial policies of *Physical Therapy* reflect a belief in the importance of sound measurements by requiring that all authors document the accuracy and relevancy of the measures they use.[1]

This chapter presents a framework for understanding and evaluating the measurements used by physical therapists. It does this by presenting several definitions of measurement, discussing scales of measurement and types of variables, introducing the statistical concepts required to understand measurement theory, and discussing types of measurement reliability and validity. Chapter 18 builds on this framework by presenting strategies for conducting research about measurement and Chapter 19 provides a sample of the measurement tools available to physical therapists.

■ DEFINITIONS OF MEASUREMENT

The broadest definition of measurement is that it is "the process by which things are differentiated."[2] A narrower definition is that measurement "consists of rules for assigning numbers to objects in such a way as to represent quantities of attributes."[3] According to the first definition, classification of patients into diagnostic groups is a form of measurement; according to the second definition, it is not. This text uses the broader definition of measurement, with the addition of one qualification: measurement is the *systematic* process by which things are differentiated. Thus, this definition emphasizes that measurement is not a random process, but one that proceeds according to rules and guidelines.

Differentiation can be accomplished with names, numerals, or numbers. For example, classifying people as underweight, normal weight, or overweight involves the assignment of names to differentiate people according to the characteristic of ideal body composition. If these groups are relabeled as Groups 1, 2, and 3 or Groups I, II, and III, then each person is assigned a numeral to represent body composition. A *numeral* is a symbol that does not necessarily have quantitative meaning[4]; it is a form of naming. Describing people not by groups but by their specific percentage of body fat (e.g., 10% or 14%) would involve the assignment of a number to represent the quantity of body fat. A *number,* then, is a numeral that has been assigned quantitative meaning.

■ SCALES OF MEASUREMENT

Four classic scales, or levels, of measurement are presented in the literature. These scales are based on the extent to which a measure has the properties of a real-number system. A real-number system is characterized by order, distance, and origin.[5(p12)] *Order* means that higher numbers represent greater amounts of the characteristic being measured. *Distance* means that the magnitude of the differences between successive numbers is equal. *Origin* means that the number zero represents an absence of the measured quality.

Nominal Scales

Nominal scales have none of the properties of a real-number system. A nominal scale provides classification without placing any value on the categories within the classification. Because there is no order, distance, or origin to the classification, the classification can be identified by name or numeral. However, it is often better to give classifications names instead of numerals so that no quantitative difference between categories is implied. Classification of patients with cerebral palsy into quadriplegic, diplegic, and hemiplegic categories is an example of a nominal measurement. The classification itself does not rank, for example, the functional impairment of the patient—that depends on intellectual functioning, level of spasticity, and a host of other factors not implied by the classification itself.

Ordinal Scales

Ordinal scales have only one of the three properties of a real-number system: order. Thus, an ordinal scale can be used to indicate whether a person or object has more or less of a certain quality. Ordinal scales do not ensure that there are equal intervals between categories or ranks. Because the intervals on an ordinal scale are either not known or are unequal, mathematical manipulations such as addition, subtraction, multiplication, or division of ordinal numbers are not meaningful.

Many functional scales are ordinal. The amount of assistance a patient needs to ambulate is often rated as maximal, moderate, minimal, standby, or independent. Is the interval between maximal and moderate assistance the same as the interval between minimal and standby assistance? Probably not. Sometimes numerals are assigned to points on an ordinal scale, but the validity of this procedure has been questioned because the numerals are often treated as if they were quantitative numbers.[6]

Figure 17–1 illustrates the phenomenon of nonequal intervals between points on an ordinal scale of gait independence. Assume that the underlying quantity represented by the assistance categories is the proportion of the total work of ambulation that is exerted by the patient. If the patient and therapist are expending equal energy to get the patient walking, then the patient is ex-

erting 50% of the total work of ambulation. If the patient is independent and the therapist does not need to expend any energy, then the patient is exerting 100% of the total work of ambulation. The top line of Figure 17–1 shows the assistance categories. The middle two lines show numerals that could be assigned to the assistance categories. Either set of numerals would meet the order criterion—higher numerals indicate higher levels of independence. The magnitude of the two sets of numerals varies greatly and shows the danger of thinking of ordinal numbers as real quantities. The bottom scale shows how the assistance categories might fall along a continuum of total work percentage. The categories "minimal," "standby," and "independent," as used by most therapists, probably fall in the top 20% of the scale. The categories "maximal" and "moderate" probably fall in the bottom 80% of the scale. Thus, the gait independence classification used by physical therapists is clearly an ordinal scale: the classification has order but does not represent equal intervals of the underlying construct that is being measured.

A second type of ordinal scale is a ranking. During the summer of 1998 two baseball players, Mark McGwire of the St. Louis Cardinals and Sammy Sosa of the Chicago Cubs, were in a race

SCALE OF GAIT INDEPENDENCE

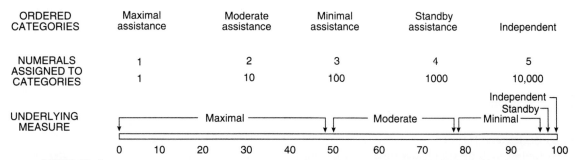

FIGURE 17–1. Level of assistance in gait as an ordinal measurement. The top row shows the assistance categories as used by many physical therapists. The bottom row shows a theoretical underlying distribution of the categories on the basis of what percentage of effort is being exerted by the patient. The middle two rows show two vastly different numbering schemes; in both schemes the numbers get larger as the amount of effort exerted by the patient increases.

for the single-season home run record. These two were clearly the best hitters of the year and the interval between the first- and second-ranked players was very slight. The difference between the second- and third-ranked players was much larger. The intervals between ranks are usually unknown and cannot be assumed to be equal.

Interval Scales

Interval scales have the real-number system properties of order and distance, but they lack a meaningful origin. A meaningful zero point represents the absence of the measured quantity. The Celsius and Fahrenheit temperature scales are examples of interval scales. The zero points on the two temperature scales are arbitrary: On the Fahrenheit scale it is the temperature at which salt water freezes, and on the Celsius scale it is the temperature at which fresh water freezes. Neither implies the absence of the basic property of heat—the temperature can go lower than zero on both scales. Both scales, however, have regular (but different) intervals. Because of the equal intervals, addition and subtraction are meaningful with interval scales. A $10°$ increase in temperature means the same thing whether the increase is from $0°$ to $10°$ or from $100°$ to $110°$. However, multiplication and division of Fahrenheit or Celsius temperature readings are not useful because these operations assume knowledge of zero quantities. A Fahrenheit temperature of $100°$ is not twice as hot as a temperature of $50°$; it is merely $50°$ hotter.

Ratio Scales

Ratio scales exhibit all three components of a real-number system: order, distance, and origin. All the arithmetic functions of addition, subtraction, multiplication, and division can be applied to ratio scales. Length, time, and weight are generally considered ratio scales because their absence is scored as zero, and the intervals between numbers are known to be equal. The Kelvin temperature scale is an example of a ratio scale because the intervals between degrees are equal and the zero point represents the absence of heat.

Determining the Scale of a Measurement

To determine the scale of a measure, the researcher must ascertain whether there is a true zero (origin), whether intervals between numbers are equal (distance), and whether there is an order to the numbers or names that constitute the measure (order). Although this sounds simple enough, there is controversy about whether some clinical measures should be considered ratio, interval, or ordinal scales.

For example, Rothstein and Echternach argue that isokinetic measures are not ratio measurements because some patients who can move their limbs are unable to register torque on an isokinetic dynamometer.[7(p17)] They argue that the zero point of an isokinetic measure does not represent the absence of torque. This question of the scale of isokinetic measures is less about the measures themselves than about the labels that are applied to the measurements. If one labels isokinetic measures as "torque," then Rothstein and Echternach's concerns are valid—there are patients who can generate torque but still register zero on an isokinetic test. If, however, isokinetic measures are labeled "speed-specific torque," then the problem disappears. If a patient is unable to generate torque at the required speed, the zero measure does, in fact, represent an absence of speed-specific torque-generating capability.

The controversy about whether isokinetic devices produce interval or ratio measures is by no means the only controversy about scales of measurement. For example, does the classification of patients as underweight, normal weight, and overweight represent a nominal or ordinal scale? The numbers are placed into classes, but these classes also have an order. As another example, do scores on the Graduate Record Examination, which purports to measure aptitude for learning in graduate school, represent ordinal or interval data? Standardized tests are often treated as interval scales even though it can be argued that the underlying construct being measured is too abstract to permit the assumption that intervals between scores are equal. Because the scale of measurement determines which mathematical manipulations are meaningful, controversy about measurement scales soon becomes controversy about which statistical tests are appropriate for which types of measures. These statistical controversies are discussed in Chapter 21.

■ TYPES OF VARIABLES

With respect to measurement, variables can be classified as continuous or discrete. A *discrete* variable is one that can assume only distinct values. Nominal scale variables are, by definition, discrete: The patients being classified must fit into a distinct category; they cannot be placed between the categories. Discrete variables that can assume only two values are called *dichotomous* variables. Examples of dichotomous variables are sex (male vs. female) or disease state (present vs. absent). Variables that are counts of behaviors or persons are discrete variables because fractional people or behaviors are not possible. If the measure of interest is the number of heel touches that occur in 10 standing trials, it is not possible to get a score of 7.5 on a single trial. Note, however, that it is possible to have an *average score* of 7.5 if the 10-trial sequence is repeated on 4 subsequent days with scores of 8, 6, 9, and 7 (8 + 6 + 9 + 7 = 30; 30/4 = 7.5). If discrete variables can assume a fairly large range of values, have the properties of a real-number system, or are averaged across trials, then they become similar to continuous variables.

A *continuous* variable is one that theoretically can be measured to a finer and finer degree.[5(p15)] Clinicians interested in the speed of patients' ambulation might record the time it takes for patients to complete a 20-m walk. Depending on the sophistication of their measurement tools, the therapists might measure time to the nearest second or to the nearest one-thousandth of a second. If the smallest increment on a therapist's watch is the second, then measurements cannot be recorded in smaller increments even though the therapist knows that the true time required for completion of a task is not limited to whole seconds. Thus, the limits of technology dictate that continuous variables will always be measured discretely.

■ STATISTICAL FOUNDATIONS OF MEASUREMENT THEORY

Seven basic concepts underlie most of measurement theory: frequency distribution, mean, variance, standard deviation, normal curve, correlation coefficient, and standard error of measurement. These concepts are introduced here and expanded on in Chapter 20.

Frequency Distribution

A *frequency distribution* is nothing more than the number of times each score is represented in the data set. If a therapist measures a patient's knee flexion 10 times during 1 day, the following scores might be obtained: 100, 100, 90, 95, 110, 110, 95, 105, 95, 100. Table 17–1 and Figure 17–2 show two ways of presenting the frequency distribution for these 10 scores.

TABLE 17-1	Frequency Distribution of 10 Knee Flexion Measurements

Score	Frequency
90	1
95	3
100	3
105	1
110	2

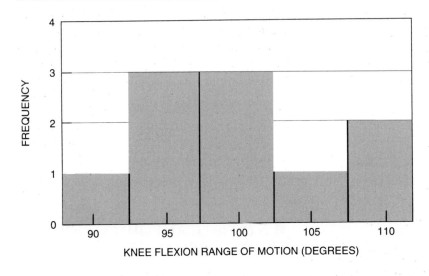

FIGURE 17–2. Histogram of the frequency distribution of hypothetical knee flexion data.

Mean

The arithmetic *mean* of a data set is the sum of the observations divided by the number of observations. Mathematical notation for the mean is

$$\overline{X} = \frac{\Sigma X}{N}$$

$\overline{X}$ is the symbol for the sample mean and is sometimes called the "X-bar." Σ is the uppercase Greek letter sigma and means "the sum of." X is the symbol for each observation. N is the symbol for the number of observations. In words, the mean equals the sum of all the observations divided by the number of observations. The mean of the data set presented earlier is calculated as follows:

$$\overline{X} = (90 + 95 + 95 + 95 + 100 + 100 + 100 + 105 + 110 + 110)/10 = 100$$

The population mean, μ, is calculated the same way, but is rarely used in practice because researchers do not have access to the entire population.

Variance

The *variance* is a measure of the variability around the mean within a data set. To calculate the variance, a researcher converts each of the raw scores in a data set to a deviation score by subtracting the mean of the data set from each raw score. In mathematical notation,

$$x = X - \overline{X}$$

The lowercase italic x is the symbol for a deviation score. The *deviation score* indicates how high or low a raw score is compared with the mean. The first two columns of Table 17–2 present the raw and deviation scores for the knee flexion data set, followed by their sums and means. Note that both the sum and the mean of the deviation scores are zero. In order to generate a nonzero index of the variability within a data set, the deviation scores must be squared. The variance is then calculated by determining the mean of the squared deviations. In mathematical notation,

$$\sigma^2 = \frac{\Sigma x^2}{N}$$

σ is the lowercase Greek sigma and when squared is the notation for the population variance. The third column in Table 17–2 shows the squared deviations from the group mean, the sum of the squared deviations, and the mean of the squared deviations. The variance is the mean

TABLE 17-2	Computation of the Variance in the 10 Knee Flexion Measurements

X	x	x^2	z score
90	−10	100	−1.59
95	−5	25	−.79
95	−5	25	−.79
95	−5	25	−.79
100	0	0	0
100	0	0	0
100	0	0	0
105	+5	25	+.79
110	+10	100	+1.59
110	+10	100	+1.59
Σ 1,000	0	400	
μ 100	0	40.0 = σ^2, variance	

of the squared deviation scores. In practice there are different symbols and slightly different formulas for the variance, depending on whether the observations represent the entire population of interest or just a sample of the population. This distinction is addressed in Chapter 20.

Although the variance is useful in many statistical procedures, it does not have a great deal of intuitive meaning because it is calculated from squared deviation scores. A measure that does have intuitive meaning is the standard deviation.

Standard Deviation

The *standard deviation* is the square root of the variance and is expressed in the units of the original measure:

$$\sigma = \sqrt{\sigma^2} = \sqrt{\frac{\Sigma x^2}{N}}$$

The mathematical notations for the standard deviation and the variance make their relationship clear: The notation for the variance (σ^2) is simply the square of the notation for standard deviation (σ). The standard deviation of the knee

flexion data presented in Table 17–2 is the square root of 40, or 6.3°.

Normal Curve

The distribution of groups of measurements frequently approximates a bell-shaped distribution known as the normal curve. The *normal curve* is a symmetric frequency distribution that can be defined in terms of the mean and standard deviation of a set of data. Any raw score within the distribution can be converted into a z *score*, which indicates how many standard deviations the raw score is above or below the mean. A z score is calculated by subtracting the mean from the raw score, creating a deviation score, and then dividing the deviation score by the standard deviation:

$$z = \frac{x}{\sigma}$$

The fourth column of Table 17–2 shows each raw score as a z score. Raw scores were transformed into z scores by dividing each of the deviation scores (x) by the standard deviation of 6.3°. The z score tells us, for example, that a measurement of 90° is 1.59 standard deviations below the mean.

In a normal distribution, 68.27% of the scores fall within 1 standard deviation above or below the mean; 95.44% of the scores fall within 2 standard deviations above or below the mean; and 99.74% of the scores fall within 3 standard deviations above or below the mean. Figure 17–3 shows a diagram of the normal curve, with the percentages of scores that are found within each standard deviation. Figure 17–4A shows the normal curve that corresponds to the knee flexion data set. The mean is 100°, and the standard deviation is 6.3°. Figure 17–4B shows that if the knee flexion scores are normally distributed, we could expect about 98% of our measurements to exceed the score of 87.4° (the shaded area in the figure). Figure 17–4C shows that we could expect about 68% of our measures to fall between 93.7° and 106.3°. Predicting the probability of

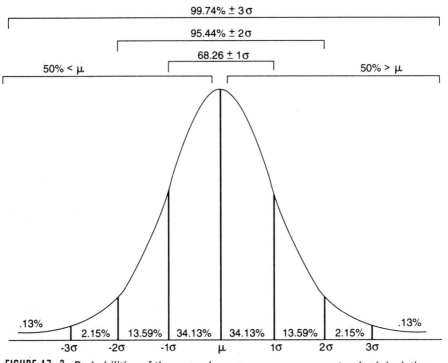

FIGURE 17–3. Probabilities of the normal curve. μ = mean; σ = standard deviation.

obtaining certain ranges of scores is one of the most basic of statistical functions.

Correlation Coefficient

A *correlation coefficient* is a statistical summary of the degree of relationship that exists between two or more measures. The relationship can be between either different variables (such as strength and range of motion) or repeated measures of the same variables (such as range-of-motion measures of the same patient taken by three different therapists). There are many different types of correlation coefficients (Table 17–3); the computational distinctions between them are discussed in Chapter 23.

A correlation coefficient of 0.0 means that there is no relationship between the variables; a correlation coefficient of 1.0 indicates that there is a perfect relationship between the variables. Values in between these two extremes indicate intermediate levels of relationship. Some correlation coefficients can also have values from 0.0 to -1.0. A negative correlation indicates an inverse relationship between variables (i.e., as the values for one variable become larger, the values for the other become smaller). In this text, r is used as a general symbol for a correlation coef-

FIGURE 17–4. Probabilities of the normal curve applied to hypothetical range-of-motion data with a mean of 100 and a standard deviation of 6.3. **A.** The range-of-motion values that correspond to 1, 2, and 3 standard deviations above and below the mean. **B.** The probability of obtaining a score greater than 87.4° (the shaded area) is 97.72%. **C.** The probability of obtaining a score between 93.7° and 106.3° (the shaded area) is 68.26%. μ = mean; σ = standard deviation.

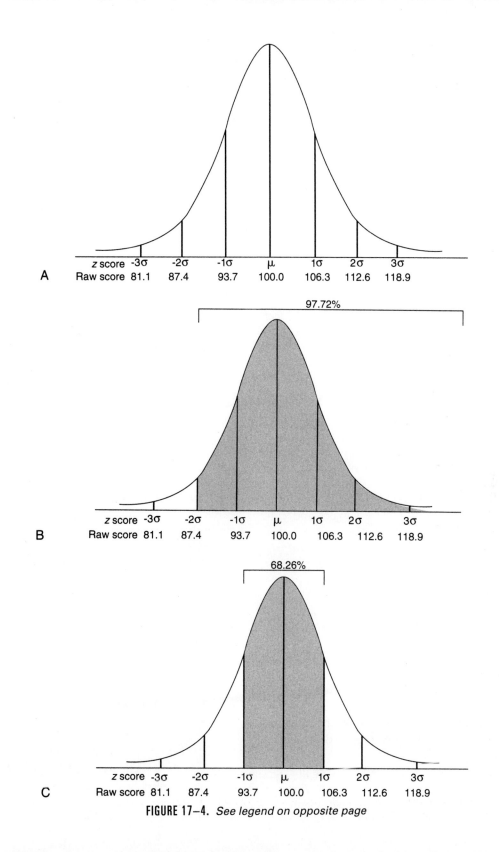

FIGURE 17–4. *See legend on opposite page*

TABLE 17-3 Correlation Coefficients		
Name of Coefficient	Type of Data Required	No. of Repeated Measures Compared
Pearson product moment correlation	Continuous	Two
Intraclass correlation	Continuous	Two or more
Spearman rank order correlation	Ranked	Two
Kendall's tau	Ranked	Two
Cohen's kappa	Nominal	Usually two; can be modified to accommodate more than two

ficient. The specific notation for each type of coefficient is introduced when needed.

Standard Error of Measurement

In addition to knowing the relationship between repeated measurements, the researcher may wish to know how much a score is likely to vary with repeated measurements of the same subject. To determine the amount of measurement error, a researcher can take many repeated measures of the same subject and calculate the standard deviation of the scores; this standard deviation is known as the *standard error of measurement* (SEM). In practice, it is difficult to determine the standard error of measurement directly. Consider the effect of measuring knee flexion up to 100 times in a patient with limited knee motion to determine the standard error of measurement. The patient's knee flexion might improve during the course of testing by virtue of the exercise associated with taking so many measurements. Conversely, the patient's knee flexion might be reduced as the knee became progressively more painful. In any event, taking so many repeated measurements would likely result in a confounding of measurement error with actual treatment effects.

Because of the difficulty in directly determining the SEM, it is often estimated as follows[8(p62)]:

$$SEM = \sigma\sqrt{1 - r}$$

Assume that a researcher takes two knee flexion measurements on each of 10 patients. If the standard deviation of the measures is 5° and the correlation between the two measures is .80, then the estimated SEM is 2.2°.

$$SEM = 5\sqrt{1 - .80} = 5\sqrt{.20} = 5(.44) = 2.2$$

The SEM is a standard deviation of measurement errors, and measurement errors are assumed to be normally distributed. Thus, by combining our knowledge of the probabilities of the normal curve with this value for the SEM, we can conclude that approximately 68% of the time, a repeated measurement of knee flexion would be within 1 standard deviation of the mean or ±2.2° of the original measurement. Approximately 96% of the time, a repeated measurement of knee flexion would be within 2 standard deviations of the mean or ±4.4° of the original measurement.

◼ MEASUREMENT FRAMEWORKS

There are two basic frameworks in which measurement is conducted and evaluated: norm referenced and criterion referenced. *Norm-referenced* measures are those used to judge individual performance in relation to group norms. The statistical concepts of the mean and standard deviation are integral to norm-referenced measures. An example of a norm-referenced measure that, in the past, was of importance to physical therapists practicing in the United States was the physical therapy licensing examination. The examination was administered and scored nationally, and each state determined the level of proficiency it required of licensees. The level of proficiency was expressed as a standard deviation from the mean; most states licensed individuals who received a score of 1.5 standard deviations below the mean or higher for a particular administration of the test. If one administration of the 200-item test resulted in a mean of 150 and a standard deviation of 10, a state with a 1.5 standard deviation requirement would license therapists who received a score of 135 or higher on that administration of the test $[\overline{X} - 1.5(\sigma) = 150 - 1.5(10) = 135]$. If a second test administration resulted in a mean of 145 and a standard deviation of 12, the same state would license therapists who scored 127 or higher on the second test $[145 - 1.5(12) = 127]$. Thus, therapists were not held to an absolute standard of performance; they were evaluated with respect to the norms of the group with whom they took the examination.

Many clinical measurements are norm referenced. Blood pressure and pulse rates are evaluated against a range of normal values, muscular performance can be compared with average performance for age- and sex-matched groups, and a patient's function after a stroke may be compared with that of patients with comparable lesions.

A *criterion-referenced* measure is one in which each individual's performance is evaluated with respect to some absolute level of achievement. When a teacher establishes 75% as the minimum passing score in a course, this is a criterion-referenced measurement. If all students exceed the 75% criterion, all pass. If only 25% exceed the criterion, only 25% pass. Therapists use a criterion-referenced framework when they set specific performance criteria that patients have to meet in order to resume athletic competition or take an assistive device home. Today, the physical therapist licensure examination is a criterion-referenced instrument and all therapists are held to the same standard, regardless of the state in which they practice or the group with whom they take the examination.

■ MEASUREMENT RELIABILITY

Reliability is the "degree to which test scores are free from errors of measurement."[9(p19)] Other terms that are similar to reliability are *accuracy, stability,* and *consistency.* This section of the chapter introduces reliability theories, components, and measures.

Two Theories of Reliability

Two basic measurement theories—classical measurement theory and generalizability theory—provide somewhat different views of reliability. *Classical measurement theory* rests on the assumption that every measurement, or obtained score, consists of a true component and an error component. In addition, each person has a single true score on the measurement of interest. Because we can never know the true score for any measure, the relationship between repeated measurements is used to estimate measurement errors. A measurement is said to be reliable if the error component is small, thus allowing consistent estimation of the true quantity of interest. With classical measurement theory, all variability within a person's score is viewed as measurement error.[10]

Classical theories of reliability have been extended into what is known as generalizability theory. *Generalizability theory* recognizes that there are different sources of variability for any measure. Measurements are studied in ways that permit the researcher to divide the measurement error into sources of variability, or *facets,* of interest to the researcher.

To understand the differences between these two approaches, consider the measurement of forward head position with a device that provides a measurement in centimeters. Classical measurement theory assumes that every person has a true value for forward head position and that variations in a person's scores are measurement errors about the true score. In contrast, generalizability theory recognizes that differences in scores may be related to any number of different facets. Facets of interest to a given researcher for this example might be the subject's level of relaxation, his or her level of comfort with the particular examiner taking the measurement, the skill of the examiner, and the accuracy of the device used to measure forward head position. The generalizability approach seems to have a great deal of promise for the study of measurements in physical therapy because it acknowledges and provides a way to quantify the many sources of variability that physical therapists see in their patients from day to day.

Components of Reliability

Several components of reliability are examined frequently: instrument, intrarater, interrater, and intrasubject reliability. Although it is often difficult to completely separate these components from one another, readers of the literature need to be able to conceptualize the different components so that they can determine which components or combinations of components are being studied.

INSTRUMENT RELIABILITY. The reliability of the instrument itself may be assessed. There are three broad categories of physical therapy measurements: biophysiological, self-report, and observational. Different instruments are used to take the different types of measurements, and the appropriate approach for determining an instrument's reliability depends on the type of instrument.

Biophysiological measurements are obtained through the use of mechanical or electrical tools such as the dynamometer, goniometer, spirometer, scale, and electromyograph. The reliability of these instruments is assessed by taking repeated measurements across the range of values expected to be found in actual use of the device. Assessment of scores on two or more administrations of a test is often called *test-retest reliability*. For example, Stratford and colleagues determined the test-retest reliability of a hand-held dynamometer by repeated application of known loads from 10 to 60 kg.[11] If the output of a device is in analog format (i.e., the tester determines the value by examining a scale on the device), then it is impossible to separate the reliability of the device from the examiner's ability to read the scale accurately. If the device output is in digital format, separation of device reliability from examiner reliability is easier because the digital reading leaves little room for examiner interpretation.

Self-report measurements are obtained through the use of instruments that require subjects to give their own account of the phenomenon under study. Written surveys, standardized tests, pain scales, and interviews are examples of self-report measures. Forms of reliability for self-report tests include test-retest reliability, in which subjects take the same test on two or more occasions; parallel-form reliability, in which similar forms of a test are each administered once; split-half reliability, in which portions of a test are compared with each other; and internal consistency, in which responses to individual items are evaluated. The reader is referred to standard texts on educational or psychological measurement for a fuller description of assessment of the reliability of written tests.[12,13]

Observational measurements require only a human instrument with systematic knowledge of what to observe. The examiner may be an unobtrusive observer or may play a more active role. The knowledge may be in the examiner's head, or the examiner may use a checklist, such as the Movement Assessment of Infants (MAI).[14] The MAI is an example of a tool that uses both active and passive observation: Some of the categories in the MAI require observation of movement without intervention; however, the tone assessment portion of the examination requires hands-on manipulation of the infant.

Manual muscle testing and placement of patients into gait independence categories are additional examples of physical therapy measures that require only a human instrument with the knowledge of what to observe. The reliability of observational scales with multiple items can be examined for internal consistency in much the same manner as are written tests. Because the tester is the instrument, determining the reliability of observational measures is linked to determining intrarater and interrater reliability, described next.

INTRARATER RELIABILITY. A strict definition of *intrarater reliability* is "the consistency with which one rater assigns scores to a single set of responses on two occasions."[15(p141)] If a researcher is using videotape analysis to determine step length, he or she can view the same videotape on two different dates. Because the behavior being assessed both times is identical, any variability in scores is, in fact, related to measurement errors of the researcher. For most of the measurements we take in physical therapy, however, we do not have the ability to exactly reproduce the movement of interest, as a videotape would. If a therapist wishes to assess intrarater reliability of knee extension performance as measured by a hand-held dynamometer, the patient will have to perform the movement two or more times. In doing so, any variability in the force measurements can be attributed to either the examiner's measurement error or the subject's inconsistent performance. It is often difficult to separate the two.

INTERRATER RELIABILITY. A strict definition of *interrater reliability* holds that it is the "consistency of performance among different raters or judges in assigning scores to the same objects or responses. . . . [It] is determined when two or more raters judge the performance of one group

of subjects at the same point in time."[15(p140)] If two therapists simultaneously observe and rate an infant's spontaneous movements as part of a developmental assessment, the comparison between their scores would be a pure measure of interrater reliability because they observed the exact same episode of movement. If they observed the child at two different times, however, it would be impossible to separate the variability attributable to differences in the examiners from the variability attributable to actual differences in the child's behavior from time to time.

A variation of intertester reliability, triangulation, is used to document the consistency of the results of qualitative research. *Triangulation* consists of comparing responses across several different sources,[16] which in effect become different raters of the phenomenon of interest. The reader is referred to the literature on qualitative research for a further discussion of reliability issues in qualitative research.[16,17]

INTRASUBJECT RELIABILITY. The final component of reliability is associated with actual changes in subject performance from time to time. Some measurements in physical therapy may appear to be unreliable simply because the phenomenon being measured is inherently variable. It may be unreasonable to think, for example, that single measurements of spasticity could be reproducible because spasticity is such a changing phenomenon. Unless one has a perfectly reliable instrument and a perfectly reliable examiner, it is impossible to derive a pure measure of subject variability. Thus, most test-retest reliability calculations reflect some combination of instrument errors, tester errors, and true subject variability. Chapter 18 presents research designs for evaluating the different reliability components or combinations of components.

Quantification of Reliability

Reliability is quantified in two ways, as either relative or absolute reliability. *Relative reliability* examines the relationship between two or more sets of repeated measures; *absolute reliability* examines the variability of the scores from measurement to measurement.[10]

RELATIVE RELIABILITY. *Relative reliability* is based on the idea that if a measurement is reliable, individual measurements within a group will maintain their position within the group on repeated measurement. For example, people who score near the top of a distribution on a first measure would be expected to stay near the top of the distribution even if their actual scores changed from time to time. Relative reliability is measured with some form of a correlation coefficient, which, as mentioned earlier in this chapter, indicates the degree of association between repeated measurements of the variable of interest. Different correlation coefficients are used with different types of data, as shown in Table 17–3.[18–20] The mathematical basis of correlation coefficients and the rationale for choosing a particular coefficient are discussed in greater detail in Chapter 23.

We know that a correlation coefficient of 1.0 indicates a perfect association between repeated measures. How much less than 1.0 can a correlation be if it is to be considered reliable? This question is not easily answered. Currier cites two different sources in which adjectives were used to describe ranges of reliability coefficients (e.g., 0.80 to 1.00 was described as "very reliable" and 0.69 and below was said to constitute "poor reliability").[21] There are problems with using adjectives to describe ranges of correlation coefficients. First, there are many different formulas for correlation coefficients, and these different formulas may result in vastly different coefficients for the same data.[22] Second, there is not universal agreement about the appropriateness of the different formulas.[23,24]

Third, the value of a correlation coefficient is greatly affected by the range of scores used to calculate the coefficient. Correlation coefficients evaluate the consistency of an individual's position within a group; if the group as a whole shows little variability on the measure of interest,

there is little mathematical basis for determining relative positions and the correlation between the repeated measurements will be low. Thus, other things being equal, the interrater reliability correlation coefficient calculated on a group of patients with knee flexion range-of-motion values between 70° and 90° would be lower than one calculated on a group with a broader range of values, say, between 30° and 90°.

Fourth, most of the correlation coefficients are not very good at detecting systematic errors. A systematic error is one that is predictable. For example, assume that on a first measurement of limb girth a researcher used one tape measure and on a second measurement used a different tape measure that was missing the first centimeter. There would be a systematic measurement error of 1 cm on the second measure. However, if each subject's position within the group were maintained, the correlation coefficients would remain high despite the absolute difference.

Because of these four problems with correlation coefficients, a rigid criterion for acceptable reliability is inappropriate. In addition, the component of reliability being studied affects the interpretation of the correlation coefficient. For example, one would ordinarily expect there to be less variability in scores recorded on a single day than in scores recorded over a longer time period. Similarly, intrarater reliability coefficients are generally higher than interrater reliability coefficients. Finally, if a researcher is deciding which of two measurement tools to use and has found that one has an intrarater reliability of .99 and the other an intrarater reliability of .80, then .80 seems unacceptable. On the other hand, if a highly abstract concept is being measured and a researcher is deciding between two instruments with intratester reliability coefficients of .45 and .60, then .60 may become acceptable.

Because of the limitations of determining relative reliability with correlation coefficients, researchers should often supplement relative information with absolute information.

ABSOLUTE RELIABILITY. *Absolute reliability* indicates the extent to which a score varies on repeated measurement. The statistic used to measure absolute reliability is the standard error of measurement, or SEM, described earlier in the chapter. Unfortunately, many researchers who report measurement studies in the physical therapy literature specify only the relative reliability of the measurement and not the absolute reliability.[25] For a physical therapist to make meaningful statements about whether a patient's or subject's condition has changed, the therapist must know how much variability in the scores could be expected solely because of measurement errors. This is illustrated in Diamond and associates' study of the reliability of diabetic foot evaluation.[26] The interrater reliability coefficients for selected foot biomechanical measurements ranged from .58 to .89. The SEM of these same measurements ranged from 1° to 4°, but the smaller SEMs were not always associated with the higher correlation coefficients! For example, the interrater reliability coefficient for tibial varum was .66 and the SEM was 1°. This indicates that approximately 96% of the time, the true value for tibial varum would be expected to fall within $\pm2°$ of the observed measurement (observed score ±2 SEMs). Conversely, a higher correlation coefficient (.89) was associated with interrater reliability for calcaneal inversion, but this measurement had an SEM of 3°. In this instance, we would expect that approximately 96% of the time the true value for calcaneal inversion would be within $\pm6°$ of the observed measurement.

Thus in Diamond and associates' study, the correlation coefficient and the SEM provided contradictory information: The correlation coefficients implied that measurement of calcaneal inversion was more reliable than tibial varum, but the SEM results implied the opposite. Because correlation coefficients and SEMs provide different and often contradictory views of reliability, it is important that researchers document both. Documenting both may prohibit straightforward interpretation of the results of a measurement study, but uncertainty based on complete information is preferable to a false sense of certainty based on incomplete information.

■ MEASUREMENT VALIDITY

Measurement validity is the "appropriateness, meaningfulness, and usefulness of the specific inferences made from test scores."[9(p9)] Reliability is a necessary, but not sufficient, condition for validity. An unreliable measure is also an invalid measurement, because measurements with a great deal of error have little meaning or utility. A reliable measure is valid only if, in addition to being repeatable, it provides meaningful information.

Earlier we defined *research validity* as the extent to which the conclusions of research are believable and useful (see Chapter 7). Note that although the two types of validity relate to different areas—measurement and research design, respectively—they are similar in that they both relate to the *utility* of findings and not to the findings themselves. Thus, measurement validity is not a quality associated with a particular instrument or test, but rather is a quality associated with the way in which test results are applied.

For example, active range-of-motion measurements may provide a valid indication of muscle performance in patients with full passive range of motion. The same active range-of-motion measures do not provide valid information about muscle performance in patients with significantly restricted passive motion. In these patients, the measure is not a meaningful indicator of muscle performance but rather an indicator of some combination of joint mobility and muscle performance.

Measurement validity is often subdivided into several categories. Construct, content, and criterion validity are discussed subsequently.

Construct Validity

Construct validity is the validity of the abstract constructs that underlie measures. For example, strength is a construct that is poorly delineated in the physical therapy literature. When physical therapists speak of strength, they may mean many different things. Strength may be conceptualized as the ability to move a body part against gravity, the ability to generate speed-specific torque, the ability to lift a certain weight a certain number of times in a certain time period, or the ability to accomplish some functional task. Manual muscle tests, isokinetic tests, work performance tests, and functional tests may all be valid measures of a particular conceptualization of strength or muscle performance.

To maximize construct validity, physical therapy researchers must first be very clear about the constructs they wish to measure. If strength is an important construct within a study, is it best conceptualized as functional strength, static strength, eccentric strength, or some other aspect of this extremely broad construct? Once the underlying construct of interest is clarified, it must be operationalized to make it measurable. An *operational definition* is a specific description of the way in which a construct is presented or measured within a study. For example, Ellison and associates studied patterns of hip rotation motions in healthy subjects and in patients with low back pain.[27] They provided operational definitions of healthy subjects (university students and staff who had no low back or hip pain that prevented them from working or attending school in the past year), patients with low back pain (patients at one clinic who were undergoing treatment for back pain at the time of the study), hip rotation measurements (a detailed description of measurements taken in the prone position), and a range-of-motion pattern classification (a detailed description of rules for placing each subject into one of four groups).

Although developing operational definitions is necessary for construct validity, it does not *guarantee* construct validity. One might argue that in Ellison and associates' study, the patient group was defined too broadly or that hip rotation measures should have been taken in the sitting position. Supplying readers with the operational definitions used in a study allows them to form their own opinion of the validity of the measurements.

Content Validity

Content validity is the extent to which a measure is a complete representation of the concept of interest. Content validity is more often a concern with self-report or observational tools than with biophysiological ones. When students come away from a test saying, "Can you believe how many questions there were on . . . ?," they are talking about the content validity of the test, because they are questioning whether the emphasis on the exam was an accurate representation of the course content.

Murney and Campbell[28] tested a form of content validity of the Test of Infant Motor Performance when they tested what they referred to as the "ecological relevance" of the test items. They found that 98% of the items in the test corresponded to environmental demands placed on the infant during normal daily activities. In a more traditional way of testing content validity, the test developers also asked a panel of experts to review the items in the test to ensure that a wide range of possible environmental demands was included within the test. When a researcher is designing a questionnaire or a functional scale, he or she should have its content validity evaluated by knowledgeable peers or evaluated in natural settings as part of the pilot testing of the instrument. These evaluation procedures may lead to the addition of items, the deletion of irrelevant or redundant items, or reassessment of the emphasis given to particular topics.

Criterion Validity

Criterion validity is the extent to which one measure is systematically related to other measures or outcomes. Whereas relative reliability compares repeated administrations of the *same* measurement, criterion validity compares administration of *different* measures. The mathematical basis for determining the degree of association between two different measures is similar to that for determining the association between repeated administrations of the same measurement. Therefore the correlation coefficients used to determine relative reliability are often used to measure criterion validity as well. The epidemiological concepts of specificity and sensitivity, described in Chapter 14, are also useful for determining criterion validity. Criterion validity can be subdivided into concurrent and predictive validity on the basis of the timing of the different measures.

Concurrent validity is at issue when one is comparing a new tool or procedure with a measurement standard. This was done when the ability of two tools to detect occult ankle fractures was determined concurrently: The new procedure was the presence of a 15-mm ankle effusion on plain radiograph and the standard was an ankle fracture detected by computed tomography.[29]

Predictive validity relates to whether a test done at one point in time is predictive of future status. Harris and associates studied the predictive validity of the MAI, described earlier in this chapter.[30] They compared the risk scores of 4-month-old infants with pediatrician assessments of their motor development at 2 years. More than 80% of the children who showed signs of cerebral palsy at 2 years had been identified as at risk by the MAI when they were 4 months old. However, there was also a 44% rate of false-positive tests, in which children rated normal at 2 years had had an abnormal MAI at 4 months. Thus, the MAI showed good sensitivity (it identified as abnormal a high percentage of children eventually determined to have cerebral palsy) but low specificity (it also identified as abnormal a high percentage of children who were apparently normal at 2 years of age). Determining the predictive validity of a screening measure such as the MAI is an essential, although obviously time-consuming, process. The premise of many screening tests is that they allow early identification of some phenomenon that is not usually apparent until some later date. The usefulness of such measures cannot be determined unless their predictive validity is known.

SUMMARY

Measurement is a systematic process by which things are differentiated. Measurements can be identified by scale (nominal, ordinal, interval, or ratio), type (discrete or continuous), and framework (norm referenced or criterion referenced). Statistical concepts of importance to measurement theory include the frequency distribution, mean, variance, standard deviation, normal curve, correlation, and standard error of measurement (SEM). Reliability is the extent to which a measure is free from error. The components of reliability include instrument, tester, and subject variability. Relative measures of reliability are correlation coefficients; the absolute measure of reliability is the standard error of measurement. Validity is the meaningfulness and utility of an application of a measurement. The components of validity include construct, content, and criterion validity.

REFERENCES

1. Information for authors. *Phys Ther.* 1998;78:526–527.
2. Hopkins KD, Stanley JC. *Educational and Psychological Measurement and Evaluation.* 6th ed. Englewood Cliffs, NJ: Prentice-Hall; 1981:3.
3. Nunnally JC. *Psychometric Theory.* 2nd ed. New York, NY: McGraw-Hill; 1978:3.
4. Kerlinger FN. *Foundations of Behavioral Research.* 3rd ed. Fort Worth, Tex: Holt, Rinehart & Winston; 1986:392.
5. Safrit MJ. An overview of measurement. In: Safrit MJ, Wood TM, eds. *Measurement Concepts in Physical Education and Exercise Science.* Champaign, Ill: Human Kinetics Books; 1989.
6. Merbitz C, Morris J, Grip JC. Ordinal scales and foundations of misinference. *Arch Phys Med Rehabil.* 1989;70:308–312.
7. Rothstein JM, Echternach JL. *Primer on Measurement: An Introductory Guide to Measurement Issues.* Alexandria, Va: American Physical Therapy Association; 1993.
8. Baumgartner TA. Norm-referenced measurement: reliability. In: Safrit MJ, Wood TM, eds. *Measurement Concepts in Physical Education and Exercise Science.* Champaign, Ill: Human Kinetics Books; 1989.
9. American Educational Research Association, American Psychological Association, and National Committee on Measurement in Education. *Standards for Educational and Psychological Testing.* Washington, DC: American Psychological Association; 1985.
10. Morrow JR. Generalizability theory. In: Safrit MJ, Wood TM, eds. *Measurement Concepts in Physical Education*

and Exercise Science. Champaign, Ill: Human Kinetics Books; 1989:74.

11. Stratford PW, Norman GR, McIntosh JM. Generalizability of grip strength measurements in patients with tennis elbow. *Phys Ther.* 1989;69:276–281.

12. Litwin MS. *The Survey Kit, Volume 7: How to Measure Survey Reliability and Validity.* Thousand Oaks, Calif: Sage Publications; 1995.

13. Cronbach LJ. *Essentials of Psychological Testing.* 5th ed. New York, NY: Harper & Row; 1990.

14. Harris SR, Haley SM, Tada WL, Swanson MW. Reliability of observational measures of the Movement Assessment of Infants. *Phys Ther.* 1989; 64:471–477.

15. Waltz CF, Strickland OL, Lenz ER. *Measurement in Nursing Research.* Philadelphia, Pa: FA Davis Co; 1984.

16. Denzin NK, Lincoln YS, eds. *Handbook of Qualitative Research.* Thousand Oaks, Calif: Sage Publications; 1994.

17. Miles MB, Huberman AM. *Qualitative Data Analysis: An Expanded Sourcebook.* 2nd ed. Thousand Oaks, Calif: Sage Publications; 1994.

18. Cohen J. A coefficient of agreement for nominal scales. *Educational and Psychological Measurement.* 1960;20:37–46.

19. Haley SM, Osberg JS. Kappa coefficient calculation using multiple ratings per subject: a special communication. *Phys Ther.* 1989;69:970–974.

20. Bartko JJ. The intraclass correlation coefficient as a measure of reliability. *Psychol Rep.* 1966;19:3–11.

21. Currier DP. *Elements of Research in Physical Therapy.* 3rd ed. Baltimore, Md: Williams & Wilkins; 1990:167.

22. Shrout PE, Fleiss JL. Intraclass correlations: uses in assessing rater reliability. *Psychol Bull.* 1979;86:420–428.

23. Bartko JJ, Carpenter WT. On the methods and theory of reliability. *J Nerv Ment Dis.* 1976;163:307–317.

24. Hart DL. Invited commentary. *Phys Ther.* 1989;69:102–103.

25. Stratford P. Reliability: consistency or differentiating among subjects? *Phys Ther.* 1989;69:299–300.

26. Diamond JE, Mueller MJ, Delitto A, Sinacore DR. Reliability of a diabetic foot evaluation. *Phys Ther.* 1989;69:797–802.

27. Ellison JB, Rose SJ, Sahrmann SA. Patterns of hip rotation range of motion: a comparison between healthy subjects and patients with low back pain. *Phys Ther.* 1990;70:537–541.

28. Murney ME, Campbell SK. The ecological relevance of the Test of Infant Motor Performance elicited scale items. *Phys Ther.* 1998;78:479–489.

29. Clark TWI, Janzen DL, Logan PM, Connell DG. Improving the detection of radiographically occult ankle fractures: positive predictive value of an ankle joint effusion. *Clin Radiol.* 1996;51:632–636.

30. Harris SR, Swanson MW, Andrews MS, et al. Predictive validity of the "Movement Assessment of Infants." *Dev Behav Pediatr.* 1984;5:336–342.

Methodological Research

Reliability Designs
  Sources of Variability
  Levels of Standardization
    Nonstandardized Approach
    Highly Standardized Approach
    Partially Standardized Approach
  Subject Selection
  Range of Scores
  Optimization Designs
    Standardization Designs
    Mean Designs

Reliability in Nonmethodological
    Studies
Validity Designs
  Construct Validation
  Content Validation
  Criterion Validation

The goals of methodological research are to document and improve the reliability and validity of clinical and research measurements. Because measurement is an integral part of clinical and research documentation, research that examines physical therapy measurements is important to the profession. In addition to the importance of measurement as a topic in its own right, documentation of the reliability and validity of the measures used within a study is a necessary component of all research. This chapter provides a framework for the design of methodological research. Reliability designs are presented first, followed by validity designs.

■ RELIABILITY DESIGNS

The reliability of a measurement is influenced by many factors, including (1) the sources of variability studied, (2) the subjects selected, and (3) the range of scores exhibited by the sample. Each of these factors is illustrated in this chapter by a hypothetical example of measurement of joint range of motion. The hypothetical example is supplemented by relevant examples from the literature. After these three general factors are discussed, two specialized types of reliability studies are considered: reliability optimization and reliability documentation within nonmethodological research.

Sources of Variability

Differences found in repeated measurements of the same characteristic can be attributed to instrument, intrarater, interrater, and intrasubject components. Within each of these four reliability components there are many additional sources of variability. When designing reliability studies, researchers must clearly delineate which of the reliability components they wish to study and which sources of variability they wish to study within each component. To assist with this task, it is helpful to list the four reliability components and all possible sources of variation for each component. Table 18–1 shows some potential sources of variability in passive range-of-motion scores as measured with a universal goniometer.

Once the sources of variability within the measurement are delineated, the researcher must determine which of the components will be the focus of his or her methodological study. As is the case with all research design, the investigator designing methodological research must identify a problem that needs to be studied. Is there a knowledge deficit about the interinstrument reliability of goniometers of different sizes or designs? Is it important to establish the degree of variation that can be expected in a particular measurement made by a single therapist? What is the magnitude of differences that could be expected if several therapists take measurements of the same person? Is subject performance consistent across days or weeks?

Each of these questions relates to one of the four components of reliability: instrument, intrarater, interrater, and intrasubject. However, in many methodological studies, more than one of the reliability components are examined, or the reliability components are intertwined and cannot be separated clearly. For example, Nussbaum and Downes[1] examined the reliability of a pressure-pain algometer by using two measurers, each taking three measurements on 3 different days. Intrarater, interrater, and intrasubject reliability are examined, although they cannot necessarily be completely separated from one another. For example, the day-to-day reliability

TABLE 18–1 Sources of Variability in Passive Range-of-Motion Measurements with a Universal Goniometer

Instrument
Loose axis (slips during measurement)
Tight axis (too difficult to move precisely)
Interinstrument differences

Intrarater
Variations in subject positioning
Inconsistent identification of landmarks
Variable end-range pressure
Inconsistent stabilization
Reading errors

Interrater
Variations in subject positioning
Inconsistent identification of landmarks
Variable end-range pressure
Inconsistent stabilization
Differing ability to gain subjects' trust
Different end-digit preference
Reading errors

Intrasubject
Varying levels of pain
Differing tolerance to end-range pressure
Mood changes
Differing activities prior to measurement
Biological variation

involves consistency of examiners across the 3 days as well as consistency across days of the subjects' perceptions of pain in response to the pressure of the instrument.

Levels of Standardization

Once the sources of variability have been determined, it is necessary to determine the degree of standardization in the measurement protocol. The degree of standardization is the number of sources of variability within a reliability component that are controlled.

Consider three different reasons to study intertester reliability of goniometric measurements. The purpose of one study might be to determine interrater reliability of goniometric measurements as they occur in the clinic, without any standardization of technique between therapists. The purpose of a second study might be to determine the upper limits of interrater reliability with a highly standardized protocol. The purpose of a third study might be to determine interrater reliability with a level of standardization that would be feasible for most clinics to achieve.

The preceding three purpose statements correspond to three general approaches to reliability that are seen in the literature: nonstandardized, highly standardized, and partially standardized. The three approaches differ in the extent to which the sources of variability are controlled within each of the reliability components under study. For intertester reliability in the measurement of passive motion with a goniometer, Table 18–1 lists seven possible sources of variability: positioning, landmark identification, end-range pressure, stabilization, patient trust in the therapist, end-digit preference (some therapists always round measurements to the nearest 5°, others round to even numbers only, and others do not round off at all), and reading errors. Let's consider how nonstandardized, highly standardized, and partially standardized studies would be applied to these sources of variability to determine intertester reliability of goniometric measurement.

NONSTANDARDIZED APPROACH. A completely nonstandardized approach would control none of these sources of variability and would establish the lower limit for the reliability component studied. The basic design of a nonstandardized study of intertester reliability would be to have each therapist take measurements privately so as not to influence the technique of the other therapists within the study.

Watkins and associates studied the reliability of goniometric measures of knee range of motion.[2] Because they wished to study reliability under typical clinical conditions, they did not train their examiners in standardized procedures. In fact, they ensured that the second therapist never saw the first therapist taking measurements, nor did they require standardized positioning of the patient or the goniometer.

HIGHLY STANDARDIZED APPROACH. In contrast to a nonstandardized approach, a highly standardized approach would control many of the possible sources of variability to determine the upper limits of the reliability of the component. Whereas a nonstandardized approach seeks to document the reliability of measurements as they commonly occur, a highly standardized approach seeks to document reliability in an ideal situation. A highly standardized approach to taking measurements may be a useful way of separating measurement error from subject variability.

In a highly standardized study of intertester goniometric reliability, positioning, stabilization, landmarks, end-range pressure, and end-digit preference would all be controlled. Positioning for shoulder internal rotation, for example, could be controlled by having all therapists take the measurements with the patient supine on the same firm plinth. Stabilization could be controlled by strapping the patient's chest to prevent substitution of scapular or trunk movements. To control inconsistent identification of landmarks, landmarks could be marked on the subjects and left in place while all therapists take their measurements. End-range pressure could be standardized by having an assistant provide a pre-determined force as documented by a hand-held dynamometer. Finally, end-digit preference could be controlled by instructing therapists to report the measurement to the nearest degree. The experimental protocol for such a study might be that one therapist positions each patient and three other therapists each take a measurement in rapid succession. Such a protocol would establish the upper limits of intertester reliability and would eliminate the effects of subject variation because the subject would not be moved between measurements.

Mayerson and Milano used a highly standardized approach to study goniometric measurement reliability.[3] A healthy subject was positioned in 22 consistent extremity joint positions; two therapists each took two measurements at each position. The protocol eliminated variability due to subject positioning, stabilization, end-range pressure, and changes in subject motion. Thus, the protocol provided a test of the reliability of goniometer placement and reading. They found that both intertester and intratester differences could confidently be expected to fall within 4° of each other in a highly standardized measurement protocol.

PARTIALLY STANDARDIZED APPROACH. The third approach to determining the sources of variability to be studied within an investigation of reliability is the partially standardized approach. As indicated by its name, this approach falls between the extremes of the nonstandardized and highly standardized approaches by standardizing a few sources of variability while leaving others non-standardized. The sources of variability that are standardized often reflect the realities of the clinic. The hypothetical highly standardized study of internal rotation range of motion described previously is probably unrealistic for routine clinical use: An assistant is not always available to position the patient, and landmarks are likely to be washed off between treatment sessions. A partially standardized measurement protocol might therefore standardize positioning and stabilization but allow landmark determination and end-range pressure to vary among therapists. The experimental protocol for a partially standardized study requires educating the examiners in the standardized methods to be employed in the study.

Youdas and colleagues used a partially standardized approach to study the reliability of cervical range-of-motion measurements taken by visual estimation, with a universal goniometer, and with a cervical range-of-motion instrument.[4] Therapists were trained in the use of a standardized protocol for positioning of the subjects; placement of the measuring devices and a warm-up protocol for subjects were also standardized.

The appropriate level of standardization for reliability studies is debated in the rehabilitation literature. Some researchers argue for the use of nonstandardized approaches applicable to clinical settings[5]; others argue for the use of highly and partially standardized approaches to isolate which aspects of measurements are unreliable.[3,6] It seems reasonable to accept that each approach is useful for specific purposes. Nonstandardized studies describe reliability as it is; highly standardized studies present idealized reliability estimates and examine the impact of limited sources of variability on reliability; partially standardized studies describe reliability with moderate levels of standardization that could be achievable in clinical settings.

Subject Selection

As is the case with all types of research, subject selection in reliability studies influences the external validity of the study; the study results can be generalized only to the types of subjects studied. Therefore, the reliability of an instrument should be determined using the individuals on whom the instrument will be used in practice. If the measure is a clinical one, it is best to determine its reliability on patients who would ordinarily require this measurement as part of their care. Watkins and associates did just this in their study of the reliability of knee range-of-motion measurements.[2] In fact, they even divided their patients into diagnostic categories to determine whether the measurements were more reliable for patients with certain types of knee dysfunction. The inappropriate use of normal subjects to establish the reliability of clinical measures has the potential to inflate reliability estimates because normal subjects may be easier to measure than patients. Pain, obliteration of landmarks because of deformity, or difficulty following directions because of neurological impairment may make it difficult to take measurements in patients.

If a researcher ultimately wishes to determine norms for certain characteristics, it is appropriate to determine the reliability of the measurements using normal subjects. If the measurement in question is part of a screening tool, such as a flexibility test that might be administered at a fitness fair, then a broad sampling of the individuals likely to be screened should be used to establish the reliability of the measurement.

Range of Scores

The reliability of a measure should be determined over the range of scores expected for that measure. There are two reasons for this. First, as discussed in Chapter 17, a restricted range of scores will lead to low reliability coefficients even in the presence of small absolute differences in repeated measurements. The use of normal subjects often restricts the range of scores within a study, thereby reducing the reliability coefficients and underestimating the reliability of the measure in clinical use. In contrast, using an extremely heterogeneous group (e.g., a mixed group of patients and nonpatients) will generally overestimate the reliability of the measure for clinical use—but might be the ideal mix of individuals for establishing the reliability of the tool for screening purposes.

Second, reliability may vary at different places in the range of scores because of difficulties unique to taking measurements at particular points in the range. For example, Nussbaum and Downes[1] found that interrater reliability was greatest when testing subjects with lower pain thresholds. Researchers need to carefully consider the characteristics of the individuals on whom the test or tool will be used and select a research sample that matches those characteristics.

Optimization Designs

In many instances, researchers have found less than satisfactory reliability for physical therapy measures, particularly as they are implemented in the clinic.[7-9] Such research is useful because it may lead to a healthy skepticism about the measurements we use. In and of itself, however, *documenting* the reliability of a clinical measure does nothing to *improve* its reliability. Improving the reliability of physical therapy measures requires that researchers study ways to optimize reliability. There are two basic designs for optimization research: standardization and mean designs.

STANDARDIZATION DESIGNS. Standardization designs compare the reliabilities of measurements taken under different sets of conditions. For example, suppose that the result of a nonstandardized reliability study was that the standard error of measurement (SEM) for passive internal rotation range of motion was 10°. Furthermore, suppose the result of a highly standardized, but clinically unfeasible, study was that the SEM was 1°. A standardization study might be developed with a goal of determining what level of standardization is needed to achieve an SEM of 3°. To do so, a researcher might determine reliability with standardized positioning. If, despite the positioning change, the SEM is still too large, both position and upper chest stabilization might be standardized. The level of standardization would be increased until the reliability goal was met. A reverse sequence could also be implemented by starting with a highly standardized procedure and eliminating standardization procedures that are not feasible in the clinic.

MEAN DESIGNS. Mean designs compare the reliabilities of single measurements and also compare the reliabilities of measurements averaged across several trials. This design is particularly appropriate for measures that are difficult to standardize for clinical use or for characteristics that are expected to show a great deal of natural variation.[10] Connelly and colleagues used a mean strategy to study the reliability of walking tests in a frail elderly population.[11] Two raters took three measures on each of 2 days. They then computed reliability coefficients comparing the means for each day between raters, the best score for each day between raters, and the first measure for each day between raters. They found that the reliability coefficients were highest when they used the mean of three measures, were worst when they used the first measure, and were intermediate when they used the best measure. Such information helps clinicians and researchers make knowledgeable decisions about whether to rely on single measures or whether to average the results of repeated measurements.

Reliability in Nonmethodological Studies

Useful research studies must be based on measurements that are reliable. Measurement reliability in nonmethodological studies should often be addressed at two times during the study: during the design phase and during the implementation phase.

In the design phase, the researcher must determine which of several possible instruments to choose, which of several possible measurement protocols to follow, and which of several raters to use. Studies of interinstrument, interrater, or intrarater reliability components may be needed to make these decisions.

When conducting a pilot reliability study, the researcher needs to simulate the research conditions as closely as possible. The same types of subjects, settings, time pressures, and the like should be employed. The results of a pilot reliability study conducted after clinic hours, when therapists and subjects have much time and few distractions, may differ from those of the actual study if the actual study takes place during clinic hours, when time is short and distractions abound.

Reliability measures should also be taken during implementation of a study. Several authors have found a decline in reliability from that seen during a training phase to that occurring during the experimental phase.[12,13] Researchers can establish reliability during the course of a study by taking repeated measures of all subjects, using pretest and posttest scores of a con-

trol group as the reliability indicator, or taking repeated measures of selected subjects at random. Which strategy is adopted depends on factors such as the expense of the measures, the risks of repeated measurements to subjects, and the number of subjects in the study.

■ VALIDITY DESIGNS

As discussed previously, the validity of a measurement is the extent to which a particular use of the measurement is meaningful. Measures are validated through argument about and research into the soundness of the interpretations made from them. To make sound interpretations, a researcher must first be confident that the measurements are reproducible, or reliable. Recall that although reliability is necessary for validity, it does not validate the meaning behind the measure. This section of the chapter presents several designs for research to determine the construct, content, and criterion validity of measurements.

Construct Validation

Constructs are artificial frameworks that are not directly observable. Strength, function, proprioception, and pain are constructs used frequently in physical therapy. Because the constructs themselves are not directly observable, there are no absolute standards against which measurements can be compared to determine if they are valid indicators of the constructs. Consider, for example, all the different measures that physical therapists use to represent the construct of strength: manual muscle testing, the number of times that a particular weight can be lifted, handheld dynamometers, and a multitude of isokinetic tests. All are appropriate for some purposes, but none is a definitive measure of strength.

In the absence of a clear-cut standard, persuasive argument becomes one means by which the construct validity of measurements is established.[14] A researcher who wishes to assess strength gains following a particular program of exercise must be prepared to defend the appropriateness of the measurements he or she used for the type of exercise program studied. Such considerations include whether the measure should test concentric or eccentric contractions, whether the test should be isometric or should sample strength throughout the range of motion, and whether the test should be conducted in an open or closed kinetic chain position.

A second way in which construct validity is established is by making predictions about the patterns of test scores that should be seen if the measure is valid.[15] One method is to examine the convergence and divergence of measures thought to represent similar and different constructs, respectively. For example, one study that sought to validate the Short Form-36 (SF-36) health survey questionnaire as a measure of general health status in the British population did so by having almost 2000 patients take both the SF-36 and the Nottingham health profile.[16] If the SF-36 was valid in this population, they predicted that the overall score would correlate fairly well with the overall score on the Nottingham health profile. In addition, they predicted that there would be higher correlations between the physical scales on the two tests than there would be between the physical and mental scales. For the most part, they found this to be true. For example, the strength of the correlation between the physical functioning scale on the SF-36 and the physical morbidity scale on the Nottingham health profile was 0.52; between the physical functioning scale on the SF-36 and the social isolation scale on the Nottingham health profile it was only 0.20. Construct validity is best supported when the scores on items thought to represent the same construct are highly associated (convergence) and when scores on items that are theoretically different have a low association (divergence).

Another set of predictions that is often used to establish construct validity relates to the performance of "extreme groups" or "known groups" on the test of interest. Ware and coworkers did this to evaluate the construct validity of the SF-12, a short form of the SF-36 health status survey.[17] Like the SF-36, the SF-12 has a "physical" health component and a "mental" health component. They predicted that the physical scales would differentiate between groups with differing levels of known physical disability, but that they would not differentiate between groups with differing levels of known mental disability. For the most part, the SF-12 was able to correctly differentiate between the groups and the groups with physical conditions showed greater deficits on the physical scale than they did on the mental scale, and vice versa. Creative researchers are able to envision the optimal performance of their tests and then set up research situations to test how close the tests come to meeting their predictions for optimal performance.

Content Validation

Content validation involves documenting that a test provides an adequate sampling of the behavior or knowledge that it is measuring. To determine the content validity of a measure, a researcher compares the items in the test against the actual practice of interest. There are four basic issues a researcher must consider when determining content validity: (1) the sample on whom the measure is validated; (2) the content's completeness; (3) the content's relevance; and (4) the content's emphasis. As an example, consider the content validity of the Clinical Performance Instrument (CPI), an assessment tool used widely to evaluate students on clinical rotations in physical therapy.[18] The CPI consists of over 40 clinical behaviors that should be exhibited by physical therapy students. If the CPI has content validity, then it should accurately represent the demands that clinical practice places on physical therapists.

To determine content validity, a researcher

needs to determine an appropriate group on whom the content can be validated. To determine the content validity of the CPI, should a random sampling of physical therapists be selected for observation of their practice? Should therapists with less than 2 years of experience constitute the sample? Should students on clinical rotations be studied? If the CPI is viewed as a tool that determines readiness for entry-level physical therapy practice, then the group of new therapists may be the most appropriate group on whom the content should be validated. If the CPI is viewed as a tool that assesses performance on clinical rotations, then the student group may be the appropriate group on whom the tool should be validated.

Once the subject group has been identified, test content can be compared with actual practice. If the validity were perfect, all activities of the observed therapists would be represented in the CPI, and all items in the CPI would be demonstrated in actual practice. In addition, more emphasis would be placed on items that are frequently performed in actual practice and less emphasis would be placed on infrequently performed items.

Criterion Validation

The criterion validation of a measure is determined by comparing it with an accepted standard of measurement. The major considerations in designing a criterion validation study are selecting the criterion; timing the administration of the tests; and selecting a sample for testing.

Three different criteria against which a test is compared are found in the literature. The first criterion is essentially *instrumentation accuracy*. The accuracy of the measurement provided by an instrument is determined by comparing the reading on the device with a standard measure. Examples in the literature include comparing the angular measurements of a goniometer with known angles[2] and testing a digitizer against known lengths.[19] Complex instruments have specific standardization procedures that allow

the investigator to check the instrument against known standards and either make adjustments until the device readings accurately reflect the standard or develop equations that can be used to correct for inaccuracies.[20]

The second criterion is a concurrent one. A concurrent criterion is applied at the same time the test in question is validated. Irrgang and colleagues determined the *concurrent validity* of their new Activities of Daily Living Scale of the Knee Outcome Survey with the Lysholm Knee Rating Scale by administering both scales multiple times for almost 400 patients with knee impairments.[21]

The third criterion is predictive. A measure has *predictive validity* if the result of its administration at one point in time is highly associated with future status. There are three difficulties in doing predictive studies: determining the criterion itself, determining the timing of administration of the criterion, and maintaining a good sample of subjects measured on both occasions. Harris and associates studied the predictive validity of the Movement Assessment of Infants (MAI) by comparing children's scores on the MAI at 4 months of age with an assessment of their motor development at 1 to 2 years.[22]

The importance of timing is also illustrated in the MAI validity study. By assessing motor development at 1 to 2 years, Harris and associates were testing relatively gross motor abilities. If status at the age of 5 years were assessed, perhaps fine motor deficits would begin to show themselves in problems with handwriting and drawing. If status at the age of 12 years were assessed, subtle coordination problems may show up as the child begins to participate in sports activities.

The third difficulty with predictive validity studies is the sample available for study. Because these studies extend over time, there may be differential loss of subjects. For example, in Harris and associates' study, only 80% of the children with 4-month MAI scores also had 1- or 2-year motor assessment scores.[22] It is possible that the majority of the children who were not followed up were normal. Differential loss of normal subjects would likely result in inflated validity estimates.

■ SUMMARY

Methodological research is conducted to document and improve measuring tools by assessing their reliability and validity. The major components of reliability are instrument, intrarater, interrater, and intrasubject reliability. Reliability research can be classified according to whether the measurement protocol used is nonstandardized, partially standardized, or highly standardized. Subjects should be selected on the basis of whether they would likely be assessed with the tool in clinical situations; in addition, subjects who demonstrate a wide range of scores should be selected. Construct validity is determined through logical argument and assessment of the convergence of similar tests and divergence of different tests. Content validity is determined by assessing the completeness, relevancy, and emphasis of the items within a test. Criterion validity is determined by comparing one measure with an accepted standard of measurement.

REFERENCES

1. Nussbaum EL, Downes L. Reliability of clinical pressure-pain algometric measurements obtained on consecutive days. *Phys Ther.* 1998;78:160–169.
2. Watkins MA, Riddle DL, Lamb RL, Personius WJ. Reliability of goniometric measurements and visual estimates of knee range of motion obtained in a clinical setting. *Phys Ther.* 1991;71:90–97.
3. Mayerson NH, Milano RA. Goniometric reliability in physical medicine. *Arch Phys Med Rehabil.* 1984;65:92–94.
4. Youdas JW, Carey JR, Garrett TR. Reliability of measurements of cervical spine range of motion—comparison of three methods. *Phys Ther.* 1991;71:98–104.
5. Riddle DL. Commentary. *Phys Ther.* 1991;71:105–106.
6. Youdas JW, Carey JR, Garrett TR. Author response. *Phys Ther.* 1991;71:106.
7. Riddle DL, Rothstein JM, Lamb RL. Goniometric reliability in a clinical setting: shoulder measurements. *Phys Ther.* 1987;67:668–673.
8. Elveru RA, Rothstein JM, Lamb RL. Goniometric reliability in a clinical setting: subtalar and ankle joint measurements. *Phys Ther.* 1988;68:672–677.
9. Potter NA, Rothstein JM. Intertester reliability for selected clinical tests of the sacroiliac joint. *Phys Ther.* 1985;65:1671–1675.
10. Stratford PW. Summarizing the results of multiple strength trials: truth or consequence. *Physiotherapy Can* 1992;44:14–18.
11. Connelly DM, Stevenson TJ, Vandervoort AA. Between- and within-rater reliability of walking tests in a frail elderly population. *Physiotherapy Can* 1996;48:47–51.
12. Mitchell SK. Interobserver agreement, reliability, and generalizability of data collected in observational studies. *Psychol Bull.* 1979;86:376–390.
13. Taplin PS, Reid JB. Effects of instructional set and experiment influence on observer reliability. *Child Dev.* 1973;44:547–554.
14. Cronbach LJ. *Essentials of Psychological Testing.* New York, NY: Harper & Row; 1990:185.
15. Streiner DL, Norman GR. *Health Measurement Scales.* 2nd ed. Oxford: Oxford University Press; 1995:152–157.
16. Brazier JE, Harper R, Jones NMB, et al. Validating the SF-36 health survey questionnaire: new outcome measure for primary care. *BMJ.* 1992;305:160–164.
17. Ware JE, Kosinski M, Keller SD. A 12-item short-form health survey: Construction of scales and preliminary tests of reliability and validity. *Med Care.* 1996;34:220–233.
18. *Clinical Performance Instrument.* Alexandria, Va: American Physical Therapy Association; 1998.
19. Norton BJ, Ellison JB. Reliability and concurrent validity of the Metrecom for length measurement on inanimate objects. *Phys Ther.* 1993;73:266–274.
20. Geddes LA, Baker LE. *Principles of Applied Biomedical Instrumentation.* 3rd ed. New York, NY: John Wiley & Sons; 1989:8–9.
21. Irrgang JJ, Snyder-Mackler L, Wainner RS, Fu FH, Harner CD. Development of a patient-reported measure of function of the knee. *J Bone Joint Surg Am.* 1998;80:1132–1145.
22. Harris SR, Swanson MW, Andrews MS, et al. Predictive validity of the "Movement Assessment of Infants." *Dev Behav Pediatr.* 1984;5:336–342.

Measurement Tools for Physical Therapy Research

Anthropometric Characteristics
  Height
  Weight
  Segmental Length
  Girth
  Volume
  Body Composition

Arousal, Mentation, and Cognition

Community and Work Integration, Self-Care, and Home Management
  Basic Activities of Daily Living
  Instrumental Activities of Daily Living
  Task-Specific Functional Assessment
  Condition-Specific Functional Assessment

Gait, Locomotion, and Balance
  Biomechanical Analysis of Gait and Locomotion
    Kinematics
    Kinetics
  Measurement of Balance
    Posturographic Methods
    Methods with a Fixed Base of Support
    Methods with a Moving Base of Support

Integumentary Integrity

Muscle Performance
  Force Generation
    Manual Muscle Testing
    Hand-Held Dynamometry
    Weights
    Cable Tensiometers and Strain Gauges
    Hand Dynamometers
    Isokinetic Dynamometers
  Electrical Activity
  Muscle Tone
  Microscopic Composition

Neuromotor Development and Sensory Integration

Pain
  Using Descriptive Words
  Assigning Numbers to Pain Intensity
  Experimentally Induced Pain

Range of Motion and Joint Integrity and Mobility
  Extrinsic Joint Motions
    Universal Goniometer
    Gravity-Referenced Goniometers
    Electrogoniometers
    Linear Measurements
  Intrinsic Joint Motions
  Joint Position and Posture

Sensory Integrity

Ventilation, Respiration, Circulation, Aerobic Capacity, and Endurance
 Cardiovascular Measures
  Heart Rate
  Blood Pressure

Fitness
Blood Flow
Pulmonary Measures
 Forced Expiratory Volume
 Oxygen Saturation
Autonomic Function

After defining a research problem, the researcher must confront the question of how to measure the constructs of interest within a study. Physical therapy researchers have a wide range of instruments from which to choose. These instruments include devices or procedures used in the clinic, instruments designed primarily for research use, observational methods that require only the skills of the researcher, and self-report instruments that require written or oral responses from subjects.

To assist physical therapists in evaluating the vast array of measurement tools available to them, the American Physical Therapy Association (APTA) has published *Standards for Tests and Measurements in Physical Therapy Practice*[1] and a *Primer on Measurement: An Introductory Guide to Measurement Issues.*[2] These documents provide a framework from which test developers, researchers, teachers, and test users can evaluate the measures they use. An additional document, published annually by the APTA is called the *Buyer's Guide*, which provides information about the suppliers of many of the measurement tools that are discussed in this chapter.[3]

This chapter introduces the wide range of measuring tools that are reported in the physical therapy literature. As mentioned in Chapters 17 and 18, the reliability of a measure depends on the way in which data are collected, and validity depends on the use to which a measurement is put rather than on the measurement itself. Therefore, in this chapter no judgments are made about the relative merits of the measurement tools presented. Instead, references that discuss the reliability, validity, and use of the various tools in physical therapy research are cited. These references provide a foundation of information on which readers can base their decision on whether to use a particular measure in their own study or in clinical practice.

This chapter is organized around the major grouping of tests and measures reported in the APTA's *Guide to Physical Therapist Practice.*[4] The Guide contains 23 groupings of tests and measures used during the physical therapy examination, as shown in Table 19–1. To eliminate duplication of tests across some of the groupings, and to limit the length of the chapter, only 11 groupings are presented in this chapter: anthropometric characteristics; arousal, mentation, and cognition; community and work integration, self-care, and home management; gait, locomotion, and balance; integumentary integrity; muscle performance; neuromotor development and sensory integration; pain; range of motion and joint integrity and mobility; sensory integrity; and ventilation, respiration, circulation, aerobic capacity, and endurance. A variety of measures are described for each grouping.

■ ANTHROPOMETRIC CHARACTERISTICS

Anthropometric measures document the size and proportions of segments of the human body. Major items assessed include height, weight, segmental length, girth, volume, and body composition.

TABLE 19-1 Tests and Measures Used by Physical Therapists	
Aerobic capacity and endurance	Muscle performance
Anthropometric characteristics	Neuromotor development and sensory integration
Arousal, mentation, and cognition	Orthotic, protective, and supportive devices
Assistive and adaptive devices	Pain
Community and work integration or reintegration	Posture
Cranial nerve integrity	Prosthetic requirements
Environmental, home, and work barriers	Range of motion
Ergonomics and body mechanics	Reflex integrity
Gait, locomotion, and balance	Self-care and home management
Integumentary integrity	Sensory integrity
Joint integrity and mobility	Ventilation, respiration, and circulation
Motor function	

Height

Height is a basic physical characteristic that is often reported in studies. Although a seemingly straightforward measurement, researchers must attend to standing posture during height measurements, whether subjects will wear shoes during the measurement, and the angle at which the horizontal measuring bar intersects the vertical measurement scale.[5]

Weight

Weight is a second basic physical characteristic that is often reported. Like height, it is a seemingly straightforward measurement that, nevertheless, requires standardization in several ways. Measurement should be standardized in relationship to the timing of eating and drinking; to the type of clothing worn during the measurement; and to the actual scale or scales used within a study.[5]

Segmental Length

Standardized procedures for determining segmental length, such as forearm or leg length, have been described by Martin and associates.[6] Accurate measurement of segmental lengths requires an anthropometric caliper set and a narrow metal tape measure.

Girth

Girth is determined by measuring the circumference of a body segment at reproducible levels. For example, calf girth might be measured at the level of the tibial tubercle and at 5, 10, 15, and 20 cm distal to the tibial tubercle. Callaway and colleagues recommend the use of a metal tape measure to prevent stretching and deformation of the tape itself, which may occur with fabric or plastic tape measures.[7] Controlled-tension tape measures may also be used. Controlled-tension tape measures have a spring on one end that allows the examiner to pull the tape to a consistent pressure at each measurement (Fig. 19–1). This reduces the variability that occurs when an examiner uses different amounts of tension on the tape on different measuring occasions or when different examiners use different amounts of tension. A controlled-tension tape measure was used by Weiss and colleagues to document circumference changes in response to heavy-resistance exercise of the triceps surae muscles.[8]

Girth has sometimes been used to document muscle hypertrophy after an exercise program or muscle atrophy after surgical procedures.[9] Use of girth in this fashion must be assessed carefully because an increase in girth caused by an increase in muscle size may be attenuated by a decrease in body fat that may accompany initiation of an exercise program.[10]

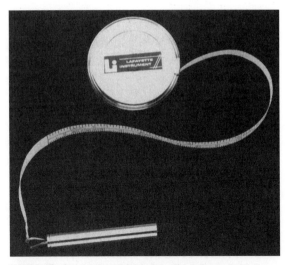

FIGURE 19–1. Controlled-tension tape measure. Photo courtesy of Lafayette Instruments, 3700 Sagamore Parkway North, Lafayette, IN 47903.

Volume

Volumeters collect and measure water displaced by immersing a limb to a certain point (Fig. 19–2). Waylett-Rendall and Seibly documented the accuracy of a commercially available volumeter.[11] Griffin and associates used a volumeter to document volume changes after intermittent compression or electrical stimulation in patients with chronic hand edema.[12] An alternate method for estimating volume of a limb uses circumferential measures that are inserted into the formula for determining the volume of a truncated cone (a cone with a flat end rather than a pointed tip).[13] The method was used by Ko and colleagues in their study of complete decongestive physiotherapy for the treatment of lymphedema.[14]

Body Composition

The proportion of lean body mass to fat is often of interest to physical therapists. The proportion may be calculated for the whole body or for a particular body segment. Subcutaneous fat thickness has been determined with skinfold calipers,[15,16] ultrasound,[17] magnetic resonance imaging,[17] and computerized axial tomography.[10] Measurements of subcutaneous fat thickness are often used as variables in equations calculated to predict body density or percentage of body fat.[15,18] Researchers must be sure that the equations they are using were developed for use with a population similar to the one they are studying.

Measures of body density that do not depend on measurement of subcutaneous fat thickness are hydrostatic weighing and body impedance analysis. Hydrostatic weighing requires that the subject be able to tolerate complete immersion in either a specially designed tank or a Hubbard tank that has been modified to include a scale.[19] Body impedance analysis is easier to accomplish because it requires only that electrodes be placed in a few limb locations.[20]

■ AROUSAL, MENTATION, AND COGNITION

Rehabilitation researchers often wish to assess arousal, mentation, and cognition, either as measures of interest within their studies or as inclusion or exclusion criteria for potential subjects.

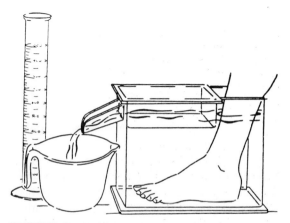

FIGURE 19–2. Foot volumeter. Courtesy of Volumeters Unlimited, 1307 Sandra Way, Redlands, CA 92374.

Two common measures include the Glasgow Coma Scale (GCS) and the Mini–Mental State Examination (MMSE).

The GCS, developed in 1974, assesses level of consciousness by observing motor and verbal responses to commands or pain stimuli. Scores range from 3 to 15, with a 15 representing someone who has his or her eyes open, follows simple commands, and is oriented to person, place, and time.[21(pp122–146)] As part of a system to "classify, triage, treat, and predict outcomes of trauma victims," [22(p429)] consistent scoring of the tool is important. However, such consistency has become increasingly problematic as advances in emergency medicine and trauma care have increased the number of patients who are intubated, sedated, or pharmacologically paralyzed at points during their care.[22] These patients are unable to provide the motor and verbal responses required for complete scoring of the GCS.

The Mini–Mental State Examination (MMSE) assesses higher-level cognitive functions by asking examinees to indicate specific times and places (date as well as time of day; city and country), subtract by 7s from 100, learn new names, repeat the objects named previously, execute three-step commands, write a sentence, and copy a figure. Scores range from 0 to 30, with 30 representing best function.[21(pp122–146)] Further information about this test can be found in Tombaugh and McIntyre's comprehensive review of measurement and administration issues related to the MMSE.[23]

A great many additional tests of arousal and cognition are available. Some tests require the expertise of a psychologist to administer, score, and interpret; others are appropriate for use by health care professionals in many disciplines. Tests of cognitive and emotional impairments that are particularly useful to physical therapists who treat patients with neurological impairments are outlined by Wade in his text on measurement in neurological rehabilitation.[21(pp59–69)] Similar psychological and cognitive tests appropriate for use with children are outlined by Shea, Towle,

and Gordon in their chapter in a text on pediatric assessment for therapists.[24] In addition, there are a great many tests of mental function that have been developed for various groups for use in a variety of settings. Although the wide range of measurement tools precludes their listing, readers are referred to volumes of the *Mental Measurements Yearbook* and its *Supplement* as comprehensive references that include test descriptions, information about obtaining tests, and reviews of literature related to the tests.[25,26]

■ COMMUNITY AND WORK INTEGRATION, SELF-CARE, AND HOME MANAGEMENT

Researchers and clinicians often wish to know the impact of their interventions on the daily lives of their subjects or patients. This emphasis is one of the chief tenets of the "outcomes" movement described earlier in Chapter 15. The areas of interest within daily life range from basic activities of daily living (BADL) such as eating and dressing, to instrumental activities of daily living (IADL) such as cooking and shopping, and social roles in the community, school, and workplace. In addition to these relatively general measures of outcome, researchers may be interested in task-specific or diagnosis- or region-specific outcomes. This section of the chapter is organized around these four types of measures: BADL, IADL, task-specific, and diagnosis- or region-specific tools. Kidd and Yoshida[27] reviewed the literature on disability measures over the last 40 years and identified three major trends: more frequent interest in IADL in addition to BADL; increasing interest in social functioning as a component of disability; and increasing recognition that client perspectives within environmental and social contexts should be considered when measuring disability. Young and Wright provide an excellent review of functional measures that have been designed for or adapted for use with children.[28]

Basic Activities of Daily Living

The state of the art in functional status assessment has been reviewed by Guccione and associates.[29] They compared several measures that assess BADL. Others have reviewed the reliability, validity, and ordinal scaling of functional status assessments.[30,31]

A frequently reported BADL assessment is the Barthel Index. The Barthel Index evaluates subjects' performance of 10 functional tasks according to the level of independence shown in each task. Scores on each task are added together to generate a single numerical score for physical function.[32] Recent studies using the Barthel Index have evaluated long-term follow-up after stroke,[33] functional status poststroke based on use of orthoses,[34] and effectiveness of home-based exercise poststroke.[35]

The Functional Independence Measure (FIM) is another widely used scale that has been assessed for reliability and validity with different examiners and with individuals with different disabilities.[36–38] Rintala and colleagues used the FIM as one measure of function in a study of pain and its relationship to function in individuals with spinal cord injury.[39] The FIM, originally developed for use with adults, now exists in a modified format for use with children, called the Functional Independence Measure for Children (WeeFIM).[40] Lepage and colleagues used the WeeFIM as one measure within their study of the association between locomotion and accomplishment of life habits in children with cerebral palsy.[41]

A different approach to measuring BADL is taken with the Physical Performance Test (PPT). This test requires timed, direct observation of individuals as they complete several BADL tasks (including writing a sentence, simulated eating, putting on a jacket, picking up a penny).[42] This is in contrast to some of the other BADL scales that can be scored by an examiner based on direct observation or through the self-report of the individual being tested. Mueller and colleagues used the PPT as one measure of function in their study of functional limitations in individuals with diabetes and transmetatarsal amputations.[43]

Instrumental Activities of Daily Living

Instrumental activities of daily living (IADL) include a variety of complex tasks necessary for independent community living. These include tasks such as using the telephone, shopping, preparing meals, doing housework, and handling money. Two of the most widely reported measures of IADL are the Lawton IADL Scale[44] and the Older Americans Resources and Services (OARS) IADL Scale.[45] These tools have been used to document the IADL status of community-dwelling elders[46] as well as individuals with particular conditions such as stroke.[35]

Task-Specific Functional Assessment

Physical therapists are often interested in a patient's ability to return to his or her previous employment setting. Assessing the ability to return to previous work depends on whether the patient can perform tasks that are specific to the work environment. Schultz-Johnson has reviewed the major tools used to evaluate the physical capacity of the hand and upper extremity.[47] Physical therapists working in occupational rehabilitation may also use more global assessments of functional capacity that determine the patient's ability to lift, push, pull, or carry certain amounts of weight; assess the patient's tolerance for standing, sitting, and walking; determine the pace at which the patient can work; and assess the patient's safety during various work-related maneuvers.[48,49] Physical therapists who work with athletes may find sport skill tests useful for the study of athletic function.[50]

Condition-Specific Functional Assessment

As noted in Chapter 15, a great many condition-specific tools have been developed to measure functional outcomes. Atherly provides an over-view of differences between condition-specific and more generic measures,[51] and Pynsent and associates provide information about a variety of condition-specific or region-specific outcome tools in orthopedics.[52] Readers should refer to Chapter 15 for a more thorough discussion of two of these many tools—the Oswestry Low Back Pain Disability Index[53] and the Lysholm Knee Rating Scale.[54] Although the general nature of this text limits the space available for a com-plete review of other instruments, readers are re-ferred to various references for tools that mea-sure outcomes for patients with cervical spine disorders,[55] after shoulder and elbow surgery,[56] after total hip arthroplasty,[57,58] after ankle frac-ture,[59] for lower extremity dysfunction,[60] and for shoulder pathology.[61]

■ GAIT, LOCOMOTION, AND BALANCE

Gait, locomotion, and balance are frequently evaluated for clinical and for research purposes. Measurements of gait, locomotion, and balance range from the very simple to the highly techni-cal, and this chapter can present only a sampling of the many available tools. This section of the chapter is divided into biomechanical analysis of gait and locomotion and measures of balance.

Biomechanical Analysis of Gait and Locomotion

Biomechanical analysis of movement is highly technical and can be divided into kinematics (the study of movement) and kinetics (the study of the forces that underlie movement). Winter's classic text on biomechanics provides basic in-formation about the various biomechanical pro-cedures.[62]

KINEMATICS

A major kinematic measurement technique is the filming of subjects in motion. Motion picture cameras (cinematography) can shoot at fast speeds to capture very fast motions. Video tech-niques sample at a slower number of frames per second and can be used for slower motions. Be-fore a subject is filmed, body landmarks are marked with tape or lights that are easily vis-ualized on the film. The coordinates of the landmarks are determined by a process called *digitizing*. Cinematographic digitizing is accom-plished by projecting each frame of the film onto a digitizing pad and identifying the landmarks with an electronic pointer that determines the coordinates for each point. An interface with a computer allows relatively efficient calculation of angles between body segments from the marked coordinates. Video digitizing is accomplished by displaying each of the video frames on a moni-tor and using a computer mouse to identify the points of interest; the coordinates are stored in a computer. Optoelectric systems use light-emitting diodes as landmarks and require no hand digitizing (Fig. 19–3).[63,64]

Blanke and Hageman used high-speed (100 frames per second) cinematography and digitiz-ing to compare the gait characteristics of young and elderly men.[65] Heriza used videotaping (60 frames per second) and digitizing to study leg movements in preterm infants.[66] Kluzik and col-leagues used an optoelectrical video system to analyze reaching movements in children with cerebral palsy.[67] Less technical approaches to kinematic studies of gait are footprint analy-sis[68,69] and direct measurement of angles from projected video images.[70]

In addition to filming, kinematic studies may use electrogoniometers and accelerometers to measure motion. Accelerometers attach to a limb segment and measure the acceleration of that segment. Like electrogoniometers, discussed later in the chapter (see Range of Motion and Joint Integrity and Mobility), accelerometers may be uniaxial or triaxial.[63,64]

KINETICS

Kinetics is the study of the forces that underlie movements. One tool of kinetic analysis is elec-

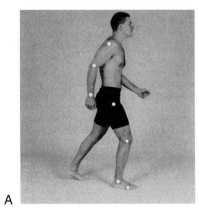

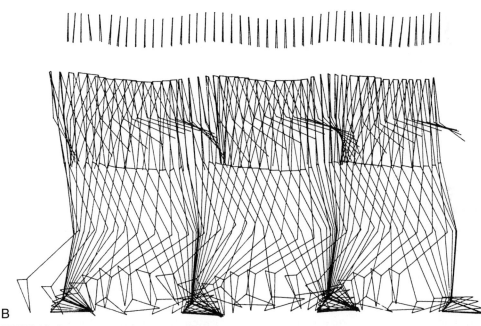

FIGURE 19–3. Video motion measurement system. **A.** Light-emitting diodes affixed to subject. **B.** Stick figures generated from video of subject with diodes.
Courtesy of Peak Performance Technologies, Suite 601, 7388 South Revere Parkway, Englewood, CO 80112.

tromyography, which is used to study patterns of muscular activation during movement, as discussed later in the chapter (see Muscle Performance). A second major kinetic measurement tool is the force platform. The force platform is typically used in gait studies to determine ground reaction forces.[70] Schuit and colleagues used a force platform to analyze the effect of heel lifts on ground reaction force patterns in subjects with leg-length discrepancies.[71] Integration of film, EMG, and force platform data can provide a very complex description of the kinetics of movement throughout a range of motion.[64,70]

Measurement of Balance

Balance is a complex phenomenon that can be measured in many different ways. Berg reviewed the literature on the measurement of balance into the late 1980s,[72] and Whitney and colleagues reviewed common tools reported during the 1990s.[73] Balance tools may be classified in many different ways; for the purpose of this chapter the tools are divided into three general categories: posturographic methods, methods with a fixed base of support, and methods with a moving base of support.

POSTUROGRAPHIC METHODS. Posturography uses computerized platforms to quantify changes in centers of pressure or magnitude of body sway during different conditions. These conditions may include standing on a stationary surface or a moving surface, standing on firm versus soft surfaces, and being surrounded with accurate or inaccurate visual information or with no visual information. A variety of systems and protocols are used in reports within the literature.[74–77]

METHODS WITH A FIXED BASE OF SUPPORT. In tests of balance from a fixed base of support, subjects do not move their feet during the test. Some of the most frequently cited measures of fixed-base balance are variations on the Romberg test. Differences in body sway are observed with subjects' eyes open and closed as they stand with their feet together, in a heel-to-toe position, or on one leg.[78,79] The length of time that subjects can maintain these positions is often determined. Bohannon and colleagues studied the timed static balance tests and determined normative values for individuals in each decade from 20 to 70 years of age.[80]

Another approach to fixed-base balance testing is to introduce many of the same variables that are introduced during high-technology posturography. One such test is the Clinical Test of Sensory Interaction and Balance, also known as the Sensory Organization Test, which measures standing time and magnitude of sway under six different conditions.[81] Three visual conditions are included: eyes open, eyes closed, and inaccurate visual input. Each visual condition is combined with two different supporting surfaces: firm and compliant. Several authors have used this test with neurologically asymptomatic adults of different ages,[82] with subjects with vestibular impairments,[82] and with individuals with hemiplegia.[83]

Another popular fixed-base balance measure is the Functional Reach developed by Duncan and colleagues.[84] This clinically accessible test measures the extent to which a subject can reach forward while maintaining a fixed stance. This measure has been found to be related to other measures of physical frailty[85] and to posturography.[86]

METHODS WITH A MOVING BASE OF SUPPORT. The balance tests that use a moving base of support are typically performance tests that require individuals to complete a series of tasks that challenge postural control mechanisms in different ways. Three of the most commonly used moving-base tests are the Berg Balance Scale, the balance portion of Tinetti's Performance Oriented Mobility Assessment (BPOMA), and the Timed Up and Go Test.

The Berg Balance Scale was developed in the late 1980s.[87,88] It consists of 14 different tasks including sitting, standing, reaching, leaning over, turning, and stepping. Each task is scored from 0 (cannot perform) to 4 (normal performance) for a total score of from 0 to 56, with 56 indicating normal performance on all tasks. This scale has been used in rehabilitation research with subjects with varying characteristics.[89,90]

Tinetti developed a performance-based mobility assessment that includes eight items related to balance. Included are tasks such as standing, sitting, turning around, maintaining stability after a sternal push, and standing with a narrow base of support.[91] A variety of studies have examined the measurement characteristics of this tool under different conditions.[92,93]

The third of the commonly reported moving-base tests is the Get-Up and Go test and its variants, originally developed by Mathias and colleagues in the late 1980s. In this test, patients perform a sequence of maneuvers including rising from a chair, walking, turning, and sitting down.[94] The original test used a subjective scoring method, which has since been modified to be scored on the length of time it takes to complete the sequence of activities.[95]

■ INTEGUMENTARY INTEGRITY

The most common reason physical therapists measure integumentary integrity is to document the size of wounds. Several authors have compared various ways of quantifying the size of wounds: through the use of transparent wound tracings; by direct measures of length, width, and depth; with photography; and by gel impressions of the wound.[96–98] Kloth and Feedar superimposed wound tracings on graph paper to document wound size in their study of the effectiveness of a high-voltage current on wound healing.[99]

■ MUSCLE PERFORMANCE

The term "muscle performance," used within the *Guide to Physical Therapist Practice*,[4] describes the very broad spectrum of qualities related to the function of the muscular system. Four different aspects of muscle performance are discussed in this section: force generation, electrical activity, muscle tone, and microscopic composition.

Force Generation

Physical therapists are often interested in the force-generating capacity of muscles: How much pressure can a subject exert? How much weight can a subject lift? How many times can a subject complete a movement? All of these questions relate either to the force generated by a muscle or to extensions of the concept of force, such as torque, work, and power. Measurements of muscular force or its extensions range from simple measures that rely on the examiner's judgment to complex instruments that cost thousands of dollars. Six types of measures are discussed: manual muscle testing, hand-held dynamometry, weights, cable tensiometers and strain gauges, hand dynamometers, and isokinetic dynamometers.

MANUAL MUSCLE TESTING. Manual muscle testing procedures are familiar to all physical therapists. Manual muscle tests do not require equipment and rely instead on therapist judgments about a subject's ability to move against gravity or against a force exerted by the examiner. In 1985, Lamb reviewed the literature on manual muscle testing and concluded that the reliability and validity of the major approaches to manual muscle testing had not been well established.[100] Studies conducted in the late 1980s evaluated the reliability of manual muscle testing as it is used in the clinic. In one study high levels of intratester reliability were found for several muscle groups that were selected because of their ease of testing[101]; in another study relatively low intertester reliability was found for nonstandardized testing of two muscles thought to be difficult to test.[102] In the 1990s, the research emphasis has been away from manual muscle testing and toward hand-held dynamometry, which is described next in this chapter. However, a limited amount of work related to manual muscle testing has been published. For manual muscle testing to be accurate, the examiner must be able to generate pushing forces greater than that of the muscles being tested. Mulroy and associates found that limitations in pushing forces would lead many clinicians to overestimate the strength of the quadriceps femoris muscle.[103] They found that female clinicians were unable to detect mild to moderate weakness in the quadriceps femoris muscles of either female or male subjects, and that male clinicians might miss moderate weakness in male subjects. In another study, Herbison and colleagues concluded that manual muscle testing missed changes in muscle strength that were detected by a hand-held dynamometer.[104] An additional limitation of manual muscle testing as a research tool is its ordinal nature; that is, the intervals between the various grades are not established.

HAND-HELD DYNAMOMETRY. Hand-held dynamometry is an instrumented extension of manual muscle testing (Fig. 19–4). However, rather than relying on the physical therapist's judgment of the external load the patient is able to withstand, hand-held dynamometers provide quantitative output of the force exerted against the instrument. The test-retest reliability of hand-held dynamometry has been determined to be relatively high for patients with brain damage,[105,106] healthy children,[107] individuals with orthopedic disor-

ders,[101,108] and individuals with neuromuscular diseases.[107,109] Other researchers have documented the intratester reliability[110] and interdevice reliability[111] of hand-held dynamometry under different conditions. Herbison and colleagues compared the use of hand-held dynamometry and manual muscle testing to evaluate changes in strength following spinal cord injury and found the hand-held dynamometer to be more sensitive to change than manual muscle testing.[104] Normative values for hand-held dynamometry are beginning to be established for the major muscle groups for different age and sex groups.[112]

WEIGHTS. The use of weights to document muscle performance was popularized by DeLorme in the 1940s.[113] Muscle performance is quantified by determining the maximum amount of weight that a subject is able to move through either a single repetition (one-repetition maximum, 1 RM) or several, typically 10, repetitions (10-repetition maximum, 10 RM). Jürimäe and colleagues used 1 RM to evaluate strength changes in the triceps brachii muscle following 12 weeks of resistance training.[114]

CABLE TENSIOMETERS AND STRAIN GAUGES. Cable tensiometers and strain gauges are mechanical and electrical versions of basically the same tool. In both, there is a device that is fixed on one end and secured to the subject's limb at the other end. When the subject exerts force against the device, quantitative output is obtained. With the cable tensiometer, a meter located along the cable measures the tension on the cable. The strain gauge measures changes in the electrical resistance of the materials that are placed under stress. Balogun and associates used a cable tensiometer to measure knee extension strength following a 6-week program of electrical stimulation.[115] Vaughan used a strain gauge to measure muscle strength in a study of the effect of immobilization on several muscle performance characteristics.[116]

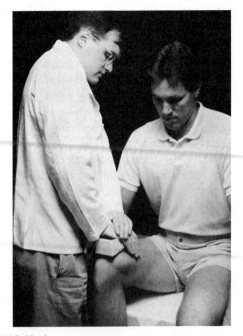

FIGURE 19–4. Hand-held dynamometer. Photo courtesy of Lafayette Instruments, 3700 Sagamore Parkway North, Lafayette, IN 47903.

HAND DYNAMOMETERS. Several different types of dynamometers are designed to measure grip or pinch strength (Fig. 19–5). Fess has reviewed the literature on the reliability and validity of hand dynamometry,[117] and more recent studies have added to the literature on reliability with these tools.[118,119] Mathiowetz and associates documented normative data for grip and pinch strength in adults,[120] and Josty and colleagues examined grip and pinch strength variations in different types of workers.[121] Jansen and Minerbo used both grip and pinch gauges in a nonexperimental research study of immobilization protocols after flexor tendon surgery.[122]

ISOKINETIC DYNAMOMETERS. Pioneered in the 1960s, isokinetic devices allow exercise and muscle testing to be conducted under constant velocity throughout the range of motion. Perrin's text on isokinetic exercise and assessment provides an overview of many of the important measurement issues involved with this form of testing.[123] Clinicians now have a choice of several different commonly available brands of isokinetic dynamometers. In addition, specialized isokinetic dynamometers have been developed for testing trunk musculature.

The dynamometers are interfaced with computers that provide many different measures of muscle performance, such as peak torque, torque to body weight ratios, endurance factors, and torque measurements at certain ranges of motion. In addition, all of these measures can be taken at different speeds. Some of the machines allow testing of eccentric as well as concentric muscle contractions. A researcher should use caution when comparing measurements taken with different brands of machines, because the measurements from different dynamometers are not interchangeable.[124,125] Recent methodological research related to isokinetic testing has compared it to hand-held dynamometry,[126,127] has examined its use with older individuals,[127–129] and has determined its relationship to functional tests.[130]

Despite the sophistication of these instruments, the validity of some of the commonly used isokinetic measures has been questioned. For example, a commonly used measure is the peak torque to body weight ratio. This ratio is calculated in an attempt to standardize peak torque values to permit comparison among individuals of different sizes. However, the correlation between peak torque and body weight has been found to be low, making the usefulness of the ratio questionable.[131] In addition, there are measurement issues related to correcting torque measurements for gravity, damping the signal, and calibrating the machines. Rothstein and associates and Winter and associates have reviewed some of the major issues involved with isokinetic testing.[132,133] In addition, a comprehensive review of the influence of subject and test design on dynamometric measurements of extremity muscles was published by Keating and Matyas in 1996.[134]

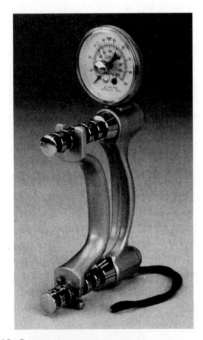

FIGURE 19–5. Hand dynamometer. Photo courtesy of Lafayette Instruments, 3700 Sagamore Parkway North, Lafayette, IN 47903.

Electrical Activity

A second aspect of muscle performance is the electrical activity of the muscle, as documented by electromyography (EMG). EMG has been used as a diagnostic tool, a biofeedback tool, and a tool for kinesiological and biomechanical research. Five characteristics of the EMG potential have been noted: duration, frequency, amplitude, characteristics of the waveform, and characteristics of the sound generated.[135] EMG potentials can be detected by both surface electrodes and fine-wire electrodes. Surface electrodes pick up more activity from large muscle masses; fine-wire electrodes are inserted into the muscle through a hollow needle and allow the study of smaller, deeper muscles (Fig. 19–6).[136]

A major concern in the interpretation of EMG results is the extent to which the EMG signal is indicative of muscle force-generating capacity. Muscular length and the type of contraction influence the relationship between EMG activity and muscular force.[137] Guidelines for human EMG research have been developed and pub-

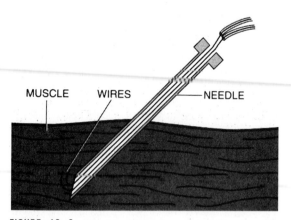

FIGURE 19–6. Bipolar fine-wire electromyographic electrode.
Redrawn from Snyder-Mackler L, Robinson AJ. *Clinical Electrophysiology, Electrotherapy, and Electrophysiologic Testing.* Baltimore, Md: Williams & Wilkins; 1989:37.

MUSCLE   WIRES   NEEDLE

lished by the Society for Psychophysiological Research.[138]

Two studies illustrate the different uses of EMG in research. In a study of postural adjustments during balance testing, Duncan and colleagues used surface EMG to determine the timing and sequence of activation of various muscle groups during postural responses.[139] Hanten and Schulthies used fine-wire electrodes to study the EMG activity of the vastus medialis oblique and vastus lateralis muscles during performance of two different exercises.[140]

Muscle Tone

Muscle tone is yet another aspect of muscle performance that interests physical therapists. A general definition of muscle tone is the "responsiveness of muscles to passive elongation or stretch."[141(p111)] A clinical manifestation of abnormal muscle tone is a disorder in the timing of different muscular actions when movement is attempted. It is difficult to measure muscle tone because it is a fluctuating phenomenon. In addition, muscle tone may change with touch and movement. Despite these difficulties, muscle tone has been quantified by description of responses to elongation and by measurement of EMG activity, range of motion, and force.

One of the simplest measures of muscle tone is the Ashworth Scale of Spasticity. This ordinal scale requires that the examiner judge resistance to movement according to descriptions of five or six grades of spasticity. This measure was used by Wright and colleagues to evaluate the impact of selective dorsal rhizotomy on spasticity in children with cerebral palsy.[142] Bohannon and Smith found their modification of the Ashworth scale to have good interrater reliability.[143] Another ordinal scale of muscle tone is the 0 to 4+ scale used to quantify the deep tendon reflexes.[144]

Range-of-motion measurements have also been used to indicate spasticity. Worley and colleagues used two different range-of-motion measures to quantify spasticity: the resting position of the joint and the position at which resistance to passive movement was encountered.[145]

An additional use of range-of-motion measures for documentation of spasticity is the pendulum test. In this test, the spasticity of the quadriceps femoris muscles is indicated by the pattern of movement after the lower leg is dropped from a position of full knee extension with the subject in a supine position and the lower legs dangling from the supporting surface. A limb with no spasticity swings rapidly to the resting position of 90° of knee flexion. The slightly spastic leg "catches" earlier in the range of motion, and the highly spastic leg may not move at all from the extended position. The points in the range of motion at which catches or oscillations occur have been documented with an electrogoniometer attached to the limb and with a goniometer incorporated within an isokinetic dynamometer.[146–148] Bajd and associates used a pendulum test to document spasticity changes in patients with spinal cord injury following electrical stimulation.[149] Variations on pendulum testing use isokinetic dynamometers to create "controlled displacements" against which the spastic forces are measured[150,151] or use hand-held or isokinetic dynamometers to quantify resistance to movement.[152]

EMG has also been used to document tone or spasticity.[153] Patterns of muscle activation may indicate changes in muscle tone, and the magnitude of muscular activity may be used to determine whether a spasticity-reducing treatment is effective. Wolf and colleagues and Dickstein and colleagues have used EMG data to document muscle activation changes with various treatments.[154,155]

Microscopic Composition

The fourth aspect of muscle performance studied by physical therapists is the microscopic composition of muscles. Ultrastructural, biochemical, and histochemical analysis of muscle tissue can determine mitochondrial and myofibril counts, the proportion of different fiber types within muscle units, the organization of motor units within a muscle, the motor units that have been fatigued by a given maneuver, and the extent of muscular degeneration or regeneration. Cress and associates used ultrastructural and histochemical analysis to determine the effects of functional training on muscle structure in older women.[156] Sinacore and colleagues used histochemical and biochemical analysis to study the order of activation of muscle fibers during electrical muscle stimulation in a human subject.[157]

■ NEUROMOTOR DEVELOPMENT AND SENSORY INTEGRATION

Many different standardized tools are used to assess children's developmental status. Tests that are reported frequently include the Bayley Scales of Infant Development[158–161] and the Peabody Developmental Motor Scales.[160,162–164] A variety of other tests appear to be reported less often in the rehabilitation literature: the Test of Infant Motor Performance,[165] the Motor Assessment of Infants,[166] the Gross Motor Function Measure,[167] and the Harris Infant Neuromotor Test.[168]

Several references provide broad-based information about various developmental tests.[169,170] The *Mental Measurements Yearbook* and its *Supplement* are comprehensive references that include test descriptions, information about obtaining the tests, and reviews of literature related to the tests.[25,26]

■ PAIN

Pain is an abstract construct that a researcher can never directly observe. Quantification of pain usually takes one of three forms: use of descriptive words, assignment of numbers to indicate intensity, or documentation of tolerance to experimentally induced pain.

Using Descriptive Words

The most frequently cited tool that uses descriptive words to document pain is the McGill Pain Questionnaire.[171] Although the questionnaire consists of four parts, the second part is the most commonly quantified. It asks patients to indicate which of up to 20 words in 20 different categories best describes their pain. A short form of the McGill Pain Questionnaire was used as one of the outcomes in a study of back school programs.[172]

Assigning Numbers to Pain Intensity

Researchers may use a visual analog scale (VAS) to quantify the nature of pain. The typical VAS is a 10-cm line with words such as "worst pain I ever felt" and "no pain" at the ends of the line. The subject marks the line at the point that represents his or her pain perception.[173] The investigator then measures the distance from the end of the line that represents no pain to the subject's mark. Price and colleagues have examined the reliability and validity of the VAS for both chronic and experimental pain.[174] Craig and colleagues used a VAS as well as the McGill Pain Questionnaire to determine the impact of an electrical modality on delayed-onset muscle soreness.[175]

Experimentally Induced Pain

Pain has been induced experimentally by electrical stimulation, thermal stimulation, or induction of extremity ischemia through use of a tourniquet.[176] In addition, exercise overloading can be used to induce delayed muscle soreness.[175] Although the previously cited scales can be used to evaluate experimentally induced pain, one variation in evaluation of such pain involves using the pain stimulus as the measurement tool. Noling and colleagues used electrical stimulation to induce pain in their study of the effect of auricular transcutaneous electrical nerve stimulation on pain threshold at the wrist. The electrical stimulation was increased in small increments until the subject identified the sensation as painful. The researchers evaluated the effectiveness of the treatment by determining changes in the amount of current tolerated before and after the treatment.[177]

■ RANGE OF MOTION AND JOINT INTEGRITY AND MOBILITY

Along with the measurement of muscle performance, the measurement of joint range of motion and position is one of the most frequently used evaluative procedures in physical therapy. These measurements can be classified into three broad categories: extrinsic joint movements, intrinsic movements within a joint, and joint or body segment position.

Extrinsic Joint Motions

Many different clinical and research tools are available for the documentation of extrinsic joint motions. The universal goniometer, gravity-referenced goniometers, electrogoniometers, and linear measurements are discussed in this section. Gajdosik and Bohannon have reviewed the literature on measurement of the extrinsic range of motion of the joints of the extremities.[178]

UNIVERSAL GONIOMETER. The universal goniometer is the most familiar clinical tool for measuring joint range of motion. Several authors have provided guidelines for using the universal goniometer.[179,180] Many authors have documented the reliability of measurements taken with the universal goniometer,[181–183] and more recent reports have compared the universal goniometer to other tools for measuring range of motion.[184–186] The universal goniometer can be used to measure both isolated joint movements and the combined movement of several segments, such as the cervical or lumbar spine and hips.

When evaluating passive range of motion, the examiner exerts a force against one of the limbs involved in the motion. Thus, the amount of force the examiner uses becomes a variable that may affect the reliability and validity of the range-of-motion measure. A measurement technique using a universal goniometer to measure range of motion and a dynamometer to standardize the force exerted for passive range-of-motion measurements has been termed *torque range of motion.*[187]

GRAVITY-REFERENCED GONIOMETERS. Gravity-referenced goniometers have some mechanism by which the measurement is referenced to either the horizontal or vertical. Some use the concept of a carpenter's level, and others use the principle of a plumb bob. The term *inclinometer* is sometimes used for gravity-referenced goniometers because they measure the degree of inclination from the vertical (Fig. 19–7). Several authors have documented reliability and validity of different inclinometers for documenting spinal and extremity motions.[188–192] Specialized goniometers have been designed for the measurement of cervical spine motions (Fig. 19–8). In addition to gravity referencing, these goniometers permit stabilization of the device on the head. Youdas and associates documented the reliability of one of the specialized cervical measurement devices.[193]

ELECTROGONIOMETERS. Electrogoniometers detect differences in electrical potential that occur when the positions of the arms of the instrument change in relation to each other. The electrogoniometer must be secured to the individual's body segment in such a way that (1) the axis of the goniometer corresponds to the axis of the joint being measured and (2) the axis and arms do not slip. Electrogoniometers may be planar (two dimensional) or triaxial (three dimensional).[62] Christensen and Nilsson used a spinal electrogoniometer to determine the reliability of and natural variation in cervical range-of-motion measurements.[194,195]

LINEAR MEASUREMENTS. The angles of some isolated or combined joint movements are so difficult to measure that a variety of linear measurement techniques have been developed. Temporomandibular joint opening is often documented by measuring the distance between the upper and lower incisors. Greater distance represents greater motion of the joint. Anterior and lateral protrusions of the jaw may also be measured by the distance between the incisors after each ma-

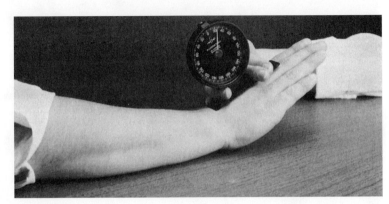

FIGURE 19–7. Inclinometer. Photo courtesy of Lafayette Instruments, 3700 Sagamore Parkway North, Lafayette, IN 47903.

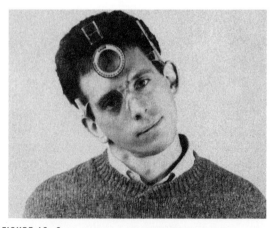

FIGURE 19–8. Cervical range-of-motion instrument. Photo courtesy of Performance Attainment Associates, 958 Lydia Drive, Roseville, MN 55113.

neuver.[180(pp216–219)] Trunk motion may be documented by the distance between the fingertips and the floor at the extremes of the range of motion or skin distraction measures that document changes in the distance between two skin markers when a patient moves from the resting position to the extreme of range of motion.[196,197] Fingertip-to-palm distance, finger abduction distance, and thumb abduction distance from the palm are frequently measured linearly.[198]

Intrinsic Joint Motions

The extent of intrinsic joint motion is frequently the judgment of the clinician, with the motion generally described as hypomobile, normal, or hypermobile. McClure and associates have studied the intertester reliability of such clinical judgments with regard to medial knee ligament integrity.[199] Global scales of joint laxity have also been developed to help identify individuals with laxity across many joints.[200] Measurement of anterior-posterior knee instability has become more objective with the introduction of knee arthrometers (Fig. 19–9).[201,202]

Joint Position and Posture

Measurement of joint position and posture is related to measurement of joint motion. However, rather than the movement of a body part, the resting position of a segment or the resting relationship between body segments is documented. Goniometers can be used to document resting positions, although there must be a relevant reference point with which the resting position can be compared. Lumbar spine position has been documented by using a flexible ruler to match

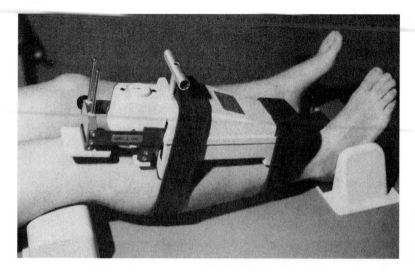

FIGURE 19–9. Knee arthrometer. Photo courtesy of MEDmetric Corporation, 7542 Trade Street, San Diego, CA 92121.

the position of the spine and then using trigonometric calculations to generate an angular measurement.[203]

SENSORY INTEGRITY

Sensation is a complex phenomenon mediated by a diverse set of mechano-, thermo-, nocio-, chemo-, and electroreceptors.[204] Of the numerous clinical tests of specific components of the sensory system that are available, measures of proprioception, two-point discrimination, and monofilament sensibility are presented.

Proprioception, or joint position sense, is often measured by having subjects reproduce various joint positions. This may be done statically by positioning a particular joint at a specific angle, returning the joint to a starting position, and asking the subject to reproduce the angle.[205,206] This may also be done by having subjects use one limb to reproduce the arc of movement that the other limb is being moved through passively.[207]

There are several different ways to test cutaneous sensation. Two-point discrimination determines the minimum distance between two points that is detectable by a patient. Nolan provides normative data for two-point discrimination in different parts of the body for young adult men and women.[208–210] The ability to detect different calibers of monofilaments, known as Semmes-Weinstein monofilaments, provides another objective view of sensation.[211] The ends of different monofilaments are pressed into the surface of the skin until they bend. The patient is asked to indicate when he or she perceives a sensation. Subjects with better cutaneous sensation are able to detect smaller monofilaments than those with impaired sensation. Compared with the tests of two-point discrimination, the monofilaments provide control of the force applied to the skin.[212] The use of monofilaments has been reported for evaluation of a wide range of disorders, including carpal tunnel syndrome,[213] diabetic peripheral neuropathy,[214] and lumbosacral radicular syndrome.[215]

VENTILATION, RESPIRATION, CIRCULATION, AEROBIC CAPACITY, AND ENDURANCE

Physical therapists often use exercise or relaxation techniques that can be expected to produce changes in cardiovascular, pulmonary, or autonomic nervous system functions. Kispert reviewed the literature related to cardiopulmonary measurements.[216]

Cardiovascular Measures

HEART RATE. Heart rate may be determined by palpation; by commercial heart rate monitors that attach to a subject's earlobe, finger, wrist, or chest; or by electrocardiographic equipment. Electrocardiographic measurement is considered the standard against which other measures of heart rate are evaluated. Sedlock and associates found a high degree of accuracy of self-determination of pulse rate after exercise in their comparison of heart rate determined through palpation of radial and carotid pulses with heart rate obtained with an electrocardiograph.[217] Araujo and associates documented the accuracy of five different heart rate monitors when subjects were at rest.[218]

Heart rate is sensitive to many factors, such as patients' activity prior to measurement, the time of day, the temperature of the room, patients' anxiety about the procedure, patients' food and drink consumption, and patients' emotional state. Researchers need to carefully control these factors, regardless of which method of measurement they choose.

BLOOD PRESSURE. Blood pressure may be determined directly with invasive measurement of pressures within arteries, or it may be determined indirectly through auscultation by an examiner or the use of an automated blood pressure device. The American Heart Association has provided guidelines for the measurement of blood pressure with sphygmomanometers.[219] Several researchers have examined a variety of measurement issues related to blood pressure monitoring equipment.[220–223]

Like heart rate, blood pressure is a labile phenomenon that may differ within an individual on the basis of the individual's emotional state, physical activity, and food and drink consumption. No matter which instrumentation a researcher uses to measure blood pressure, he or she must carefully control extraneous factors that may alter blood pressure.

FITNESS. Maximum oxygen consumption ($\dot{V}O_2$max) is the standard against which other measures of fitness are compared. $\dot{V}O_2$max is measured by analyzing the exhaled gases of a person who exercises in graded increments until oxygen consumption levels off or begins to decrease.[224] Such measures may be obtained manually through systems that collect expired gases or automatically by systems that analyze expired gases continuously (Fig. 19–10).[225] Nelson and colleagues used automated oxygen consumption measurement in a study of changes in fitness during training.[226] Gussoni and associates used manual oxygen consumption measurement in a study of the energy cost of walking with hip joint impairment.[227]

In addition to *direct* measurements of oxygen consumption, numerous tests *estimate* oxygen consumption by determining the distance a subject can run or walk in a specified period of time or the heart rate a subject achieves during a submaximal bout of bicycling, walking or jogging on a treadmill, or ascending and descending a step.[224,228] Amundsen and associates used a step test to estimate the fitness of elderly women before and after an exercise program.[229]

BLOOD FLOW. Because several physical therapy techniques are purported to work by increasing local blood flow, physical therapy researchers may have an interest in measuring the blood flow to an area before and after a given treatment. Doppler flowmeters provide a noninvasive way of determining blood flow. The hand-held Doppler device contains transmitting and receiving ultrasound crystals that are placed over the

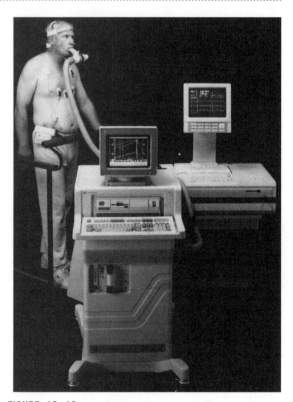

FIGURE 19–10. Automatic gas analysis system for evaluating maximum oxygen consumption. Photo courtesy of Sensormedics, 22705 Savi Ranch Parkway, Yorba Linda, CA 92687.

vessel in which blood flow is being measured. The blood flow pattern can be printed on a chart recorder, providing both quantitative measures of flow and qualitative interpretations based on the shape of the curve.[230] Walker and associates used a Doppler flowmeter to study the effect of high-voltage pulsed electrical stimulation on blood flow.[231] Skin temperature changes have also been used as an indirect measure of blood flow.[232]

Pulmonary Measures

The measures of pulmonary function can be grossly divided into those that assess the mechanics of breathing and those that assess physiological function. One of each type of test is described.

FORCED EXPIRATORY VOLUME. Forced expiratory volume (FEV) is measured to assess a person's ability to move air out of the lungs. A spirometer measures the volume of air expired after a maximal inspiration. FEV_1 is a variant of FEV that documents the proportion of air that is expelled in the first second of a forced exhalation. Cerny used FEV, FEV_1, and related measures to document pulmonary function in children with cystic fibrosis.[233]

OXYGEN SATURATION. Noninvasive oximeters can be used to measure the level of oxygen saturation in the blood. Because oxygen saturation is related to arterial oxygenation, oximetry provides a useful measure of physiological function. Cerny used an ear oximeter that clips to the earlobe to measure saturation in children with cystic fibrosis.[233] Kelly and colleagues used a pulse oximeter attached to the foot to determine saturation levels in preterm infants.[234]

Autonomic Function

Physical therapists are often interested in whether the goal of relaxation has been achieved. However, few investigators have effectively quantified changes in autonomic function that should indicate relaxation. Measures that have been used include heart rate,[232] blood pressure,[232] galvanic skin response,[232] skin temperature,[232] and respiratory sinus arrhythmia.[235] Galvanic skin response is related to sweat gland activity, which in turn is related to autonomic arousal.[236] Respiratory sinus arrhythmia—the rhythmic increase in heart rate associated with inspiration and the decrease associated with expiration—is thought to be an indication of vagal, or parasympathetic, tone.[232]

■ SUMMARY

A vast array of measurement tools are available to physical therapists. Tools for the measurement of 11 major categories within physical therapy were reviewed: anthropometric characteristics; arousal, mentation, and cognition; community and work integration, self-care, and home management; gait, locomotion, and balance; integumentary integrity; muscle performance; neuromotor development and sensory integration; pain; range of motion and joint integrity and mobility; sensory integrity; and ventilation, respiration, circulation, aerobic capacity, and endurance. Physical therapy clinicians must critically evaluate the measures they use to document patient status, readers of the literature need to critically examine the measurement tools described in research reports, and researchers must critically evaluate their measurement options to determine which tool is most appropriate for the study at hand.

REFERENCES

1. *Standards for Tests and Measurements in Physical Therapy Practice.* Alexandria, Va: American Physical Therapy Association; 1990.
2. Rothstein JM, Echternach JL. *Primer on Measurement: An Introductory Guide to Measurement Issues.* Alexandria, Va: American Physical Therapy Association; 1993.
3. The 1999 Buyer's Guide. *PT—Magazine of Physical Therapy.* 1998;6(8).
4. Guide to physical therapist practice. *Phys Ther.* 1997;77: 1163–1650.
5. Gordon CC, Chumlea WC, Roche AF. Stature, recumbent length, and weight. In: Lohman TG, Roche AF, Martorell R, eds. *Anthropometric Standardization Reference Manual.* Champaign, Ill: Human Kinetics Publishers; 1988:3–8.
6. Martin AD, Carter JEL, Handy KC, Malina RM. Segment lengths. In: Lohman TG, Roche AF, Martorell R, eds. *Anthropometric Standardization Reference Manual.* Champaign, Ill: Human Kinetics Publishers; 1988:9–26.
7. Callaway CW, Chumlea WC, Bouchard C, et al. Circumference. In: Lohman TG, Roche AF, Martorell R, eds. *Anthropometric Standardization Reference Manual.* Champaign, Ill: Human Kinetics Publishers; 1988:39–54.
8. Weiss LW, Clark FC, Howard DG. Effects of heavy-resistance triceps surae muscle training on strength and muscularity of men and women. *Phys Ther.* 1987; 67:1359–1364.
9. Ross M, Worrell TW. Thigh and calf girth following knee

injury and surgery. *J Orthop Sports Phys Ther.* 1998; 27:9–15.

10. Cureton KJ, Collins MA, Hill DW, McElhannon FM Jr. Muscle hypertrophy in men and women. *Med Sci Sports Exerc.* 1988;20:338–344.

11. Waylett-Rendall J, Seibly DS. A study of the accuracy of a commercially available volumeter. *J Hand Ther.* 1991;4:10–13.

12. Griffin JW, Newsome LS, Stralka SW, Wright PE. Reduction of chronic posttraumatic hand edema: a comparison of high voltage pulsed current, intermittent pneumatic compression, and placebo treatments. *Phys Ther.* 1990;70:279–286.

13. Casley-Smith JR. Measuring and representing peripheral oedema and its alterations. *Lymphology.* 1994;27:56–70.

14. Ko DSC, Lerner R, Klose G, Cosimi AB. Effective treatment of lymphedema of the extremities. *Arch Surg.* 1998;133:452–458.

15. Jackson AS, Pollack ML. Practical assessment of body composition. *Physician Sportsmedicine.* 1985;13(5): 76–90.

16. Harrison GG, Buskirk ER, Carter JEL, et al. Skinfold thicknesses and measurement technique. In: Lohman TG, Roche AF, Martorell R, eds. *Anthropometric Standardization Reference Manual.* Champaign, Ill: Human Kinetics Publishers; 1988:55–70.

17. Hayes PA, Sowood PJ, Belyavin A, Cohen JB, Smith FW. Subcutaneous fat thickness measured by magnetic resonance imaging, ultrasound, and calipers. *Med Sci Sports Exerc.* 1988;20:303–309.

18. Oppliger RA, Spray JA. Skinfold measurement variability in body density prediction. *Res Q Exerc Sport.* 1987;58.178–183.

19. Williams D, Anderson T, Currier D. Underwater weighing using the Hubbard tank vs the standard tank. *Phys Ther.* 1984;64:658–664.

20. Caton JR, Mole PA, Adams WC, Heustis DS. Body composition analysis by bioelectrical impedance: effect of skin temperature. *Med Sci Sports Exerc.* 1988;20: 489–491.

21. Wade DT. *Measurement in Neurological Rehabilitation.* Oxford, England: Oxford University Press, 1992.

22. Buechler CM, Blostein PA, Koestner A, Hurt K, Schuur M, McKernan J. Variation among trauma centers' calculation of Glasgow Coma Scale score: results of a national survey. *J Trauma.* 1998;45:429–432.

23. Tombaugh TN, McIntyre NJ. The Mini–Mental State Examination: a comprehensive review. *J Am Geriatr Soc.* 1992;40:922–935.

24. Shea V, Towle PO, Gordon BN. Psychological and cognitive tests. In: King-Thomas L, Hacker BJ, eds. *A Therapist's Guide to Pediatric Assessment.* Boston, Mass: Little, Brown & Co; 1987.

25. Impara JC, Plake BS, eds. *The Thirteenth Mental Measurements Yearbook.* Lincoln, Neb: Buros Institute of Mental Measurements of the University of Nebraska–Lincoln; 1998.

26. Impara JC, Conoley JC, eds. *Supplement to the Twelfth Mental Measurements Yearbook.* Lincoln, Neb: Buros Institute of Mental Measurements of the University of Nebraska–Lincoln; 1996.

27. Kidd T, Yoshida K. Critical review of disability mea-

sures: conceptual developments. *Physiotherapy Can.* 1995;47:108–119.

28. Young NL, Wright JG. Measuring pediatric physical function. *J Pediatr Orthop.* 1995;15:244–253.

29. Guccione AA, Cullen KE, O'Sullivan SB. Functional assessment. In: O'Sullivan SB, Schmitz TJ, eds. *Physical Rehabilitation: Assessment and Treatment.* 3rd ed. Philadelphia, Pa: FA Davis Co; 1994:193–207.

30. Merbitz C, Morris J, Grip JC. Ordinal scales and foundations of misinference. *Arch Phys Med Rehabil.* 1989;70:308–312.

31. Kaufert JM. Functional ability indices: measurement problems in assessing their validity. *Arch Phys Med Rehabil.* 1983;64:260–267.

32. Shah S, Vanclay F, Cooper B. Improving the sensitivity of the Barthel Index for stroke rehabilitation. *J Clin Epidemiol.* 1989;42:703–709.

33. Wilkinson PR, Wolfe CDA, Warburton FG, et al. A long-term follow-up of stroke patients. *Stroke.* 1997;28: 507–512.

34. Kakurai S, Akai M. Clinical experiences with a convertible thermoplastic knee-ankle-foot orthosis for post-stroke hemiplegic patients. *Prosthet Orthot Int.* 1996;20:191–194.

35. Duncan P, Richards L, Wallace D, et al. A randomized, controlled pilot study of a home-based exercise program for individuals with mild and moderate stroke. *Stroke.* 1998;29:2055–2060.

36. Whiteneck GG, Charlifue SW, Gerhart KA, Overholser JD, Richardson GN. Quantifying handicap: a new measure of long-term rehabilitation outcomes. *Arch Phys Med Rehabil.* 1992;73:519–526.

37. Heinemann AW, Linacre JM, Wright BD, Hamilton BB, Granger CV. Relationships between impairment and physical disability as measured by the functional independence measure. *Arch Phys Med Rehabil.* 1993;74: 566–573.

38. Linacre JM, Heinemann AW, Wright BD, Granger CV, Hamilton BB. The structure and stability of the functional independence measure. *Arch Phys Med Rehabil.* 1994;75:127–132.

39. Rintala DH, Loubser PG, Castro J, Hart KA, Fuhrer MJ. Chronic pain in a community-based sample of men with spinal cord injury: prevalence, severity, and relationship with impairment, disability, handicap, and subjective well-being. *Arch Phys Med Rehabil.* 1998;79:604–614.

40. Msall ME, DiGaudio K, Rogers BT, et al. The Functional Independence Measure for Children (WeeFIM): conceptual basis and pilot use in children with developmental disabilities. *Clin Pediatr.* 1994;33:421–430.

41. Lepage C, Noreau L, Bernard P-M. Association between characteristics of locomotion and accomplishment of life habits in children with cerebral palsy. *Phys Ther.* 1998;78:458–469.

42. Reuben DB, Siu AL. An objective measure of physical function of elderly outpatients: the Physical Performance Test. *J Am Geriatr Soc.* 1990;38:1105–1112.

43. Mueller MJ, Salsich GB, Strube MJ. Functional limitations in patients with diabetes and transmetatarsal amputations. *Phys Ther.* 1997;77:937–943.

44. Lawton MP, Brody EM. Assessment of older people:

self-maintaining and instrumental activities of daily living. *Gerontologist.* 1969;9:179–186.

45. Fillenbaum GG. Screening the elderly: a brief instrumental activities of daily living measure. *J Am Geriatr Soc.* 1985;33:698–706.

46. Reuben DB, Valle LA, Hays RD, Siu AL. Measuring physical function in community-dwelling older persons: a comparison of self-administered, interviewer-administered, and performance-based measures. *J Am Geriatr Soc.* 1995;43:17–23.

47. Schultz-Johnson K. Upper extremity functional capacity evaluation. In: Hunter JM, Macklin EJ, Callahan AD, eds. *Rehabilitation of the Hand: Surgery and Therapy.* Vol 2. 4th ed. St. Louis, Mo: CV Mosby Co; 1995:1739–1774.

48. King PM, Tuckwell N, Barrett TE. A critical review of functional capacity evaluations. *Phys Ther.* 1998;78: 852–866.

49. Isernhagen SJ. Industrial physical therapy. In: Malone TR, McPoil TG, Nitz AJ, eds. *Orthopedic and Sports Physical Therapy.* 3rd ed. St. Louis, Mo: Mosby–Year Book; 1997.

50. Bosco JS, Gustafson WF. *Measurement and Evaluation in Physical Education, Fitness, and Sports.* Englewood Cliffs, NJ: Prentice-Hall; 1983:227–272.

51. Atherly A. Condition-specific measures. In: Kane RL, ed. *Understanding Health Care Outcomes Research.* Gaithersburg, Md: Aspen Publishers; 1997:53–66.

52. Pynsent P, Fairbank J, Carr A. *Outcome Measures in Orthopaedics.* Oxford: Butterworth-Heinemann; 1993.

53. Fairbank J, Couper J, Davies J, O'Brien J. Oswestry low back pain disability index. *Physiotherapy.* 1980;66: 271–273.

54. Tegner Y, Lysholm J. Rating systems in the evaluation of knee ligament injuries. *Clin Orthop.* 1985;190:43–49.

55. Riddle DL, Stratford PW. Use of generic versus region-specific functional status measures on patients with cervical spine disorders. *Phys Ther.* 1998;78:951–963.

56. Barrett WP, Franklin JL, Jackins SE, Wyss CR, Matsen FA. Total shoulder arthroplasty. *J Bone Joint Surg Am.* 1987; 69:865–872.

57. Harris WH. Traumatic arthritis of the hip after dislocation in acetabular fractures: treatment by mould arthroplasty. *J Bone Joint Surg Am.* 1969;51:737–755.

58. Kavanagh BF, Fitzgerald RH. Clinical and roentgenographic assessment of total hip arthroplasty: a new hip score. *Clin Orthop.* 1985;193:133–140.

59. Olerud C, Molander H. A scoring scale for symptom evaluation after ankle fracture. *Arch Orthop Trauma Surg.* 1984;103:190–194.

60. Öberg U, Öberg B, Öberg T. Validity and reliability of a new assessment of lower-extremity dysfunction. *Phys Ther.* 1994;74:861–871.

61. Roach KE, Budiman-Mak E, Songsiridej N, Lertratanakul Y. Development of a shoulder pain and disability index. *Arthritis Care Res.* 1991;4:143–149.

62. Winter DA. *Biomechanics and Motor Control of Human Movement.* 2nd ed. New York, NY: John Wiley & Sons; 1990.

63. Robertson G, Sprigings E. Kinematics. In: Dainty DA, Norman RW, eds. *Standardized Biomechanical Testing in Sport.* Champaign, Ill: Human Kinetics Publishers; 1987.

64. Dainty D, Gagnon M, Lagasse P, Norman R, Robertson G, Sprigings E. Recommended procedures. In: Dainty DA, Norman RW, eds. *Standardized Biomechanical Testing in Sport.* Champaign, Ill: Human Kinetics Publishers; 1987.

65. Blanke DJ, Hageman PA. Comparison of gait of young men and elderly men. *Phys Ther.* 1989;69:144–148.

66. Heriza CB. Organization of leg movements in preterm infants. *Phys Ther.* 1988;68:1340–1346.

67. Kluzik J, Fetters L, Coryell J. Quantification of control: a preliminary study of effects of neurodevelopmental treatment on reaching in children with spastic cerebral palsy. *Phys Ther.* 1990;70:65–76.

68. Rose-Jacobs R. Development of gait at slow, free, and fast speeds in 3- and 5-year-old children. *Phys Ther.* 1983;63:1251–1259.

69. Burdett RG, Borello-France D, Blatchly C, Potter C. Gait comparison of subjects with hemiplegia walking unbraced, with ankle-foot orthosis, and with Air-Stirrup ® brace. *Phys Ther.* 1988;68:1197–1203.

70. Gagnon M, Robertson G, Norman R. Kinetics. In: Dainty DA, Norman RW, eds. *Standardized Biomechanical Testing in Sport.* Champaign, Ill: Human Kinetics Publishers; 1987.

71. Schuit D, Adrian M, Pidcoe P. Effect of heel lifts on ground reaction force patterns in subjects with structural leg-length discrepancies. *Phys Ther.* 1989;69: 663–670.

72. Berg K. Balance and its measure in the elderly: a review. *Physiotherapy Can.* 1989;41:240–246.

73. Whitney SL, Poole JL, Cass SP. A review of balance instruments for older adults. *Am J Occup Ther.* 1998;52: 666–671.

74. Nashner LM, Peters JF. Dynamic posturography in the diagnosis and management of dizziness and balance disorders. *Neurol Clin.* 1990;8:331–349.

75. Perrin PP, Jeandel C, Perrin CA, Béné MC. Influence of visual control, conduction, and central integration on static and dynamic balance in healthy older adults. *Gerontology.* 1997;43:223–231.

76. Camicioli R, Panzer VP, Kaye J. Balance in the healthy elderly: posturography and clinical assessment. *Arch Neurol.* 1997;54:976–981.

77. Baloh RW, Spain S, Socotch TM, Jacobson KM, Bell T. Posturography and balance problems in older people. *J Am Geriatr Soc.* 1995;43:638–644.

78. Briggs RC, Gossman MR, Birch R, Drews JE, Shaddeau SA. Balance performance among noninstitutionalized elderly women. *Phys Ther.* 1989;69:748–756.

79. Iverson BD, Gossman MR, Shaddeau SA, Turner ME Jr. Balance performance, force production, and activity levels in noninstitutionalized men 60 to 90 years of age. *Phys Ther.* 1990;70:348–355.

80. Bohannon RW, Larkin PA, Cook AC, Gear J, Singer J. Decrease in timed balance test scores with aging. *Phys Ther.* 1984;64:1067–1070.

81. Shumway-Cook A, Horak FB. Assessing the influence of sensory interaction on balance: suggestion from the field. *Phys Ther.* 1986;66:1548–1550.

82. Cohen H, Blatchly CA, Gombash LL. A study of the clinical test of sensory interaction and balance. *Phys Ther.* 1993;73:346–354.

83. Di Fabio RP, Badke MB. Relationship of sensory organization to balance function in patients with hemiplegia. *Phys Ther.* 1990;70:542–548.

84. Duncan PW, Weiner DK, Chandler J, Studenski S. Functional reach: a new clinical measure of balance. *J Gerontol.* 1990;45:M192–M197.

85. Weiner DK, Duncan PW, Chandler J, Studenski SA. Functional reach: a marker of physical frailty. *J Am Geriatr Soc.* 1991;40:203–207.

86. Fishman MN, Colby LA, Sachs LA, Nichols DS. Comparison of upper-extremity balance tasks and force platform testing in persons with hemiparesis. *Phys Ther.* 1997;77:1052–1062.

87. Berg K, Wood-Dauphinee S, Williams JI, Gayton D. Measuring balance in the elderly: preliminary development of an instrument. *Physiotherapy Can.* 1989;41:304–311.

88. Berg KO, Wood-Dauphinee SL, Williams JI, Maki B. Measuring balance in the elderly: validation of an instrument. *Can J Public Health.* 1992;83(suppl 2):S7–S11.

89. Shumway-Cook A, Baldwin M, Polissar NL, Gruber W. Predicting the probability of falls in community-dwelling older adults. *Phys Ther.* 1997;77:812–819.

90. Harada N, Chiu V, Fowler E, Lee M, Reuben DB. Physical therapy to improve functioning of older people in residential care facilities. *Phys Ther.* 1995;75:830–839.

91. Tinetti ME. Performance-oriented assessment of mobility problems in elderly patients. *J Am Geriatr Soc.* 1986;34:119–126.

92. Cipriany-Dacko LM, Innerst D, Johannsen J, Rude V. Interrater reliability of the Tinetti balance scores in novice and experienced physical therapy clinicians. *Arch Phys Med Rehabil.* 1997;78:1160–1164.

93. Harada N, Chiu V, Damron-Rodriguez J, Fowler E, Sui A, Reuben DB. Screening for balance and mobility impairment in elderly individuals living in residential care facilities. *Phys Ther.* 1995;75:462–469.

94. Mathias S, Nayak USL, Isaacs B. Balance in elderly patients: the "get-up and go" tests. *Arch Phys Med Rehabil.* 1986;67:387–389.

95. Podsiadlo D, Richardson S. The Timed "Up & Go": a test of basic functional mobility for frail elderly persons. *J Am Geriatr Soc.* 1991;39:142–148.

96. Majeske C. Reliability of wound surface area measurements. *Phys Ther.* 1992;72:138–141.

97. Cutler NR, George R, Seifert RD, et al. Comparison of quantitative methodologies to define chronic pressure ulcer measurements. *Decubitus.* 1993;6(6):22–30.

98. Griffin JW, Tolley EA, Tooms RE, Reyes RA, Clifft JK. A comparison of photographic and transparency-based methods for measuring wound surface area. *Phys Ther.* 1993;73:117–122.

99. Kloth LC, Feedar JA. Acceleration of wound healing with high voltage, monophasic, pulsed current. *Phys Ther.* 1988;68:503–508.

100. Lamb RL. Manual muscle testing. In: Rothstein JM, ed. *Measurement in Physical Therapy.* New York, NY: Churchill Livingstone; 1985:47–55.

101. Wadsworth CT, Krishnan R, Sear M, Harrold J, Nielsen DH. Intrarater reliability of manual muscle testing and hand-held dynametric muscle testing. *Phys Ther.* 1987;67:1342–1347.

102. Frese E, Brown M, Norton BJ. Clinical reliability of manual muscle testing: middle trapezius and gluteus medius muscles. *Phys Ther.* 1987;67:1072–1076.

103. Mulroy SJ, Lassen KD, Chambers SH, Perry J. The ability of male and female clinicians to effectively test knee extension strength using manual muscle testing. *J Orthop Sports Phys Ther.* 1997;26:192–199.

104. Herbison GJ, Isaac Z, Cohen ME, Ditunno JF Jr. Strength post–spinal cord injury: myometer vs manual muscle test. *Spinal Cord.* 1996;34:543–548.

105. Bohannon RW. Test-retest reliability of hand-held dynamometry during a single session of strength assessment. *Phys Ther.* 1986;66:206–209.

106. Riddle DL, Finucane SD, Rothstein JM, Walker ML. Intrasession and intersession reliability of hand-held dynamometer measurements taken on brain-damaged patients. *Phys Ther.* 1989;69:182–189.

107. Stuberg WA, Metcalf WK. Reliability of quantitative muscle testing in healthy children and in children with Duchenne muscular dystrophy using a hand-held dynamometer. *Phys Ther.* 1988;68:977–982.

108. Kwoh CK, Petrick MA, Munin MC. Inter-rater reliability of function and strength measurements in the acute care hospital after elective hip and knee arthroplasty. *Arthritis Care Res.* 1997;10:128–134.

109. Brinkmann JR. Comparison of a hand-held and fixed dynamometer in measuring strength of patients with neuromuscular disease. *J Orthop Sports Phys Ther.* 1994;19:100–104.

110. Horvat M, Croce R, Roswal G. Intratester reliability of the Nicholas manual muscle tester on individuals with intellectual disabilities by a tester having minimal experience. *Arch Phys Med Rehabil.* 1994;75:808–811.

111. Trudelle-Jackson E, Jackson AW, Frankowski CM, Long KM, Meske NB. Interdevice reliability and validity assessment of the Nicholas hand-held dynamometer. *J Orthop Sports Phys Ther.* 1994;20:302–306.

112. Andrews AW, Thomas MW, Bohannon RW. Normative values for isometric muscle force measurements obtained with hand-held dynamometers. *Phys Ther.* 1996;76:248–259.

113. Spielholz NI. Scientific bases of exercise programs. In: Basmajian JV, Wolf SL, eds. *Therapeutic Exercise.* 5th ed. Baltimore, Md: Williams & Wilkins; 1990:58.

114. Jürimäe J, Abernathy PJ, Blake K, McEniery MT. Changes in the myosin heavy chain isoform profile of the triceps brachii muscle following 12 weeks of resistance training. *Eur J Appl Physiol.* 1996;74:287–292.

115. Balogun JA, Onilari OO, Akeju OA, Marzouk DK. High voltage electrical stimulation in the augmentation of muscle strength: effects of pulse frequency. *Arch Phys Med Rehabil.* 1993;74:910–916.

116. Vaughan VG. Effects of upper limb immobilization on isometric muscle strength, movement time, and triphasic electromyographic characteristics. *Phys Ther.* 1989;69:119–129.

117. Fess EE. Documentation: essential elements of an upper extremity assessment battery. In: Hunter JM, Macklin EJ, Callahan AD, eds. *Rehabilitation of the Hand: Surgery and Therapy.* Vol 1. 4th ed. St. Louis, Mo: CV Mosby Co; 1995:185–214.

118. Hamilton A, Balnave R, Adams R. Grip strength testing reliability. *J Hand Ther.* 1994;7:163–170.

119. Stephens JL, Pratt N, Parks B. The reliability and validity of the Tekdyne hand dynamometer: part I. *J Hand Ther*. 1996;9:10–17.

120. Mathiowetz V, Kashman N, Volland G, Weber K, Dowe M, Rogers S. Grip and pinch strength: normative data for adults. *Arch Phys Med Rehabil*. 1985;66:69–74.

121. Josty IC, Tyler MPH, Shewell PC, Roberts AHN. Grip and pinch strength variations in different types of workers. *J Hand Surg Br*. 1997;22:266–269.

122. Jansen CWS, Minerbo G. A comparison between early dynamically controlled mobilization and immobilization after flexor tendon repair in zone 2 of the hand: preliminary results. *J Hand Ther*. 1990;3:20–25.

123. Perrin DH. *Isokinetic Exercise and Assessment*. Champaign, Ill: Human Kinetics Publishers; 1993.

124. Francis K, Hoobler T. Comparison of peak torque values of the knee flexor and extensor muscle groups using the Cybex II and Lido 2.0 isokinetic dynamometers. *J Orthop Sports Phys Ther*. 1987;8:481–483.

125. Thompson MC, Shingleton LG, Kegerreis ST. Comparison of values generated during testing of the knee using the Cybex II Plus and Biodex Model B-2000 isokinetic dynamometers. *J Orthop Sports Phys Ther*. 1989;11:108–115.

126. Deones VL, Wiley SC, Worrell TW. Assessment of quadriceps muscle performance by a hand-held dynamometer and an isokinetic dynamometer. *J Orthop Sports Phys Ther*. 1994;20:296–301.

127. Reed RL, Den Hartog R, Yochum K, Pearlmutter L, Ruttinger AC, Mooradian AD. A comparison of hand-held isometric strength measurement with isokinetic muscle strength measurement in the elderly. *J Am Geriatr Soc*. 1993;41:53–56.

128. Frontera WR, Hughes VA, Dallal GE, Evans WJ. Reliability of iskoinetic muscle strength testing in 45- to 78-year-old men and women. *Arch Phys Med Rehabil*. 1993;74:1181–1185.

129. Madsen OR, Lauridsen UB. Knee extensor and flexor strength in elderly women after recent hip fracture: assessment by the Cybex 6000 dynamometer of intra-rater inter-test reliability. *Scand J Rehabil Med*. 1995;27:219–226.

130. Li RCT, Maffulli N, Hsu YC, Chan KM. Isokinetic strength of the quadriceps and hamstrings and functional ability of anterior cruciate deficient knees in recreational athletes. *Br J Sports Med*. 1996;30:161–164.

131. Brown M, Kohrt WM, Delitto A. Peak torque to body weight ratios in older adults: a re-examination. *Physiotherapy Can*. 1991;43:7–11.

132. Rothstein JM, Lamb RL, Mayhew TP. Clinical uses of isokinetic measurements: critical issues. *Phys Ther*. 1987;67:1840–1844.

133. Winter DA, Wells RP, Orr GW. Errors in the use of isokinetic dynamometers. *Eur J Appl Physiol*. 1981;46:397–404.

134. Keating JL, Matyas TA. The influence of subject and test design on dynametric measurements of extremity muscles. *Phys Ther*. 1996;76:866–889.

135. Echternach JL. Measurement issues in nerve conduction velocity and electromyographic testing. In: Rothstein JM, ed. *Measurement in Physical Therapy*. New York, NY: Churchill Livingstone; 1985:281–304.

136. Soderberg GL, Cook TM. Electromyography in biomechanics. *Phys Ther*. 1984;64:1813–1820.

137. Portney LG. Electromyography and nerve conduction velocity tests. In: O'Sullivan SB, Schmitz TJ, eds. *Physical Rehabilitation: Assessment and Treatment*. 3rd ed. Philadelphia, Pa: FA Davis Co; 1994:133–165.

138. Fridlund AJ, Cacioppo JT. Guidelines for human electromyographic research. *Psychophysiology*. 1986;23:567–589.

139. Duncan PW, Studenski S, Chandler J, Bloomfeld R, LaPointe LK. Electromyographic analysis of postural adjustments in two methods of balance testing. *Phys Ther*. 1990;70:88–96.

140. Hanten WP, Schulthies SS. Exercise effect on electromyographic activity of the vastus medialis oblique and vastus lateralis muscles. *Phys Ther*. 1990;70:561–565.

141. O'Sullivan SB. Motor control assessment. In: O'Sullivan SB, Schmitz TJ, eds. *Physical Rehabilitation: Assessment and Treatment*. 3rd ed. Philadelphia, Pa: FA Davis Co; 1994:111–131.

142. Wright V, Sheil EMH, Drake JM, Wedge JH, Naumann S. Evaluation of selective dorsal rhizotomy for the reduction of spasticity in cerebral palsy: a randomized controlled trial. *Dev Med Child Neurol*. 1998;40:239–247.

143. Bohannon RW, Smith MB. Interrater reliability of a modified Ashworth scale of muscle spasticity. *Phys Ther*. 1987;67:206–207.

144. Rothstein JM, Roy SH, Wolf SL. *The Rehabilitation Specialist's Handbook*. 2nd ed. Philadelphia, Pa: FA Davis Co; 1998:368.

145. Worley JS, Bennett W, Miller G, Miller M, Walter B, Harmon C. Reliability of three clinical measures of muscle tone in the shoulders and wrists of poststroke patients. *Am J Occup Ther*. 1991;45:50–58.

146. Bajd T, Vodovnik L. Pendulum testing of spasticity. *J Biomed Eng*. 1984;6:9–16.

147. Bohannon RW, Larkin PA. Cybex II isokinetic dynamometer for the documentation of spasticity: suggestion from the field. *Phys Ther*. 1985;65:46–47.

148. Bohannon RW. Variability and reliability of the pendulum test for spasticity using a Cybex II isokinetic dynamometer. *Phys Ther*. 1987;67:659–661.

149. Bajd T, Gregoric M, Vodovnik L, Benko H. Electrical stimulation in treating spasticity resulting from spinal cord injury. *Arch Phys Med Rehabil*. 1985;66:515–517.

150. Perell K, Scremin A, Scremin O, Kunkel C. Quantifying muscle tone in spinal cord injury patients using isokinetic dynamometric techniques. *Paraplegia*. 1996;34:46–53.

151. Wang R-Y, Tsai M-W, Chan R-C. Effects of surface spinal cord stimulation on spasticity and quantitative assessment of muscle tone in hemiplegic patients. *Am J Phys Med Rehabil*. 1998;77:282–287.

152. Boiteau M, Malouin F, Richards CL. Use of a hand-held dynamometer and a Kin-Com dynamometer for evaluating spastic hypertonia in children: a reliability study. *Phys Ther*. 1995;75:796–802.

153. Corcos DM. Strategies underlying the control of disordered movement. *Phys Ther*. 1991;71:25–38.

154. Wolf SL, LeCraw DE, Barton LA. Comparison of motor copy and targeted biofeedback training techniques for

restitution of upper extremity function among patients with neurologic disorders. *Phys Ther.* 1989;69:719–735.

155. Dickstein R, Pillar T, Shina N, Hocherman S. Electromyographic responses of distal ankle musculature of standing hemiplegic patients to continuous anterior-posterior perturbations during imposed weight transfer over the affected leg. *Phys Ther.* 1989;69:484–491.

156. Cress ME, Conley KE, Balding SL, Hansen-Smith F, Konczak J. Functional training: muscle structure, function, and performance in older women. *J Orthop Sports Phys Ther.* 1996;24:4–10.

157. Sinacore DR, Delitto A, King DS, Rose SJ. Type II fiber activation with electrical stimulation: a preliminary report. *Phys Ther.* 1990;70:416–422.

158. Case-Smith J, Butcher L, Reed D. Parents' report of sensory responsiveness and temperament in preterm infants. *Am J Occup Ther.* 1998;52:547–555.

159. Karmel BZ, Gardner JM, Freedland RL. Neonatal neurobehavioral assessment and Bayley I and II scores of CNS-injured and cocaine-exposed infants. *Ann NY Acad Sci.* 1998;846:391–395.

160. Skranes J, Vik T, Nilsen G, Smevik O, Andersson HW, Brubakk AM. Can cerebral MRI at age 1 predict motor and intellectual outcomes in very-low-birthweight children? *Dev Med Child Neurol.* 1998;40:256–262.

161. Chiarello LA, Palisano RJ. Investigation of the effects of a model of physical therapy on mother-child interactions and the motor behaviors of children with motor delay. *Phys Ther.* 1998;78:180–194.

162. Gebhard AR, Ottenbacher KJ, Lane SJ. Interrater reliability of the Peabody Developmental Motor Scales: fine motor scale. *Am J Occup Ther.* 1994;48:976–981.

163. Palisano RJ, Kolobe TH, Haley SM, Lowes LP, Jones SL. Validity of the Peabody Developmental Gross Motor Scale as an evaluative measure of infants receiving physical therapy. *Phys Ther.* 1995;75:939–951.

164. Kolobe THA, Palisano RJ, Stratford PW. Comparison of two outcome measures for infants with cerebral palsy and infants with motor delays. *Phys Ther.* 1998;78:1062–1072.

165. Murney ME, Campbell SK. The ecological relevance of the Test of Infant Motor Performance elicited scale items. *Phys Ther.* 1998;78:479–489.

166. Harris SR, Haley SM, Tada WL, Swanson MW. Reliability of observational measures of the Movement Assessment of Infants. *Phys Ther.* 1989;64:471–477.

167. Nordmark E, Hägglund G, Jarnlo G-B. Reliability of the Gross Motor Function Measure in cerebral palsy. *Scand J Rehabil Med.* 1997;29:25–28.

168. Harris SR, Daniels LE. Content validity of the Harris Infant Neuromotor Test. *Phys Ther.* 1996;76:727–737.

169. Campbell SK. The child's development of functional movement. In: Campbell SK, ed. *Physical Therapy for Children.* Philadelphia, Pa: WB Saunders Co; 1994:3–37.

170. King-Thomas K, Hacker BJ, eds. *A Therapist's Guide to Pediatric Assessment.* Boston, Mass: Little, Brown & Co; 1987.

171. Melzack R. The McGill Pain Questionnaire: major properties and scoring methods. *Pain.* 1975;1:277–299.

172. Bonaiuti D, Fontanella G. The affective dimension of low-back pain: its influence on the outcome of back school. *Arch Phys Med Rehabil.* 1996;77:1239–1242.

173. Materson RS. Techniques for assessing and diagnosing pain. In: Weiner RS, ed. *Pain Management: A Practical Guide for Clinicians.* Vol 1. 5th ed. Boca Raton, Fla: St. Lucie Press; 1998:45–57.

174. Price DD, McGrath PA, Rafii A, Buckingham B. The validation of visual analogue scales as ratio scale measures for chronic and experimental pain. *Pain.* 1983;17:45–56.

175. Craig JA, Cunningham MB, Walsh DM, Baxter GD, Allen JM. Lack of effect of transcutaneous electrical nerve stimulation upon experimentally induced delayed onset muscle soreness in humans. *Pain.* 1996;67:285–289.

176. Echternach JL. Evaluation of pain in the clinical environment. In: Echternach JL, ed. *Pain.* New York, NY: Churchill Livingstone; 1987.

177. Noling LB, Clelland JA, Jackson JR, Knowles CJ. Effect of transcutaneous electrical nerve stimulation at auricular points on experimental cutaneous pain threshold. *Phys Ther.* 1988;68:328–332.

178. Gajdosik RL, Bohannon RW. Clinical measurement of range of motion: review of goniometry emphasizing reliability and validity. *Phys Ther.* 1987;67:1867–1872.

179. American Academy of Orthopaedic Surgeons. *Joint Motion: Method of Measuring and Recording.* Chicago, Ill: American Academy of Orthopaedic Surgeons; 1965.

180. Norkin CC, White DJ. *Measurement of Joint Motion: A Guide to Goniometry.* 2nd ed. Philadelphia, Pa: FA Davis Co; 1995:216–219.

181. Boone DC, Azen SP, Lin C-M, Spence C, Baron C, Lee L. Reliability of goniometric measurements. *Phys Ther.* 1978;58:1355–1360.

182. Rothstein JM, Miller PJ, Roettger RF. Goniometric reliability in a clinical setting: elbow and knee measurements. *Phys Ther.* 1983;63:1611–1615.

183. Mayerson NH, Milano RA. Goniometric reliability in physical medicine. *Arch Phys Med Rehabil.* 1984;65:92–94.

184. Rome K, Cowieson F. A reliability study of the universal goniometer, fluid goniometer, and electrogoniometer for the measurement of ankle dorsiflexion. *Foot Ankle Int.* 1996;17:28–32.

185. Youdas JW, Bogard CL, Suman VJ. Reliability of goniometric measurements and visual estimates of ankle joint active range of motion obtained in a clinical setting. *Arch Phys Med Rehabil.* 1993;74:1113–1118.

186. Brosseau L, Tousignant M, Budd J, et al. Intratester and intertester reliability and criterion validity of the parallelogram and universal goniometers for active knee flexion in healthy subjects. *Physiother Res Int.* 1997;2:150–166.

187. Breger-Lee D, Bell-Krotoski J, Brandsma JW. Torque range of motion in the hand clinic. *J Hand Ther.* 1990;1:7–13.

188. Mayer TG, Kondraske G, Beals SB, Gatchel RJ. Spinal range of motion: accuracy and sources of error with inclinometric measurement. *Spine.* 1997;22:1976–1984.

189. Chen S-PC, Samo DG, Chen EH, et al. Reliability of three lumbar sagittal motion measurement methods: surface inclinometers. *J Occup Envrion Med.* 1997;39:217–223.

190. Samo DG, Chen S-PC, Crampton AR. Validity of three lumbar sagittal motion measurement methods: surface inclinometers compared with radiographs. *J Occup Environ Med.* 1997;39:209–216.

191. Stude DE, Goertz C, Gallinger MC. Inter- and intraexaminer reliability of a single, digital inclinometric range of motion measurement technique in the assessment of lumbar range of motion. *J Manipulative Physiol Ther.* 1994;17:83–87.

192. Green S, Buchbinder R, Forbes A, Bellany N. A standardized protocol for measurement of range of movement of the shoulder using the Plurimeter-V inclinometer and assessment of its intrarater and interrater reliability. *Arthritis Care Res.* 1998;11:43–52.

193. Youdas JW, Carey JR, Garrett TR. Reliability of measurement of cervical spine range of motion—comparison of three methods. *Phys Ther.* 1991;71:98–104.

194. Christensen HW, Nilsson N. The reliability of measuring active and passive cervical range of motion: an observer-blinded and randomized repeated-measures design. *J Manipulative Physiol Ther.* 1998;21:341–347.

195. Christensen HW, Nilsson N. Natural variation of cervical range of motion: a one-way repeated-measures design. *J Manipulative Physiol Ther.* 1998;21:383–387.

196. Merritt JL, McLean TJ, Erickson RP, Offord KP. Measurement of trunk flexibility in normal subjects: reproducibility of three clinical methods. *Mayo Clin Proc.* 1986;61:192–197.

197. Burdett RG, Brown KE, Fall MP. Reliability and validity of four instruments for measuring lumbar spine and pelvic positions. *Phys Ther.* 1986;66:677–684.

198. Cambridge-Keeling CA. Range-of-motion measurement of the hand. In: Hunter JM, Macklin EJ, Callahan AD, eds. *Rehabilitation of the Hand: Surgery and Therapy.* Vol 1. 4th ed. St. Louis, Mo: CV Mosby Co; 1995:93–107.

199. McClure PW, Rothstein JM, Riddle DL. Intertester reliability of clinical judgments of medial knee ligament integrity. *Phys Ther.* 1989;69:268–275.

200. Acasuso-Díaz M, Collantes-Estévez E. Joint hypermobility in patients with fibromyalgia syndrome. *Arthritis Care Res.* 1998;11:39–42.

201. Neuschwander DC, Drez D, Paine RM, Young JC. Comparison of anterior laxity measurements in anterior cruciate deficient knees with two instrumented testing devices. *Orthopedics.* 1990;13:299–302.

202. Ballantyne BT, French AK, Heimsoth SL, Kachingwe AF, Lee JB, Soderberg GL. Influence of examiner experience and gender on interrater reliability of KT-1000 arthrometer measurements. *Phys Ther.* 1995;75:898–906.

203. Schenk RJ, Doran RL, Stachura JJ. Learning effects of a back education program. *Spine.* 1996;21:2183–2189.

204. Schmitz TJ. Sensory assessment. In: O'Sullivan SB, Schmitz TJ, eds. *Physical Rehabilitation: Assessment and Treatment.* 3rd ed. Philadelphia, Pa: FA Davis Co; 1994;83–95.

205. Petrella RJ, Lattanzio PJ, Nelson MG. Effect of age and activity on knee joint proprioception. *Am J Phys Med Rehabil.* 1997;76:235–241.

206. Lattanzio P-J, Chess DG, MacDermid JC. Effect of the posterior cruciate ligament in knee-joint proprioception in total knee arthroplasty. *J Arthroplasty.* 1998;13:580–585.

207. McNair PJ, Marshall RN, Maguire K, Brown C. Knee joint effusion and proprioception. *Arch Phys Med Rehabil.* 1995;76:566–568.

208. Nolan MF. Two-point discrimination assessment in the upper limb in young adult men and women. *Phys Ther.* 1982;62:965–969.

209. Nolan MF. Limits of two-point discrimination ability in the lower limb in young adult men and women. *Phys Ther.* 1983;63:1424–1428.

210. Nolan MF. Quantitative measure of cutaneous sensation: two-point discrimination values for the face and trunk. *Phys Ther.* 1985;65:181–185.

211. Holewski JJ, Stess RM, Graf PM, Grunfeld C. Aesthesiometry: quantification of cutaneous pressure sensation in diabetic peripheral neuropathy. *J Rehabil Res Dev.* 1988;25(2):1–10.

212. Bell-Krotoski JA. Sensibility testing: current concepts. In: Hunter JM, Macklin EJ, Callahan AD, eds. *Rehabilitation of the Hand: Surgery and Therapy.* Vol 1. 4th ed. St. Louis, Mo: CV Mosby Co; 1995:109–128.

213. Marx RG, Hudak PL, Bombardier C, Graham B, Goldsmith C, Wright JG. The reliability of physical examination for carpal tunnel syndrome. *J Hand Surg Br.* 1998;23:499–502.

214. Mueller MJ. Identifying patients with diabetes mellitus who are at risk for lower-extremity complications: use of Semmes-Weinstein monofilaments. *Phys Ther.* 1996; 76:68–71.

215. Peeters GG, Aufdemkampe G, Oostendorp RA. Sensibility testing in patients with a lumbosacral radicular syndrome. *J Manipulative Physiol Ther.* 1998;21:81–88.

216. Kispert CP. Clinical measurements to assess cardiopulmonary function. *Phys Ther.* 1987;67:1886–1890.

217. Sedlock DA, Knowlton RG, Fitzgerald PI, Tahamont MV, Schneider DA. Accuracy of subject-palpated carotid pulse after exercise. *Physician Sportsmedicine.* 1983; 11(4):106–116.

218. Araujo, J, Born DG, Thomas TR. An evaluation of five portable heart monitors [abstract]. *Med Sci Sports Exerc.* 1981;13:124.

219. Kirkendall WM, Feinleib M, Freis ED, Mark AL. Recommendations for human blood pressure determination by sphygmomanometers. *Hypertension.* 1981;3:510A–519A.

220. Mion D, Pierin AM. How accurate are sphygmomanometers? *J Hum Hypertens.* 1998;12:245–248.

221. Kroke A, Fleischhauer W, Mieke S, Klipstein-Grobusch K, Willich SN, Boeing H. Blood pressure measurement in epidemiological studies: a comparative analysis of two methods. Data from the EPIC-Potsdam Study. European Prospective Investigation into Cancer and Nutrition. *J Hypertens.* 1998;16:739–746.

222. Dobbin KR. Noninvasive blood pressure monitoring. *Crit Care Nurs.* 1998;18:101–102.

223. Lightfoot JT, Tankersley C, Rowe SA, Freed AN, Fortney SM. Automated blood pressure measurements during exercise. *Med Sci Sports Exerc.* 1989;21:698–707.

224. McArdle WD, Katch FI, Katch VL. *Exercise Physiology: Energy, Nutrition, and Human Performance.* 4th ed. Baltimore, Md: Williams & Wilkins; 1996:198–200.

225. Wasserman K, Hansen JE, Sue DY, Whipp BJ, Casaburi R. *Principles of Exercise Testing and Interpretation.* 2nd ed. Philadelphia, Pa: Lea & Febiger; 1994:440–442.

226. Nelson AG, Arnall DA, Loy SF, Silvester LJ, Conlee RK. Consequences of combining strength and endurance training regimens. *Phys Ther.* 1990;70:287–294.

227. Gussoni M, Margonato V, Ventura R, Veicsteinas A. Energy cost of walking with hip joint impairment. *Phys Ther.* 1990;70:295–301.

228. American College of Sports Medicine. *ACSM's Guidelines for Exercise Testing and Prescription.* 5th ed. Baltimore, Md: Williams & Wilkins; 1995:68–75.

229. Amundsen LR, DeVahl JM, Ellingham CT. Evaluation of a group exercise program for elderly women. *Phys Ther.* 1989;69:475–483.

230. Hurley JJ, Woods JJ, Hershey FB. Noninvasive testing: practical knowledge for evaluating diabetic patients. In: Levin ME, O'Neal LW, Bowker JH, eds. *The Diabetic Foot.* St. Louis, Mo: Mosby–Year Book; 1993:321–340.

231. Walker DC, Currier DP, Threlkeld AJ. Effects of high voltage pulsed electrical stimulation on blood flow. *Phys Ther.* 1988;68:481–485.

232. Reed BV, Held JM. Effects of sequential connective tissue massage on autonomic nervous system of middle-aged and elderly adults. *Phys Ther.* 1988;68:1231–1234.

233. Cerny FJ. Relative effects of bronchial drainage and exercise for in-hospital care of patients with cystic fibrosis. *Phys Ther.* 1989;69:633–639.

234. Kelly MK, Palisano RJ, Wolfson MR. Effects of a developmental physical therapy program on oxygen saturation and heart rate in preterm infants. *Phys Ther.* 1989;69:467–474.

235. Watkins LL, Grossman P, Krishnan R, Sherwood A. Anxiety and vagal control of heart rate. *Psychosom Med.* 1998;60:498–502.

236. Marcer D. *Biofeedback and Related Therapies in Clinical Practice.* Rockville, Md: Aspen Systems Corp; 1986:14.

SECTION 6

Data Analysis

Statistical Reasoning

Data Set	**Sampling Distribution**
Frequency Distribution	Confidence Intervals of the
Frequency Distribution with	Sampling Distribution
Percentages	**Significant Difference**
Grouped Frequency Distribution	Null Hypothesis
with Percentages	Alpha Level
Frequency Histogram	Probability Determinants
Stem-and-Leaf Plot	*Between-Groups Difference*
Central Tendency	*Within-Group Variability*
Mean	*Sample Size*
Median	**Errors**
Mode	**Power**
Variability	**Statistical Conclusion Validity**
Range	Low Power
Variance	Lack of Clinical Importance
Standard Deviation	Error Rate Problems
Normal Distribution	Violated Assumptions
z Score	
Percentages of the Normal	
Distribution	

Statistics has a bad name. Consider this tongue-in-cheek sampling from the irreverent *Journal of Irreproducible Results*:

> We all know that you can prove anything with statistics. So I recently proved that nobody likes statistics, except for a few professors. If you don't believe that, just ask the person on the street. I did. The first person I saw referred to the subject as "sadistics." The second person, an old gentleman along the Mississippi River, muttered something about "liars, damned liars, and statisticians." [1(p13)]

Although quips about statistics are amusing, the discipline of statistics should not be confused with the conclusions that researchers draw from statistical analyses. Statistics is a discipline in which mathematics and probability are applied in ways that allow researchers to make sense of their data. Although there are many different statistical tests and procedures—too many to include even in textbooks devoted solely to statistics—there are remarkably few central concepts that underlie all of the tests.

In this chapter, the central concepts of statistics are introduced. Readers should be prepared to read this chapter, and Chapters 21 through 24, which cover particular statistical tests, very slowly. Careful reading, examination of the tables and figures, and independent calculation of the examples in this chapter should provide a strong basis for understanding not only the following chapters but, more important, the data analysis and results portions of research articles in the physical therapy literature.

The chapter begins by presenting a data set that is used for all of the statistical examples in this and the following two chapters. Next, the concepts of frequency distribution, central tendency, variability, and normal distribution, which were introduced in Chapter 17, are reviewed and expanded. Then the new concepts of sampling distribution, significant difference, and power are explained. Finally, the concepts are integrated by a discussion of statistical conclusion validity.

DATA SET

Achieving a conceptual understanding of statistical reasoning is greatly enhanced by performing simple computational examples. Thus, a small hypothetical data set has been developed for use throughout this and the following two chapters. Our data set consists of 30 hypothetical patients, 10 at each of three clinics, who have undergone rehabilitation for a total knee arthroplasty. Eighteen pieces of information are available for each patient:

Case number

Clinic attended

Sex

Age

Three-week knee flexion range of motion (ROM)

Six-week knee flexion ROM

Six-month knee flexion ROM

Six-month knee extensor torque

Six-month knee flexor torque

Six-month gait velocity

Four 6-month activities of daily living (ADL) indexes

Four 6-month deformity indexes

The ADL and deformity indexes were adapted for the purposes of this data set from a knee-rating system used at Brigham and Women's Hospital in Boston.[2] Table 20–1 provides an outline of the data set, indicating abbreviations for each variable, the unit of measurement when appropriate, and the meaning of any numerical coding. Table 20–2 presents the actual data set.

FREQUENCY DISTRIBUTION

A *frequency distribution* is a tally of the number of times each score is represented in a data set. There are four ways of presenting a frequency distribution: frequency distribution with percentages, grouped frequency distribution with percentages, frequency histogram, and stem-and-leaf plot.

Frequency Distribution with Percentages

Table 20–3 shows a frequency distribution with percentages for the variable 3-week ROM. The first column lists the scores that were obtained. The second column, absolute frequency, lists the number of times that each score was obtained. For example, two subjects had 3-week ROM values of 67°. The third column, relative frequency, lists the percentage of subjects who received each score. This is calculated by dividing the number of subjects with that score by the total number of subjects. From this column we find that the four subjects who had scores of 81 represent 13.3% of the sample [(4/30) $\times$ 100 = 13.3%]. The fourth column, cumulative frequency, is formed by adding the relative fre-

TABLE 20-1 Data Set Specifications for Patients Who Underwent Rehabilitation After Total Knee Arthroplasty

Variable Code	Variable Name	Variable Values
CASE	Case number	01–30
CN	Clinic number	1 = Community Hospital
		2 = Memorial Hospital
		3 = Religious Hospital
SEX	Patient sex	0 = male
		1 = female
AGE	Patient age	In years at last birthday
W3R	Three-week range of motion (ROM) at each clinic	To nearest degree
W6R	Six-week ROM	To nearest degree
M6R	Six-month ROM	To nearest degree
E	Six-month extension torque	To nearest Newton • meter (N•m)
F	Six-month flexion torque	To nearest N•m
V	Gait velocity	To nearest cm/sec
DFC	Deformity: flexion contracture	1 = >15°
		2 = 6–15°
		3 = 0–5°
DVV	Deformity: varus/valgus angulation in stance	1 = >10° valgus
		2 = >5° varus or 6–10° valgus
		3 = 5° varus to 5° valgus
DML	Deformity: mediolateral stability	1 = marked instability
		2 = moderate instability
		3 = stable
DAP	Deformity: anteroposterior stability with knee at 90° flexion	1 = marked instability
		2 = moderate instability
		3 = stable
ADW	Activities of daily living (ADL): distance walked	5 = unlimited
		4 = 4–6 blocks
		3 = 2–3 blocks
		2 = indoors only
		1 = transfers only
AAD	ADL: assistive device	5 = none
		4 = cane outside
		3 = cane full-time
		2 = two canes or crutches
		1 = walker or unable to walk
ASC	ADL: stair climbing	5 = reciprocal, no rail
		4 = reciprocal, with rail
		3 = one at a time, with or without rail
		2 = one at a time, with rail and assistive device
		1 = unable to climb stairs
ARC	ADL: rising from a chair	5 = no arm assistance
		4 = single arm assistance
		3 = difficult with two-arm assistance
		2 = needs assistance of another
		1 = unable to rise

TABLE 20-2 Data Set for Patients Who Underwent Rehabilitation After Total Knee Arthroplasty

Case	CN	Sex	Age	W3R	W6R	M6R	E	F	V	DFC	DVV	DML	DAP	ADW	AAD	ASC	ARC
01	1	1	50	95	90	100	170	100	165	2	1	2	1	5	5	5	5
02	1	0	87	32	46	85	100	60	100	2	2	1	1	3	4	4	2
03	1	0	66	67	78	100	130	70	130	1	1	2	2	4	5	5	4
04	1	0	46	92	85	105	175	95	170	2	2	1	2	5	5	5	5
05	1	0	53	87	85	105	157	86	150	1	2	2	2	5	4	5	5
06	1	0	76	58	50	95	88	52	135	2	1	2	2	4	4	4	4
07	1	1	43	92	95	110	120	75	153	1	1	1	1	5	5	5	5
08	1	1	46	88	90	100	130	90	145	2	3	3	2	4	5	5	5
09	1	1	43	84	80	95	132	92	147	1	1	1	2	5	5	5	4
10	1	1	48	81	90	105	156	98	145	2	2	3	2	5	5	4	5
11	2	0	92	34	63	90	87	53	95	3	2	2	2	3	3	3	3
12	2	0	65	56	71	90	160	95	150	2	3	2	2	4	4	5	5
13	2	0	76	45	63	78	92	60	120	1	2	1	2	4	3	3	4
14	2	0	92	27	35	65	85	49	85	3	3	3	3	2	1	1	2
15	2	1	68	76	70	95	170	102	165	2	3	2	2	4	3	5	5
16	2	1	79	49	55	98	81	37	93	2	2	2	1	3	2	3	2
17	2	1	85	47	58	84	87	46	70	3	2	2	2	2	1	2	2
18	2	1	82	50	60	80	93	63	94	1	1	2	2	3	2	2	2
19	2	0	81	40	40	83	96	58	101	2	2	2	2	3	2	2	2
20	2	1	90	67	70	95	103	63	103	1	1	3	2	2	2	2	3
21	3	0	66	32	67	105	180	105	180	1	2	1	1	5	5	5	5
22	3	0	72	50	67	105	150	85	150	2	3	3	2	5	4	5	4
23	3	0	68	60	65	95	154	89	156	2	3	3	2	4	4	4	4
24	3	0	77	84	30	105	141	83	146	2	2	2	1	3	3	4	3
25	3	0	60	81	35	100	168	93	178	3	3	3	2	4	5	5	5
26	3	1	75	81	94	110	146	84	135	2	1	3	3	5	5	5	5
27	3	1	73	84	90	100	120	74	134	2	2	2	3	4	4	4	4
28	3	1	72	81	95	103	110	68	120	2	1	2	3	4	5	3	4
29	3	1	72	82	90	104	116	74	126	3	2	3	1	4	3	4	3
30	3	1	63	91	95	106	137	86	131	2	1	3	3	4	5	5	5

Note: All variables are identified in Table 20-1.

TABLE 20-3	Frequency Distribution of Three-Week Range-of-Motion Values		

Score (°)	Absolute Frequency	Relative Frequency (%)	Cumulative Frequency (%)
27	1	3.3	3.3
32	2	6.7	10.0
34	1	3.3	13.3
40	1	3.3	16.7
45	1	3.3	20.0
47	1	3.3	23.3
49	1	3.3	26.7
50	2	6.7	33.4
56	1	3.3	36.7
58	1	3.3	40.0
60	1	3.3	43.3
67	2	6.7	50.0
76	1	3.3	53.3
81	4	13.3	66.6
82	1	3.3	70.0
84	3	10.0	80.0
87	1	3.3	83.3
88	1	3.3	86.6
91	1	3.3	90.0
92	2	6.7	96.7
95	1	3.3	100.0
Total	30	100.0	

quencies of the scores up to and including the score of interest. For example, a researcher might be interested in the percentage of patients who had ROM scores of less than 50° 3 weeks postoperatively. From the cumulative frequency column one finds that 26.7% of the sample had ROM values of 49° or less.

A variation of this basic display is needed if there are missing values in the sample. Suppose that Patients 3 through 5 missed their 3-week evaluation appointments. Table 20–4 presents a revised frequency distribution that accounts for these three missing pieces of data. Note that another column, adjusted frequency, has been added. The adjusted frequency is calculated by dividing the number of observations for each score by the number of valid scores for each

variable, rather than by the number of subjects. In this case, there are 27 valid scores. The relative frequency of a ROM score of 81° is now 14.8% [(4/27) × 100 = 14.8%]. The cumulative frequency is the sum of the adjusted frequencies. If many data points are missing, it is often misleading to present the frequencies as percentages of the total sample; use of adjusted frequencies corrects the problem.

Grouped Frequency Distribution with Percentages

The grouped frequency distribution is another way frequency information is commonly presented. When there are many individual scores in a distribution, the characteristics of the distribution may be grasped more easily if scores are placed into groups. Table 20–5 presents a grouped frequency distribution for the 3-week ROM values. From this grouped distribution it is readily apparent that the group with the highest frequency is that with scores from 80° to 89°.

A disadvantage of the grouped frequency distribution is that information is lost. Table 20–5 indicates that there are three subjects whose scores range from 30° to 39°. But what does this mean? This could mean all three patients had scores of 39, three patients had scores of 30, or the three had a variety of scores within this range.

Frequency Histogram

Another way to present a grouped frequency distribution is a histogram. A histogram presents each grouped frequency as a bar on a graph. The height of each bar represents the frequency of observations in the group. Figure 20–1 shows a histogram of the 3-week ROM data. As with the grouped frequency distribution from which the histogram is generated, information is lost because one does not know how the scores are distributed within each group.

| TABLE 20-4 | Frequency Distribution of Three-Week Range-of-Motion Scores, Modified for Missing Values | | | |

Score (°)	Absolute Frequency	Relative Frequency (%)	Adjusted Frequency (%)	Cumulative Frequency (%)
27	1	3.3	3.7	3.7
32	2	6.7	7.4	11.1
34	1	3.3	3.7	14.8
40	1	3.3	3.7	18.5
45	1	3.3	3.7	22.2
47	1	3.3	3.7	25.9
49	1	3.3	3.7	29.6
50	2	6.7	7.4	37.0
56	1	3.3	3.7	40.7
58	1	3.3	3.7	44.4
60	1	3.3	3.7	48.1
67	1	3.3	3.7	51.8
76	1	3.3	3.7	55.5
81	4	13.3	14.8	70.3
82	1	3.3	3.7	74.3
84	3	10.0	11.1	85.1
88	1	3.3	3.7	88.8
91	1	3.3	3.7	92.5
92	1	3.3	3.7	96.2
95	1	3.3	3.7	100.0
Missing	3	10.0	Missing	
Total	30	100.0	100.0	

| TABLE 20-5 | Grouped Frequency Distribution for Three-Week Range of Motion Values | | |

Scores (°)	Frequency	Relative Frequency (%)	Cumulative Frequency (%)
20–29	1	3.3	3.3
30–39	3	10.0	13.3
40–49	4	13.3	26.7
50–59	4	13.3	40.0
60–69	3	10.0	50.0
70–79	1	3.3	53.3
80–89	10	33.3	86.7
90–99	4	13.3	100.0
Total	30	100.0	

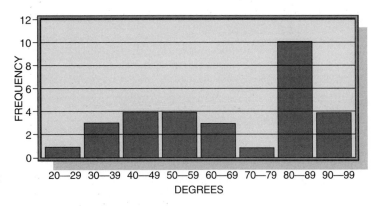

FIGURE 20–1. Histogram of 3-week range-of-motion scores.

Stem-and-Leaf Plot

A final way of presenting frequency data is the stem-and-leaf plot. This plot presents data concisely, without losing information in the grouping process. Each individual score is divided into a "stem" and a "leaf," as shown in Table 20–6. In this instance the stem is the digit representing the multiple of 10 (20, 30, 40, etc.), and the leaf is the digit representing the multiple of 1 (1, 2, 3, 4, etc.). The row with the stem of 5 has leaves of 0, 0, 6, 8. The stems and leaves together represent the four scores of 50, 50, 56, and 58. The stem-and-leaf plot, like the histogram, provides a good visual picture of the frequency distribution.

TABLE 20-6	Stem-and-Leaf Plot of Three-Week Range-of-Motion Frequency Distribution

Stem	Leaf	Total
2	7	1
3	2 2 4	3
4	0 5 7 9	4
5	0 0 6 8	4
6	0 7 7	3
7	6	1
8	1 1 1 1 2 4 4 4 7 8	10
9	1 2 2 5	4
Total		30

■ CENTRAL TENDENCY

Researchers often wish to collapse a set of data into a single score that represents the whole set. In other words, the researcher is interested in the central tendency of the data. The three commonly used measures of central tendency are the mean, the median, and the mode. If a distribution is perfectly symmetric, then the mean, median, and mode are all identical. If the distribution is asymmetric, they differ.

Mean

The arithmetic *mean* of a data set is the sum of the observations divided by the number of observations. Recall from Chapter 17 that mathematical notation for the mean is as follows:

$$\bar{X} = \frac{\Sigma X}{N}$$

In words, this equation says the mean is the sum of all the observations divided by the number of observations. The mean of the 3-week ROM scores for Clinic 1 is 77.6° [(95 + 32 + 67 + 92 + 87 + 58 + 92 + 88 + 84 + 81)/10 = 77.6]. The mean is a versatile measure of central tendency because it uses information from all the scores in the distribution. However, extreme values can distort the mean. In this example, seven of the 10 scores are greater than 80°, but the very low score of 32° pulls the mean down to 77.6°.

Median

The *median* is the "middle" score of a distribution, or the score above which half of the distribution lies. To calculate the median, a researcher must first rank the scores. When the distribution has an odd number of scores, the middle score is easy to locate: (N + 1)/2 = the middle-ranked score. Thus, in a sample of 987 scores, the 494th ranked score is the median. When the number of scores in a distribution is even, as in our example, the median is calculated by finding the mean of the two middle scores: [N/2] and [(N/2) + 1]. In a sample with 988 scores, the median is the mean of the 494th and 495th ranked scores. Table 20–7 presents the frequency distribution for the 10 3-week measurements we are considering. The median, as shown, is 85.5°. The median is a useful measure of central tendency when the distribution contains a few extreme values that distort the mean. The disadvantage of the median is that it does not include information from all of the scores in the distribution.

Mode

The *mode* is the score that occurs most frequently in a distribution. If there are two modes, the distribution is termed *bimodal.* Our example of 3-week ROM scores has a mode of 92, as shown in Table 20–7. The mode is often used to describe nominal data, which have neither the property of order nor the property of distance and therefore cannot provide a median and mean (see Chapter 17).

■ VARIABILITY

The variability of a data set is the amount of spread in the data. Two different groups might have the same mean score, yet have very different characteristics. For example, a sample of female college athletes might have the same mean weight as a sample of female nonathletes at the school. However, the athletes would be expected to have a relatively narrow range of weights, whereas the nonathletes would be ex-

---

| TABLE 20-7 | Median and Mode Calculations for Three-Week Range-of-Motion Values for Clinic 1 | | | |

Score (°)	Absolute Frequency	Cumulative (%)	Median*	Mode†
32	1	10.0		
58	1	20.0		
67	1	30.0		
81	1	40.0		
84	1	50.0		
			85.5	
87	1	60.0		
88	1	70.0		
92	2	90.0		92
95	1	100.0		

* Median is the "middle" score. When there is an even number of scores, the two middle scores are averaged. In this example, the median is (84 + 87)/2 = 85.5.
† Mode is the score that occurs most frequently.

pected to range in weight from the very under-weight to the very overweight. The three measures of variability are range, variance, and standard deviation.

Range

The *range* is the difference between the highest and lowest values in the distribution. In the group of 10 patients from Clinic 1, the range is 63° (95 − 32 = 63). Although the range is technically a single score, it is often reported by presenting both the high and low scores so that readers will understand not only the range but also the magnitude of the scores in the distribution.

Variance

The *variance* is a measure of variability that, like the mean, requires that every score in the distribution be used in its calculation. Although the calculation of the variance was presented in Chapter 17, it is reviewed here with our 3-week ROM data from Clinic 1. To calculate the variance, we convert each of the raw scores in the data set to a *deviation score* by subtracting the mean of the data set from each raw score. In mathematical notation,

$$x = X - \overline{X}$$

Recall from Chapter 17 that the lowercase, italic x is the symbol for a deviation score. The deviation score indicates how high or low a raw score is compared with the mean. The first two columns of Table 20–8 present the raw and deviation scores for the knee flexion data set and, below them, their sums and means. Note that both the sum and the mean of the deviation scores are zero. To generate a nonzero index of the variability within a data set, we must square the deviation scores. We can then calculate the

population variance by determining the mean of the squared deviations. In mathematical notation,

$$\sigma^2 = \frac{\Sigma x^2}{N}$$

We know from Chapter 17 that σ is the lowercase Greek sigma and when squared is the notation for the variance. The third column in Table 20–8 shows the squared deviations from the group mean and, below them, their sum and mean. The population variance is used when all of the members of a population are known. In practice this rarely occurs, so the *sample variance* is used to *estimate* the population variance. The sample variance is calculated by dividing the sum of the squared deviations by N − 1, as follows:

$$s^2 = \frac{\Sigma x^2}{N - 1}$$

The symbol for the sample variance is s^2. In our example, the sample variance is calculated by dividing 3542.40 (the sum of the squared deviations) by 9 (N − 1), as shown in Table 20–8.

The rationale for dividing the sum of the squared deviations by N − 1 rests on the concept of *degrees of freedom*. Although an abstract concept, degrees of freedom can be understood in a general sense through the use of an illustration. In a sample of 10 values with a known mean, 9 of the values are "free" to fluctuate, as long as the investigator has control over the final value. We know that for our sample of 10 observations with a mean of 77.6°, the sum of those 10 observations adds up to 776. If we wanted to generate another sample with a mean of 77.6°, we could select 9 numbers randomly as long as we could manipulate the 10th value. If 9 randomly selected numbers happen to each have a value of 100, then they add to a total of 900. The sample can still have a mean value of 77.6° if the 10th value is manipulated to be −124 (900 −

TABLE 20-8	Computation of the Variance, z Scores, and Probabilities for Three-Week Range-of-Motion Scores at Clinic 1			
X	**x**	**x^2**	**z score**	**p**
32	−45.6	2,079.36	−2.30	.011
58	−19.6	384.16	−.99	.161
67	−10.6	112.36	−.53	.298
81	3.4	11.56	.17	.433
84	6.4	40.96	.32	.374
87	9.4	88.36	.47	.319
88	10.4	108.16	.52	.302
92	14.4	207.36	.73	.233
92	14.4	207.36	.73	.233
95	17.4	302.76	.88	.189

$\Sigma =$ 776 0 3,542.40

$\overline{X} =$ 77.6 0 354.24 = population variance (σ^2)

18.82 = population standard deviation (σ)

$s^2 = \dfrac{\Sigma x^2}{N - 1}$ 393.60 = sample variance (s^2)

19.84 = sample standard deviation (s)

124 = 776; 776/10 = 77.6). This phenomenon is termed degrees of freedom, or the number of items that are free to fluctuate. Thus, for the mean, there are always N − 1 degrees of freedom. Statisticians have found that using the degrees of freedom for the mean as the denominator of the sample variance formula leads to an unbiased estimation of the population variance. The degrees of freedom concept is used in the computation of many different statistical tests.

Standard Deviation

As just defined, the population variance is the mean of the squared deviation from the mean, and the sample variance is the sum of the squared deviations from the mean, divided by

the degrees of freedom for the mean. Although the variance is useful in many statistical procedures, it does not have a great deal of intuitive meaning because it is calculated from squared deviation scores. A measure that has such meaning is the *standard deviation*. The standard deviation is the square root of the variance and is expressed in the units of the original measure. The population standard deviation is the square root of the population variance; the sample standard deviation is the square root of the sample variance:

$$s = \sqrt{s^2}$$

The mathematical notations for the sample standard deviation and the sample variance make their relationship clear: The notation for the variance (s^2) is simply the square of the notation for standard deviation (s). In practice, the entire population is not usually measured, so the sample standard deviation is used as an estimate of the population standard deviation. The sample standard deviation of the knee flexion data presented in Table 20–8 is the square root of 393.60, or 19.84°.

Taken together, the measures of central tendency and variability are referred to as descriptive measures. When these measures are used to describe a population, they are known as *parameters;* when they are used to describe a sample, they are known as *statistics.* Because researchers can rarely measure all the subjects within a population, they use sample statistics such as the mean and standard deviation as estimates of the corresponding population parameters.

■ NORMAL DISTRIBUTION

The normal distribution is central to many of the statistical tests that are presented in subsequent chapters. Groups of measurements frequently approximate a bell-shaped distribution known as the normal curve. The *normal curve* is a symmetric frequency distribution that can be defined in terms of the mean and standard deviation of a set of data.

z Score

Any score within a distribution can be standardized with respect to the mean and standard deviation of the data. That is, each score can be expressed in terms of how many standard deviations it is above or below the mean. The result of such a standardization procedure is called a z score. A z score is calculated by dividing the deviation score ($x = X - \overline{X}$) by the standard deviation:

$$z = \frac{x}{s}$$

When a normally distributed set of data is converted to z scores, the distribution of the z scores is known as the *standard normal distribution.* The standard normal distribution has a mean of zero and a standard deviation of 1.0. The fourth column of Table 20–8 shows our 10 raw 3-week ROM scores as z scores. This was done by dividing each of the deviation scores (x) by the standard deviation (s) of 19.84°. The magnitude and sign of the z score tell us, for example, that a measurement of 32° is 2.30 standard deviations below the mean.

Percentages of the Normal Distribution

In a normal distribution the percentage of scores that fall within a certain range of scores is known. Approximately 68% of scores fall within 1 standard deviation above or below the mean. Approximately 96% of the scores fall within 2 standard deviations of the mean, and almost 100% of the scores fall within 3 standard deviations of the mean. Figure 20–2 shows a diagram of the normal curve, with the exact percentages

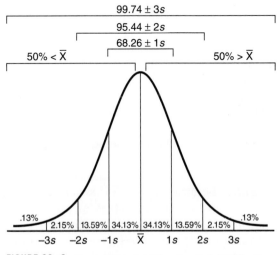

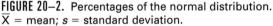

FIGURE 20–2. Percentages of the normal distribution. $\overline{X}$ = mean; s = standard deviation.

of scores that are found within each standard deviation.

Figure 20–3A shows the normal curve that corresponds to our 3-week ROM data for Clinic 1. The sample mean is 77.6°, and the sample standard deviation is 19.84°. The x axis is labeled with both z scores and the raw scores that correspond to 1, 2, and 3 standard deviations above and below the mean. Figure 20–3B shows that if the knee flexion scores are normally distributed, we would estimate that 98% of our measurements would exceed the score of 37.92°; Figure 20–3C shows that we could expect 68% of our measurements to fall between 57.76° and 97.44°. Predicting the probability of obtaining certain ranges of scores is basic to most of the statistical testing presented in Chapters 21 and 22.

We know from the preceding paragraphs the approximate probability of obtaining scores within 1, 2, and 3 standard deviations of the mean. A table of z scores can provide exact probabilities of achieving scores at any level within the distribution. Earlier we calculated that 32° of ROM at 3 weeks postoperatively was 2.30 standard deviations below the mean for patients at Clinic 1. Without a table, we know only that the probability of obtaining scores outside the second standard deviation is approximately 2%. Consulting a z table tells us the exact probability of obtaining scores that are less than or equal to 2.30 standard deviations below the mean. Appendix D provides a z table.

To identify the z score of 2.30 in Appendix D, look in the far left-hand column for the stem 2.3, and then read across the uppermost row to the leaf .00. The intersection of the row and column gives a value of .011 or, if stated as a percentage, 1.1%. The picture of the normal curve above the table shows that the proportion indicated is either at the upper or lower tail of the curve, depending on whether the z score is positive or negative. Because the curve is symmetric, there is no need for separate tables of positive and negative z scores; researchers simply need to know that the probabilities associated with positive z scores lie in the upper portion of the

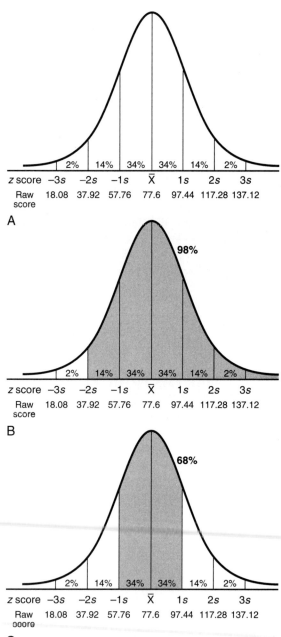

FIGURE 20–3. A. Percentages of the normal distribution for 3-week range-of-motion scores at Clinic 1. **B.** Shaded area represents approximately 98% of the distribution. **C.** Shaded area represents approximately 68% of the distribution. $\overline{X}$ = mean; s = standard deviation.

curve and the probabilities associated with negative z scores lie in the lower portion of the curve. The final column of Table 20–8 gives the probabilities associated with each z score. Readers may wish to use the z table in Appendix B to confirm that they understand how these probabilities were obtained.

■ SAMPLING DISTRIBUTION

To understand statistical testing, it is extremely important to understand sampling distributions. The sampling distribution is a specific type of normal distribution. Imagine that you had access to the entire population of individuals who had total knee arthroplasties in a given year. If we drew a random sample of 10 individuals from this large population and examined their 3-week ROM values, we might get a sample with a mean of 77.6°, as in the example from Clinic 1. If we drew another random sample of 10 individuals, we might get a mean of 98.2°. If we drew another random sample, we might get a mean of 59.1°. Assume that we drew 10 samples and obtained means of 77.6°, 98.2°, 59.1°, 84.5°, 78.9°, 45.6°, 89.5°, 64.3°, 68.7°, and 75.4°. Using each of these mean scores to represent each sample, we can calculate both a mean of the sample means (74.18°) and a standard deviation of the sample means (15.37°).

Table 20–9 shows the calculations that provide this mean and standard deviation. The calculations are the same as those presented in Table 20–8; the only difference is that each score in the distribution in Table 20–9 represents a group rather than an individual, as in Table 20–8. The distribution of the means of several samples drawn from the same population is called a *sampling distribution*. The mean of the sampling distribution is assumed to be the mean of the population. The standard deviation of the sampling distribution is called the *standard error of the mean*, or the SEM. Note that SEM is also the abbreviation for the standard error of measurement (see Chapter 17). When this abbrevia-

| TABLE 20–9 | Computation of the Mean, Sample Variance (s^2), and Sample Standard Deviations (s) for the Sampling Distribution of Three-Week Range-of-Motion Scores |

X	x	x^2
98.2	24.02	576.96
89.5	15.32	234.70
84.5	10.32	106.50
78.9	4.72	22.28
77.6	3.42	11.70
75.4	1.22	1.48
68.7	− 5.48	30.03
64.3	− 9.88	97.61
59.1	− 15.08	227.41
45.6	− 28.58	816.82

$\Sigma \quad = \quad 741.8 \qquad 0 \qquad 2125.49$

$\overline{X} \quad = \quad 74.18 \qquad 0$

$s^2 \quad = \quad \dfrac{\Sigma x^2}{N - 1} \quad = \quad 236.16$

$s \quad = \quad 15.37$

tion is used, it should be made clear whether it refers to the standard error of the mean or the standard error of measurement. The term "error" does not refer to a mistake made by the researcher. Rather, "error" denotes the inevitable differences that are found between a population and the samples that are drawn from the population.

The SEM varies with sample size. When we draw sample sizes of 10, the presence of just one extremely low or high value alters the mean greatly. For example, assume that we have 9 scores of 75° and one score of 115°; the mean is 79°—4° away from the modal score of 75°. Do the same to a sample of 100 with 99 scores of 75° and one score of 115°. The mean in this case is 75.4°—less than half a degree higher than the majority of scores. Thus, the means of large samples are more stable than means of small samples because they are less influenced by extreme scores. This stability is reflected in the magnitude of the SEM: The SEM of a sample distribution generated from a large sample is small; the SEM of a sampling distribution generated from a small sample is large.

Researchers often do not have the time or resources to draw repeated samples from a population to determine the SEM of the resulting sampling distribution. Therefore, the SEM is usually estimated from a single sample drawn for study. As just noted, the sample size greatly affects the variability of mean scores, so the SEM estimation formula takes sample size into account:

$$SEM = \frac{s}{\sqrt{N}}$$

The estimate of the SEM is found by dividing the sample standard deviation (s) by the square root of the number in the sample. This estimated SEM, or one of several mathematical variations, is used in the calculation of many of the statistical tests discussed in Chapters 21 and 22. For our single sample with a mean of 77.6°, a standard deviation of 19.84°, and a sample size of 10, the estimated SEM is 6.27° (19.84/$\sqrt{10}$ = 6.27).

Confidence Intervals of the Sampling Distribution

Because the sampling distribution is a normal distribution, we can find the probability of obtaining a sample with a certain range of mean scores by consulting a z table. The procedure is the same as discussed earlier, except that the scores now represent sample means rather than individual scores. Earlier we started with a particular z score and determined the probability of obtaining scores that either equaled or exceeded the selected score. We can also use the z table in reverse by specifying a particular probability in which we are interested and determining the z score that corresponds to that probability. This reverse process is used to determine *confidence intervals* (CIs) about the mean.

Recall that the sample mean of 3-week ROM scores at Clinic 1 is 77.6°, the standard deviation is 19.84°, and the SEM is 6.27°. We recognize that the obtained sample mean is only an estimate of the population mean because of the phenomenon of sampling error. We can use the probabilities of the sampling distribution to identify a range of mean scores that is likely to include the true population mean. If we take the mean score (77.6) and subtract and add one SEM (77.6 − 6.27 = 71.33; 77.6 + 6.27 = 82.87), we get a range of means from 71.33° to 82.87°. From our knowledge of the probabilities of the normal distribution we know that approximately 68% of the scores in a distribution fall within the first standard deviation from the mean. Thus, there is an approximately 68% chance that the true population mean lies somewhere between 71.33° and 82.87°. This is known as the 68% CI.

In practice, researchers usually report a 90%, 95%, or 99% CI. To generate these intervals, we need to determine what z scores correspond to them. For the 90% CI, 10% is excluded—5% (.05) in the upper tail of the distribution and 5% in the lower tail of the distribution. For the 95% and 99% CIs, the percentages excluded in each tail are 2.5% (.025) and 0.5% (.005), respectively. Refer to the z table in Appendix B to confirm that the z scores that correspond to .05 and .025 are 1.645 and 1.960, respectively. The z table included in this text was selected for its simplicity and conciseness. However, this simplicity is at the expense of some precision in the very low probability ranges. Thus, we cannot determine from the concise z table of Appendix B the exact z score that corresponds to .005. From a more complete z table printed elsewhere the value is found to be 2.575.[3(p309)] Thus, the desired CI of the mean is determined by adding and subtracting the appropriate number of SEMs to and from the mean. In mathematical notation,

90% CI = $\overline{X}$ ± 1.645 (SEM)

95% CI = $\overline{X}$ ± 1.960 (SEM)

99% CI = $\overline{X}$ ± 2.575 (SEM)

Inserting the values of 77.6° ($\overline{X}$) and 6.27° (SEM), we find the following:

90% CI = 67.3° to 87.9°

95% CI = 65.3° to 89.9°

99% CI = 61.4° to 93.7°

We are 90% confident that the true population mean is somewhere between 67.3° and 87.9°; we are 99% confident that it lies somewhere between 61.4° and 93.7°. The computations given here are for the simplest calculation of a CI for the population mean. CIs can also be calculated for population proportions, for the difference between population proportions, and for the difference between population means.[3(pp123–129)]

■ SIGNIFICANT DIFFERENCE

Researchers often wish to do more than describe their data. They wish to determine whether there are differences between groups who have been exposed to different treatments. The branch of statistics that is used to determine whether, among other things, there are significant differences between groups is known as *inferential statistics*. The theoretical basis of inferential statistics is that population parameters can be inferred from sample statistics. The determination of whether two sample means are significantly different from one another is actually a determination of the likelihood that the two sample means are drawn from populations with the same means. The sampling distribution of the mean is used as the basis for making these inferential statements—it is the link between the observed samples and the theorized population.

When we compare two groups who have received different experimental treatments, we almost always find that there is some difference between the means of the two groups. For example, assume that we wish to determine the effect of continuous passive motion on 3-week ROM in our patients who have had total knee arthroplasty. Assume that the patients at Clinic 1

received continuous passive motion postoperatively and that the patients at Clinic 3 did not. The mean 3-week ROM score for Clinic 1 is 77.6°; for Clinic 3, it is 72.6°. This is a difference of 5.0°. We wonder whether this difference is a true difference between the two groups or chance variation due to sampling error.

If it is highly likely that the difference was due to sampling error, then we conclude that there is *no significant difference* between the two group means. In other words, if sampling errors are a likely explanation for the difference between the means of the groups, then it is likely that the two groups were drawn from populations with the same means. Conversely, if it is highly unlikely that the difference between the groups was the result of sampling errors, then we conclude that there is a *significant difference* between the groups. If sampling error is not a likely explanation for differences between the groups, then it is likely that the two groups come from populations with different means. To determine whether the difference between groups is significant, we test a null hypothesis at a particular alpha level, as described next.

Null Hypothesis

The seemingly convoluted language needed to describe the meaning of a statistically significant difference derives from the fact that the statistical hypothesis that is tested is the hypothesis of "no difference." This hypothesis is referred to as the *null hypothesis*, or H_0. The formal null hypothesis for determining whether there are different mean 3-week ROM scores between Clinics 1 and 3 is as follows:

$$H_0: \mu_1 = \mu_3$$

Thus, the null hypothesis is that the population mean for Clinic 1 (μ_1) is equal to the population mean for Clinic 3 (μ_3). For now we will assume that the alternative hypothesis, or H_1, is that the population mean of Clinic 1 is greater than the population mean of Clinic 3:

$H_1: \mu_1 > \mu_3$

Other alternative hypotheses are possible and are addressed later with specific statistical tests. In statistical testing, we determine the probability that the null hypothesis is true. If the probability is sufficiently low, we conclude that the null hypothesis is false, accept the alternative hypothesis, and conclude that there are significant differences between the groups. If the probability that the null hypothesis is true is high, we conclude that the null hypothesis is true, accept the null hypothesis, and conclude that there are no significant differences between the groups.

Alpha Level

Before conducting a statistical analysis of differences, researchers must determine how much of a probability of drawing an incorrect conclusion they are willing to tolerate. To use null hypothesis terminology, how low is the "sufficiently low" probability needed to detect a significant difference? The conventional level of chance that is tolerated is 5%, or .05. This is referred to as the *alpha* (α) *level*. If a difference in means is significant at the .05 level, this means that 5% of differences of this magnitude would have been the result of chance fluctuations caused by sampling errors. That is, 95% of the time the difference would represent a true difference and 5% of the time the difference would represent sampling error. Occasionally the more stringent level of .01 is used, as is the more permissive level of .10.

There are two twists that occur with alpha levels as they are reported in research. The first is the distinction between the alpha level and the obtained probability; the second is inflation and correction of the alpha level during performance of multiple statistical tests.

The distinction between the alpha level and the obtained probability (p) level is the distinction between what the researcher is willing to accept as chance and what the actual results are. The alpha level is specified before the data analysis is conducted; the probability level is a product of the data analysis. Researchers may set the alpha level at .05, meaning that they are willing to accept a 5% chance that significant findings may actually be the result of sampling error. In studies in which significant differences are found, the actual probability that a given result will occur by chance may be much less than the alpha level set by the researcher.

Assume that the result of a statistical test comparing two group means is that the probability that the difference will occur by chance is .001. This means that in only one of 1000 instances would a difference of this magnitude likely be the result of sampling error. Now that computers are available to calculate statistics, such precise probability levels are often reported. Because the obtained probability level of .001 is less than the present alpha level of .05, the researcher concludes that there is a significant difference between the groups. Does the reporting of the obtained probability level of .001 somehow indicate that the researcher changed the alpha level during the course of the data analysis? No. The reporting of a specific probability level simply indicates to the reader the extent to which the obtained probability was lower or higher than the alpha set by the researcher.

The second twist that is given to an alpha level in a study is called *alpha level inflation*. This occurs when researchers conduct many statistical tests within a given study. Using an alpha level of 5%, we know that the probability that differences occurred by chance is 5% for each test. If we conduct many tests, the overall probability of obtaining chance significant differences increases. This increase is alpha level inflation. When researchers conduct multiple tests, they may correct for alpha level inflation by using a more stringent alpha level for each individual test. They may obtain a more stringent alpha by using, for example, the *Bonferroni adjustment*. This adjustment divides the total alpha level for the experiment, called the experiment-wise alpha, by the number of statistical tests conducted to determine a test-wise alpha level.[4(p128)] For example, a researcher may set the experiment-wise alpha at .05 and conduct 10 tests, each with a test-wise alpha level of .005 (.05/10 = .005). Some researchers consider this adjustment too stringent and compensate by setting a higher experiment-wise alpha level. For example, if a researcher sets the experiment-wise alpha at .15 and conducts seven tests, the adjusted test-wise alpha level would be .0214. Although the Bonferroni adjustment is commonly used, statisticians do not always agree on when to adjust for alpha inflation, nor do they all agree that the Bonferroni adjustment is the best procedure to use when an adjustment is desired.[5,6]

An example of the use of the Bonferroni adjustment is found in Mueller and colleagues' study of functional status after transmetatarsal amputation.[7] One of the measures, the physical performance test, can have a total score as well as be subdivided into eight subscores. Mueller chose to conduct a statistical test on the total score at an alpha level of .05. Then, he conducted eight more tests on the subscores, each at a divided alpha level of .006 (.05/8 = .006).

Statistical analysis requires that the researcher set an alpha level. If the statistical test results in an obtained probability that is less than the predetermined alpha level, the result is deemed statistically significant. Whether a result is statistically significant or not often depends on the way in which the researcher sets the alpha level. Thus, tests of statistical significance do not provide absolute conclusions about the meaning of data. Rather, these tests provide the researcher with information about the probability that the obtained results occurred by chance. The researcher then draws statistical conclusions about whether a statistically significant difference exists. Researchers and readers then need to interpret the statistical conclusions in light of their knowledge of the subject being studied.

Probability Determinants

Three pieces of information are essential to the determination of statistical probabilities: the magnitude of the differences *between* groups (or between levels of the independent variable when there is only one group); variability, or differences *within* a group; and sample size. In this section, the effect of each of these determinants is illustrated conceptually, without determination of actual probabilities. Actual probabilities are determined in subsequent chapters when specific statistical tests are discussed.

BETWEEN-GROUPS DIFFERENCE. To illustrate the influence of the size of the difference between two groups, let us compare the differences in mean 3-week ROM scores between Clinics 1 through 3. Clinic 1 has a mean of 77.6°, Clinic 2 a mean of 49.1°, and Clinic 3 a mean of 72.6°. If within-group variability and sample size are held constant, then a larger between-groups difference is associated with a smaller probability that the difference occurred by chance. Thus, there is a relatively low probability that the large 28.5° difference in the 3-week ROM means for Clinics 1 and 2 occurred by chance. Conversely, there is a relatively high probability that the smaller 5.0° difference in the 3-week ROM means for Clinics 1 and 3 did occur by chance.

WITHIN-GROUP VARIABILITY. The second piece of information used to determine the probability that a difference is a true difference is the variability within a group. If the between-groups difference and sample size are held constant, the differences between groups with lower within-group variability have a lower probability of occurring by chance than difference between groups with high within-group variability. Assume that we have two groups of 100 with means of 72.6° and 77.6°. If the groups have high within-group variability—say, standard deviations of 30.0°—curves representing their sampling distributions would look like those drawn in Figure 20–4A. The sampling distributions, which each have an SEM of 3 ($30/\sqrt{100} = 3$), overlap a great deal.

Because of the overlap in sampling distributions, there is a high probability that the two samples came from populations that have the same mean. Because this probability is high, we conclude that the difference in means occurred by chance; that is, the difference between the means of the two groups is not significant.

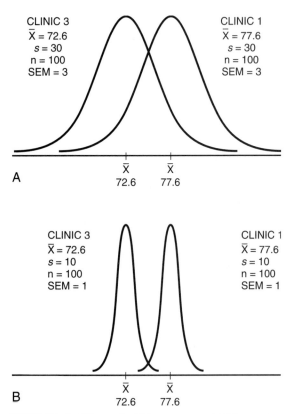

A

B

FIGURE 20–4. Effect of within-group variability on the overlap of sampling distributions. **A.** High variability leads to overlap of sampling distributions. **B.** Low variability leads to minimal overlap of sampling distributions. $\overline{X}$ = mean; s = standard deviation; n = number of subjects; SEM = standard error of the mean.

Contrast Figure 20–4A and B. Figure 20–4B illustrates the same between-groups difference, 5.0°. However, the within-group variability has been reduced sharply. In this example, each group standard deviation is set at 10.0°, meaning that the SEM is 1° ($10/\sqrt{100} = 1$). With a SEM of only 1°, the two curves overlap very little. Because they do not overlap very much, there is a low probability that the samples could have been drawn from populations with the same mean. Because this probability is low, we can conclude that the difference in means did not occur by chance; that is, the difference between the means of the two groups is a significant one.

Even small differences between groups can be statistically significant if the within-group variability is sufficiently low.

SAMPLE SIZE. The third piece of information used to determine the probability that a difference is a true difference is the sample size. We already know that the mean of a large sample is more stable than a mean of a small sample. Assume that we have two groups of 100, each with a standard deviation of 10.0°, and a mean difference between the groups of 5.0°. Because of the large sample sizes, we are confident that the mean values are stable indicators of the means of the populations from which the samples are drawn. The estimated SEM for each group's sampling distribution is 1.0° ($10/\sqrt{100} = 1$); Figure 20–5A shows the minimal overlap between the two sampling distributions. This minimal overlap leads us to conclude that it is unlikely that the differences between the two groups are due to chance; in other words, there is a significant difference between the groups.

Now assume that we have two groups of 10 subjects each. The mean difference between the groups is the same as the previous example (5.0°), as is the standard deviation of each group (10.0°). Because we know that sample sizes of only 10 are sensitive to extreme values, we know that the mean of a sample of 10 is considerably less stable than a mean from a sample of 100. This is reflected in the calculation of the estimated SEM. With a standard deviation of 10° and a sample size of 10, the SEM becomes 3.16° ($10/\sqrt{10} = 3.16$). Figure 20–5B shows the curves that correspond to the sampling distributions of our smaller samples. The curves overlap considerably, leading us to conclude that the samples might well have been drawn from populations with the same mean; that is, there is no significant difference between the means of the two groups. Thus, if the sample size is large enough, even small between-groups differences may be statistically significant and, conversely, if the sample size is too small, even large between-groups differences may not be statistically significant.

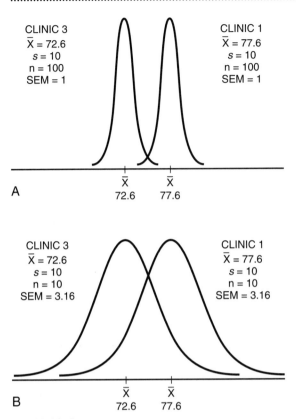

FIGURE 20–5. Effect of sample size on the overlap of sampling distributions. **A.** Large sample size leads to low overlap. **B.** Small sample size leads to extensive overlap. $\overline{X}$ = mean; s = standard deviation; n = number of subjects; SEM = standard error of the mean.

■ ERRORS

Because researchers determine statistical differences by making probability statements, there is always the possibility that the statistical conclusion has been reached in error. Unfortunately, researchers never know when an error has been made, they only know the probability of making that error. There are two types of statistical errors, labeled simply Type I and Type II. Figure 20–6 shows the difference between them. The columns represent the two possible states of reality: there is or is not a difference between groups. The rows represent the two statistical conclusions that can be drawn: there is or is not

a difference between groups. The intersection of the columns and rows creates four different combinations of statistical conclusions and reality. If the statistical conclusion is that there is no difference between groups and there is in fact no difference, then we have made a correct statistical conclusion. If the statistical conclusion is that there is a difference between groups and this is in fact the case, then we have also come to a correct statistical conclusion.

However, if the statistical conclusion is that there is a difference between groups when in fact there is no difference, then we have come to an erroneous statistical conclusion. This error is called a *Type I error*. The probability of making a Type I error is alpha. Recall that researchers set alpha according to the amount of chance they are willing to tolerate. An alpha level of .05 means that the researcher is willing to accept a 5% chance that significant results occurred by chance. Thus, alpha is the probability that significant results will be found when in fact no significant difference exists. Researchers never know when they have committed a Type I error; they only know the probability that one occurred. If researchers wish to decrease the probability of making a Type I error, they simply reduce alpha.

A *Type II error* occurs when the statistical conclusion is that there is no difference between the groups when in reality there is a difference. The probability of making a Type II error is beta.

	REALITY	
	No difference	Difference
STATISTICAL CONCLUSION — No difference	Correct	Type II error
STATISTICAL CONCLUSION — Difference	Type I error	Correct

FIGURE 20–6. Type I and Type II errors reflect the relationship between statistical conclusions and reality.

Beta is related to alpha but is not as easily obtained. Figure 20–7 shows the relationship between alpha and beta.

For this example we assume samples of 25 with standard deviations of 10°, giving us an SEM of 2.0° (10/$\sqrt{25}$ = 2). We also assume that Clinic 3, with a mean of 72.6°, is the standard against which Clinic 1, with a mean of 77.6°, is being compared. Our null hypothesis is that $\mu_1 = \mu_3$. Our alternative hypothesis is that $\mu_1 > \mu_3$. In words, we wish to determine whether the mean of Clinic 1 is significantly greater than the mean of Clinic 3. Alpha is set at 5% in Figure 20–7A.

To determine beta, we first must determine the point on the Clinic 3 curve above which only 5% of the distribution lies. From the z table we find that .05 corresponds to a z score of 1.645. A z score of 1.645 corresponds in this case to a raw score of 75.9° [through algebraic rearrangement, $\overline{X}$ + (z)(SEM) = X; 72.6 + (1.645)(2) = 75.9]. Thus, if Clinic 1's mean is greater than 75.9° (1.645 SEM above Clinic 3's mean), it would be considered significantly different from Clinic 3's mean of 72.6° at the 5% level. The dark shading at the upper tail of Clinic 3's sampling distribution corresponds to the alpha level of 5% and is the probability of making a Type I error. This darkly shaded area is sometimes referred to as the *rejection region* because the null hypothesis of no difference between groups would be rejected if a group mean within this area were obtained. Any group mean less than 75.9° would not be identified as statistically different from the group mean of 72.6°.

The entire part of the curve below the rejection region (including the parts that are lightly shaded) is termed the *acceptance region* because the null hypothesis of no difference between groups would be accepted if a group mean within this area were obtained.

Shift your attention now to the lightly shaded lower tail of the sampling distribution of Clinic 1. Using the z table, we can determine the probability of obtaining sample means less than 75.9°, if the population mean was actually 77.6°. To do so, we convert 75.9 to a z score in relation to 77.6°: z = (X − $\overline{X}$)/SEM; (75.9 − 77.6)/2 = −.85. Using the z table, we find that 19.77% of Clinic 1's sampling distribution will fall below a z score of .85. This percentage is the probability of making a Type II error. If Clinic 1, in reality, has a mean that is significantly greater than Clinic 3's mean, we would fail to detect this difference almost 20% of the time because of the overlap in the sampling distributions. Almost 20% of Clinic 1's sampling distribution falls within the acceptance region of Clinic 3's sampling distribution.

There is an inverse relationship between the probability of making Type I and II errors. When the probability of one increases, the probability of the other decreases. Figure 20–7B shows that, for this example, when the probability of making a Type I error is decreased to 1%, the Type II error increases to 43%. Thus, in setting the alpha

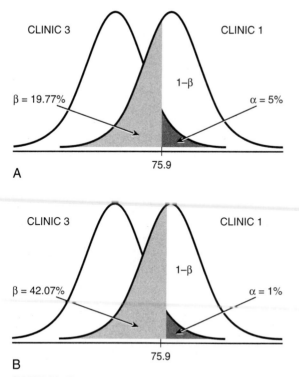

A

B

FIGURE 20–7. Relationship between Type I and Type II errors. **A.** α (probability of making a Type I error) is 5% and β (probability of making a Type II error) is 19.77%. **B.** α is 1% and β is 42.07%.

level for an experiment, the researcher must find a balance between the likelihood of detecting chance differences (Type I error—alpha) and the likelihood of ignoring important differences (Type II error—beta).

■ POWER

The *power* of a test is the likelihood that it will detect a difference when one exists. Recall that beta was the probability of ignoring an important difference when one existed. The probability of detecting a true difference, or power, is therefore $1 - \beta$, as shown in the Clinic 1 curves in Figure 20–7. Recall that the size of the between-groups difference, the size of the sample, and the variability within the sample are the factors that determine whether significant differences between groups are detected. When the sampling distributions of the groups have minimal overlap, the power of a test is high. Factors that contribute to nonoverlapping sampling distributions are large between-groups differences, small within-group differences, and large sample sizes.

Ottenbacher and Barrett[8] have shown that power is often lacking in rehabilitation research, as other have found within their respective disciplines.[9] This is because between-groups differences are often small, sample sizes are usually small, and within-group variability is often large. This lack of statistical power in our literature may mean that promising treatment approaches are not pursued because research has failed to show a significant advantage to the approaches. The power of a given statistical test can be determined by consulting published power tables.[10,11]

Researchers may increase a test's statistical power in three ways. First, they can maximize between-groups differences by carefully controlling extraneous variables and making sure they apply experimental techniques consistently. Note, however, that rigid controls may reduce a study's external validity by making the condi-

tions under which it was conducted very different from the clinical situation to which the researcher wishes to generalize the results.

Second, researchers can reduce within-group variability by studying homogeneous groups of subjects or by using subjects as their own controls in repeated measures designs. Note that these strategies also may reduce external validity by narrowing the group of patients to whom the results can be generalized.

Third, researchers can increase sample size. Increasing sample size does not have the negative impact on external validity that the other two solutions have. However, the increased cost of research with more subjects is an obvious disadvantage to this strategy.

Published power tables can also be used to determine what sample size is needed to achieve a particular power rating. The variables needed to determine sample size requirements are:

- Desired power (Ottenbacher and Barrett recommend a power level of .80[8])
- The alpha level that will be used in the research
- An estimate of the size of the between-groups difference that would be considered clinically meaningful
- An estimate of the within-group variability expected

A researcher can obtain these values from previous research or from a pilot study. In some instances it is difficult to determine sample size because there is no previous information on which to base one's estimates.

■ STATISTICAL CONCLUSION VALIDITY

Readers have previously been introduced to the research design concepts of internal, external, and construct validity (see Chapter 7). The final type of design validity that a researcher must consider when evaluating a research report is statistical conclusion validity. Four threats to statistical conclusion validity, modified from Cook and Campbell, are presented in this section.[12]

Low Power

When statistically insignificant results are reported, readers must ask whether the nonsignificant result is a true indication of no difference or the result of a Type II error. Researchers who give power estimates provide their readers with the probability that their analysis could detect differences and, in doing so, provide information readers need to make a decision about the potential usefulness of further study in the area. The editors of the *Journal of Bone and Joint Surgery,* for example, encourage authors to analyze or discuss power when they report p values between .05 and .15.[6]

Whether or not a power analysis is provided, readers should examine nonsignificant results to determine whether any of the nonsignificant changes were in the desired direction or of a clinically important magnitude. If the nonsignificant differences seem clinically useful and the probability of making a Type II error seems high (sample size was small, the within-group variability was large, or an analysis showed less than 80% power), then readers should be cautious about dismissing the results altogether. Studies with promising nonsignificant results should be replicated with more powerful designs.

An example of a study with low power is Palmer and associates' report of the effects of two different types of exercise programs in patients with Parkinson's disease.[13] Seven patients participated in each exercise program. No significant changes were found in measures of rigidity, although some showed nonsignificant changes in the desired direction. A power analysis of this study reveals that it had, at most, a 50% power level.[8] Because the probability of making a Type II error was so high, the nonsignificant findings should not necessarily be taken to mean that exercise was not useful for these patients. A logical next step in investigat-

ing the effects of exercise for patients with Parkinson's disease is to replicate this study with a more powerful design.

Lack of Clinical Importance

If the power of a test is sufficiently great, it may detect differences that are so small that they are not clinically meaningful. This occurs when samples are large and groups are homogeneous. Just as readers need to examine the between-groups differences of statistically insignificant results to determine whether there is promise in the results, they must also use their clinical reasoning skills to examine statistically significant between-groups differences to determine whether they are clinically meaningful.

Error Rate Problems

Inflation of alpha when multiple tests are conducted within a study is referred to as an error rate problem because the probability of making a Type I error rises with each additional test. As discussed earlier, some researchers compensate for multiple tests by dividing an experiment-wise alpha among the tests to be conducted. Although division of alpha controls the experiment-wise alpha, it also dramatically reduces the power of each test. Readers must determine whether they believe that researchers who have conducted multiple tests have struck a reasonable balance between controlling alpha and limiting the power of their statistical analyses.

A study of balance function in elderly people illustrates alpha level inflation.[14] In this study, three groups were tested: nonfallers, recent fallers, and remote fallers. Five different measures of balance function were obtained on each of two types of supporting surfaces for each of two types of displacement stimuli. The combination of all these factors produced 20 measures for each subject. In the data analysis nonfallers were compared with recent fallers, recent fallers were compared with remote fallers, and nonfallers were compared with remote fallers on each of the 20 measures. This yielded a total of 60 different tests of statistical significance. With this many tests, the overall probability that a Type I error was committed was far higher than the .05 level set for each analysis. Statistical techniques that would have permitted comparison of more than two groups or more than one dependent variable simultaneously could have been used to prevent this alpha level inflation; these techniques are presented in Chapters 21 and 22.

Violated Assumptions

Each of the statistical tests that are presented in Chapters 21 through 24 is based on certain assumptions that should be met for the test to be valid. These assumptions include whether the observations were made independently of one another, whether subjects were randomly sampled, whether the data were normally distributed, and whether the variance of the data was approximately equal across groups. These assumptions, and the consequences of violating them, are discussed in detail in Chapters 21 through 24.

■ SUMMARY

All statistical analyses are based on a relatively small set of central concepts. Descriptive statistics are based on the concepts of central tendency (mean, median, or mode) and variability (range, variance, and standard deviation) within a data set. The distribution of many variables forms a bell-shaped curve known as the normal distribution. The percentage of scores that fall within a certain range of the normal distribution is known and can be used to predict the likelihood of obtaining certain scores. The sampling distribution is a special normal distribution that consists of a theoretical distribution of sample means.

Inferential statistical tests use sampling distributions to determine the likelihood that different samples came from populations with the same characteristics. A significant difference between groups indicates that the probability that the samples came from populations with the same characteristics is lower than a predetermined level, alpha, that is set by the researcher. There is always a probability that one of two statistical errors will be made: a Type I error occurs when a significant difference is found when in fact there is no difference; a Type II error occurs when a difference actually exists but is not identified by the test. The power of a test is the probability that it will detect a true difference. The validity of statistical conclusions is threatened by low power, results that are not clinically meaningful, alpha level inflation with multiple tests, and violation of statistical assumptions.

REFERENCES

1. Chottiner S. Statistics: toward a kinder, gentler subject. *Irreproducible Results*. 1990;35(6):13–15.
2. Ewald FC, Jacobs MA, Miegel RE, Walker PS, Poss R, Sledge CB. Kinematic total knee replacement. *J Bone Joint Surg Am*. 1984;66:1032–1040.
3. Elston RC, Johnson WD. *Essentials of Biostatistics*. Philadelphia, Pa: FA Davis Co; 1994.
4. Shott S. *Statistics for Health Professionals*. Philadelphia, Pa: WB Saunders Co; 1990.
5. Aickin M, Gensler H. Adjusting for multiple testing when reporting research results: the Bonferroni vs Holm methods. *Am J Public Health*. 1996;86:726–727.
6. Senghas RE. Statistics in the *Journal of Bone and Joint Surgery:* suggestions for authors. *J Bone Joint Surg Am*. 1992;74:319–320.
7. Mueller MJ, Salsich GB, Strube MJ. Functional limitations in patients with diabetes and transmetatarsal amputations. *Phys Ther*. 1997;77:937–943.
8. Ottenbacher KJ, Barrett KA. Statistical conclusion validity of rehabilitation research: a quantitative analysis. *Am J Phys Med Rehabil*. 1990;69:102–107.
9. Polit DF, Sherman RE. Statistical power in nursing research. *Nurs Res* 1990;39:365–369.
10. Kraemer HC, Thiemann S. *How Many Subjects? Statistical Power Analysis in Research*. Newbury Park, Calif: Sage Publications; 1987.
11. Cohen J. *Statistical Power Analysis for the Behavioral Sciences*. 2nd ed. Hillsdale, NJ: Lawrence Erlbaum Associates; 1988.
12. Cook TD, Campbell DT. *Quasi-experimentation: Design and Analysis Issues for Field Settings*. Chicago, Ill: Rand McNally College Publishing Co; 1979:37–94.
13. Palmer SS, Mortimer JA, Webster DD, Bistevins R, Dickinson GL. Exercise therapy for Parkinson's disease. *Arch Phys Med Rehabil*. 1986;67:741–745.
14. Ring C, Nayak USL, Isaacs B. Balance function in elderly people who have and who have not fallen. *Arch Phys Med Rehabil*. 1988;69:261–264.

Statistical Analysis of Differences: The Basics

Distributions for Analysis of Differences
 t Distribution
 F Distribution
 Chi-Square Distribution

Assumptions of Tests of Differences
 Random Selection from a Normally
  Distributed Population
 Homogeneity of Variance
 Level of Measurement

Independence or Dependence of Samples

Steps in the Statistical Testing of Differences

Statistical Analysis of Differences
 Differences Between Two
  Independent Groups

 Independent t Test
 Mann-Whitney or Wilcoxon Rank Sum Test
 Chi-Square Test of Association
Differences Between Two or More
 Independent Groups
 One-Way ANOVA
 Kruskal-Wallis Test
 Chi-Square Test of Association
Differences Between Two
 Dependent Samples
 Paired-t Test
 Wilcoxon Signed Rank Test
 McNemar Test
Differences Between Two or More
 Dependent Samples
 Repeated Measures ANOVA
 Friedman's ANOVA

Researchers use statistical tests when they wish to determine whether a significant difference exists between two or more sets of numbers. In this chapter, the general statistical concepts presented in Chapter 20 are applied to specific statistical tests of differences commonly reported in the physical therapy literature. The distributions most commonly used in statistical testing are presented first, followed by the general assumptions that underlie statistical tests of differences. The sequence of steps common to all statistical tests of differences is then outlined. Finally, specific tests of differences are presented. In this chapter, basic tests using one independent variable are presented. Each is illustrated with an example from the hypothetical knee arthroplasty data set presented in Chapter 20 as well as an example from the literature. In Chapter 22 more advanced tests using two independent variables are presented, as are a variety of specialized techniques for analyzing differences.

■ DISTRIBUTIONS FOR ANALYSIS OF DIFFERENCES

In Chapter 20 the rationale behind statistical testing was developed in terms of the standard normal distribution and its z scores. Use of this distribution assumes that the population standard deviation is known. Because the population standard deviation is usually *not* known, we cannot ordinarily use the standard normal distribution and its z scores to draw statistical conclusions from samples. Therefore, researchers conduct most statistical tests using distributions that resemble the normal distribution but are altered somewhat to account for the errors that are made when population parameters are estimated. The three most common distributions

used for statistical tests are the t, F, and chi-square (χ^2) distributions, shown in Figure 21–1. Just as we determined the probability of obtaining certain z scores based on the standard normal distribution, we can determine the probability of obtaining certain t, F, and chi-square statistics based on their respective distributions. The exact shapes of the distributions vary with the degrees of freedom associated with the test statistic. The degrees of freedom are calculated in different ways for the different distributions, but in general are related to the number of subjects within the study or the number of levels of the independent variable, or both. When test statistics are reported within the literature, they often include a subscript that indicates the degrees of freedom.

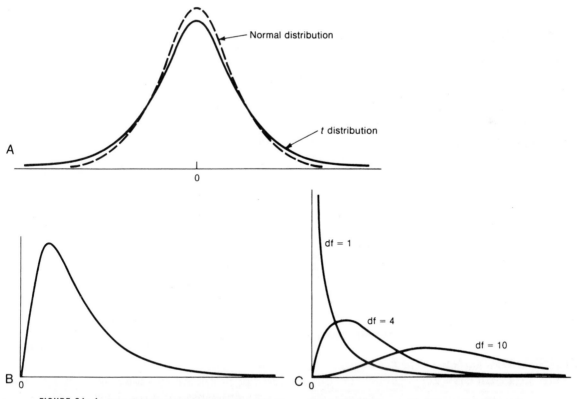

FIGURE 21–1. Distribution of test statistics. **A.** The solid t distribution with 5 degrees of freedom (df) compared with the dashed normal distribution. **B.** F distribution with 6 and 12 degrees of freedom. **C.** Chi-square distribution with 1, 4, and 10 degrees of freedom.
Reprinted with permission from Shott S. *Statistics for Health Professionals.* Philadelphia, Pa: WB Saunders Co; 1990:75, 148, 208.

t Distribution

The *t* distribution is a symmetric distribution that is essentially a "flattened" *z* distribution (Fig. 21–1A). Compared with the *z* distribution, a greater proportion of the *t* distribution is located in the tails and a lesser proportion in the center of the distribution. The *z* distribution is spread to form the *t* distribution to account for the errors that are introduced when population parameters are estimated from sample statistics. The shape of a *t* distribution varies with its degrees of freedom, which is based on sample size. Because estimation of population parameters is more accurate with larger samples, *t* distributions become more and more similar to *z* distributions as sample size and degrees of freedom increase.

F Distribution

The *F* distribution is a distribution of squared *t* statistics (Fig. 21–1B). It is asymmetric and, because it is generated from squared scores, consists only of positive values. The actual shape of a particular *F* distribution depends on two different degrees of freedom—one associated with the number of groups being compared and one associated with the sample size.

Chi-Square Distribution

The chi-square distribution is a distribution of squared *z* scores (Fig. 21–1C). As is the case with the *t* and *F* distributions, the shape of the chi-square distribution varies with its degrees of freedom.

■ ASSUMPTIONS OF TESTS OF DIFFERENCES

Statistical tests of differences are either parametric or nonparametric. *Parametric tests* are based on specific assumptions about the distribution of populations. They use sample statistics such as the mean, standard deviation, and variance to estimate differences between population parameters. The two major classes of parametric tests are *t* tests and analyses of variance (ANOVAs).

Nonparametric tests are not based on specific assumptions about the distribution of populations. They use rank or frequency information to draw conclusions about differences between populations.[1] Parametric tests are usually assumed to be more powerful than nonparametric tests and are often preferred to nonparametric tests.[2(p100)] However, parametric tests cannot always be used because the assumptions on which they are based are more stringent than the assumptions for nonparametric tests. Two parametric assumptions are commonly accepted: random selection and homogeneity of variance. A third assumption is controversial and relates to the measurement level of the data.

Random Selection from a Normally Distributed Population

The first basic assumption of parametric testing is that the subjects are randomly selected from normally distributed populations. However, this assumption may be violated as long as the data sets used in the analysis are relatively normally distributed. Even when the data sets are not normally distributed, statistical researchers have shown that the various statistical tests are *robust,* meaning that they usually still provide an appropriate level of rejection of the null hypothesis. The extent to which a data set is normally distributed may be tested; however, the details are beyond the scope of this text.[2(pp41–43)]

When data are extremely nonnormal, one data analysis strategy is to convert, or *transform,* the data mathematically so that they become normally distributed. Squaring, taking the square root of, or calculating a logarithm of raw data are common transformations. Parametric tests can then be conducted on the transformed scores. A second strategy for dealing with nonnormality is to use nonparametric tests, which do not require normally distributed data.

Homogeneity of Variance

The second basic assumption of parametric testing is that the population variances of the groups being tested are equal, or *homogeneous*. Homogeneity of variance may be tested statistically.[3(p264)] If homogeneity of variance is tested and the variances of the groups are found to differ significantly, then nonparametric tests must be used. When the sample sizes of the groups being compared are the same, then differences in the variances of the groups become less of a concern.[4(p131)] Therefore, researchers generally design their studies to maximize the chance of having equal, or nearly equal, samples sizes across groups.

Level of Measurement

The third, and most controversial, assumption for parametric testing concerns the measurement level of the data. As noted earlier, one distinction between the parametric and nonparametric tests is that the two types of tests are used with different types of data. Nonparametric tests require rankings or frequencies—nominal and ranked ordinal data meet this need, and interval and ratio data can be converted into ranks or grouped into categories to meet this need. Parametric tests require data from which means and variances can be calculated—interval and ratio data clearly meet this need; nominal data clearly do not. The controversy, then, surrounds the use of parametric statistics with ordinal measurements.

The traditional belief that parametric tests can be conducted only with interval or ratio data is no longer considered valid.[5,6(p24)] Although ordinal-scaled variables do not have the property of equal intervals between numerals, the distribution of ordinal data is often approximately normal. As long as the data themselves meet the parametric assumptions, regardless of the origin of the numbers, then parametric tests can be conducted. As is the case with all statistical tests of differences, the researcher must interpret parametric statistical conclusions that are based on ordinal data in light of their clinical or practical implications.

For example, a common type of ordinal measurement used by physical therapists is a scale of the amount of assistance a patient needs to accomplish various functional tasks. The categories maximal, moderate, minimal, standby, and no assistance could be coded numerically from 1 to 5, with 5 representing no assistance. Assume that four different groups have mean scores of 1.0, 2.0, 4.0, and 5.0 and that these group means have been found to be significantly different from one another. If the researchers believe that the "real" interval between maximal and moderate assistance is greater than the interval between standby and no assistance, they might interpret the difference between the groups with means of 1.0 and 2.0 to be more clinically important than the difference between the groups with means of 4.0 and 5.0. It is reasonable to conduct parametric tests with ordinal data as long as interpretation of the tests accounts for the nature of the ordinal scale.

■ INDEPENDENCE OR DEPENDENCE OF SAMPLES

Another important consideration for either parametric or nonparametric testing concerns whether the different sets of numbers being compared are independent or dependent. Sets are independent when values in one set tell nothing about values in another set. When two or more groups consist of different, unrelated individuals, the observations made about the samples are independent. For example, the 3-week range-of-motion (ROM) scores for patients in Clinics 1 through 3 in our hypothetical knee arthroplasty study are independent of one another. Knowing the 3-week ROM values for patients at Clinic 1 provides us with no information about 3-week ROM values of the different patients being seen at Clinic 2 or Clinic 3.

When the sets of numbers consist of repeated measures on the same individuals, they are said to be dependent. The 3-week, 6-week, and 6-

month ROM scores for patients across the three clinics are dependent measures. A patient's 6-week score is expected to be related to the 3-week score. Repeated measures taken on the same individual are not the only type of dependent measures, however. If we compare male and female characteristics by using brother-sister pairs, we have dependent samples. If we study pairs or trios of individuals matched for factors such as income, education, age, height, and weight, then we also have dependent samples.

Different statistical tests are used with independent versus dependent samples, and the assumption of either independence or dependence must not be violated. The researcher must select the correct test according to whether the samples are independent or dependent.

■ STEPS IN THE STATISTICAL TESTING OF DIFFERENCES

The statistical testing of differences can be summarized in 10 basic steps, regardless of the particular test used. A general assumption of these steps is that researchers plan to perform parametric tests and resort to the use of nonparametric tests only if the assumptions for parametric testing are not met. The steps are as follows:

1. State the null and alternative hypotheses in parametric terms.
2. Decide on an alpha level for the test.
3. Determine whether the samples are independent or dependent.
4. Determine whether parametric assumptions are met. If they are not met, revise hypotheses for nonparametric testing.
5. Determine the appropriate statistical test, given the above information.
6. Calculate the test statistic.
7. Determine the degrees of freedom for the test statistic.
8. Determine the probability of obtaining the calculated test statistic, taking into account the degrees of freedom. Computer statistical packages generate the precise

probability of obtaining a given test statistic for the given degrees of freedom.
9. Compare the probability obtained in Step 8 with the alpha level established in Step 2. If the obtained probability is less than the alpha level, the test has identified a statistically significant difference; that is, the null hypothesis is rejected. If the obtained probability is equal to or greater than the alpha level, the test has failed to identify a statistically significant difference; that is, the null hypothesis is not rejected.
10. Evaluate the statistical conclusions in light of clinical knowledge. If the result is statistically significant but the differences between groups do not seem to be important from a clinical perspective, this discrepancy should be discussed. If the result is statistically insignificant but the differences between groups appear clinically important, a power analysis should be conducted and discussed in light of the discrepancy between the statistical and clinical conclusions.

Table 21–1 lists these steps. The first column shows how the steps are implemented when a computer program is used for the statistical analysis, the second column shows how the steps are implemented in the increasingly rare instances when calculators and tables are used to perform the statistical analysis. Steps that are common to both computation methods cross the two columns. The remainder of this chapter illustrates how these 10 steps are implemented for several different statistical tests of differences.

■ STATISTICAL ANALYSIS OF DIFFERENCES

The hypothetical total knee arthroplasty data set presented in Chapter 20 is used in the rest of this chapter to illustrate 10 different statistical tests of differences. All analyses were conducted with

| TABLE 21-1 | Ten Steps in the Statistical Testing of Differences |

	Computation Method	
Step	**Computer Package**	**Calculator and Tables**
1	State hypotheses.	
2	Determine alpha level.	
3	Determine whether samples are independent or dependent.	
4	Run frequency and descriptive programs to determine whether parametric assumptions are met.	Plot frequencies and calculate descriptive statistics to determine whether parametric assumptions are met.
5	Determine appropriate test.	
6	Use appropriate programs to calculate test statistic.	Use appropriate formulas to calculate test statistic.
7	Program calculates the degrees of freedom.	Calculate the degrees of freedom.
8	Program calculates the probability of obtaining the test statistic given the degrees of freedom.	Determine the critical value of the test statistic given the degrees of freedom and predetermined alpha level.
9	Compare the obtained probability with the alpha level to draw statistical conclusion. When the obtained probability is less than alpha, a statistically significant difference has been identified.	Compare the obtained test statistic with the critical value of the test statistic to draw statistical conclusion. When the obtained test statistic is greater than the critical value, a statistically significant difference has been identified.
10	Evaluate the statistical conclusions in light of clinical knowledge.	

the Statistical Package for the Social Sciences (SPSS).[7,8] Formulas and computations are included with the first few examples to illustrate how the test statistics are calculated. However, the purpose of this chapter is to enable readers to understand the results of tests, not to perform statistical analyses. Researchers who wish to analyze small data sets by hand can refer to any number of good biostatistical references for the formulas and tables needed to do so.[2–4,9–11]

The 10 tests presented in this chapter are organized by the type of difference being analyzed, rather than by statistical technique. For each type of difference being analyzed, both a parametric and a nonparametric test are given. Although the number of tests may seem daunting, there are actually only a few basic tests that are varied according to the number of groups being compared, whether the samples are independent or dependent, the nature of the data, and whether parametric assumptions are met.

Table 21–2 presents an overview of the tests presented in this chapter.

Differences Between Two Independent Groups

Assume that Clinics 1 and 2 have different postoperative activity protocols for their patients who have had total knee arthroplasty. We wonder whether there are differences in 3-week ROM results between patients at Clinic 1 and Clinic 2. The null and alternative hypotheses we intend to test are as follows:

$$H_0: \mu_1 = \mu_2$$

$$H_1: \mu_1 \neq \mu_2$$

We set alpha at 5% and determine that we have independent samples because different, unrelated patients make up the samples from the two

| TABLE 21-2 | Basic Statistical Tests for Analyzing Differences | | | |

	Independent Levels of the Independent Variable		Dependent Levels of the Independent Variable	
Design	*Parametric*	*Nonparametric*	*Parametric*	*Nonparametric*
One independent variable with two levels; dependent variables analyzed one at a time	Independent t test	Mann-Whitney (ranks) Wilcoxon rank sum (ranks) Chi-square (frequencies)	Paired-t test	Wilcoxon signed rank (ranks) McNemar (frequencies)
One independent variable with two or more levels; dependent variables analyzed one at a time	One-way analysis of variance (ANOVA)	Kruskal-Wallis (ranks) Chi-square (frequencies)	Repeated measures ANOVA	Friedman's ANOVA (ranks)

clinics. Now we have to determine whether our data meet the assumptions for parametric testing. Table 21–3 shows the descriptive statistics and stem-and-leaf plots for the 3-week ROM data for the two groups. The variances, although not identical, are at least of similar magnitude. The ratio of the larger variance to the smaller variance is 1.85, which is less than the 2.0 maximum recommended for meeting the homogeneity-of-variance assumption for the independent t test [11(p117)] The plot for Clinic 1 is negatively *skewed;* that is, it has a long tail of lower numbers. The plot for Clinic 2 looks fairly symmetric. Under these conditions some researchers would proceed with a parametric test, and others would use a nonparametric test because of the nonnormal shape of the Clinic 1 data. The parametric test of differences between two independent sample means is the independent t test; the nonparametric test is either the Mann-Whitney test or the Wilcoxon rank sum test.

INDEPENDENT t TEST

Like most test statistics, the test statistic for the independent t test is the ratio of the differences

between the groups to the differences within the groups. The pooled formula for the independent t is presented at the bottom of Table 21–3. The numerator is simply the difference between the two sample means. The denominator is a form

TABLE 21-3	Independent t Test	
Clinic	1	2
Data	3 2	2 7
	5 8	3 4
	6 7	4 0579
	8 1478	5 06
	9 225	6 7
		7 6
Mean	$\bar{X}_1 = 77.6$	$\bar{X}_2 = 49.1$
Variance	$s_1^2 = 393.62$	$s_2^2 = 212.58$
Standard deviation	$s_1 = 19.84$	$s_2 = 14.58$

$$t = \frac{\bar{X}_1 - \bar{X}_2}{\left(\sqrt{\dfrac{(n_1 - 1)s_1^2 + (n_2 - 1)s_2^2}{n_1 + n_2 - 2}}\right)\left(\sqrt{\dfrac{1}{n_1} + \dfrac{1}{n_2}}\right)}$$

$$= \frac{28.5}{(17.4)(.447)} = 3.66$$

of a standard error of the mean created by pooling the standard deviations of the samples and dividing by the square root of the pooled sample sizes. When the *t* formula is solved by inserting the values from our example, a value of 3.66 is obtained. A separate variance formula is available for use if the difference between the two group variances is too great to permit pooling.[2(p125)] The computer-generated two-tailed probability of obtaining a *t* statistic of 3.66 with 18 degrees of freedom ($n_1 + n_2 - 2$) is .002. Because .002 is less than the predetermined alpha level of .05, we reject the null hypothesis. We conclude that the mean 3-week ROM scores of the populations from whom the Clinic 1 and Clinic 2 patients are drawn are significantly different from one another. The difference between the means of the two groups is 28.5°. Because this difference seems clinically important, our statistical and clinical conclusions concur.

In determining our statistical conclusions in the paragraph above, a two-tailed probability was used. The *t* test is one of only a few statistical tests that require the researcher to differentiate between directional and nondirectional hypotheses before conducting the test. The alternative hypothesis given at the beginning of this section, $\mu_1 \neq \mu_2$, is *nondirectional,* meaning that we are open to the possibility that Clinic 1's mean ROM is either greater than *or* less than Clinic 2's mean ROM. If Clinic 1's mean is greater than Clinic 2's mean, as in our example, the *t* statistic would be positive. If, however, Clinic 2's mean is greater than Clinic 1's mean, the value of *t* would be negative. Because our research hypothesis allows for either a positive or a negative *t,* the probability that *t* will be greater than +3.66 *and* the probability that *t* will be less than −3.66 must both be accounted for. The two-tailed probability of .002 is the sum of the probability that *t* will exceed +3.66 and the probability that *t* will be less than −3.66.

A *directional hypothesis* is used occasionally as the alternative to the null hypothesis. A directional hypothesis specifies which of the means is expected to be greater than the other. Use of a directional hypothesis is justified only if there is

existing evidence of the direction of the effect or when only one outcome is of interest to the researcher. Researchers who use a directional hypothesis are interested in only one tail of the *t* distribution. Because the two-tailed probability is the sum of the probabilities in the upper and lower tails of the distribution, the one-tailed probability is determined by dividing the two-tailed probability in half. Thus, for our example, the two-tailed probability of .002 becomes a one-tailed probability of .001.

In this example both the one- and two-tailed probabilities are so low that both lead to the same statistical conclusion. Imagine, though, if the two-tailed probability for a test were .06. If we set alpha at .05 and conduct a two-tailed test, there is no significant difference between groups. However, if we conduct a one-tailed test we divide the two-tailed probability in half to get a one-tailed probability of .03. This is less than our alpha level of .05; thus with the one-tailed test we conclude that there is a significant difference between groups. As can be seen, the one-tailed test is more powerful than the two-tailed test. Researchers should not be tempted to abuse this power by conducting one-tailed tests unless they have an appropriate rationale for doing so.

Independent *t* tests are often used to analyze pretest-posttest designs when there are only two groups and two measurements on each subject. One strategy is to perform an independent *t* test on the pretest data; if there is no significant difference between groups at pretest, then an independent *t* test is run on the posttest data to determine whether there was a significant treatment effect. A second strategy is to create gain scores by subtracting the pretest value from the posttest value for each subject. An independent *t* test is then run on the gain scores to determine whether one group had a significantly greater change than the other. Egger and Miller provide a useful description of different options for analyzing pretest-posttest designs, along with guidelines for making decisions among the options.[12]

An independent *t* test would typically be summarized in a journal article as follows:

DATA ANALYSIS

An independent t test was used to determine whether there was a significant difference between mean 3-week range-of-motion (ROM) values at Clinics 1 and 2. A two-tailed test was conducted with alpha set at .05.

RESULTS

The mean 3-week ROM at Clinic 1 was 28.5° greater than at Clinic 2; this difference was statistically significant (Table 1).

Table 1. Three-Week Range-of-Motion Difference Between Clinics

Clinic	N	$\bar{X}$	s	t	p
1	10	77.6°	19.84°	3.66	.002
2	10	49.1°	14.58°		

Dean and Shepherd used independent t tests to determine whether there were significant differences between experimental and control groups on a variety of dependent variables.[13] The subjects were at least 1 year poststroke and participated in either a task-specific seated reaching training program or a sham training program. They used independent t tests to determine whether there were significant differences between experimental and control groups for the following dependent variables: change in maximum distance reached during seated reaching tasks, change in hand movement time during seated reaching tasks, and change in ground reaction forces (GRF) through the affected foot during seated forward-reaching tasks.

MANN-WHITNEY OR WILCOXON RANK SUM TEST

The Mann-Whitney and Wilcoxon rank sum tests are two equivalent tests that are the nonparametric alternatives to the independent t test. If the assumptions for the independent t test are vi-

olated, researchers may choose to analyze their data with one of these tests. When nonparametric tests are employed, the hypotheses need to be stated in more general terms than the hypotheses for parametric tests.

H_0: The populations from which Clinic 1 and Clinic 2 samples are drawn are identical.

H_1: One population tends to produce larger observations than the other population.[11(p238)]

To perform the Mann-Whitney test, a researcher ranks the scores from the two groups, irrespective of original group membership. Table 21–4 shows the ranking of 3-week ROM scores for Clinics 1 and 2. When a number occurs more than once, its ranking is the mean of the multiple ranks it occupies. For example, the two 67s are the 11th and 12th ranked scores in this distribution, so each receives a rank of 11.5. The next-ranked number, 76, receives the rank of 13. The sum of the Clinic 1 ranks is 142.5; the sum of the Clinic 2 ranks is 67.5.

To understand the logic behind the Mann-Whitney, imagine that our two clinics have vastly different scores that do not overlap at all. The

TABLE 21–4	**Mann-Whitney or Wilcoxon Rank Sum Test**
Clinic 1	**Clinic 2**
Score (Rank)	*Score (Rank)*
32 (2)	27 (1)
58 (10)	34 (3)
67 (11.5)	40 (4)
81 (14)	45 (5)
84 (15)	47 (6)
87 (16)	49 (7)
88 (17)	50 (8)
92 (18.5)	56 (9)
92 (18.5)	67 (11.5)
95 (20)	76 (13)
Rank sum (142.5)	(67.5)

Clinic 2 ranks would be 1 through 10, which add up to 55; the Clinic 1 ranks would be 11 through 20, which add up to 155. Now suppose the opposite case, in which the scores are very similar. The Clinic 2 scores might get all the odd ranks, which add up to 100; the Clinic 1 scores might get all the even ranks, which add up to 110. When the two samples are similar, their rank sums will be similar. When the samples differ greatly, the rank sums will be very different. The rank sums (67.5 and 142.5) of our two samples of patients with total knee arthroplasty fall between the two extremes of (a) 55 and 155 and (b) 100 and 110. To come to a statistical conclusion, we need to determine the probability of obtaining the rank sums of 67.5 and 142.5 if in fact the populations from which the samples are drawn are identical. To do so, we transform the higher rank sum into a z score and calculate the probability of obtaining that z score.

An alternative form of the Mann-Whitney test uses a U statistic, which is converted into a z score. In this example, the computer-generated z score is 2.84 and the associated two-tailed probability is .0046. We conclude from this that there is a significant difference between the scores from Clinic 1 and the scores from Clinic 2. Given the 28.5° difference in the means and the 37.5° difference in the medians between the clinics, this difference seems clinically important. Once again, our statistical and clinical conclusions concur.

The results of a Mann-Whitney test might be written up as follows in a journal article:

DATA ANALYSIS

Because the distribution of Clinic 1's range-of-motion (ROM) scores was nonnormal, we chose to analyze differences between the two groups with a nonparametric Mann-Whitney test. The 5% significance level was used for hypothesis testing.

RESULTS

A significant difference between the 3-week ROM scores for the two groups was found. Table 1 shows descriptive measures and rank sums for both groups.

Table 1. Three-Week Range-of-Motion Difference Between Clinics

Clinic	Median	X̄	s	Rank Sum[*]
1	85.5°	77.6°	19.84°	142.5
2	48.0°	49.1°	14.58°	67.5

[*] Significant at $p < .05$.

Dean and Shepherd, whose study was cited earlier as an example of the independent t test, also used a Mann-Whitney test within their data analysis.[13] They used the Mann-Whitney test to determine whether there were significant differences between experimental and control groups in the percentage of trials in which various muscles were activated. Although the authors do not give an explicit rationale for choosing the Mann-Whitney test for the electromyographic (EMG) data, a review of their results shows that the experimental group members often had very high percentages of trials during which the desired muscle was activated. Thus, the data for the experimental group were probably not normally distributed and the experimental group variances were probably much lower than the control group variances. Thus, the EMG data likely did not meet the normality and homogeneity of variance assumptions needed for parametric testing.

CHI-SQUARE TEST OF ASSOCIATION

Assume that we still wish to determine whether there are differences in the 3-week ROM scores of Clinics 1 and 2. However, let us further assume that previous research has shown that the ultimate functional outcome after total knee arthroplasty depends on having regained at least 90° of knee flexion by 3 weeks postsurgery. If such evidence existed, we might no longer be interested in the absolute 3-week ROM scores at our clinics. We might instead be interested in the proportion of patients who achieve 90° of knee flexion 3 weeks postoperatively. In this case, we would convert the raw ROM scores into categories: "less than 90°" and "greater than or equal to 90°." Then we would use a chi-square test of association to determine whether the two clinics had similar proportions of patients with and without 90° of knee flexion at 3 weeks postoperatively. A complete chi-square example is presented in the next section on analysis of differences among two or more independent groups.

Differences Between Two or More Independent Groups

If Clinics 1 through 3 all have different postoperative protocols for their patients who have undergone total knee arthroplasty, we might wonder whether there are significant differences in mean 3-week ROM scores among the three clinics. To test this question statistically, we develop the following hypotheses:

H_0: $\mu_1 = \mu_2 = \mu_3$

H_1: At least one of the population means is different from another population mean.

We shall set alpha at .05 for the analysis. The samples are independent because they consist of different, unrelated subjects. The descriptive measures and stem-and-leaf plots for all three clinics are presented in Table 21–5. The scores for both Clinics 1 and 3 appear to be nonnormal; the variances are similar. If we believe that the parametric assumptions have been met, we test the differences with a one-way ANOVA. If we do not believe that the parametric assumptions have been met, the comparable nonparametric test is the Kruskal-Wallis test. A chi-square test of association can be used to test differences between groups when the dependent variable consists of nominal-level data.

ONE-WAY ANOVA

ANOVA techniques partition the variability in a sample into between-groups and within-group

TABLE 21–5	Frequencies and Descriptive Statistics for Three-Week Range-of-Motion at Clinics 1 Through 3		
Clinic	1	2	3
Data		2 7	
	3 2	3 4	3 2
	4	4 0579	4
	5 8	5 06	5 0
	6 7	6 7	6 0
	7	7 6	7
	8 1478		8 111244
	9 225		9 1
$\overline{X}$	77.6	49.1	72.6
s^2	393.62	212.58	357.38
s	19.84	14.58	18.90

variability. A ratio is created with between-groups variability as the numerator and within-group variability as the denominator. This ratio is an F statistic, which is distributed as shown in Figure 21–1B, discussed earlier. Because the F distribution is a squared t distribution, F cannot be negative. This means that all the extreme values for F are in the upper tail of the distribution, eliminating the need to differentiate between one- and two-tailed tests. The ANOVA is a very versatile statistical technique, and many different variations of it are available. All of the ANOVA techniques are based on partitioning variability to create an F ratio that is evaluated against the probabilities of the F distribution.

The ANOVA required in our example is known as a *one-way ANOVA*. "One-way" refers to the fact that only one independent variable is examined. In this case, the independent variable is clinic, and it has three levels—Clinic 1, Clinic 2, and Clinic 3. Table 21–6 shows the calculations needed to determine the F statistic. Although time-consuming, the calculations presented here are not difficult. To compute the F statistic, we must first know the individual group means as well as the grand mean. The *grand mean* is the mean of all of the scores across the

TABLE 21-6 **One-Way Analysis of Variance Calculations of Sum of Squares Total (SST), Within Group (SSW), and Between Groups (SSB)**

Clinic No.	Raw Score	Deviation from Grand Mean	Deviation^2	Deviation from Group Mean	Deviation^2
1	32	−34.4	1183.36	−45.6	2079.36
1	58	−8.4	70.56	−19.6	384.16
1	67	.6	.36	−10.6	112.36
1	81	14.6	213.16	3.4	11.56
1	84	17.6	309.76	6.4	40.96
1	87	20.6	424.36	9.4	88.36
1	88	21.6	466.56	10.4	108.16
1	92	25.6	655.36	14.4	207.36
1	92	25.6	655.36	14.4	207.36
1	95	28.6	817.96	17.4	302.76
2	27	−39.4	1552.36	−22.1	488.41
2	34	−32.4	1049.76	−15.1	228.01
2	40	−26.4	696.96	−9.1	82.81
2	45	−21.4	457.96	−4.1	16.81
2	47	−19.4	376.36	−2.1	4.41
2	49	−17.4	302.76	−.1	.01
2	50	−16.4	268.96	.9	.81
2	56	−10.4	108.16	6.9	47.61
2	67	.6	.36	17.9	320.41
2	76	9.6	92.16	26.9	723.61
3	32	−34.4	1183.36	−40.6	1648.36
3	50	−16.4	268.96	−22.6	510.76
3	60	−6.4	40.96	−12.6	158.76
3	81	14.6	213.16	8.4	70.56
3	81	14.6	213.16	8.4	70.56
3	81	14.6	213.16	8.4	70.56
3	82	15.6	243.36	9.4	88.36
3	84	17.6	309.76	11.4	129.96
3	84	17.6	309.76	11.4	129.96
3	91	24.6	605.16	18.4	338.56
Σ			13,303.40 (SST)		8671.70 (SSW)

SSB − (77.6 − 66.4)^2 (10) + (49.1 − 66.4)^2 (10) + (72.6 − 66.4)^2 (10) = 4631.7

Note: Clinic 1 mean = 77.6°, Clinic 2 mean = 49.1°, and Clinic 3 mean = 72.6°.

groups; for our three samples the grand mean is 66.4°.

The total variability within the data set is determined by calculating the sum of the squared deviations of each individual score from the grand mean. This is called the *total sum of squares* (SST). The SST calculation is shown in the fourth column of Table 21–6. The second column shows the raw scores; the third column, the deviation of each raw score from the grand mean; and the fourth column, the squared deviations. The sum of these squared deviations across all 30 subjects is the SST.

The within-group variability is determined by calculating the sum of the squared deviations of the individual scores from the group mean. This is known as the *within-group sum of squares* (SSW). The second column of Table 21-6 shows the raw scores; the fifth column, the deviations of each raw score from its group mean; and the final column, the squared deviations. The sum of all of the 30 squared deviation scores in the sixth column is the SSW.

The between-groups variability is determined by calculating the sum of the squared deviations of the group means from the grand mean, with each deviation weighted according to sample size. This is known as the *between-groups sum of squares* (SSB) and is shown at the bottom of Table 21–6.

The SST is the sum of the SSB and the SSW. Conceptually, then, the total variability in the sample is partitioned into variability attributable to differences between the groups and variability attributable to differences within each group.

The next step in calculating the F statistic is to divide the SSB and SSW by appropriate degrees of freedom to obtain the mean square between groups (MSB) and the mean square within each group (MSW), respectively. The degrees of freedom for the SSB is the number of groups minus 1; the degrees of freedom for the SSW is the total number of subjects minus the number of groups. The F statistic is the MSB divided by the MSW. Thus, for our example, the MSB is 2315.85:

$$MSB = \frac{SSB}{(groups - 1)} = \frac{4631.7}{2} = 2315.85$$

The MSW is 321.17:

$$MSW = \frac{SSW}{(N - groups)} = \frac{8671.7}{27} = 321.17$$

The F statistic is 7.21:

$$F = \frac{MSB}{MSW} = \frac{2315.85}{321.17} = 7.21$$

Large F values indicate that the differences between the groups are large compared with the differences within groups. Small F values indicate that the differences between groups are small compared with the differences within groups. The computer-generated probability for our F of 7.21 with 2 and 27 degrees of freedom is .0031. Because this is less than our predetermined alpha level of .05, we can conclude that there is at least one significant difference among the three means that were compared.

If a one-way ANOVA does not identify a significant difference among means, then the statistical analysis is complete. If, as in our example, a significant difference is identified, the researcher must complete one more step. Our overall, or *omnibus*, F test tells us that there is a difference among the means. It does not tell us whether Clinic 1 is different from Clinic 2, whether Clinic 2 is different from Clinic 3, or whether Clinic 1 is different from Clinic 3. To determine the sources of the differences identified by the omnibus F, we must make multiple comparisons between pairs of means.

Conceptually, conducting multiple-comparison tests is similar to conducting t tests between each pair of means, but with a correction to prevent inflation of the alpha level. A comparison of two means is called a *contrast*. Common multiple-comparison procedures, in order of decreasing power, are

- Planned orthogonal contrasts
- Newman-Keuls test
- Tukey test
- Bonferroni test
- Scheffé test[3(p386)]

The more powerful tests identify smaller differences between means as significant. Various assumptions must be met for the different multiple-comparison procedures to be valid.

Using a Newman-Keuls procedure on our example, the mean ROM scores for Clinic 1 (77.6°) and Clinic 3 (72.6°) were not found to be significantly different, and the mean ROM score for

Clinic 2 (49.1°) was found to differ significantly from the mean ROM scores for both Clinics 1 and 3. From a clinical viewpoint, it seems reasonable to conclude that the 5° difference between Clinics 1 and 3 is not important but the difference of more than 20° between Clinic 2 and Clinics 1 and 3 is.

There are two additional twists to the multiple-comparison procedure: (1) whether the contrasts are planned or post hoc and (2) whether the multiple-comparison results are consistent with the omnibus test.

In *planned contrasts*, the researcher specifies which contrasts are of interest before the statistical test is conducted. If, for some reason, the researcher is not interested in differences between Clinics 2 and 3, then only two comparisons need to be made: Clinic 1 versus Clinic 3 and Clinic 1 versus Clinic 2.

If planned contrasts are not specified in advance, all possible multiple comparisons should be conducted as post hoc tests. As more multiple comparisons are conducted, each contrast becomes more conservative to control for alpha inflation.

Occasionally, the omnibus *F* test identifies a significant difference among the means, but the multiple-comparison procedure fails to locate any significant contrasts. One response to these conflicting results is to believe the multiple-comparison results and conclude that despite the significant *F* there is no significant difference among the means. Another response is to believe the *F*-test results and use progressively less conservative multiple-comparison procedures until the significant difference between means is located. A one-way ANOVA might be reported in the literature as follows:

DATA ANALYSIS

One-way analysis of variance (ANOVA) was used to determine whether there were significant 3-week range-of-motion (ROM) differences among the three clinics. Alpha was set at .05; Newman-Keuls post hoc comparisons were conducted.

RESULTS

Tables 1 and 2 show the descriptive statistics and ANOVA summary for the tests of differences between the 3-week ROM means at the three clinics. The omnibus test identified a significant difference among the means. The post hoc analysis showed that the differences of greater than 20° between Clinic 2 and both Clinics 1 and 3 were significant, but that the 5° difference between Clinics 1 and 3 was not.

Table 1. Three-Week Range of Motion at Clinics 1, 2, and 3

Clinic	N	$\bar{X}$	s
1	10	77.6°	19.8°
2	10	49.1°	14.6°
3	10	72.6°	18.9°

Table 2. Summary of Analysis of Variance for Three-Week Range of Motion at Clinics 1, 2, and 3

Source	Sum of Squares	Degrees of Freedom	Mean Square	F
Between groups	4631.7	2	2315.8	7.21[*]
Within group	8671.7	27	321.2	
Total	13,303.4	29		

[*] $p = .0031$.

A one-way ANOVA was used to analyze differences between a treatment and a control group in Weiss's study of the effects of heavy-resistance exercise on triceps surae muscularity.[14] This example shows that although an ANOVA can be used to analyze differences between many groups simultaneously, it is equally appropriate when only two groups are being compared.

KRUSKAL-WALLIS TEST

The Kruskal-Wallis test is the nonparametric equivalent of the one-way ANOVA. If the assumptions of the parametric test are not met, the nonparametric test should be performed. The hypotheses for the nonparametric test must be stated in more general terms than the hypotheses for the parameteric test:

H_0: The three samples come from populations that are identical.

H_1: At least one of the populations tends to produce larger observations than another population.[11(p241)]

To conduct the Kruskal-Wallis test, a researcher ranks the scores, irrespective of group membership. The ranks for each group are then summed and plugged into a formula to generate a Kruskal-Wallis (KW) statistic. The distribution of the KW statistic approximates a chi-square distribution. The computer-generated value of the KW statistic for our example is 11.10; the respective probability is .0039. Because .0039 is less than the alpha level of .05 that we set before conducting the test, we conclude that there is a significant difference somewhere among the groups.

An appropriate multiple-comparison procedure to use when a Kruskal-Wallis test is significant is the Mann-Whitney test with a Bonferroni adjustment of alpha. We have three comparisons to make, and each is tested at an alpha of .017. The probabilities associated with the three Mann-Whitney tests are as follows: For Clinic 1 compared with Clinic 2, $p = .0046$; for Clinic 1 compared with Clinic 3, $p = .2237$; and for Clinic 2 compared with Clinic 3, $p = .0072$. Thus, the multiple comparisons tell us that there is no significant difference between Clinics 1 and 3 and that Clinic 2 is significantly different from both Clinics 1 and 3. In this example the nonparametric conclusions are the same as the parametric conclusions. The results of a Kruskal-Wallis test might be reported in a journal article as follows:

DATA ANALYSIS

Three-week range-of-motion (ROM) differences among the three clinics were studied with a Kruskal-Wallis (KW) analysis of variance with an alpha level of .05. A nonparametric test was used because the data at Clinics 1 and 3 were not normally distributed. Post hoc comparisons were made with three Mann-Whitney tests. The Bonferroni adjustment was used to set alpha at .017 (.05/3 = .017) for each post hoc comparison to compensate for the alpha level inflation that occurs with multiple tests.

RESULTS

A significant difference among the 3-week ROM scores at the three clinics was found (KW = 11.10, $p = .0039$). Clinics 1 and 3, with medians of 85.5° and 81.0°, respectively, were not significantly different from one another ($p = .2237$). Both were significantly different from Clinic 2, which had a median of 48.0° (for Clinic 1 vs. 2, $p = .0046$; for Clinic 2 vs. 3, $p = .0072$).

Rothweiler and colleagues used several Kruskal-Wallis tests to analyze differences in psychosocial functioning among different age groups of subjects with head injury.[15] The independent variable, age, had five levels: 18 to 29 years, 30 to 39 years, 40 to 49 years, 50 to 59 years, and 60+ years. There were several dependent variables: the Glasgow Outcome Scale, postinjury living situation, and postinjury employment status.

CHI-SQUARE TEST OF ASSOCIATION

Assume that we still wish to determine whether there are differences in the 3-week ROM scores of the three clinics. However, let us assume, as we did when the chi-square test was introduced earlier, that previous research has shown that the ultimate functional outcome after total knee arthroplasty depends on having regained at least 90° of knee flexion by 3 weeks postsurgery. In light of such evidence we might no longer be interested in the absolute 3-week ROM scores at our three clinics. Our interest, instead, would be in the relative proportions of patients with at least 90° of motion across the three clinics. Our hypotheses would be as follows:

H_0: There is no association between the clinic and ROM category proportions.

H_1: There is an association between the clinic and ROM category proportions.

Table 21–7 presents the data in the contingency table format needed to calculate chi-square. A *contingency table* is simply an array of data organized into a column variable and a row variable. In this table, clinic is the row variable and consists of three levels. ROM category is the column variable and consists of two levels. Calculation of the chi-square statistic is based on differences between observed frequencies and frequencies that would be expected if the null hypothesis were true.

To determine the observed frequencies, we need to examine the raw data and place each subject in the appropriate ROM category. To de-

termine the expected frequencies, we need to determine the distribution of scores if the proportion in each ROM category were equal across the clinics. In our example, 26 of the 30 subjects overall have ROM scores less than 90°. If these patients were equally distributed among the clinics, each clinic would be expected to have 8.7 (26/3 = 8.7) patients with ROM less than 90° There are four subjects with ROM greater than or equal to 90°. If these four subjects were equally distributed among clinics, each clinic would be expected to have 1.3 (4/3 = 1.3) subjects with ROM greater than or equal to 90°. In this example, the expected frequencies are easy to calculate because there is an equal number of patients in each group. If there are unequal numbers, the expected frequencies are proportionate to the numbers in each group.

An alternative test, the *chi-square test of goodness of fit,* compares the observed frequencies with hypothesized expected frequencies. For example, if we knew of previous research results that indicated that 80% of patients with total knee arthroplasty achieved 90° of motion by 3 weeks postoperatively, then we might test each of our clinic proportions against this hypothesized proportion.

To compute the chi-square statistic, the squared deviation of each expected cell frequency from the observed frequency is divided by the expected frequency for that cell; this is done for every cell, and the values are added together, as shown at the bottom of Table 21–7. If the dependent variable consists of only two categories, then a variation of chi-square called *Fisher's exact test* is sometimes used. If the expected frequencies are below five in a number of the cells of the table, the chi-square statistic is sometimes modified with *Yates' correction.*[3(p288)]

Table 21–7 shows the chi-square calculation for our example. The chi-square of 4.04, with 2 degrees of freedom (the number of columns − 1 × number of rows − 1), is associated with a probability of .1327. Because this probability is higher than the .05 we set as our alpha level, we conclude that there is no significant dif-

---

TABLE 21-7 **Chi-Square χ^2 Test of Association**

Clinic No.	Three-Week Knee Flexion Range-of-Motion Category	
	$<$**90°**	$\geq$**90°**
1	7 (8.67)	3 (1.33)
2	10 (8.67)	0 (1.33)
3	9 (8.67)	1 (1.33)
Total	26	4

$$\chi^2 = \Sigma \frac{(O - E)^2}{E} = (.32) + (.20) + (.01) + (2.10)$$
$$+ (.01) + (.08) + 4.04*$$

Note: Values are actual frequencies. Expected frequencies are in parentheses.

* $p = .1327$.

ference in the proportions of patients in the two ROM categories across the three clinics.

Note that the statistical conclusions of the chi-square analysis differ from those of the ANOVA and Kruskal-Wallis test. The ANOVA, which used all the original values of the data for the analysis, detected a difference among groups. The Kruskal-Wallis test, based on a ranking of the original data, also detected a difference. The chi-square test of association, however, using only nominal data, which eliminated much of the information in the original data set, failed to detect a difference among the groups.

In general, if ratio or interval data exist, it is not wise to convert them to a lower measurement level unless there is a strong theoretical rationale for doing so. Given the hypothetical rationale that was used to set up this chi-square example, we would conclude that patients at all three clinics are likely to have equally poor functional outcomes because of the low proportion of patients at any of the clinics who achieved 90° of motion by 3 weeks postoperatively. Chi-square results might be written up in a journal article as follows:

DATA ANALYSIS

Patients at each clinic were placed into one of two 3-week range-of-motion (ROM) categories. The limited-progress category included those with less than 90° of flexion; the normal-progress category included those with ROM greater than or equal to 90°. The chi-square test of association (alpha = .05) was used to determine whether patients in the two categories were equally distributed across the three clinics.

RESULTS

Chi-square analysis showed no significant difference in the distribution of 3-week ROM categories across the clinics (Table 1).

Table 1. Frequency and Percentage of Three-Week Range-of-Motion Categories Across Clinics*

Clinic	<90°		≥90°	
	Frequency	%	Frequency	%
1	7	70.0	3	30.0
2	10	100.0	0	0.0
3	9	90.0	1	10.0

*$\chi^2_2 = 4.04$, $p = .133$.

Mayer and colleagues used the chi-square test of association within their study of return-to-work patterns of injured workers. They used the chi-square test to determine whether there were significant differences in the rate of returning to work for patients who had completed a functional restoration program versus patients who had dropped out of the program and patients who had not entered a program.[16]

Differences Between Two Dependent Samples

Suppose that we are interested in whether there is a change in ROM from 3 weeks postoperatively to 6 weeks postoperatively for patients across all three of our clinics. The hypotheses we test are as follows:

H_0: $\mu_{3\text{-week ROM}} = \mu_{6\text{-week ROM}}$

H_1: $\mu_{3\text{-week ROM}} \neq \mu_{6\text{-week ROM}}$

We shall set the alpha level at .05. In this example, the two levels of the independent variable of interest are dependent—they are repeated measures taken on the same individuals. When determining whether the data are suitable for parametric testing, remember that the relevant data are the differences between the pairs, rather than the raw data. Table 21–8 presents the distributions of the differences for the entire sample. The differences were calculated by subtracting the 3-week ROM values from the 6-week ROM values given in Table

TABLE 21–8	Difference Between Six-Week and Three-Week Range-of-Motion Scores Across Clinics

−0	8 7 6 5 4 4 2
0	0 2 3 3 4 4 5 6 7 8 8 9
1	0 1 1 3 4 4 5 7 8
2	9
3	5

Mean of the differences: 7.0°
Standard deviation of the differences: 10.03°

$$t = \frac{\bar{X}_d}{\frac{S_d}{\sqrt{n}}} = \frac{7.0}{\frac{10.03}{\sqrt{30}}} = 3.82$$

20–2. A positive difference therefore indicates an improvement in ROM over the 3-week time span. The distribution of difference scores is asymmetric, with a greater proportion of scores in the lower end of the range. The parametric test of differences for two dependent samples is the paired-t test. The corresponding nonparametric test is the Wilcoxon signed rank test. The test of differences between two dependent samples for nominal data is the McNemar test.

PAIRED-t TEST

To calculate the paired-t test, we first determine the difference between each pair of measurements. The mean difference and standard deviation of the differences are calculated, and then the mean is compared with a mean difference of zero. The mean of our example differences is 7.0°; the standard deviation of the differences is 10.03°. We calculate the t statistic for paired samples by dividing the mean difference by the standard error of the mean differences, as shown at the bottom of Table 21–8. The probability associated with the t statistic of 3.82 with 29 degrees of freedom (number of pairs − 1) is .001. Because .001 is less than the alpha level of .05, we conclude that there is a significant difference be-

tween 3-week and 6-week ROM scores. Clinically, an average 7.0° difference in motion over 3 weeks seems modest for this population, particularly considering that few patients are even close to achieving the maximal mechanical ROM of their new knee joints. Therefore, the statistical conclusion must be tempered with a statement about the relatively small size of the difference. Paired-t test results might be reported in a journal article as follows:

DATA ANALYSIS

The difference between 6-week and 3-week range-of-motion (ROM) values was analyzed with a paired-t test. A two-tailed test with alpha at .05 was conducted.

RESULTS

The difference between the 6-week and 3-week ROM scores ranged from −8° to +35°, with a mean of 7.0° and a standard deviation 10.03°. A positive difference indicates an improvement in ROM score from Week 3 to Week 6. Twenty-two subjects improved in the 3-week time span; eight either did not change or experienced a decrease in ROM. The difference in motion was statistically significant. $t_{29} = 3.82$, $p = .001$.

DISCUSSION

Although the difference in ROM between the 3-week and 6-week measurements was statistically significant, the clinical importance of an average 7.0° change over 3 weeks must be questioned, particularly because so few subjects were close to the mechanical flexion limits of their prostheses. Because we had anticipated much larger changes, we conclude that the postoperative progress of these subjects, although statistically significant, is limited.

Roach and associates used paired-t tests to determine whether there were significant differences in Acute Care Index of Function scores from initial evaluation to discharge in a single group of inpatients referred to physical therapy for lower extremity orthopedic problems.[17]

WILCOXON SIGNED RANK TEST

The Wilcoxon signed rank test is the nonparametric version of the paired-t test. The nonparametric hypotheses relate to the median:

H₀: The difference between the population medians is equal to zero.

H₁: The difference between the population medians is not equal to zero.

To conduct the Wilcoxon signed rank test, we calculate the difference between each pair of numbers. We rank the nonzero differences according to their absolute value and then separate them into the ranks associated with positive and negative differences. If there is no difference from one time to the next, then the sum of the positive ranks should be approximately equal to the sum of the negative ranks. Table 21–9 shows the sums of the positive and negative ranks for this example. As is the case with the Mann-Whitney procedures for analyzing differences between independent samples, the ranked information is transformed into a z score. The computer-generated z score and probability for this example are 3.298 and .001, respectively. This probability being less than our alpha of .05, we conclude that there is a significant difference between 3-week and 6-week ROM.

To determine the clinical importance of the difference, we examine the median of the difference between the two samples. The median difference for this example is 6.5.° This seems a fairly modest gain for a 3-week period. Once again, we should temper our statistical conclusion with a statement about the relatively small size of the median difference. Wilcoxon signed rank test results might be reported in a journal article as follows:

DATA ANALYSIS

The Wilcoxon signed rank procedure was used to analyze the difference in range-of-motion (ROM) scores from 3 weeks to 6 weeks. This nonparametric test was selected because the distribution of the difference scores was positively skewed and did not meet parametric assumptions. A nondirectional test was performed with alpha set at .05.

RESULTS

The median difference between 3-week and 6-week ROM was 6.5°, with a range from −8° to +.35°. A positive difference indicates an improvement over time. This difference was statistically significant (z = 3.298, p = .001).

DISCUSSION

Although the difference in ROM between the 3-week and 6-week measurements was statistically significant, the clinical importance of a median 6.5° change over 3 weeks must be questioned, particularly because so few subjects were close to the mechanical flexion limits of their prostheses. Because we had anticipated much larger changes, we conclude that the postoperative progress of these subjects, although statistically significant, is limited.

Griffin and colleagues used a Wilcoxon signed rank test to determine whether there was a significant change in hand volume from the time that patients with chronic hand edema entered the clinic to after they rested for 10 minutes with the hand elevated.[18]

McNEMAR TEST

The McNemar test is the nominal-data analogue to the paired-t test and the Wilcoxon signed rank test. It can also be viewed as the dependent sam-

TABLE 21-9	Wilcoxon Signed Rank Test		
Difference	**Rank by Absolute Value**	**Positive Difference Rank**	**Negative Difference Rank**
0			
−2	1.5		1.5
2	1.5	1.5	
3	3.5	3.5	
3	3.5	3.5	
−4	6.5		6.5
−4	6.5		6.5
4	6.5	6.5	
4	6.5	6.5	
−5	9.5		9.5
5	9.5	9.5	
−6	11.5		11.5
6	11.5	11.5	
7	13.5	13.5	
−7	13.5		13.5
−8	16		16.0
8	16	16.0	
8	16	16.0	
9	18	18.0	
10	19	19.0	
11	20.5	20.5	
11	20.5	20.5	
13	22.0	22.0	
14	23.5	23.5	
14	23.5	23.5	
15	25	25.0	
17	26	26.0	
18	27	27.0	
29	28	28.0	
35	29	29.0	
Σ signed ranks		370	65

ples version of the chi-square test. In fact, a review of rehabilitation research showed that chi-square tests were often used inappropriately for dependent samples when the McNemar test would have been more appropriate.[19] The McNemar test can only be used to analyze 2 × 2 contingency tables, and thus its usefulness is limited. Suppose we want to determine whether there is a predictable change in ROM from 3 weeks to 6 weeks and are interested not in absolute range scores, but only in whether patients

have greater than or less than 90° of motion. Our hypotheses are as follows:

H_0: The proportion of patients with less than 90° of motion at 3 weeks postoperatively is identical to the proportion of patients with less than 90° of motion at 6 weeks postoperatively.

H_1: The population proportions are not equal at the two time intervals.

To perform the McNemar test, we generate a 2 × 2 table of frequencies, as shown in Table 21–10. Each subject is represented only once in the table. For example, a subject who had less than 90° of motion at 3 weeks and still had less than 90° of motion at 6 weeks is one of the 20 individuals indicated in the upper left corner of the table. If the proportion of patients in each category stays the same from 3 weeks to 6 weeks, we would expect that (1) some patients will not change categories (upper left and lower right cells) and (2) the number of patients who change categories will be evenly distributed between those moving from less than to greater than 90° and those moving from greater than to less than 90° (lower left and upper right cells). Table 21–10 shows that 23 patients did not change ROM categories, 6 improved from less than to greater than 90°, and only 1 had a decline in motion from greater than to less than 90°.

The probability of such an occurrence, if in fact there is no difference in proportions, is .1250, as generated by the computer program. Thus, we conclude that the change in proportions from 3 weeks to 6 weeks is not significant. Clinically, a change of categories in only seven of 30 patients seems to indicate minimal effectiveness of the intervention over the 3-week time span. Thus, the statistical conclusion of an insignificant difference in proportions concurs with our clinical impression. Our McNemar test might be reported in a journal article as follows:

DATA ANALYSIS

To determine whether there was a significant change in range of motion (ROM) from 3 weeks to 6 weeks postoperatively, we compared the proportion of patients with less than 90° of motion (limited progress) or greater than or equal to 90° of motion (normal progress) at 3 weeks and 6 weeks. Because the 3-week and 6-week categories are repeated measures, we made the comparison with a McNemar test, setting alpha at .05.

RESULTS

Twenty-three of 30 subjects did not change ROM categories over the time span studied: 20 had limited motion at both occasions, and 3 had acceptable ROM at both occasions. Of the 7 subjects who changed ROM categories over the 3-week time span, 6 moved from the limited- to the normal-progress category, and 1 moved from the normal- to the limited-progress category. This change in proportions was not statistically significant (p = .1250).

Calkins and colleagues used a McNemar test to analyze differences in perceptions of patient and physician communication about postdischarge treatment plans.[20] The McNemar test identified a significant difference, with almost all the physicians believing that patients understood when to resume normal activities after discharge, although only about half of the patients thought they understood postdischarge treatment.

Differences Between Two or More Dependent Samples

We wish now to determine whether patients show a pattern of ROM improvement from 3 weeks postoperatively, to 6 weeks postoperatively, to 6 months postoperatively. Our hypotheses for such a question are as follows:

TABLE 21-10 **McNemar Test**		
	Six-Week Range of Motion	
Three-Week Range of Motion	*Limited Progress* *(<90°)*	*Normal Progress* *(≥90°)*
Limited progress (<90°)	20	6
Normal progress (≥90°)	1	3

H_0: $\mu_{3\text{-week ROM}} = \mu_{6\text{-week ROM}} = \mu_{6\text{-month ROM}}$

H_1: At least one population mean does not equal another population mean.

We set alpha at .05. The samples are dependent because each subject is measured three times. Table 21–11 shows the stem-and-leaf displays for the ROM scores at all three time periods; none is symmetric. Additional assumptions about the variances and covariances of the measures must be met, but a full discussion of these is beyond the scope of this text. The parametric test of differences between more than two dependent means is the repeated measures ANOVA. The corresponding nonparametric test is Friedman's ANOVA.

REPEATED MEASURES ANOVA

Just as the one-way ANOVA is the extension of the independent t test from two groups to more than two groups, the repeated measures ANOVA is the extension of the paired-t test to more than three dependent samples. There are three different approaches to a repeated measures ANOVA: multivariate, univariate, and adjusted univariate. The assumptions for the univariate approach are more stringent than those for the multivariate approach; statistical packages provide a test (Mauchly test of sphericity) of the assumptions to guide researchers in deciding which approach to use.[11(p169)] The univariate approach is similar to the one-way ANOVA and is discussed here.

Recall the procedure used for the paired-t test. We started with a group of subjects with ROM scores ranging from 32° to 95°. To determine the test statistic, we calculated the difference between the 3-week and 6-week measures. Taking the difference of the paired scores effectively eliminated the widespread variability between subjects in the sample and allowed us to focus on the changes within subjects with time. Like the paired-t test, the repeated measures ANOVA mathematically eliminates between-subjects variability to focus the analysis on within-subject variability.

Recall that the one-way ANOVA partitioned the variability in the data set into between-groups and within-group categories. The univariate repeated measures ANOVA first partitions the variability in the data set into *between-subjects* and *within-subject* categories. The within-subject variability is then subdivided into between-treatments and error (or residual) components (Table 21–12). Two F ratios can be generated from a repeated measures ANOVA: One is the ratio of between-subjects to within-subject variability; the other is the ratio of between-treatments to residual variability. The first ratio is sometimes reported but is not relevant to the research question we are addressing here. A significant between-subjects F ratio would merely tell us that there is substantial variability between individual subjects, and a nonsignificant between-subjects F ratio would tell us that subjects are fairly homogeneous. Neither result is relevant to the question of whether there are differences between *treatments*. Thus the between-treatments F ratio is the one that is relevant to our research question. It is the ratio of the between-treatments variability to the variability that is left after the variability due to differences between subjects is removed. Thus, the variability that makes up the denominator of the F ratio is called the *residual*. It is also referred to

| TABLE 21–11 | Stem-and-Leaf Displays of Range-of-Motion Data at Three Times |

Stem	Week 3	Week 6	Month 6
2	7		
3	224		
4	0579	06	
5	0068	0568	
6	077	033577	5
7	6	0018	8
8	1111244478	00555	0345
9	1225	000004555	00555558
10			00000345555556
11			00

TABLE 21-12	Summary of a Repeated Measures Analysis of Variance				

Source	Sum of Squares	Degrees of Freedom	Mean Square	F	p
Between subjects	20,710.46	29	714.15	2.23	.0047
Within subject	19,244.67	60	320.74		
Between treatments	14,709.42	2	7354.71	94.06	.0001
Residual	4535.24	58	78.19		
Total	39,955.12	89			

as *error* because this represents random differences in subjects due to sampling errors.

If a repeated measures ANOVA identifies a significant difference among the means, the next step is to make multiple comparisons between pairs of means to determine which time frames are significantly different from one another. The multiple-comparison procedures for repeated measures must be based on assumptions of dependence between the pairs being compared. Maxwell recommends the use of paired-*t* tests with a Bonferroni adjustment of alpha.[21]

In our example, a significant difference between treatments was identified: $F_{2,58} = 94.06$, $p = .0001$. Three paired-*t* tests are used as the multiple comparisons to determine where the differences lie. Because three comparisons are needed, the overall alpha level of .05 becomes .017 (.05/3 = .017). The results of the paired-*t* tests are as follows: For 3-week versus 6-week scores, $t_{29} = 3.83$, $p = .001$; for 3-week versus 6-month scores, $t_{29} = 10.38$, $p = .000$; and for 6-week versus 6-month scores, $t_{29} = 11.51$, $p = .000$. (Note that the probability is never actually zero, but in this case it is low enough that it can be rounded off to zero.)

To determine the clinical relevance of these differences, we need to examine the means for the different time periods: 3 weeks—66.4°, 6 weeks—73.4°, and 6 months—96.4°. As noted previously, the average 7.0° difference between Weeks 3 and 6 seems small, but the 23.0° difference between Week 6 and Month 6 seems highly important. A repeated measures ANOVA might be reported in the literature as follows:

DATA ANALYSIS

Differences in range-of-motion (ROM) scores at the three time periods were analyzed with a univariate approach to repeated measures analysis of variance since the Mauchly test of sphericity showed that the required assumptions were met ($p = .642$). Post hoc comparisons were made with paired-*t* tests. The alpha level for the ANOVA was set at .05; the Bonferroni correction was used to set alpha at .017 for each of the multiple comparisons.

RESULTS

The means and standard deviations for ROM scores at 3 weeks, 6 weeks, and 6 months, respectively, are 66.4° ± 21.4°, 73.4° ± 17.3°, and 96.4° ± 10.5°. Repeated measures ANOVA demonstrated a significant difference among the means, $F_{2,58} = 94.06$, $p = .000$. All three means were significantly different from one another at $p \leq .001$.

Harada and colleagues used a repeated measures ANOVA to examine differences in gait and balance outcomes at three different times (baseline, following physical therapy, and 1 month after the completion of physical therapy) in a group of elderly individuals receiving individualized physical therapy in a mobility training program.[22]

FRIEDMAN'S ANOVA

Friedman's ANOVA is the nonparametric equivalent of the repeated measures AVOVA. Hypotheses are as follows:

H_0: All possible rankings of the observations for any subject are equally likely.

H_1: At least one population tends to produce larger observations than another population.[11(p245)]

Calculation is based on rankings of the repeated measures for each subjects. Two different formulas can be used to calculate either a Friedman's F or a Friedman's chi-square. The computer-generated chi-square for the differences in ROM at 3 weeks, 6 weeks, and 6 months postoperatively is 48.75, and the associated probability is .0000. Because .0000 is less than our present alpha of .05, we conclude that at least one time frame is different from another. An appropriate nonparametric multiple-comparison procedure is the Wilcoxon signed rank test with a Bonferroni adjustment of the alpha level for each test. All three multiple comparisons show significant differences: For 3-week ROM versus 6-week ROM, $p = .001$; for 3-week ROM versus 6-month ROM, $p = .000$; and for 6-week ROM versus 6-month ROM, $p = .000$. Thus, for this example, the nonparametric and parametric results agree. These results might be written in a journal article as follows:

DATA ANALYSIS

Friedman's analysis of variance (ANOVA) was used to assess the differences in range of motion (ROM) 3 weeks, 6 weeks, and 6 months postoperatively. This nonparametric test was chosen because the distribution of scores at each time was not normal. Alpha was set at .05 for Friedman's ANOVA. Multiple comparisons were conducted between the paired time frames with Wilcoxon signed rank procedures with alpha set at .017 (.05/3 tests = .017) to compensate for alpha inflation with multiple testing.

RESULTS

The median ROM scores for each time frame are as follows: 3 weeks, 71.5°; 6 weeks, 74.5°; and 6 months, 100.0°. The Friedman's ANOVA revealed a significant difference among the groups, $\chi^2 = 48.75$, $p = .0000$; the post hoc analysis showed that all three groups were significantly different from one another at $p \leq .001$.

MacKean and associates used a Friedman's ANOVA to determine whether there was a significant difference in rankings of ankle orthoses during performance of a battery of basketball skills tests.[23]

■ SUMMARY

Statistical testing of differences between samples is based on 10 steps: (1) stating the hypotheses; (2) deciding on the alpha level; (3) examining the frequency distribution and descriptive statistics to determine whether the assumptions for parametric testing are met; (4) determining whether samples are independent or dependent; (5) determining the appropriate test; (6) using the appropriate software or formulas to determine the value of a test statistic; (7) determining the degrees of freedom; (8) determining the probability of obtaining the test statistic for the given degrees of freedom if the null hypothesis is true; (9) evaluating the obtained probability against the alpha level to draw a statistical conclusion; and (10) evaluating the statistical conclusions in light of clinical knowledge.

The independent t, Mann-Whitney or Wilcoxon rank sum, and chi-square tests are used to evaluate differences between two independent samples; the one-way ANOVA, Kruskal-Wallis, and chi-square tests can be used for two or more independent samples. The paired-t, Wilcoxon signed rank, and McNemar tests are used to evaluate differences between two dependent samples; the repeated measures ANOVA and Friedman's ANOVA can be used for two or more dependent samples.

REFERENCES

1. Siegel S, Castellan NJ. *Nonparametric Statistics for the Behavioral Sciences*. 2nd ed. New York, NY: McGraw-Hill; 1988.
2. Munro BH. *Statistical Methods for Health Care Research*. 3rd ed. Philadelphia, Pa: JB Lippincott; 1997.
3. Glass GV, Hopkins KD. *Statistical Methods in Education and Psychology*. 2nd ed. Englewood Cliffs, NJ: Prentice-Hall; 1984.
4. Dawson-Saunders B, Trapp RG. *Basic and Clinical Biostatistics*. 2nd ed. Norwalk, Conn: Appleton & Lange; 1994.
5. Gaito J. Measurement scales and statistics: resurgence of an old misconception. *Psychol Bull*. 1980;87:564–567.
6. Nunnally JC, Bernstein IH. *Psychometric Theory*. 3rd ed. New York, NY: McGraw-Hill; 1994.
7. *SPSS® Base 7.5 for Windows® User's Guide*. Chicago, Ill: SPSS Inc; 1997.
8. *SPSS Advanced Statistics™ 7.5*. Chicago, Ill: SPSS Inc; 1997.
9. Polit DF. *Data Analysis and Statistics for Nursing Research*. Stamford, Conn: Appleton & Lange; 1996.
10. Elston RC, Johnson WD. *Essentials of Biostatistics*. 2nd ed. Philadelphia, Pa: FA Davis; 1994.
11. Shott S. *Statistics for Health Professionals*. Philadelphia, Pa: WB Saunders Co; 1990.
12. Egger MJ, Miller JR. Testing for experimental effects in the pretest-posttest design. *Nurs Res*. 1984;33:306–312.
13. Dean CM, Shepherd RB. Task-related training improves performance of seated reaching tasks after stroke. *Stroke*. 1997;28:722–728.
14. Weiss LW, Clark FC, Howard DG. Effects of heavy-resistance triceps surae muscle training on strength and muscularity of men and women. *Phys Ther*. 1988;68:208–213.
15. Rothweiler B, Temkin NR, Dikmen SS. Aging effect on psychosocial outcome in traumatic brain injury. *Arch Phys Med Rehabil*. 1998;79:881–887.
16. Mayer TG, Gatchel RJ, Mayer H, Kishino ND, Keeley J, Mooney V. A prospective two-year study of functional restoration in industrial low back injury. *JAMA*. 1987;258:1763–1767.
17. Roach KE, Ally D, Finnerty B, et al. The relationship between duration of physical therapy services in the acute care setting and change in functional status in patients with lower-extremity orthopedic problems. *Phys Ther*. 1998;78:19–24.
18. Griffin JW, Newsome LS, Stralka SW, Wright PE. Reduction of chronic posttraumatic hand edema: a comparison of high voltage pulsed current, intermittent pneumatic compression, and placebo treatments. *Phys Ther*. 1990;70:279–286.
19. Ottenbacher KJ. The chi-square test: its use in rehabilitation research. *Arch Phys Med Rehabil*. 1995;76:678–681.
20. Calkins DR, Davis RB, Reiley P, et al. Patient-physician communication at hospital discharge and patients' understanding of the postdischarge treatment plan. *Arch Intern Med*. 1997;157:1026–1030.
21. Maxwell SE. Pairwise multiple comparisons in repeated measures designs. *J Educ Stat*. 1980;5:269–287.
22. Harada N, Chui V, Fowler E, Lee M, Reuben DB. Physical therapy to improve functioning of older people in residential care facilities. *Phys Ther*. 1995;75:830–839.
23. MacKean LC, Bell G, Burnham RS. Prophylactic ankle bracing vs. taping: effects on functional performance in female basketball players. *J Orthop Sports Phys Ther*. 1995;22:77–81.

Statistical Analysis of Differences: Advanced and Special Techniques

Advanced ANOVA Techniques
    Differences Between More Than
      One Independent Variable
    Between-Subjects Two-Way ANOVA
    Mixed-Design Two-Way ANOVA
    Differences Across Several
      Dependent Variables
    Effect of Removing an Intervening
      Variable
Analysis of Single-System Designs
    Celeration Line Analysis
    Level, Trend, and Slope Analysis
    Two Standard Deviation Band
      Analysis

Survival Analysis
    Survival Curves
    Differences Between Survival
      Curves
Hypothesis Testing with
Confidence Intervals
    Review of Traditional Hypothesis
      Testing
    Foundations for Confidence Interval
      Testing
    Interpretation and Examples
Power Analysis and Effect Size
    Power Analysis—Design Phase
    Power Analysis—Analysis Phase

The analyses presented in Chapter 21 provide broad coverage of the most commonly reported statistical tests of differences. Readers will, however, find articles of interest that include a variety of advanced or special data analysis techniques. It seems likely that the use of these advanced techniques will increase because the widespread availability of sophisticated statistical analysis software eliminates the computational burden of these techniques. This chapter provides an overview of these more advanced or specialized techniques. First, the following ad-

vanced analysis of variance (ANOVA) techniques are covered: factorial ANOVA (including between-subjects and mixed-design models), multivariate ANOVA (MANOVA), and analysis of covariance (ANCOVA). Second, three specialized techniques for analyzing single-system data are presented: celeration lines; analysis of level, trend, and slope; and two standard deviation band approach. Third, the concept of survival analysis and determining differences between survival curves are introduced. Fourth, the use of confidence intervals for hypothesis testing is discussed. Finally, the related concepts of power analysis and effect size are presented.

ADVANCED ANOVA TECHNIQUES

From Chapter 21 we know that ANOVA is a powerful statistical technique that can be used to evaluate differences among two or more independent or dependent groups by partitioning the variance in the data set in different ways. The same general process can be extended to analyze differences between more than one independent variable at a time, between more than one dependent variable simultaneously, and when it is desirable to mathematically remove the impact of an intervening variable.

Differences Between More Than One Independent Variable

There are several instances in which researchers wish to determine the impact of more than one independent variable on a dependent variable. Different forms of advanced ANOVA techniques are used for such analysis, depending on the nature of the independent variables selected for analysis. Using the data set presented in Chapter 20, we might wish to know whether there are differences in 3-week range-of-motion (ROM) values between clinics and between the sexes. This particular question involves two between-subjects factors, meaning that neither factor consists of repeated measures on the same subjects. A different research question is whether ROM differences between clinics (a between-subjects factor) are consistent across time (a repeated, within-subject factor). The first research question is analyzed with a two-factor ANOVA for two between-subjects factors; the second is analyzed with a two-factor ANOVA for one between-subjects and one within-subject factor. The second analysis is sometimes referred to as a mixed-design ANOVA.

Whenever we examine the influence of more than one independent variable on a dependent variable, we must also examine whether there is an *interaction* between the independent variables. In the between-subjects example, the interaction question is whether the responses of men and women to treatment depend on the clinic at which they are treated. In the mixed design, the interaction question is whether changes across time are consistent across the clinics. Each of these two variations on two-factor ANOVA is discussed subsequently.

BETWEEN-SUBJECTS TWO-WAY ANOVA

The statistical hypotheses are as follows:

H_0: There is no interaction between clinic and sex.

H_1: There is an interaction between clinic and sex.

H_0: $\mu_{C1} = \mu_{C2} = \mu_{C3}$

H_C: At least one clinic population mean is different from another clinic population mean.

H_0: $\mu_W = \mu_M$

H_S: The population mean for women is different from the population mean for men.

TABLE 22–1 **Three-Week Range-of-Motion Data for Two-Factor Between-Subjects Analysis of Variance**

Clinic	Sex	
	Men	*Women*
1	32, 67, 92, 87, 58	95, 92, 88, 84, 81
	$\overline{X}_{1M} = 67.2$	$\overline{X}_{1W} = 88.0$
2	34, 56, 45, 27, 40	76, 49, 47, 50, 67
	$\overline{X}_{2M} = 40.4$	$\overline{X}_{2W} = 57.8$
3	32, 50, 60, 84, 81	81, 84, 81, 82, 91
	$\overline{X}_{3M} = 61.4$	$\overline{X}_{3W} = 83.8$

TABLE 22-2	**Summary of a Two-Factor Between-Subjects Analysis of Variance**				
Source	**Sum of Squares**	**Degrees of Freedom**	**Mean Square**	**F**	**p**
Clinic	4631.667	2	2315.833	9.963	.001
Sex	3060.300	1	3060.300	13.165	.001
Clinic × Sex	32.600	2	16.300	.070	.932
Residual	5578.800	24	232.450		
Total	13,303.367	29			

There are null and alternative hypotheses for the interaction between clinic and sex, for the main effect of clinic, and for the main effect of sex. The overall alpha level is set at .05. This particular test is known as a two-way or two-factor ANOVA because two independent variables are examined. It can also be described as a 3 × 2 ANOVA, describing the number of levels of each of the factors. Three- and four-way ANOVAs are also possible. Table 22–1 shows the data and Table 22–2 summarizes the ANOVA for this example.

Because interpretation of two-way ANOVAs depends on the interaction result, let's examine the interaction first. The F ratio for interaction (the Clinic × Sex row in Table 22–2) is only .070,

and the probability is .932. Because the probability exceeds the .05 alpha level we set prior to the analysis, we conclude that there is no interaction between sex and clinic. This means that men and women respond the same across the clinics. Interactions can be interpreted best if the cell means are graphed as shown in Figure 22–1.

Note that although the means for men and women are different, the pattern of response is the same across clinics: Both men and women do best at Clinic 1, slightly worse at Clinic 3, and worst at Clinic 2. The nearly parallel lines between the means of the men and women across clinics provide a visual picture of what is meant by no interaction.

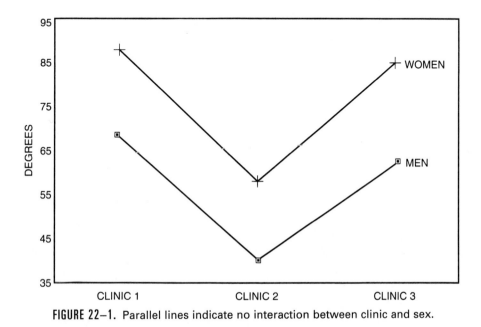

FIGURE 22-1. Parallel lines indicate no interaction between clinic and sex.

Because no interaction has been identified, we now examine the main effects for clinic and sex. The main effect for clinic is determined by comparing the means of all subjects at each clinic, regardless of whether they are men or women. The main effect for sex is calculated by determining the sum of squares for men and women, regardless of the clinic at which they are treated. Analysis of the main effects depends on the assumption that the factors do not interact and that therefore each factor can be examined independently, without concern for the other factors. In this example, the main effects for both clinic and sex are significant: $F_{2,24} = 9.96$, $p = .001$, and $F_{1,24} = 13.16$, $p = .001$, respectively (Table 22–2). Because the sex variable has only two levels, we do not need to conduct post hoc testing to locate the difference. Because the clinic variable has three levels, multiple comparisons are needed, as described in the one-way ANOVA example in Chapter 21.

When an interaction is present the data analysis proceeds much differently. To illustrate this the data presented previously have been altered to create a significant interaction between clinic and sex. Table 22–3 shows the new data, Table 22–4 summarizes the ANOVA, and Figure 22–2 shows the modified graph of the cell means. The lines in Figure 22–2 are not parallel, indicating an interaction. Although women do better than men at Clinics 2 and 3, men do better than women at Clinic 1.

When a significant interaction is present, the

TABLE 22-3 Three-Week Range-of-Motion Data for Two-Factor Analysis of Variance Revealing an Interaction

| Clinic | Sex | |
	Men	Women
1	95, 92, 87, 92, 88 $\bar{X}_{1M} = 90.8$	32, 67, 58, 84, 81 $\bar{X}_{1W} = 64.4$
2	34, 56, 45, 27, 40 $\bar{X}_{2M} = 40.4$	76, 49, 47, 50, 67 $\bar{X}_{2W} = 57.8$
3	32, 50, 60, 84, 81 $\bar{X}_{3M} = 61.4$	81, 84, 81, 82, 91 $\bar{X}_{3W} = 83.8$

main effects for the individual variables cannot be interpreted. For example, although Table 22–4 indicates that the main effect for clinic is significant, it would be erroneous for us to make any general statements about differences between clinics because these differences are not uniform across men and women. Likewise, the main effect for sex would lead us to conclude that there are no differences between men and women. However, it is clear that there are differences between the sexes at each clinic—the opposite directions of these differences cancel out any main effect and erroneously make it appear that there are no differences between the sexes.

When a significant interaction is identified, the researcher must analyze simple main effects, rather

TABLE 22-4 Summary of a Two-Factor Analysis of Variance Revealing an Interaction with Simple Main Effects for Clinic Within Sex

Source	Sum of Squares	Degrees of Freedom	Mean Square	F	p
Clinic	4631.66	2	2315.83	11.301	.000
Sex	149.63	1	149.63	.730	.401
Clinic × Sex	3604.06	2	1802.03	8.794	.001
Clinic within sex (Women)	1826.53	2	913.27	4.457	.023
Clinic within sex (Men)	6409.20	2	3204.60	15.639	.000
Residual	4918.00	24	204.91		
Total	13,303.36	29			

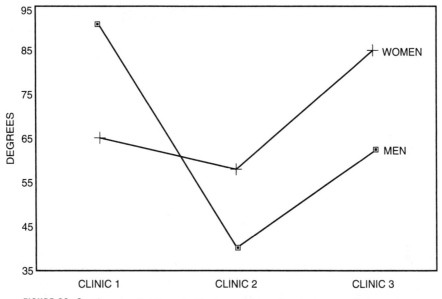

FIGURE 22–2. Nonparallel lines indicate an interaction between clinic and sex.

than overall main effects. A simple main effect is one in which the differences among the levels of one factor are assessed separately for each level of the other factor. In this example, there are significant differences between clinics for the men and for the women (Table 22–4). These results might be summarized in a journal article as follows:

DATA ANALYSIS

A two-way analysis of variance was used to determine whether there were significant differences between clinics and sexes for 3-week range of motion and whether there was a significant interaction between clinic and sex. Identification of a significant interaction led to further analysis of a simple main effect for clinic and post hoc analysis of significant simple main effects with the Newman-Keuls procedure. Alpha was set at .05 for each analysis.

RESULTS

As shown in Figure 22–2, there was a significant interaction between clinic and sex ($F_{2,24} = 8.794$,

$p = .001$). For both the men and the women the simple main effect of clinic was significant, as shown in Table 22–4. Post hoc analysis revealed that all clinics were significantly different for the men, whereas only Clinics 2 and 3 were significantly different for the women.

An example of a two-factor ANOVA can be found in Magalhaes and colleagues' study of differences in motor coordination on three different tasks based on age and sex.[1] The age variable had five levels: 5, 6, 7, 8, and 9 years old. The sex variable had two levels: boys and girls. In this study, no interactions were found, so the main effects were interpreted for each of the analyses.

MIXED-DESIGN TWO-WAY ANOVA

We are now interested in determining whether there are differences in ROM across the three clinics and across the three times that measurements are taken: 3 weeks, 6 weeks, and 6 months. Clinic is a between-subjects factor because different subjects are measured at each clinic. Time is a within-subject factor because ROM measures are repeated on each of the subjects across the time intervals in the study. The hypotheses for our test are as follows:

H_0: There is no interaction between clinic and time.

H_I: There is an interaction between clinic and time.

H_0: $\mu_{C1} = \mu_{C2} = \mu_{C3}$

H_C: At least one clinic population mean is different from another clinic population mean.

H_0: $\mu_{3\text{-week ROM}} = \mu_{6\text{-week ROM}} = \mu_{6\text{-month ROM}}$

H_T: At least one time population mean is different from another time population mean.

Interpretation of a mixed-design ANOVA follows the same sequence of analysis as the two-factor, between-subjects ANOVA. Table 22–5 presents the means for our example, and Table 22–6 presents the F ratios and p levels associated with each comparison. As shown in Figure 22–3, there is no interaction between clinic and time. This indicates that all the clinics had the same pattern of change across time. Because there is no interaction, the main effects for clinic and time are examined, and there is a significant effect for each. Post hoc analysis shows that all three clinics are significantly different from one another and that all three time periods are significantly different from one another.

TABLE 22–5	Mean Range of Motion over Time at Clinics 1 Through 3		
Clinic	Three Weeks	Six Weeks	Six Months
1	77.6°	78.9°	100.0°
2	49.1°	58.6°	85.8°
3	72.6°	82.8°	103.3°

The mixed-design ANOVA is frequently used to analyze pretest-posttest control-group designs. In the simplest design, there is a treatment factor with two levels (treatment group and control group) and a time factor with two levels (pretest and posttest). The ideal results for such a study would be for the two groups to be essentially the same at the pretest, the control group to remain unchanged at posttest, and the treatment group to be improved considerably at posttest. Figure 22–4 shows a graph of these ideal results. A significant interaction is illustrated—the treatment group responded differently over time than did the control group. Thus, when a mixed-design two-factor ANOVA is used to analyze a pretest-posttest design, the research question is answered by examining the interaction between the group factor and the time factor. These results might be summarized in a journal article as follows:

DATA ANALYSIS

A 3×3 analysis of variance with one between-subjects factor (clinic) and one within-subject fac-

TABLE 22–6	Summary of Two-Factor Mixed Design Analysis of Variance				
Source	Sum of Squares	Degrees of Freedom	Mean Square	F	p
Clinic	9138.76	2	4569.38	10.66	.000
Error	11,571.70	27	428.58		
Time	10,709.42	2	7354.71	100.89	.000
Clinic × Time	598.64	4	149.66	2.05	.100
Error	3936.60	54	72.90		

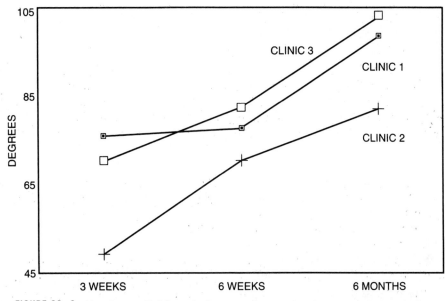

FIGURE 22–3. Nearly parallel lines indicate no interaction between clinic and time.

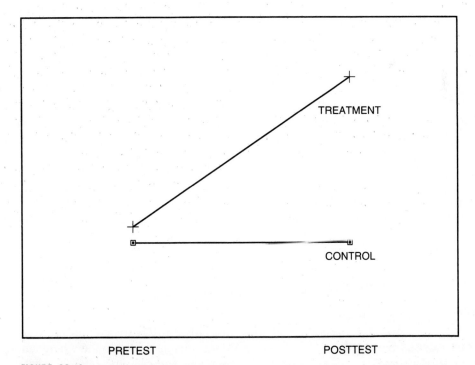

FIGURE 22–4. Ideal pretest-posttest results. The two groups are almost equal at pretest, the control group does not change at posttest, and the treatment group shows significant improvement at posttest. The nonparallel lines indicate a significant interaction between group and time.

tor (time) was used to analyze differences between range-of-motion (ROM) means at an alpha level of .05. Post hoc comparisons were made for the clinic factor, with Newman-Keuls tests at alpha = .05, and for the time factor, with paired-t tests at alpha = .017.

RESULTS

The mean ROM for each group at each point in time is presented in Table 22–5. There was no sigificant interaction between clinic and time ($F_{4,54}$ = 2.05, p = .100). There were significant main effects for both clinic ($F_{2,27}$ = 10.66, p = .000), and time ($F_{2,54}$ = 100.89, p = .000). Overall means for Clinic 1 (85.5°) and Clinic 3 (86.2°) were not significantly different; Clinic 2's mean (64.5°) was significantly different from those of Clinics 1 and 3. Means for all three time periods were significantly different from one another (3-week mean = 66.4°, 6-week mean = 73.4°, and 6-month mean = 96.4°).

Bandy and Irion[2] used a mixed-design two-factor ANOVA to test the effect of stretching technique (four levels: none, 15-, 30-, and 60-second stretches) and time (two levels: pretest and posttest) on hamstring flexibility. The interaction between group and time was significant, indicating a difference in response over time for the four groups. The researchers then explored differences among the groups. They found no difference between the groups that stretched for 30 and 60 seconds, and no difference between the group that did not stretch and the group that stretched for 15 seconds. They did, however, determine that the "short-stretch" cluster of levels (0- and 15-second groups) was different from the "long-stretch" cluster of levels (30- and 60-second groups).

Differences Across Several Dependent Variables

Researchers are often interested in the effects of their treatments on several different dependent variables. In our sample data set, we are now interested in whether several 6-month outcomes are different between clinics: ROM, knee extensor strength, knee flexor strength, and gait velocity. One analysis approach is to run a one-way ANOVA for each dependent variable. There are two potential problems with this approach. The first is the alpha level inflation that results from conducting multiple tests. The second is the possibility that although no single variable exhibits significant differences across clinics, small, consistent differences across several dependent variables are present. Because an ANOVA can handle only one dependent variable at a time, a cumulative effect over several dependent variables would be undetected.

Multivariate procedures solve these problems by analyzing several dependent variables simultaneously. Multivariate analyses should not be confused with multifactor analyses: The former analyze several *dependent* variables simultaneously; the latter analyze several *independent* variables simultaneously. Although the mathematical basis for multivariate testing of differences is beyond the scope of this text, the interpretation of multivariate results is simply an extension of what has already been learned about ANOVA procedures.

A multivariate analysis of variance (MANOVA) uses an omnibus test to determine whether there are significant differences on the factor of interest (in our case, clinic) when the dependent variables of interest are combined mathematically. The multivariate test statistic used most frequently is Wilks' lambda, although several others are often reported by computer statistical packages. Wilks' lambda is usually converted to an estimated F statistic, and the probability of this estimated F is determined to test the null hypothesis.[3(p387)]

If the omnibus F level is significant, then a univariate ANOVA is conducted for each dependent variable to determine where among the dependent variables the differences lie. Once the dependent variables that are significantly different are identified, multiple-comparison procedures can be conducted to determine which levels of the independent variable are different on the dependent variables for which significant differences have been identified.

For our total knee arthroplasty example, the omnibus F is 3.53 and is significant at the .003 level. Table 22–7 presents univariate and post hoc results for each of the dependent variables. This analysis might be reported in a journal article as follows:

DATA ANALYSIS

Differences in 6-month status across clinics were examined with a multivariate analysis of variance (MANOVA) for the following dependent variables: 6-month range of motion, extension torque, flexion torque, and gait velocity. Univariate F tests with Newman-Keuls post hoc analyses were conducted to determine the sources of any difference identified by the MANOVA.

RESULTS

The multivariate F of 3.53 was significant at the .003 level. Table 22–7 shows the mean for each dependent variable for each clinic, the F and p values for the test for differences across clinics for each dependent variable, and an indication of which

multiple comparisons showed significant differences between clinics. All four dependent variables were significantly different across clinics. In addition, all four dependent variables showed the same pattern of pairwise differences among clinics: None of the dependent variable means were significantly different between Clinics 1 and 3; all were significantly different between Clinics 1 and 2 and between Clinics 2 and 3.

Worrell and colleagues used a MANOVA to analyze their study of health outcomes in subjects with patellofemoral pain.[4] One research question was whether there were significant differences in outcomes across the four treatment years included within the study (1993 through 1996). The outcomes that were measured included self-rated global function, a functional score, satisfaction, and stress. Rather than performing four separate ANOVAs—one each for each of the dependent variables—Worrell and colleagues analyzed all of the dependent variables simultaneously with a MANOVA technique. They found significant differences among years for all of the dependent variables combined. Having found this overall difference, they then searched for specific differences among years for the individual dependent variables.

TABLE 22-7 **Multivariate Analysis of Variance for Four Dependent Variables**

Dependent Variable	Independent Variable			Statistic		Multiple Comparisons		
	Clinic 1	Clinic 2	Clinic 3	F	p	1/2	1/3	2/3
Six-month range of motion(°)	100.0	85.8	103.3	15.63	.000	*		*
Extension torque (N·m)	135.8	105.4	142.2	4.90	.015	*		*
Flexion torque (N·m)	81.8	62.6	84.1	5.12	.013	*		*
Gait velocity (cm/s)	144.0	107.6	145.6	8.25	.002	*		*

Note: Asterisk indicates a significant difference between the means of the indicated pair of clinics.

Effect of Removing an Intervening Variable

In our examples we have identified significant differences between clinics. However, scrutiny of patient characteristics at the three clinics shows that Clinic 2 has a patient population that is much older ($\overline{X}$ = 81.0 years) than the patients at Clinic 1 ($\overline{X}$ = 55.8 years) and Clinic 3 ($\overline{X}$ = 69.8 years). If younger patients tend to gain ROM faster than older patients, perhaps the age difference between the clinics, rather than differences in the quality of care, explains the difference in early ROM results.

A procedure known as analysis of covariance (ANCOVA) uses the overall relationship between a dependent variable and an intervening variable, or *covariate*, to adjust the dependent variable scores in light of the covariate scores. For example, let us reexamine the differences between clinics on the 3-week ROM variable by using age as a covariate. In our example, there is a strong negative correlation between age and 3-week ROM; that is, younger patients tend to

have higher scores, and older patients tend to have lower scores (Fig. 22–5).

An ANCOVA essentially takes each subject's 3-week ROM score and adjusts it to a predicted value as if the subject's age were the same as the mean age of the sample. In our total sample of 30 patients, the mean age is 68.8 years. Thus, the 3-week ROM scores of subjects who are younger than 68.8 years are reduced and those of subjects who are older than 68.8 years are increased. Once this mathematical adjustment has taken place, an ANOVA is run on the adjusted data. Figure 22–6 shows this adjustment graphically. The ANCOVA is summarized in Table 22–8. Once age is accounted for, the differences between the groups disappear—the F value of 1.88 is not significant (p = .173).

The preceding example used a patient characteristic (age) as the covariate. Another typical use of an ANCOVA is to test for differences between posttest scores using pretest scores as covariates. If pretest scores between groups are significantly different, as is common in clinical research when random assignment to groups has

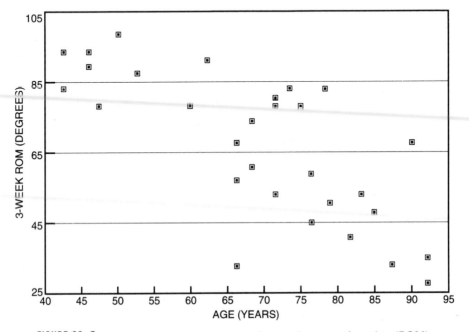

FIGURE 22–5. Relationship between age and 3-week range of motion (ROM).

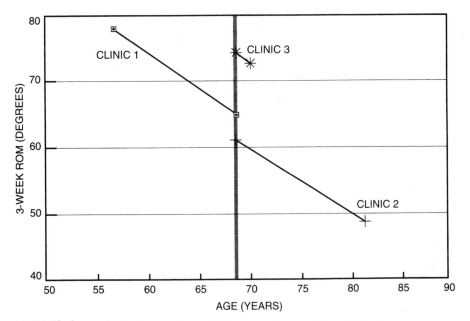

FIGURE 22–6. Analysis of covariance with age as the covariate. Original group means are adjusted to predicted values as if the mean age of each group is equal to the overall mean age of 68.8 years, represented by the vertical line. ROM = range of motion.

not been possible, then posttest scores can be adjusted to mathematically eliminate the pretest differences.[5] However, it is preferable to have equivalent groups at the start of the study, because there are any number of assumptions that must be met before an ANCOVA can be used legitimately. The ANCOVA results in our total knee arthroplasty example might be reported in a journal article as follows:

TABLE 22–8	Analysis of Covariance of Three-Week Range of Motion (ROM)

Clinic	Mean Age	Actual Three-Week ROM	Adjusted Three-Week ROM[*]
1	55.8 yr	77.6°	64.54°
2	81.0 yr	49.1°	61.22°
3	69.8 yr	72.6°	73.53°

* No significant differences among clinics, $F_{2,26}$ = 1.88, p = .173.

DATA ANALYSIS

An analysis of covariance was used to determine whether there were significant differences between clinics once the effect of subject age was removed. Alpha was set at .05.

RESULTS

Table 22–8 shows the mean values for age, actual 3-week range of motion (ROM), and adjusted 3-week ROM across the three clinics. The difference among the adjusted means was not statistically significant.

Mackay and colleagues studied the impact of early, formalized rehabilitation after traumatic brain injury on a variety of outcomes.[6] The groups they were comparing, those whose did and did not undergo a formalized rehabilitation program in the acute care hospital, exhibited some subtle differences in acute admission status as measured by the Glasgow Coma Scale (GCS) and the Rancho Los Amigos Scale of Cognitive Functioning (RLA). To adjust for these differences among groups, Mackay and colleagues performed two sets of ANCOVAs within their study: one set examined differences between groups after controlling for GCS score and another set examined differences after controlling for RLA score. In this example, then, patient characteristics that might represent severity of injury were used as the intervening variables.

A second ANCOVA example illustrates the use of a pretest score as the covariate. Wessling and associates studied the effect of three different stretching protocols on triceps surae extensibility.[7] They used a repeated measures design in which subjects were given a different treatment at each of three different sessions. Because differences in pretreatment dorsiflexion ROM measures were found, an ANCOVA was used to adjust each subject's posttest value in light of his or her pretest value.

■ ANALYSIS OF SINGLE-SYSTEM DESIGNS

Thus far, most of our analyses have examined group differences by making inferences to the populations from which the groups were drawn. This approach is not satisfactory for single-system designs, in which our interest is in whether an individual has changed over time. Let us assume that we have a patient who has extremely limited ROM 10 weeks after total knee arthroplasty. After treating the patient for 10 weeks with manual stretching and exercise, the therapist decides that more drastic measures are needed and implements a new treatment for 10 weeks, which has the results shown in Figure 22–7. It appears that the new treatment results in an improvement over the baseline, but is there any way to express this more quantitatively? There are, in fact, many different techniques that can be used to analyze single-system data. Many of these techniques are described by

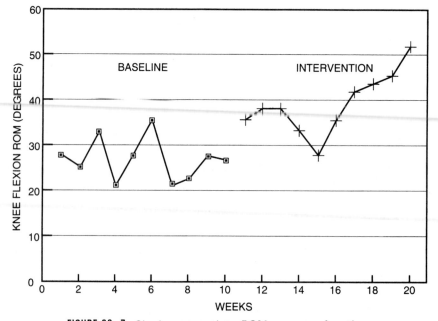

FIGURE 22–7. Single-system data. ROM = range of motion.

Ottenbacher and his colleagues in several different articles and a book.[8–11] Readers are referred to these references for specific calculation details and for discussion of when to use which of the analyses. In this chapter, three of the more commonly used techniques are summarized: celeration line analysis; analysis of level, trend, and slope; and two standard deviation band analysis.

Celeration Line Analysis

In celeration line analysis, a researcher compares data in different phases by generating a line or lines based on the median of subsets of data in each phase (Fig. 22–8). To determine the celeration line through the baseline data, the researcher splits the data in half and splits each half in half again. The median of each of the halves is plotted on vertical lines (the points in Fig. 22–8 represent these two medians). A line is

drawn through these two points and is extended into the intervention area. The number of data points in the intervention phase and the number exceeding the celeration line are counted. The probability of having a certain proportion of scores above the celeration line can be generated from a table based on the binomial distribution.[11(p184)] The table indicates that in a one-tailed test at an alpha level of .05, nine or 10 intervention-phase numbers must be above the celeration line for a significant difference to have occurred. Because all 10 intervention-phase points are above the celeration line, we can conclude that significant improvement occurred during the treatment phase. A basic assumption of the celeration line approach is that the baseline data do not exhibit serial dependency, a phenomenon associated with the ability to predict the next point from the previous point.[11(p170)] An example analysis with celeration lines is presented with the example analysis in the next section of the chapter.

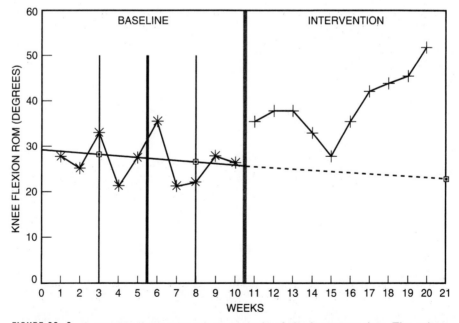

FIGURE 22–8. Celeration line approach to analysis of single-system data. The celeration line determined for the baseline phase (*solid line*) is extrapolated into the intervention phase (*dotted line*). ROM = range of motion.

Level, Trend, and Slope Analysis

In addition to the results related to the extended celeration line, quantification of changes in level, trend, and slope of the data may facilitate the description of the patterns seen across time (Fig. 22–9). To evaluate these changes, a researcher calculates a celeration line for each phase of the study. *Level* is the difference between the numerical value of observations in one phase and the numerical value of observations in a subsequent phase. A change in level is quantified by calculating the difference between the end of one celeration line and the beginning of the celeration line in the subsequent phase. There is a difference of +4° in level between the baseline and intervention phases of our example.

Trend is the direction of change in the pattern of results. In our example there has been a reversal of the trend: It was downward in the baseline phase and is upward in the intervention

phase. Trend can be quantified by calculating the slopes of the lines. *Slope* is the amount that the Y value changes for each unit change in X. To calculate slope, we select two data points on the celeration line. The slope is the difference between the two Y values divided by the difference between the X values. In our example, the data points used to generate the baseline celeration line are (3, 28) and (8, 27). The slope is calculated as follows: $(27 - 28) / (8 - 3) = -1 / 5 = -0.2$. This means that, on average, the patient loses 0.2° of motion each week during the baseline phase. The slope of the intervention-phase celeration line is calculated similarly and is +1.8. On average, the patient gained 1.8° of motion each week in the intervention phase. Thus, not only does the trend reversal indicate a positive treatment effect, but the difference in the magnitude of the slopes indicates that treatment led to a fairly rapid improvement in ROM in the intervention phase compared with the

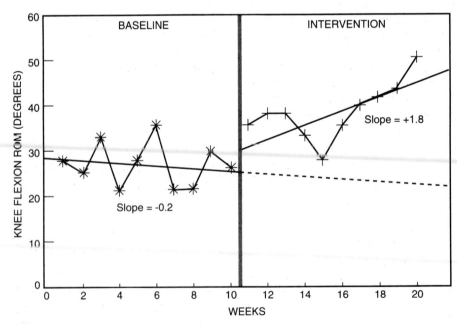

FIGURE 22–9. Level, trend, and slope analysis of single-system data. Celeration lines are calculated for each phase. There is a 4° level change, indicated by the intersections of the celeration lines in each phase with the vertical line separating the phases. There is a change in trend from downward to upward and a change in slope from −0.2 to +1.8. ROM = range of motion.

baseline phase. The results of this example analysis might be reported in a journal article as follows:

DATA ANALYSIS

Celeration lines for the baseline and intervention phases were developed using the split-middle approach. Differences between phases were described through calculation of trend, slope, and level changes from phase to phase. To determine whether the difference between the baseline and intervention phase was statistically significant, we extended the celeration line for the baseline phase into the intervention phase and evaluated the distribution of scores above and below the line in the intervention phase against a tabled value based on binomial probabilities. Alpha was set at .05.

RESULTS

Figure 22–9 shows the data and celeration lines for each phase of the study. The baseline trend was downward and the intervention trend upward, as indicated by the slopes of −0.2 and +1.8, respectively. The change in level, or the extent of discontinuity between the celeration lines where they intersect the vertical line separating the two phases, was +4°. All 10 data points in the intervention phase fall above the extended baseline celeration line; this indicates a statistically significant treatment effect at $p <.05$.

Goodman and Bazyk used extended celeration lines to analyze the effects of a thumb splint on hand function for a child with cerebral palsy.[12] Embrey and colleagues determined level, trend, and slope to evaluate the celeration lines generated during multiple treatment and baseline phases of a study of the effect of neurodevelopmental treatment on the gait of a child with diplegia.[13]

Two Standard Deviation Band Analysis

A third way to analyze single-system data is to calculate the mean and standard deviation of the baseline points. Using this information, a horizontal line representing the mean is drawn across the baseline and intervention phases that are being compared. Two other horizontal lines are drawn in at two standard deviations above and below the mean. The area between the two new lines is the "two standard deviation (2-SD)" band. This band represents the "likely" scores for the patient if there is no change as a result of the treatment. If there is a change, one would expect that several scores during the intervention phase would fall outside of the 2-SD band. In fact, Ottenbacher, citing earlier authors, indicates that a general rule of thumb is that when two successive points fall outside of the 2-SD band a statistically significant (at an alpha of .05) difference has been detected between the baseline and intervention points.[11(p188)] Figure 22–10 shows that the 2-SD band method of analysis leads to the conclusion that a significant different does exist between the baseline and intervention scores. The results of this example analysis might be reported in a journal article as follows:

DATA ANALYSIS

The two standard deviation (2-SD) band analysis technique was used to determine whether there was a significant difference between baseline and intervention scores. The mean and standard deviation of the baseline data were calculated and a 2-SD band around the baseline data was plotted across both the baseline and intervention phases (Fig. 22–10). Our statistical decision rule was that a significant difference between baseline and intervention phases would be identified if two successive intervention points fell outside the 2-SD band.[11(p188)]

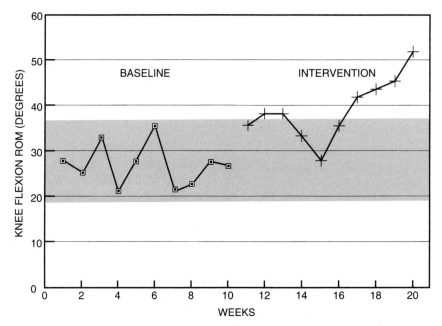

FIGURE 22–10. Two standard deviation band method of analyzing single-system data. The shaded band shows two standard deviations above and below the mean of the baseline data. ROM = range of motion.

RESULTS

Figure 22–10 shows that more than two successive intervention points fell outside the 2-SD band, indicating a statistically significant difference between the baseline and intervention phases.

Mulcahey and colleagues used a 2-SD band method to analyze their study of outcomes after tendon transfer surgery and occupational therapy for a child with a spinal cord injury.[14] Significant differences were found between phases for several variables including pinch strength and grasp and release activities.

■ SURVIVAL ANALYSIS

Survival analysis, as its name implies, is a mathematical tool that was initially used to analyze the changing proportion of survivors over time after some naturally occurring initial event (e.g.,

survival after stroke) or after some manipulation (e.g., survival after heart transplant surgery). Just as the outcomes movement in health care research, discussed in Chapter 15, has led to widespread use of dependent variables other than mortality, there is now expanded use of survival analysis for outcomes other than death.

Survival Curves

The basic elements needed for survival analysis are two defined events that form the basis for a survival curve: the event that qualifies a patient for inclusion in the analysis and the event that removes the patient from the analysis. In classic survival analysis, for example, a patient would enter the analysis when he or she received a heart transplant and exit the analysis when he or she died. With contemporary survival analysis, the exit event might be one of many outcomes other than death: failure of a prosthetic joint replacement, resumption of independent ambulation after surgery, admission to an extended care facility, return to a health care practitioner for further consultation for a condition presumed to be resolved, return to sport following injury, or loss of a job following successful placement after completion of a work conditioning program. The exit event may be negative or positive as long as it separates the proportion of individuals who have not yet experienced the event from those who have.

Determining the proportion of patients who have and have not experienced the exit event across time is easier to conceptualize than it is to actually calculate. First, the calculations depend on whether a new proportion is calculated at specified time intervals (actuarial or life table analysis) or each time a patient changes status (Kaplan-Meier analysis).[15(pp188–209)] Second, the calculations depend on the handling of subjects who are lost to follow-up or who must leave the study because of an event other than the specified exit event. For example, assume that the exit event is admission to an extended care facility after returning home following an intensive post-stroke rehabilitation program. Researchers need to know how to account for patients who die shortly after completing the rehabilitation program but who remained independent in their homes until their death. Computation details and information about the use of statistical analysis programs for survival analysis are beyond the scope of this text but can be found in other resources.[15(pp188–209),16(pp261–310)]

Differences Between Survival Curves

Although researchers may be interested in a single survival curve for subjects who have experienced a single event or procedure, they are often more interested in whether there is a significant difference in survival curves for subjects who have experienced different events or procedures. Hoenig and associates[17] made such a comparison when they sought to determine whether there were differences in the timing of ambulation after surgical repair of a hip fracture,

based on the timing of the surgical repair (early, defined as within 2 days of hospital admission, versus late) and the frequency of physical and occupational therapy (high frequency, defined as more than five sessions per week, versus low frequency). Readers can refer to Chapter 15 and Figure 15–2 for a more complete presentation of their findings.

There are several statistical methods, each using different mathematical principles, that can be used to compare survival curves.[15(pp196–203)] The Wilcoxon rank sum test, introduced in Chapter 21, can be used to determine differences in the survival time ranking between two groups. The log-rank test, sometimes referred to with the addition of either or both the Cox and Mantel names, uses chi-square test principles, also introduced in Chapter 21, to compare the observed survivors in each group with the expected survivors based on the combined groups. The Mantel-Haenszel test uses odds ratios, introduced in Chapter 14, to compare the odds of survival for both groups. A final type of test for differences in survival is known as a proportional hazards, or Cox regression, model.[15(p221)] This model is based on regression analysis techniques, which are presented in Chapters 23 and 24. Clearly, additional details about these methods are beyond the scope of this text. However, readers should take from this brief discussion two central ideas. First, the array of tests and the varied naming conventions make it difficult for even sophisticated readers to make judgments about the appropriateness of the test chosen. Second, despite the wide variety of tests of differences between survival curves, all of the tests rest on the basic statistical foundations presented elsewhere in this text.

■ HYPOTHESIS TESTING WITH CONFIDENCE INTERVALS

Up to this point, the process of testing differences between groups or levels has been presented in terms of comparisons between an obtained probability level (p) and a predetermined probability of error set by the researcher, the alpha (α) level. Recall that the determinants of the p value in any statistical test of differences are (1) the size of the difference in the dependent variable between levels of the independent variable, (2) the amount of variability on the dependent variable within levels of the independent variable, and (3) the sample size. In traditional hypothesis testing these factors are used within a specific formula for a statistic such as t or F. The t or F value is found and computerized statistical analysis programs are used to determine the probability (p) associated with the particular value of t or F. If this p value is less than the preset alpha level, then a statistically significant finding has been identified.

Critics of this traditional approach note that the emphasis on p and alpha levels leads to "lazy thinking"[18(p746)] because each decision about the meaningfulness of data is reduced to a dichotomy of "significant" versus "nonsignificant." Put into terms of the steps of statistical analysis that were presented in Chapter 21, these critics believe that an emphasis on p values leads many researchers to stop the analysis process with Step 9 (comparing the obtained probability with the alpha level to draw statistical conclusion) instead of proceeding to the final Step 10 (evaluating the statistical conclusions in light of clinical knowledge). These critics believe that presentation of statistical results in the form of confidence intervals rather than p values facilitates the higher level of evaluation that they believe is important to the proper interpretation of research results.

Review of Traditional Hypothesis Testing

Understanding the basis of the argument for using confidence intervals for hypothesis testing requires that we revisit some of the statistical principles originally introduced in Chapter 20. Readers who have difficulty following the greatly abbreviated discussion of these principles should review the appropriate sections of Chapters 20 and 21.

Recall that the mean is a sample statistic. Further, remember that sample statistics are not precise values in and of themselves; rather, they are estimates of population parameters. As estimates, sample means contain a certain amount of error. The magnitude of this error depends on the variability within the data and the size of the sample. Specifically, this error is known as the standard error of the mean (SEM) and can be calculated for each group by dividing the group's standard deviation by the square root of the size of the group. *Confidence intervals* (CIs) around the mean can be computed by adding and subtracting standard errors to and from the mean. The error that the researcher is willing to tolerate is based on the number of standard deviations above and below the mean that are included in the confidence interval. With large groups of normally distributed data, adding and subtracting 1.645 SEMs yields a 90% CI; 1.96 SEMs yields a 95% CI; and 2.576 SEMs yields a 99% CI.

We have earlier used an independent t test to compare the 3-week range of motion values between Clinic 1 ($\overline{X} = 77.6°$, $s = 19.84$) and Clinic 2 ($\overline{X} = 49.1°$, $s = 14.58$). The independent t formula, presented in Table 21–3, is the difference between the means divided by the standard error of the difference between the means ($t = 28.5 / 7.78 = 3.66$). The computer-generated probability of obtaining this t value was .002, which was less than the preset alpha of .05, so a statistically significant difference was identified.

Foundations for Confidence Interval Testing

As noted in the previous section, in traditional hypothesis testing we compute a probability and reach our statistical conclusion when we compare the obtained p to a preset alpha level. In hypothesis testing with confidence intervals we calculate a confidence interval for the difference of interest and reach our statistical conclusion by determining whether the confidence interval includes the value that corresponds to the null hypothesis. For most purposes this value is zero ("0") because the null hypothesis proposes that there will be "no difference" between groups. If the confidence interval contains "0" then we conclude that there is no statistically significant difference between groups. If the confidence interval does not contain "0" then we conclude that there is a statistically significant difference between groups. When using confidence intervals to determine the significance of odds ratios and relative risk ratios, a significant difference is identified when the interval does not contain the number one ("1"). This is because a ratio of "1" means that the risks for the groups being compared are equal.

Using confidence intervals for hypothesis testing means that the concept of confidence intervals for each group must be extended to the concept of a confidence interval for the difference between groups. Doing so involves rearranging the mathematical concepts of the t test.[18(p749)] The general confidence interval (CI) formula for the difference between two independent group means is

CI = (difference between the means) ± (appropriate multiplier) (standard error of the difference)

For this example, the computations given in Chapter 21 (Table 21–3) give us two of the three values we need for computing the confidence interval:

CI = 28.5 ± (appropriate multiplier) (7.78)

The third value cannot be determined directly from the information in this text, because it depends on access to a complete t table, commonly found in texts solely devoted to statistics. However, the conceptual basis for this value can be identified easily. Recall that when determining the confidence interval for a single, normally distributed group, the appropriate multiplier for a 95% confidence interval, based on the normal z distribution, was 1.96. Further, recall that the t distribution is a slightly flattened z distribution.

The appropriate multiplier for a 95% confidence interval for the difference between two means is based on the t distribution rather than the z distribution, and is slightly further toward the tail of the distribution at 2.101. Inserting 2.101 into our formula, we find that the 95% confidence interval for the difference between these two means is 12.15° to 44.85°:

95% CI = 28.5 ± (2.101) (7.78)

95% CI = 28.5 ± 16.35

95% CI = 12.15 to 44.85

Because this confidence interval does not contain "0" we conclude that there is a significant difference between the means of Clinics 1 and 2. This statistical conclusion matches the conclusion we reached with the independent t test in Chapter 21. This is not surprising since the two methods depend on algebraic rearrangement of the same formula.

Sim and Reid believe that confidence intervals are underutilized within the physical therapy literature.[19] They recommend that confidence intervals be used (1) when sample statistics are used as estimates of population parameters; (2) in addition to or instead of the results of hypothesis testing; (3) as a means to assess the clinical importance of research results; (4) with adjusted confidence levels when multiple intervals are calculated (the equivalent to controlling for alpha inflation); and (5) when reporting the results of individual studies that are included within meta-analyses.

Interpretation and Examples

With the traditional method, the reader is tempted to believe that in our hypothetical example the "true" difference between the means is 28.5° and that the difference between the means is "really" significant because the p value of .002 is so much less than the alpha of .05. With the confidence interval presentation, the reader is reminded that 28.5° is only an estimate of a difference between the means. The confidence interval tells us that there is a 95% chance that the population difference in mean 3-week ROM values is between approximately 12° and approximately 45°. With this information the researcher or reader has a sound basis on which to judge the clinical importance of the finding.

Van der Windt and colleagues used confidence intervals to supplement their traditional hypothesis testing in a study of the effectiveness of corticosteroid injections versus physical therapy for treatment of painful stiff shoulders.[20] For example, they found a difference of 31% in success rates between groups: 77% of patients treated with the corticosteroid injections were "successes" at 7 weeks compared with only 46% of those treated with physical therapy. The confidence interval for this difference in percentage was 14% to 48%. Since this interval does not contain "0," it corresponds to a statistically significant difference in percentage of treatment successes between groups after 7 weeks of treatment. Prencipe and coworkers used confidence intervals to test the significance of the odds ratio for dementia in elderly, community-dwelling individuals with and without stroke.[21] The odds ratio for dementia was 5.8 with a 95% confidence interval from 3.1 to 10.8. Since this interval does not contain "1," the authors concluded that there was a significant increase in the odds of dementia for individuals who have had stroke compared with those without stroke. Further, there is a 95% chance that the population of individuals with stroke is 3.1 to 10.8 times more likely to have dementia compared with the population of individuals without stroke.

■ POWER ANALYSIS AND EFFECT SIZE

Power is the ability of a statistical test to detect a difference when it exists, as discussed in Chapter 20. Maximizing power within a research design involves (1) maximizing the size of the difference in the dependent variable between levels of the independent variable; (2) minimizing the amount of variability on the dependent variable within levels of the independent variable; and (3) maximizing the sample size. In addition, the alpha level selected by the researcher influences power, with higher power associated with larger alpha levels. Power analysis is used at two very different points in the research process: in the design phase and after the analysis phase.

Power Analysis—Design Phase

During the design phase of a research project power analysis is used to help the researcher design a study that has "enough" power, typically 80%, to detect differences that exist. To do so, the researchers could estimate the size of the between-group difference that they would consider to be important, the variability they would expect to see within the groups being studied, and the sample size that is reasonable given the constraints of the research setting. From this information a "dry run" statistical analysis can be done and the power of the analysis can be calculated. If the power is less than 80%, then the researchers need to reconsider some of the elements of the design. Could treatment be extended to maximize the chance of a large between-group difference? Could a more homogeneous group of subjects be studied to minimize the within-group variability? Could another clinic be involved to increase the sample size?

In the preceding paragraph the between-group difference, within-group variability, and sample size were given and the power was calculated based on those givens. When power analysis is used in the design phase of a study, however, it is usually run in "reverse." Rather than solving for "power," researchers usually specify power at 80% and solve for one of the other factors that they can control. Because the nature of the treatment and the characteristics of the subjects are often dictated by the research question, sample size is generally seen to be the most controllable factor related to power. Therefore, power analysis in the design phase is most often used to help estimate the sample size for the study.

When power analysis is used to estimate sample size, researchers must specify their desired power level, as well as the anticipated between-group differences and within-group variability. In practice, estimating these two factors may be difficult, particularly in topic areas for which little previous research exists. When this is the case, researchers may use the concept of *effect size* to help them plan their sample sizes. The effect size is a ratio of the difference between the means to the pooled standard deviation of the groups being compared. For a comparison of two group means, an effect size of .20 is considered small, .50 is considered medium, and .80 is considered large.[22] Using these conventions, researchers who do not have reliable estimates of the between-group differences and within-group variability can determine what sample sizes would be required to detect effect sizes that would be considered small, medium, and large.

Without going into computational details, for power of 80% and an alpha level of .05, the sample size requirements for a two-sample independent *t* test can be shown to be 25 per group to detect a large effect of .80, 63 per group to detect a medium effect of .50, and 392 per group to detect a small effect of .20.[23] This means that a total of 50, 126, or 784 subjects would be required to detect large, medium, and small effects, respectively. Of 100 rehabilitation studies reviewed by Ottenbacher and Barrett[24] the maximum number of subjects in a study was 126. In addition, 76 of the 100 studies had fewer than 50 subjects. If we assume that all 100 studies were two-group studies, this means that none of the 100 studies had enough subjects to detect a small effect, only 1 could detect a medium effect, and only 23 studies could detect a large effect. Clearly, rehabilitation researchers who use group designs should work to design more powerful studies.

Power Analysis—Analysis Phase

The second use of power analysis is to compute the power of a statistical test after it has failed to identify a statistically significant difference. When a difference is not identified, the researcher and the reader wonder whether a correct conclusion has been reached or whether a Type II error has been committed. A correct conclusion is assured when the finding of no difference between the samples corresponds with the reality of no difference between the populations from which the samples were drawn. A Type II error is committed when the finding of no difference between the samples is at odds with a true difference between the populations. Since the entire populations are generally not available for study, researchers never know whether they are correct or whether they have committed a Type II error. The probability of making a Type II error is known as beta, or β (power is $1 - \beta$). Because of this relationship between power and Type II errors, low probabilities of Type II errors are associated with high power values. Power may be expressed as a percentage by moving the decimal two places to the right. By convention, 80% power is desirable. As noted earlier, rehabilitation research often lacks power. Thus, lack of power, or a Type II error, is often a likely explanation for a nonsignificant result in rehabilitation research. Editorial policies for journals often indicate when researchers should present power analyses in the face of nonsignificant findings. For the *Journal of Bone and Joint Surgery* power analyses are requested when *p* is between .05 and .15.[25] The policies of the *Archives of Physical Medicine and Rehabilitation*[26] and *Physical Therapy*[27] specify that power calculations be provided within articles that report nonsignificant findings.

■ SUMMARY

Basic ANOVA techniques can be extended to factorial ANOVA (analyzing more than one independent variable simultaneously, including between-subjects and mixed-design models), multivariate ANOVA, or MANOVA (analyzing more than one dependent variable simultaneously), and analysis of covariance, or ANCOVA (removing the effect of an intervening variable). Three specialized techniques for analyzing single-system data are used frequently. Celeration line analysis extrapolates a baseline celeration line into the treatment phase and determines whether the distribution of data points in the treatment phase reflects a significant difference. Level, trend, and slope analysis compares the characteristics of the celeration lines from different phases of the study. Two standard deviation band analysis compares actual values in the treatment phase with values that would be expected if there were no difference between treatment and baseline phases. Actuarial and Kaplan-Meier survival analysis methods are used to determine the proportion of patients who have and have not experienced a defined event at different points in time. Differences in survival curves can be determined by Wilcoxon rank sum, log rank, Mantel-Haenszel, and proportional hazards methods. Some researchers prefer to present their statistical findings in terms of confidence intervals rather than p values. Doing so involves algebraic rearrangements of traditional hypothesis testing formulas. Power analysis can be used in the design phase of a study to determine the sample size needed to detect different effect sizes or used in the analysis phase to look for possible explanations of nonsignificant findings.

REFERENCES

1. Magalhaes LC, Koomar JA, Cermak SA. Bilateral motor coordination in 5- to 9-year-old children: a pilot study. *Am J Occup Ther.* 1989;43:437–443.
2. Bandy WD, Irion JM. The effect of time on static stretch on the flexibility of the hamstring muscles. *Phys Ther.* 1994;74:845–852.
3. Tabachnick BG, Fidell LS. *Using Multivariate Statistics.* 2nd ed. New York, NY: Harper & Row; 1989.
4. Worrell TW, Guenin J, Huse L, et al. Health outcomes in subjects with patellofemoral pain. *J Rehabil Outcomes Meas.* 1998;2(4):10–19.
5. Egger MJ, Miller JR. Testing for experimental effects in the pretest-posttest design. *Nurs Res.* 1984;33:306–312.
6. Mackay LE, Bernstein BA, Chapman PE, Morgan AS, Milazzo LS. Early intervention in severe head injury: long-term benefits of a formalized program. *Arch Phys Med Rehabil.* 1992;73:635–641.
7. Wessling KC, DeVane DA, Hylton CR. Effects of static stretch and static stretch and ultrasound combined on triceps surae muscle extensibility in healthy women. *Phys Ther.* 1987;67:674–679.
8. Ottenbacher KJ. Analysis of data in idiographic research. *Am J Phys Med Rehabil.* 1992;71:202–208.
9. Nourbakhsh MR, Ottenbacher KJ. The statistical analysis of single-subject data: a comparative examination. *Phys Ther.* 1994;74:768–776.
10. Bobrovitz CD, Ottenbacher KJ. Comparison of visual inspection and statistical analysis of single-subject data in rehabilitation research. *Am J Phys Med Rehabil.* 1998; 77:94–102.
11. Ottenbacher KJ. *Evaluating Clinical Change: Strategies for Occupational and Physical Therapists.* Baltimore, Md: Williams & Wilkins; 1986.
12. Goodman G, Bazyk S. The effects of a short thumb opponens splint on hand function in cerebral palsy: a single-subject study. *Am J Occup Ther.* 1991;45:726–731.
13. Embrey DG, Yates L, Mott DH. Effects of neuro-developmental treatment and orthoses on knee flexion during gait: a single-subject design. *Phys Ther.* 1990;70:626–637.
14. Mulcahey MJ, Smith BT, Betz RR, Weiss AA. Outcomes of tendon transfer surgery and occupational therapy in a child with tetraplegia secondary to spinal cord injury. *Am J Occup Ther.* 1995;49:607–617.
15. Dawson-Saunders B, Trapp RG. *Basic and Clinical Biostatistics.* 2nd ed. Norwalk, Conn: Appleton & Lange; 1994.
16. *SPSS Advanced Statistics 7.5.* Chicago, Ill: SPSS Inc; 1997.
17. Hoenig H, Rubenstein LV, Sloane R, Horner R, Kahn K. What is the role of timing in the surgical and rehabilitative care of community-dwelling older persons with acute hip fracture? *Arch Intern Med.* 1997;157:513–520.
18. Gardner MJ, Altman DG. Confidence intervals rather than P values: estimation rather than hypothesis testing. *BMJ.* 1986;292:746–750.
19. Sim J, Reid N. Statistical inference by confidence intervals: issues of interpretation and utilization. *Phys Ther.* 1999;79:186–195.
20. van der Windt DA, Koes BW, Deville W, Boeke AJP, de Jong BA, Bouter LM. Effectiveness of corticosteroid injections versus physiotherapy for treatment of painful stiff shoulder in primary care: randomised trial. *BMJ.* 1998;317:1292–1296.
21. Prencipe M, Ferretti C, Casini AR, Santini M, Giubilei F, Culasso F. Stroke, disability, and dementia. *Stroke.* 1997; 28:531–536.
22. Cohen J. *Statistical Power Analysis for the Behavioral Sciences.* 2nd ed. Hillsdale, NJ: Lawrence Erlbaum Associates; 1988.
23. Polit DF. *Data Analysis and Statistics for Nursing Research.* Stamford, Conn: Appleton & Lange; 1996.
24. Ottenbacher KJ, Barrett KA. Statistical conclusion validity of rehabilitation research: a quantitative analysis. *Am J Phys Med Rehabil.* 1990;69:102–107.
25. Senghas RE. Statistics in the *Journal of Bone and Joint Surgery:* suggestions for authors. *J Bone Joint Surg Am.* 1992;74:319–320.
26. Information for authors. *Arch Phys Med Rehabil.* 1999; 78:i–xv.
27. Information for authors. *Phys Ther.* 1999;79:86–87.

Statistical Analysis of Relationships: The Basics

Correlation
    Calculation of the Pearson Product
        Moment Correlation
    Alternative Correlation Coefficients
    Assumptions of the Correlation
        Coefficients
    Interpretation of Correlation
        Coefficients

Strength of the Coefficient
Variance Shared by the Two Variables
Statistical Significance of the Coefficient
Confidence Intervals Around the Coefficient
Limits of Interpretation
    Literature Examples
Linear Regression

Researchers often wish to know the extent to which variables are related to one another. For example, in Chapter 11, a study is cited in which the relationship between lower extremity muscle force and gait characteristics is examined for individuals with transtibial amputations.[1] This is an example of the use of relationship analysis to determine the extent to which different concepts, in this case muscle force and gait characteristics, are related to one another. In Chapter 18, several studies are cited in which the reliability of a measure was determined by documenting the relationship between repeated measurements of scores taken across time or by different therapists.[2–4] For example, Nussbaum and Downes[2] examined the reliability of a pressure-pain algometer by using two measurers, each taking three measurements on 3 different days. This study demonstrates that the analysis of relationships is not always between different concepts but may be between different conditions under which a single concept is measured.

Relationship analysis studies are generally nonexperimental, with the researcher observing different phenomena rather than manipulating groups of subjects, as is done in experimental studies. Recall from Chapters 21 and 22 that the analysis of differences centers on determining whether there are mean differences between groups or between repeated administrations of a test to a single group. In contrast, the analysis of relationships centers on determining the *association* between scores on two or more variables that are available for each individual in a single group.

This chapter introduces the major ways in which relationships among variables are analyzed. As in Chapters 21 and 22, the purpose of this chapter is not to enable readers to conduct their own statistical analyses, but to enable them to understand relationship analysis as it is presented in the physical therapy literature. Simple correlation and linear regression are presented in this chapter. The more advanced topics of multiple and logistic regression techniques, the uses of relationship analysis for documenting reliability, and factor analysis are deferred until Chapter 24.

■ CORRELATION

When two variables are correlated, the value an individual exhibits on one variable is related to the value he or she exhibits on another variable. The magnitude and direction of the relationship between variables are expressed mathematically as a correlation coefficient. The presence of relationships among variables does not enable researchers to draw causal inferences about the variables: Correlation is not causation. For example, although there is an obvious relationship between the amount of corn grown in a particular locale and the flatness of the land on which it is grown, reasonable people do not conclude that growing corn causes the land to become flat.[5]

This section begins with calculation of the most frequently used correlation coefficient, the Pearson product moment correlation. This is followed by discussion of alternative correlation coefficients, the assumptions that underlie corre-

lation coefficients, the ways in which correlation coefficients are interpreted, and examples of the use of correlation from the literature.

Calculation of the Pearson Product Moment Correlation

Calculation of the Pearson product moment correlation is mathematically tedious, although relatively simple conceptually: The Pearson product moment correlation, or r, is the average of the cross-products of the z scores for the X and Y variables. In mathematical notation,

$$r = \frac{\Sigma Z_x Z_y}{N}$$

Suppose we are interested in determining the extent of the relationship between a functional variable such as gait velocity and a physical impairment variable such as knee flexion range of motion (ROM) in patients who have undergone total knee arthroplasty. Table 23–1 shows the calculation of the correlation between 6-month ROM and gait velocity in patients at Clinic 1. In the calculation of the Pearson r value, either

TABLE 23-1	Calculation of Pearson r: Relationship Between Six-Month Range of Motion and Gait Velocity at Clinic 1						
Subject	X	x	Y	y	z_x	z_y	$z_x z_y$
01	100	0	165	21	0.00	1.13	0.00
02	85	−15	100	−44	−2.24	−2.37	5.31
03	100	0	130	−14	0.00	−0.75	0.00
04	105	5	170	26	0.75	1.40	1.05
05	105	5	150	6	0.75	0.32	0.24
06	95	−5	135	−9	−0.75	−0.48	0.36
07	110	10	153	9	1.49	0.48	0.72
08	100	0	145	1	0.00	0.05	0.00
09	95	−5	147	3	−0.75	0.16	−0.12
10	105	5	145	1	0.75	0.05	0.04
Σ	1000.0		1440.0				7.6
N	10.0		10.0				10.0
Mean	100.0		144.0				$r = .76$
σ	6.71		18.60				

variable may be designated X or Y, and neither is considered independent or dependent. The X and Y scores for each subject are converted to z scores, and the product of z_x and z_y (called the *crossproduct*) is determined for each subject. The mean of the crossproducts is the Pearson product moment correlation coefficient.

The values that r may take range from -1.0 to $+1.0$. A correlation coefficient of -1.0 indicates a perfect negative, or inverse, relationship: A higher value on one variable is associated with a lower value on the other variable. A correlation coefficient of $+1.0$ indicates a perfect positive, or direct, relationship: A higher value on one variable is associated with a higher value on the other variable. In this example $r = .76$, indicating a fairly strong direct relationship between the two variables. Figure 23–1 shows a scatterplot of the 10 pairs of scores. They fall rather loosely around an imaginary diagonal line running from the bottom left corner of the graph to the top right corner. This indicates that as ROM scores increase, so do gait velocity values.

Researchers often collect many variables within a single study and are interested in which of the variables are most related to one another. When a researcher calculates many correlation coefficients in a study, he or she usually displays them in a correlation matrix, as shown in Table 23–2. In this table, all the variables of interest are listed as both columns and rows, and the correlation between each pair of variables is presented at the intersection of the row and column of interest. For example, the Pearson r between flexion torque and extension torque is .9524 and can be found in two places on the table (the intersection of Row 2 and Column 3 and the intersection of Row 3 and Column 2). A full correlation matrix like this includes redundant information because each correlation coefficient between two different variables is listed twice. It also includes unnecessary information because the correlation between each variable and itself is known (1.000), and these correlations form the diagonal. In articles, therefore, most researchers display only the nonredundant portion of the correlation matrix, which lies either above or below the diagonal.

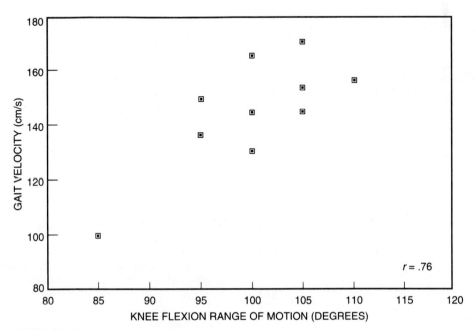

FIGURE 23–1. Relationship between 6-month knee flexion range of motion and gait velocity.

TABLE 23-2 Correlation Matrix for Six-Month Variables

	Range of Motion	Flexion Torque	Extension Torque	Gait Velocity
Range of motion	1.0000	.5610	.5947	.6399
Flexion torque	.5610	1.0000	.9524	.8921
Extension torque	.5947	.9524	1.0000	.9014
Gait velocity	.6399	.8921	.9014	1.0000

Alternative Correlation Coefficients

Correlation coefficients other than the Pearson product moment correlation have been developed for a variety of uses beyond that of quantifying the degree of relationship between two interval or ratio variables. Several are listed in Chapter 17, where correlation is introduced as a concept related to measurement theory, and Table 23–3 lists the characteristics of several additional correlation measures.

Spearman's rho (ρ) and Kendall's tau (τ) correlations are designed for use when both variables are ranked. The point-biserial correlation is used with one continuous and one dichotomous variable. The Spearman rho and point-biserial formulas are simply shortcut versions of the Pearson r.[6(pp237,238)] Correlation coefficients for use with nominal data are the phi (φ) and kappa (κ) coefficients. Phi is another shortcut version of the Pearson r, applicable when both variables are dichotomous, such as in determining the relationship between sex and the answer to a yes/no question.[6(p237)] Kappa, discussed in more detail in Chapter 24, is a reliability coefficient that can be used when nominal variables consist of more than two categories.

Correlation coefficients for more than two variables are also available. The *intraclass* correlation coefficients (ICCs), discussed more fully in Chapter 24, are a family of reliability coefficients that can be used when two or more repeated measures have been collected. *Kappa* can also

TABLE 23-3 Characteristics of Different Correlation Coefficients

Coefficient	Characteristics
Pearson product moment correlation	Two continuous variables
Spearman's rho (ρ)	Two ranked variables; shortcut calculation of Pearson
Point biserial	One continuous variable, one dichotomous variable
Kendall's tau (τ)	Two ranked variables
Phi (ϕ)	Two dichotomous variables; shortcut calculation of Pearson
Kappa (κ)	Two or more nominal variables with two or more categories; a reliability coefficient
Intraclass correlation	Two or more continuous variables; a reliability coefficient
Partial correlation	Two variables, with effects of a third held constant
Multiple correlation	More than two variables
Canonical correlation	Two sets of variables

be used with more than two nominal repeated measures. *Partial* correlation is used to assess the relationship between two variables with the effect of a third variable eliminated. *Multiple* correlation is used to assess the variability shared by three or more variables. *Canonical* correlation is a technique for assessing the relationships between two sets of variables.

Assumptions of the Correlation Coefficients

Calculation of the Pearson product moment and related correlation coefficients depends on three major assumptions. First, the relationships between variables are assumed to be *linear*. Analysis of a scatterplot of the data must show that the relationship forms a straight line. Curvilinear relationships (those that do not follow a straight line) may be analyzed, but this requires more advanced techniques than are discussed in this text. Figure 23–2 shows the scatterplot of our hy-

pothetical total knee arthroplasty data showing the relationship between age and a new variable, length of acute care hospital stay postoperatively. There is an obvious relationship between variables, but it is not linear. Both the young and very old patients have short lengths of stay, possibly because the young reach their ROM goals quickly and the old are transferred to a skilled nursing facility for continued rehabilitation. Those of intermediate age stay in the hospital somewhat longer, presumably to achieve their ROM goals in the acute care hospital, without transfer to a skilled nursing facility. The Pearson *r* for this relationship is .3502, indicating a minimal degree of linear relationship between these two variables. If researchers rely solely on Pearson *r* values to guide their conclusions, they may mistakenly conclude that no relationship exists when in fact a strong *nonlinear* relationship exists.

The second assumption is *homoscedasticity*. As shown in Figure 23–3A, homoscedasticity means that for each value of one variable, the other vari-

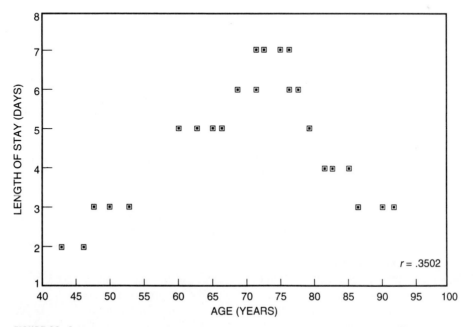

FIGURE 23–2. Relationship between age and length of stay. There is a strong nonlinear relationship between the two variables. The low *r* value is deceptive because it is designed to detect linear relationships only.

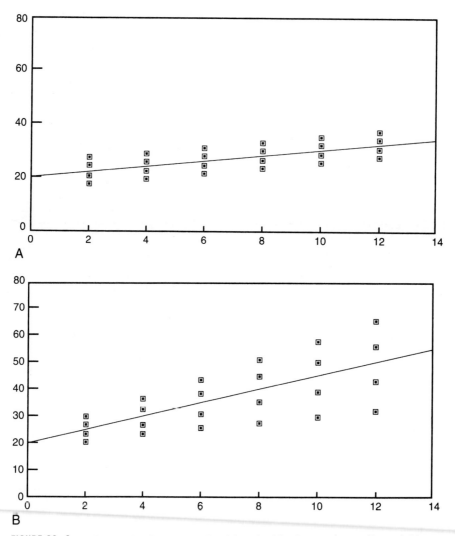

FIGURE 23–3. A. Example of homoscedasticity; the Y values are equally variable at each level of X. **B.** Example of nonhomoscedasticity; the Y values are not equally variable at each level of X.

able has equal variability. Nonhomoscedasticity is illustrated in Figure 23–3B. Because the calculation of Pearson r is based on z scores, whose calculation in turn depends on standard deviations for each variable, widely varying variances at different levels will distort the calculated value of r.

The third assumption is that both variables have enough *variability* to demonstrate a relationship. If either or both variables have a restricted range, then the correlation coefficient will be artificially low and uninterpretable. Figure 23–4A shows the scatterplot of Clinic 3's data for 6-month ROM and gait velocity. There appears to be little relationship between the two, because the data cluster in the top right corner of the graph and the Pearson r is $-.2673$. However, the range of ROM values is very restricted, with all subjects showing close to full ROM of their prosthetic knees.

Figure 23–4B shows the scatterplot of 6-month

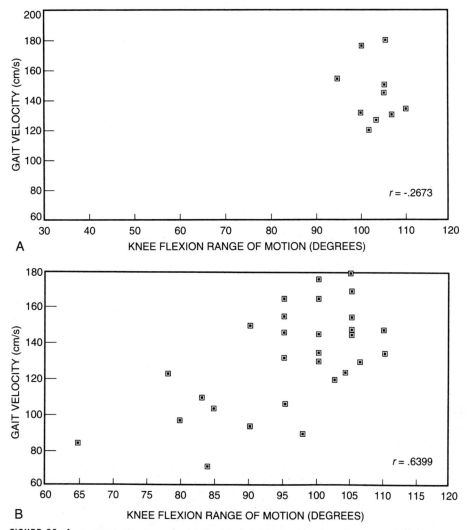

FIGURE 23–4. A. Restricted range of the X variable results in a low correlation coefficient. **B.** The addition of a broader range of X values reveals a pattern that was not apparent in **A.**

ROM and gait velocity for the entire sample of 30 patients. In this example each variable takes a fairly wide range of values, and the relationship between 6-month ROM and gait velocity is obvious. The Pearson *r* for this set of data is .6399.

Thus, the restricted-range data yielded a correlation coefficient that was different in both magnitude and direction from the coefficient calculated on data with a greater range of values.

Interpretation of Correlation Coefficients

There are four major ways in which correlation coefficients are interpreted: (1) the strength of the coefficient itself; (2) the variance shared by the two variables, as calculated by the coefficient of determination; (3) the statistical significance of the correlation coefficient; and (4) the confidence intervals about the correlation coefficient. Regardless of which method is chosen, the interpretation should not be extrapolated beyond the range of the data used to generate the correlation coefficient.

STRENGTH OF THE COEFFICIENT. The first way to interpret the coefficient is to examine the strength of the relationship, which is independent of the direction (direct or inverse) of the relationship. This method of interpretation is exemplified by Munro's descriptive terms for the strength of correlation coefficients[6(p235)]:

.00–.25	Little, if any correlation
.26–.49	Low correlation
.50–.69	Moderate correlation
.70–.89	High correlation
.90–1.00	Very high correlation

Such a system of descriptors assumes that the meaningfulness of a correlation is the same regardless of the context in which it is used. This assumption is not necessarily valid. For example, if one is determining the reliability of a strength measure from one day to the next, an r of .70 may be considered unacceptably low for the purpose of documenting day-to-day changes in status. However, if one is determining the relationship between abstract constructs such as self-esteem and motivation that are difficult to measure, then a correlation of .50 may be considered very strong.

VARIANCE SHARED BY THE TWO VARIABLES. The second way to evaluate the importance of the correlation coefficient is to calculate what is called the *coefficient of determination*. The coefficient of determination, r^2, is the square of the correlation coefficient, r. The coefficient of determination is an indication of the percentage of variance that is shared by the two variables. For the relationship between 6-month ROM and gait velocity at Clinic 1 (Table 23–1), the coefficient of determination is approximately .58 ($.76^2 = .5776$). This means that 58% of the variability within one variable can be accounted for by the other variable. The remaining 42% of the variability is due to variables not yet considered, perhaps height, leg length, pain, age, or sex. Using the coefficient of determination, we find, for example, that a "high" correlation coefficient of .70 accounts for only 49% of the variance among the variables, and a "low" correlation of .30 accounts for an even lower 9% of the variance between the variables.

STATISTICAL SIGNIFICANCE OF THE COEFFICIENT. The third method of interpreting correlation coefficients is to statistically determine whether the coefficient calculated is significantly different from zero. In other words, we determine the probability that the calculated correlation coefficient would have occurred by chance if in fact there was no relationship between the variables. A special form of a t test is used to determine this probability. The problem with this approach is that very weak correlations may be statistically different from zero even though they are not very meaningful. This is particularly likely to occur with large samples. For example, Sellers studied the relationship between antigravity control and postural control in 107 children.[7] Correlations as low as .11 were found to be statistically different from zero at the .05 level. Although statistically significant, correlations of this magnitude probably do not describe clinically meaningful relationships.

CONFIDENCE INTERVALS AROUND THE COEFFICIENT. The fourth way to determine the meaningfulness of a correlation coefficient is to calculate a confidence interval about the correlation coefficient. To do so, a researcher converts the r values into z scores, calculates confidence intervals with the z scores, and transforms the z-score intervals back into a range of r scores. Using steps outlined by Munro, the 95% confidence interval for an r of .76 for 6-month ROM and gait velocity at Clinic 1 is .17 to .94.[6(pp236,237)] The confidence interval is very large because the sample is small (n = 10) and does not permit accurate estimation. Using the same procedures, the 95% confidence interval for the same r calculated for a sample of

100 subjects is approximately .65 to .83, a far smaller interval. As is the case for the confidence intervals calculated in the analysis of differences, larger samples permit more accurate estimation of true population values.

LIMITS OF INTERPRETATION. A consideration common to all four interpretation methods is that the interpretation of correlation coefficients should not extend beyond the range of the original data. For example, Figure 23–5 shows the fairly strong relationship between the 6-month ROM and gait velocity data (asterisks). The line showing the trend of the data is extrapolated to a ROM of 0°. At this ROM, the trend line indicates that the gait velocity would be estimated to be approximately *negative* 38 cm/s, an impossible figure! Rather than being a linear relationship throughout the ROM, it is likely that the relationship becomes curvilinear as ROM becomes closer to 0° with gait velocity bottoming out at some low level

(crosses). Knowing that the relationship between ROM and gait velocity is strong and linear in the top half of the usual values does not permit us to extrapolate these conclusions to values outside the ranges encountered in the original data collection. A full interpretation of the correlation between 6-month ROM and gait velocity might be written in a journal article as follows:

DATA ANALYSIS

A Pearson product moment correlation *(r)* was used to quantify the relationship between 6-month range of motion (ROM) and gait velocity for the sample of 30 subjects. Interpretation of the coefficient was through significance testing at the 5% level, calculation of r^2, and construction of a 95% confidence interval around the correlation coefficient.

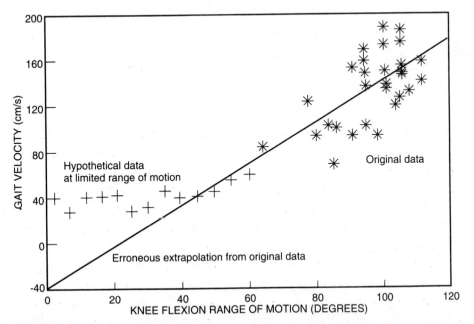

FIGURE 23–5. Extending interpretation of regression beyond the original data results in invalid conclusions. Original data (*asterisks*) extrapolated past the X and Y values predict that patients with no flexion range of motion will have a negative gait velocity. Crosses indicate the more likely relationship between the two variables in their lower ranges.

RESULTS

The Pearson r between 6-month ROM and gait velocity was .6399. This was significantly different from zero at a level of $p < .01$. The coefficient of determination (r^2) was .41, indicating that about 40% of the variability in gait velocity can be attributed to differences in 6-month ROM. The 95% confidence interval for r was .365 to .812.

DISCUSSION

The moderate correlation of approximately .64 between 6-month ROM and gait velocity seems important clinically because it provides evidence that those patients with less physical impairment (i.e., those with good ROM) also have less functional disability, as measured by gait velocity. The confidence interval for r is large, because of the moderate sample size within this study. On the basis of the strength of the correlation found in this study, we recommend further data collection on a larger sample to provide a more accurate estimation of the true relationship between these two variables.

Literature Examples

Powers and colleagues studied the relationship of muscle force and gait characteristics of individuals with transtibial amputation.[1] They examined the strength of seven different lower extremity muscle groups (bilateral hip extensors, bilateral hip abductors, bilateral knee extensors, and unilateral ankle plantar flexors) for three different gait characteristics (velocity, cadence, and stride length) at two walking speeds (free and fast). They calculated 42 Pearson product moment correlation coefficients within their study: there was a coefficient for each muscle group correlated with each of the gait characteristics for each speed. The importance of each correlation was evaluated by testing it for statistical significance and calculating the coefficient of determination to see how much of the variability in one variable could be accounted for by the other variable. To simplify the reporting of results, p values and coefficients of determination were reported for only those correlation coefficients that were found to be statistically different from zero.

Andrews and colleagues studied the relationship between muscle force for many muscle actions and a variety of other variables.[8] Because these other variables had different measurement characteristics, different correlation coefficients were used as appropriate. The Pearson product moment correlation was used between the continuous muscle force variables and the continuous variables of weight, age, and height. The Spearman rank correlation was used between the muscle force variables and ordinal activity level variables. The point-biserial correlation was used between the muscle force variables and the dichotomous gender variable. The importance of the various correlations was evaluated in this study by examining both the strength and the statistical significance of the correlations.

■ LINEAR REGRESSION

Correlational techniques, as discussed earlier, are used to describe the relationships among two or more variables. When the researcher's purpose extends beyond description of relationships to include prediction of future characteristics from previously collected data, then the statistical analysis extends from correlation to regression techniques.

Suppose we wish to predict a patient's eventual gait velocity on the basis of an early postoperative indicator such as 3-week ROM. The Pearson product moment correlation between these two variables is .5545, indicating a moderate degree of correlation in which 31% of the variability in gait velocity ($r^2 = .3075$) can be accounted for by variability in 3-week ROM. Unlike correlation techniques, regression techniques require that variables be defined as independent or dependent. In this example, the independent variable is 3-week ROM and is used to predict the dependent variable, gait velocity.

Figure 23–6 shows a scatterplot of 3-week ROM and gait velocity scores, with a line showing the best fit between these two variables. This line is generated by using the data to solve the general equation for a straight line:

$$Y = bX + a$$

where b is the slope of the line and a is the intercept (i.e., the Y value at the point at which the line intersects the Y axis). The slope, b, is found by multiplying the Pearson r value by the ratio of the standard deviation of Y to the standard deviation of X: [$b = r(S_y/S_x)$]. The intercept, a, is found by subtracting the product of the slope and the mean of X from the mean of Y: ($a = \overline{Y} - \overline{X}b$). As with most statistical analyses today, computer programs can generate regression equations quickly and easily without the need for hand calculations. The formula for the regression line of gait velocity on 3-week ROM is $Y = 0.75X + 82.56$. Although this equation defines the best-fitting line through the data, most of the points do not fall precisely on the line.

The vertical distance from each point to the line is known as the *residual,* and the mean of the residuals is zero. The standard deviation of the residuals is known as the *standard error of the estimate* (SEE).

Once the regression equation is generated, it can be used to predict the gait velocity of future patients by solving for Y (gait velocity) on the basis of the patient's X (3-week ROM) score. For example, suppose that a patient has 70° of ROM 3 weeks postoperatively. The predicted gait velocity for this patient is 135.06 cm/s [0.75(70) + 82.56 = 135.06]. Because we know that this prediction is unlikely to be precise, we can provide additional useful information by generating a confidence interval around the predicted value. The confidence interval around the predicted value is created by using the SEE. A 95% confidence interval, for example, is created by adding and subtracting 1.96 SEEs from the regression line, as shown graphically in Figure 23–7. In this example, the SEE generated by the computer is 24.54 cm/s and the 95% confidence interval would be found by adding and subtracting 48.09 cm/s

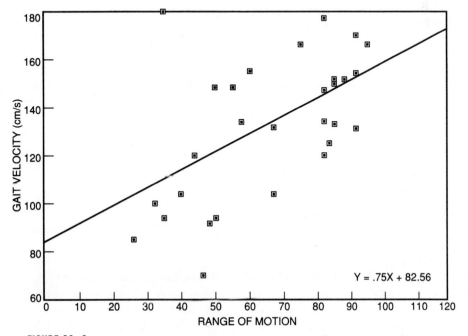

FIGURE 23–6. Regression of gait velocity on 3-week knee flexion range of motion.

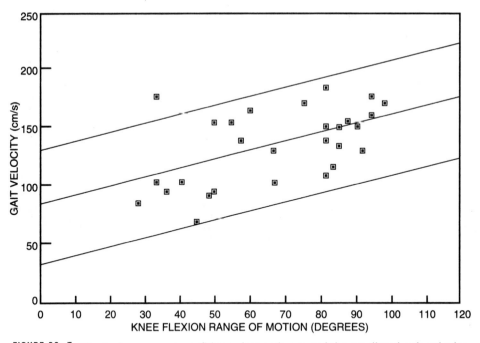

FIGURE 23–7. Ninety-five percent confidence intervals around the predicted gait velocity.

to and from the predicted Y value. For patients with 3-week ROM of 70°, we therefore are 95% certain that their gait velocity at 6 months will be between 86.96 and 183.16 cm/s. Ideally, the dependent variable is highly correlated with the independent variable, resulting in small residuals, a small SEE, and a more precise prediction.

The statistical significance of a regression equation is usually determined with an F test to evaluate whether r^2, the amount of variance in Y predicted by X, is significantly different from zero. As is the case with statistical testing of the correlation coefficient using a t test, r^2 may be statistically different from zero without being terribly meaningful. In our example, the r^2 of .3075 is significantly different from zero at $p = .0015$. Despite this statistical significance, we know that the 95% confidence interval for predicting a single score is quite large and may not allow for clinically useful prediction. For instance, the gait velocity needed to cross most streets safely is approximately 130 cm/s.[9] The range of the confidence interval is great enough that for most

patients we could not predict whether their eventual velocity would enable them to be community ambulators. This reflects the fact that there is only a moderate correlation between the two variables in question.

In practice, then, this regression equation would not likely be perceived to be very useful, and the researchers would search for additional independent variables that would allow for more precise prediction of the dependent variable. When more than one variable is used to predict another variable, the simple linear regression technique is extended to multiple regression, as discussed in Chapter 24.

■ SUMMARY

Relationship analysis studies are generally non-experimental, with the researcher observing different phenomena rather than manipulating groups of subjects. The magnitude and direction of relationships between variables are expressed mathematically as Pearson product moment correlations or a variety of alternative correlation coefficients. Assumptions for use of the correlation coefficients include linearity, homoscedasticity, and an adequate range of values for each variable. Correlation coefficients are interpreted in several ways: by the strength of the coefficient itself, by the coefficient of determination, by the statistical significance of the correlation coefficient, and by confidence intervals about the correlation coefficient. When the researcher's purpose extends beyond description of relationships to include prediction, then the statistical analysis extends from correlation to regression techniques.

REFERENCES

1. Powers CM, Boyd LA, Fontaine CA, Perry J. The influence of lower-extremity muscle force on gait characteristics in individuals with below-knee amputations secondary to vascular disease. *Phys Ther.* 1996;76:369–377.
2. Nussbaum EL, Downes L. Reliability of clinical pressure-pain algometric measurements obtained on consecutive days. *Phys Ther.* 1998;78:160–169.
3. Watkins MA, Riddle DL, Lamb RL, Personius WJ. Reliability of goniometric measurements and visual estimates of knee range of motion obtained in a clinical setting. *Phys Ther.* 1991;71:90–97.
4. Mayerson NH, Milano RA. Goniometric reliability in physical medicine. *Arch Phys Med Rehabil.* 1984;65:92–94.
5. Swartz HM, Flood AB. The corntinental theory of flat and depressed areas: on the relationship between corn and topography. *Irreproducible Results.* 1990;35(5):16–17, 19.
6. Munro BH. *Statistical Methods for Health Care Research.* 3rd ed. Philadelphia, Pa: JB Lippincott; 1997.
7. Sellers JS. Relationship between antigravity control and postural control in young children. *Phys Ther.* 1988;68:486–490.
8. Andrews AW, Thomas MW, Bohannon RW. Normative values for isometric muscle force measurements obtained with hand-held dynamometers. *Phys Ther.* 1996;76:248–259.
9. Lerner-Frankiel MB, Vargas S, Brown M, Krusell L, Schoneberger W. Functional community ambulation: what are your criteria? *Clin Manage Phys Ther.* 1986;6(2):12–15.

Statistical Analysis of Relationships: Advanced and Special Techniques

Reliability Analysis
  Pearson Product Moment
    Correlation with Extensions
  Intraclass Correlation Coefficients
  Kappa
Multiple Regression
  Variable Entry in Multiple
    Regression
  Interpretation of the Multiple
    Regression Equation

  Literature Example
Logistic Regression
  Rationale for Logistic Regression
  Literature Examples
Factor Analysis
  Factor Analysis Steps
  Literature Example

Chapter 23 introduced basic correlation and regression techniques by emphasizing bivariate procedures, that is, those in which just two variables are involved. In addition, the techniques presented in Chapter 23 were used to analyze relationships between distinctly different variables such as age and gait velocity. In this chapter, which covers more advanced correlation and regression techniques, these basic concepts are extended in two ways. First, specialized reliability correlation coefficients, in which repeated measures of the same variable are analyzed, are examined. Second, procedures that examine the complex interrelationships among many variables are introduced. These procedures include multiple regression, logistic regression, and factor analysis.

■ RELIABILITY ANALYSIS

A specialized type of relationship analysis is used to assess the reliability of a measure. As discussed in Chapter 17, there are two major classes of reliability measures: those that document relative reliability and those that document absolute reliability. It is the measures of relative reliability that depend on correlational techniques. In some instances, the correlational technique does not provide all of the desired reliability information, and regression or difference analysis techniques are used to supplement the correlational technique. Three techniques used for reliability analysis are presented here: the Pearson product moment correlation with regression and difference analysis extensions, the intraclass correlation coefficients, and the kappa correlations.

Pearson Product Moment Correlation with Extensions

The Pearson product moment correlation is a measure of relative reliability: A high, positive Pearson value indicates that high scores on one measure are associated with high scores on another measure and that low scores on one measure are associated with low scores on another measure. When we compare two different variables, such as 3-week range of motion (ROM) and gait velocity, the strength of the relationship is the only information we desire, so the Pearson correlation is ideal.

When we are comparing paired measurements for the purpose of determining their reliability, however, we are concerned with both the relationship between the two measures and the magnitude of the differences between the two measures. These two forms of reliability are called *relative reliability* and *absolute reliability* (also *association* and *concordance*), respectively. Alone, the Pearson product moment correlation (introduced in Chapter 23) is not a complete tool for documenting reliability because it assesses association and not concordance.

There are three strategies used by physical therapy researchers to supplement the information gained from the Pearson correlation coefficient: paired-*t* test, slope and intercept documentation, and determination of the standard error of measurement. They are all demonstrated in this section using a data sample representing repeated measures of 3-week ROM made by Therapists A and B at Clinic 3, as shown in Table 24–1. Therapist B consistently rates subjects higher than Therapist A—in fact, an average of 10.8° higher. The subject who scores highest for Therapist A also scores highest for Therapist B, even though the actual ROM scores differ on the basis of which therapist took the measure. Thus, the relative reliability is high, with a Pearson *r* of .977. However, to assume that the scores are interchangeable would clearly be incorrect given the 10.8° difference between therapist measures.

The first way to extend the reliability analysis beyond the Pearson measure of relative reliability is to conduct a paired-*t* test on the data. For our data, *t* is 8.11, with an associated probability of .000. This means that there is a very small chance that the difference between therapists scores occurred by chance, so we conclude that there is a significant difference between the

TABLE 24–1	Reliability Data for Three-Week Range-of-Motion Measurements by Therapists A and B		
Subject	Therapist A	Therapist B	Difference (B − A)
01	32	38	6
02	50	64	14
03	60	73	13
04	84	90	6
05	81	87	6
06	81	93	12
07	84	94	10
08	81	98	17
09	82	98	16
10	91	99	8
Σ	726.0	834.0	108.0
$\overline{X}$	72.6	83.4	10.8

scores of Therapist A and Therapist B. The scores from the two therapists are highly associated but lack concordance.

The second way to extend the reliability analysis beyond the Pearson measure is to generate a regression equation for the data and document the slope and intercept. If a measure is absolutely reliable, the slope will be close to 1.0 and the intercept will be close to 0.0.[1] In Figure 24–1, the dotted line represents perfect concordance between the two repeated measures, with a slope of 1.0 and an intercept of zero. The solid line represents a proportionate bias on the part of Rater 2. The intercept is still zero, but the slope exceeds 1.0. In Figure 24–2, the dotted line again represents perfect concordance between the two repeated measures, with a slope of 1.0 and an intercept of zero. The solid line represents an additive bias on the part of Rater 2, with scores consistently 5 points higher than Rater 1. The slope of this regression line is still 1.0, but the intercept is now 5.0.

For the Therapist A and B data, the slope is 1.0156 and the intercept is 9.666, as shown in Figure 24–3. This indicates the presence of a largely additive bias on the part of one of the therapists.

The third way to add to the usefulness of the Pearson product moment correlation for documenting reliability is to also report the standard error of measurement for the paired data. Using the formula presented in Chapter 17, we find that the standard error of measurement for this data is 2.96, meaning that a 95% confidence interval would be $\pm 5.8°$ (2.96×1.96), permitting us to be 95% confident that repeated measures would fall within 11.6° of one another.

The results of an extended Pearson reliability analysis might be written up as follows:

DATA ANALYSIS

To assess the association between the two therapists' scores, the Pearson product moment correlation was calculated. The concordance of the scores was assessed by calculation of the slope and intercept of the regression equation of one therapist's

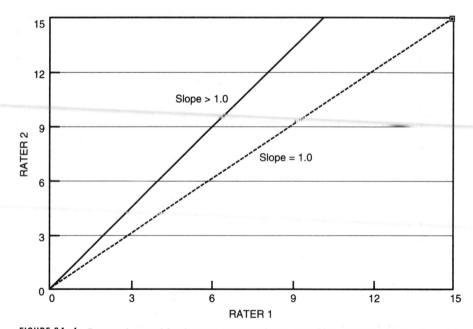

FIGURE 24–1. Proportionate bias between raters is revealed by a slope greater than 1.0. Dotted line represents perfect agreement with a slope of 1.0 and an intercept of 0.0.

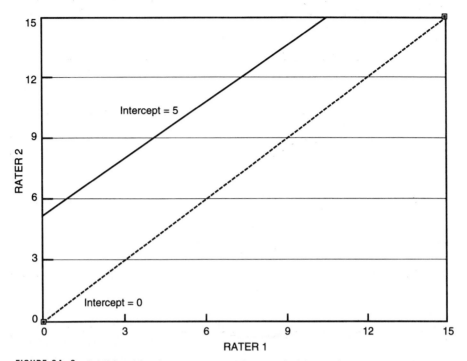

FIGURE 24–2. Additive bias between raters is revealed by an intercept equal to 5.0. Dotted line represents perfect agreement with a slope of 1.0 and an intercept of 0.0.

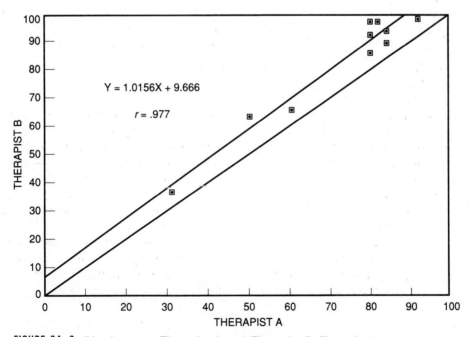

FIGURE 24–3. Bias between Therapist A and Therapist B. There is almost no proportionate bias (slope = 1.0156), but there is a large additive bias (intercept = 9.666°).

scores on the other, determination of the standard error of measurement (SEM), and calculation of a paired-t test.

RESULTS

The Pearson r was found to be .977, indicating a high degree of association between the scores of the two therapists. However, the slope was 1.02 and the intercept was 9.67. The SEM was ±5.8°. The paired-t test revealed that the 10.8° mean difference between therapist scores was statistically significant at the .000 level.

DISCUSSION

Despite the high degree of association between the measures taken by Therapist A and Therapist B, the absolute difference between scores means that the interrater reliability is too low to permit viewing the measures of the two therapists as interchangeable.

Readers should recognize that researchers would probably not use all three extensions in a single study. Any one of these extensions in this case

would be sufficient to cast doubt on the absolute reliability of the measures.

Intraclass Correlation Coefficients

The intraclass correlation coefficients (ICCs) are a family of coefficients that allow comparison of two or more repeated measures. The technique depends on repeated measures analysis of variance (ANOVA). There are at least six different ICC formulas, and the issue of which one to use in a particular calculation has generated considerable confusion.[2,3] Table 24–2 provides two of the formulas and indications for their use, based on the work of Shrout and Fleiss.[4] In addition to being able to handle more than two repeated measures, the ICC is said by some to be a better measure than the Pearson r because it accounts for absolute as well as relative reliability. Delitto and Strube believe that the ICCs take into account "level" differences, but are not true measures of concordance.[1] Thus, researchers who report reliability on the basis of an ICC should still report the results of an absolute reliability indicator such as the SEM or the repeated measures ANOVA.

For our example of the interrater reliability between Therapists A and B at Clinic 3, the ICC (2,1)

TABLE 24–2 Calculations of Intraclass Correlation Coefficients (ICCs)

Source of Variation	Degrees of Freedom	Mean Square (MS)
Between subjects	$N^* - 1$	Between subjects (BMS)
Within subject	$N(K^\dagger - 1)$	Within subject (WMS)
Between judges	$K - 1$	Between judges (JMS)
Error	$(N - 1)(K - 1)$	Error (EMS)

Formula	Appropriate Use
$ICC\,(1,1) = \dfrac{BMS - WMS}{BMS + (K - 1)\,WMS}$	Each subject is rated by different randomly selected judges.
$ICC\,(2,1) = \dfrac{BMS - EMS}{BMS + (K - 1)\,EMS + \dfrac{K(JMS - EMS)}{N}}$	Each subject is rated by the same randomly selected judges.

*Subjects.
†Judges.

may be most appropriate because the two therapists in question were selected from a larger group of therapists at the clinic, both measured each patient, and the results are to be generalized to other randomly selected judges rather than just applied to the two therapists in question. Table 24–3 shows the ICC (2,1) calculation to be .854. This is less than the .977 that was calculated with the Pearson product moment correlation, but it still would generally be interpreted to be a fairly high level of correlation. Thus, it is useful to examine the results of a repeated measures ANOVA, which shows that there is a significant difference between the measures of the two therapists, $F_{1,9} = 65.7$, $p = .000$. Using the repeated measures ANOVA results with an ICC is analogous to using a paired-t test to extend the results of a Pearson product moment correlation reliability analysis.

Although this example of an ICC used only two raters to compare the results with those found with the Pearson product moment correlation analysis in the previous section, the ICC, like the ANOVA it is based on, extends easily to accommodate more than two raters. When only two raters are present, the researcher has a choice between the Pearson and an ICC; when three or more raters measure each subject, an ICC must be used.

Watkins and associates studied intertester reliability of measurements of knee ROM.[5] Fourteen different raters were involved in the study, with each subject being measured by a randomly selected pair of raters. The ICC (1,1) they used for analysis seems appropriate for their design, in which raters for each subject were selected randomly.

Diamond and associates studied intertester reliability of diabetic foot evaluation.[6] In this study, only two raters were involved; each measured every subject. Thus, the ICC (2,1) they used seems appropriate because their design meets the criterion that each subject be assessed by the same raters.

Kappa

Kappa is a reliability coefficient designed for use with nominal data. Suppose that we wanted to determine whether Therapists A and B at Clinic 3 agreed with each other on the stair-climbing ability of their patients. Table 24–4 shows the cross-tabulation of the data of Therapists A and B. For 6 of the 10 patients, the therapists gave identical scores. For 4 of the 10 patients, the therapists differed by one category. The simplest

---

TABLE 24–3	ICC (2,1) Calculation for Three-Week Range of Motion for Therapists A and B			
Source of Variation	Degrees of Freedom	Mean Square (MS)	F	p
Between subjects	9	734.78 (RMS)		
Within subjects	10	66.30 (WMS)		
Between judges	1	583.20 (JMS)	65.7	.000
Error	9	8.87 (EMS)		

$$\text{ICC (2,1)} = \frac{\text{BMS} - \text{EMS}}{\text{BMS} + (\text{K} - 1)\ \text{EMS} + \dfrac{\text{K}^\dagger(\text{JMS} - \text{EMS})}{\text{N}^*}}$$

$$\text{ICC (2,1)} = \frac{734.78 - 8.87}{734.78 + (2 - 1)\ 8.87 + \dfrac{(2)\ (583.20 - 8.87)}{10}} = .854$$

*Subjects.
†Judges.

TABLE 24-4	**Kappa Correlation Calculation**				
	Therapist A				
Therapist B	**5**	**4**	**3**	**2**	**Total**
5	2 (.20) [.12]	1			3 (.30)
4	2	3 (.30) [.20]			5 (.50)
3			1 (.10) [.02]		1 (.10)
2				1	1 (.10)
Total	4 (.40)	4 (.40)	2 (.20)		10 (1.0)

$$\kappa = \frac{p_0 - p_c}{1 - p_e} = \frac{.60 - .34}{1 - .34} = .3939$$

p_0 = sum of the observed probabilities in perfect agreement = .60
p_c = sum of the chance probabilities for perfect agreement = .34

Note: Numbers are the number of observations in the cell. Numbers in parentheses are the proportion of observations in the cell. Numbers in brackets are the proportion of observations expected by chance in the cell. The proportion expected by chance is calculated by multiplying the marginal proportion (total row or column) for the corresponding row and column.

way to express the degree of concordance between the therapists' observations is to calculate the percentage of patients on whose ability the two therapists agreed completely. For this example, the agreement is 60%. However, because there are only a few nominal categories, there is a high probability that some of the agreements occurred by chance. The kappa correlation coefficient adjusts the agreement percentage to account for chance agreements, as shown in the formula at the bottom of Table 24–4.[7] The kappa for this example is .3939.

Kappa can also be weighted to account for the seriousness of the discrepancy.[8] Consider one disagreement in which one rater scores the patient as a 5 in stair climbing (reciprocal, no railing) and the other scores the patient as a 4 (reciprocal, with rail). Contrast this with a disagreement between a 4 and a 3 (one at a time, with or without rail). Some therapists might believe that disagreement on the use of a rail is a less serious reliability problem than disagreement about whether the patient can maneuver the stairs reciprocally. A weighted kappa allows

the researcher to establish different weights for different disagreements. In addition to occurring in weighted and nonweighted forms, kappa can be extended to more than two raters.[9]

Van Dillen and colleagues studied the reliability of physical examination items used for classification of patients with low back pain.[10] Many of the items required patients to report whether their symptoms were the same, decreased, or increased in response to a particular movement. Other items described alignment and movement, scoring the items as "yes" or "no" based on whether a patient exhibited the various alignment or movement patterns. Because these scoring systems are nominal, the authors used kappa to determine reliability. For the symptom behavior items the agreement percentage ranged from 98% to 100% and the corresponding kappas ranged from .87 to 1.00. For the alignment and movement variables the agreement percentage ranged from 55% to 100% and the corresponding kappas ranged from .00 to .78. Landis and Koch described the strength of agreement of kappa to be slight for kappas between .00 and .20, fair for kappas between .21 and .40, moderate for between .41 and .60, substantial between .61 and .80, and almost perfect for .81 to 1.00.[11] According to these descriptors, Van Dillen and colleagues found almost perfect correlations for the symptom behavior items, but wide variation in the strengths of agreement (from slight to substantial) for the alignment and movement variables.

MULTIPLE REGRESSION

Multiple regression techniques are designed to analyze complex relationships among many different variables. The classic use of multiple regression uses numerical independent variables to predict a numerical dependent variable.[12] In our example, gait velocity is a continuous numerical variable that is appropriate for analysis with multiple regression. Many of the independent variables we might use in this equation would also be numerical variables such as age, height, leg length, and weight. In addition to these variables, however, we might also wish to include some nominal independent variables such as gender (male, female) or postoperative complications (yes, no). Even though multiple regression techniques were designed for use with numerical variables, they can accommodate nominal independent variables if a different number is assigned to each of the nominal levels. For example, the presence of a postoperative complication might be entered as a "1" whereas the absence of a complication would be entered as a "0." This process of assigning arbitrary numbers to nominal independent variables is called *dummy coding*.

In Chapter 23 simple linear regression was used to predict 6-month gait velocity (the dependent variable) from 3-week ROM of patients after total knee arthroplasty. A regression equation was calculated, but it was not very precise, with 3-week ROM accounting for only 31% of the variability in gait velocity. Clearly, there are factors other than 3-week ROM that must account for the gait velocity of these patients.

Because the prediction of gait velocity from 3-week ROM is not precise enough to be useful clinically, the next logical step is to add an additional variable or variables to the equation to determine whether the prediction can be made more precise. For example, suppose we add patients' age to the equation. The general prediction equation for multiple regression is

$$Y = b_1X_1 + b_2X_2 + b_iX_i + a$$

For each independent variable there is a corresponding slope, which is referred to in multiple regression as a *b-weight*. For the entire equation there is one intercept, which is referred to as the *constant*. The computer-generated regression equation for 3-week ROM and age as predictors of gait velocity is

(velocity) = .04 (3-week ROM) − 1.41 (age) + 227.04

A 65-year-old patient with 70° of motion 3 weeks postoperatively would be predicted to have a gait velocity of 138.19 cm/s 6 months postoperatively:

.04 (70) − 1.41 (65) + 227.04 = 138.19

The correlation between all the independent variables and the dependent variable in a multiple regression equation is represented by R, to distinguish it from r, the correlation between the two variables in a simple linear regression equation. For this equation the multiple correlation, R, is .77483 and the R^2 is .55477. This means that the combination of 3-week ROM and age accounts for 55% of the variability in gait velocity. Recall that 3-week ROM alone accounted for only 31% of the variability in gait velocity. The addition of age to the equation has greatly improved its predictability.

Variable Entry in Multiple Regression

When performing a multiple regression, researchers often specify various decision rules to guide the computer in generating the regression equation. The rules are generally constructed so that the method of variable entry maximizes the accuracy of predictions while minimizing the number of variables in the equation. Variables are retained in the equation if they improve the R^2 by a specified amount or if they are associated with a probability of some specified amount.

In a forward regression strategy, a researcher adds one variable at a time and stops when additional variables do not contribute the preset amount. In a backward regression strategy, the researcher begins with all the possible variables of interest in the equation and deletes them one at a time if their presence does not contribute the preset amount. A stepwise regression strategy combines forward and backward procedures to generate the equation. If any of these strategies were used in our example, the age variable would be entered first, and the 3-week ROM variable would not be entered because it contributes so little beyond that of age. For example, the R^2 associated with age alone is .55432; for age and 3-week ROM combined, it is only .55477, an increase of only .00045. This means that the addition of 3-week ROM to the equation adds only .045% of additional predictability for gait velocity. Clinically, this means that if our interest is primarily in predicting gait velocity, we can eliminate the possibly inconvenient and expensive measurement of 3-week ROM and substitute the inexpensive, easily obtained age value.

Interpretation of the Multiple Regression Equation

The meaningfulness of the multiple regression equation can be assessed in several ways. First, an F test of R^2 can be conducted to determine whether it is significantly different from zero. For our example the computer-generated significance of the F test is .0000, indicating that there is a very low probability that the R^2 of .55477 was obtained by chance.

The second way to assess the meaningfulness of a multiple regression equation is to generate a confidence interval. The computer-generated standard error of the estimate (SEE) for the multiple regression equation is 20.03 cm/s, and a 95% confidence interval would add and subtract 39.27 cm/s to the predicted Y value [±1.96 (SEE)]. Thus, we could be 95% certain that our 65-year-old patient with 70° of knee flexion 3 weeks postoperatively would have a 6-month gait velocity of 98.92 to 177.46 cm/s. Recall that the 95% confidence interval for the simple regression of gait velocity on range of motion was 86.96 to 183.16 cm/s, as presented in Chapter 23. Because a greater proportion of the variability in gait velocity is accounted for by the multiple regression compared with the simple regression, this multiple regression interval is somewhat narrower than the simple regression interval.

A third way to evaluate the regression equation is to determine the relative contribution of each of the variables to the equation. This can be done by either conducting a t test of the contribution of each variable or dividing the R^2 into the components attributable to each variable. This division is done through beta (β)-weights, which are standardized versions of b-weights. The beta-weight for each variable is multiplied by the correlation coefficient between that variable and the dependent variable. For our example, the mathematical notation is

$$R^2 = (\beta_{\text{3-week ROM}})\,(r_{\text{3-week ROM, velocity}}) + (\beta_{\text{age}})\,(r_{\text{age, velocity}})$$

Using computer-generated beta-weights and correlation coefficients, we find the following:

$$.5547 = (.0305)\,(.5545) + (-.7224)\,(-.7445) = .0169 + .5378$$

This means that of the 55% of the variability in gait velocity predicted by the equation, almost 54% is due to the relationship between age and gait velocity and less than 2% is due to the relationship between 3-week ROM and velocity. The *t* tests of the contribution of variables yield significance levels of .8711 for 3-week ROM and .0006 for age. Both the division of R^2 and the *t* tests indicate that age is a much more important predictor of gait velocity than is 3-week ROM.

Recall that in the simple linear regression of gait velocity on 3-week ROM, the ROM variable accounted for approximately 31% of the variability in gait scores. How is it that it now accounts for only 2% of that variability? The answer can be found in an examination of the interrelationships among all three variables. The Venn diagrams in Figure 24–4 illustrate this principle. Independently, 3-week ROM accounts for about 31% of the variability in gait velocity, as shown in Figure 24–4A. Independently, age accounts for

about 55% of the variability in gait velocity, as shown in Figure 24–4B. In addition, age and 3-week ROM are highly related, with one variable accounting for approximately 53% ($r_{\text{age, 3-week ROM}} = -.7253$) of the variability in the other, as shown in Figure 24–4C. When all three are examined together, almost all of the variability in velocity that is accounted for by 3-week ROM is also accounted for by the relationship between age and velocity. Thus, in the regression of gait velocity on both age and 3-week ROM, the latter assumes much less importance than when it is the sole variable used to predict gait velocity. The results of this multiple regression analysis might be written up in a journal article as follows:

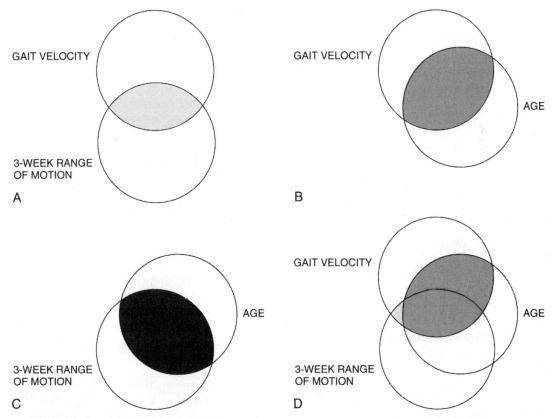

FIGURE 24–4. **A.** Relationship between gait velocity and 3-week range of motion. **B.** Relationship between gait velocity and age. **C.** Relationship between 3-week range of motion and age. **D.** Relationship of both age and 3-week range of motion to gait velocity. Most of the variability in gait velocity accounted for by 3-week range of motion is also accounted for by age.

DATA ANALYSIS

Simple linear regression of gait velocity on 3-week range of motion (ROM) was used initially to test whether early ROM status could be used to predict eventual function as measured by gait velocity. Multiple regression was used to add the variable of age to the prediction equation when 3-week ROM proved to be an inadequate independent predictor. The significance of each variable was determined with a t test, the significance of R^2 was determined with an F test, and alpha was set at .05. In addition, confidence intervals around the predicted Y value were generated.

RESULTS

For the simple regression of gait velocity on 3-week ROM, the r was only .5545. Although significantly different from zero ($p = .0015$), this means that only 30.75% of the variance in gait velocity was accounted for by 3-week ROM. The 95% confidence interval around the predicted gait velocity score for a given individual would require that 48.09 cm/s be added to and subtracted from the predicted score.

To enhance predictability, a multiple regression equation was developed to predict gait velocity from both 3-week ROM and age. The equation developed from the two predictor variables was Velocity = .04 (3-week ROM) − 1.41 (age) + 227.04. The R^2 for this equation was .5547 and was significant at $p = .0000$. The contribution of age was .5378 and was significant at $p = .0006$, the contribution of 3-week ROM was only .0169 and was not significant at $p = .8711$. For this equation, the 95% confidence interval around the predicted gait velocity score for a given individual would require that 39.27 cm/s be added to and subtracted from the predicted score.

DISCUSSION

The simple regression of gait velocity on 3-week ROM did not confirm the clinical observation that early ROM status is a good predictor of eventual gait outcome. When age was added to the equation, prediction of gait velocity improved. However, the very strong relationship between age and gait velocity meant that the contribution of 3-week ROM to prediction of gait velocity became insignificant when age was included in the equation. Thus, for this group of patients, eventual gait velocity can be predicted almost as well by age alone as by the combination of age and 3-week ROM.

Literature Example

Andrews and associates used stepwise multiple regression to develop prediction equations for muscle force for dominant and nondominant sides.[13] The independent variables they used for these predictions were gender, weight, and age. Because gender is a nominal variable, dummy codes (0 = male, 1 = female) were assigned so that it could be included in the analysis. The multiple R^2 associated with the different muscle groups ranged from .389 for ankle dorsiflexion on the nondominant side to .770 for shoulder medial rotation on the nondominant side. Thus, they found that they could predict between 39% and 77% of the variability in muscle force on the basis of these three easily collected variables (gender, weight, and age).

■ LOGISTIC REGRESSION

Multiple regression procedures, as described previously, can provide useful information for predicting numerical dependent variables. However, therapists are often interested in predicting dichotomous outcomes, such as whether or not a patient achieves independence or whether or not a patient returns home following rehabilitation. For example, we might be interested in determining what factors predict the need for an assistive device 6 months after total knee arthroplasty surgery.

Rationale for Logistic Regression

Using the data set originally presented in Chapter 20, we find that almost 100% of patients in their 40s and 50s, 57% in their 60s, 22% in their 70s, and 0% in their 80s and 90s are independent in gait without an assistive device. Figure 24–5 illustrates these data conceptually with a smoothed line representing the approximate relationship between age and use of gait devices 6 months after total knee arthroplasty. It is obvious that the relationship between these two factors is not linear. Rather, it remains at a high level in the younger age ranges, drops off rapidly for the intermediate ages, and then bottoms out at a low level for the older age ranges.

This S-shaped curve is typical of the relationship between a dichotomous variable and a continuous variable. Because the relationship is nonlinear, standard linear correlation and re-

gression techniques are not appropriate and techniques that use logarithmic and exponential transformations of the data are used instead.[14] The general technique that is used to predict dichotomous outcomes from numerical independent variables is called *logistic regression*.

Literature Examples

In the rehabilitation literature logistic regression has been used to examine the factors that predict falls among the elderly. Because of the complex mathematical transformations involved in logistic regression, the presentation of results can be confusing and a full discussion is beyond the scope of this text. However, readers should know that there are two common ways of presenting the results of logistic regression: with odds ratios for the variables within the logistic regression equation or by presenting the equation itself.

For example, Berg and associates used logistic regression to determine the extent to which a variety of factors could predict multiple falls versus single or no falls (over a 12-month period of time) in a group of elderly individu-

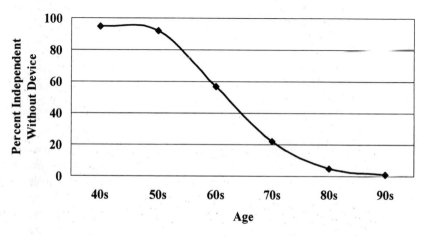

FIGURE 24–5. Graph illustrates the nonlinear, S-shaped curve that describes the relationship between a continuous variable (age) and a dichotomous variable (independence without an assistive device).

als.[15] The analysis showed that Berg Balance Scale scores, a history of falls in the 3 months prior to the initiation of the study, and visual problems were significant predictors of fall status during the study. By reporting the odds ratios associated with each independent variable and the dependent variable of fall status, the authors showed that individuals with a history of falls in the past 3 months were 5.75 times as likely to have multiple falls as those without such a history and individuals with visual problems were 2.80 times as likely to have multiple falls as those without visual problems. The odds ratio for the Berg Balance Scale scores, .90, was less than 1.0, indicating an inverse relationship. That is, individuals with lower Berg Balance Scale scores were more likely to sustain multiple falls.

Shumway-Cook and her colleagues also used logistic regression to analyze the relationships among falls and a variety of other factors.[16] Rather than presenting their results as odds ratios, they chose to provide readers with the actual logistic regression equation and with some sample predictions from the equations. By doing so, they help readers get past the complex equation that results from any logistic regression to see the implications of the equation. They showed that solving the equation for an individual without a history of imbalance and a Berg Balance Scale score of 54 would result in a prediction of a 5% probability of falling. They also solved their equation for an individual with a history of imbalance and a Berg Balance Scale score of 42 to show a predicted 91% probability of falling.

■ FACTOR ANALYSIS

Factor analysis is a tool whereby correlational techniques are used to discover which of many variables cluster together as a related unit, separate from other, unrelated clusters. It is a data reduction technique in which many variables are grouped into a smaller number of related groups.

Factor analysis is generally done for one of three reasons: test development, theory development, or theory testing. In test development, factor analysis is often used to help reduce a great number of items into a smaller number. Factor analysis groups items that are related to one another, and the test developer can then select certain questions from each factor for inclusion in the final version of the test. In theory development, factor analysis is used to examine the underlying structure of a set of variables about which the researcher has not developed a conceptual framework. The factors that emerge are then examined and named by the researcher, who then develops hypotheses about interrelationships among the factors. In theory testing, items thought to be representative of certain constructs are factor analyzed to determine whether the items load as hypothesized.

In our sample data set, 12 different pieces of data are recorded for each patient at 6 months postoperatively:

One ROM measure

Two muscle strength measures

Four deformity measures

Four activities of daily living (ADL) measures

One gait velocity measure

A theoretical grouping of these variables might be according to impairment and disability, as defined by the World Health Organization.[17] The impairment variables relate to abnormal structures and would include the ROM measure, the strength measures, and the deformity measures. The disability variables relate to abnormal performance of activities and in this example would include the ADL measures and gait velocity. Researchers might hypothesize that if impairment and disability are truly different constructs, then a factor analysis of the 12 variables would yield one factor that consists of the impairment variables and one factor that consists of the disability variables.

Factor Analysis Steps

The result of a factor analysis of these 12 variables is presented here. The mathematical basis of factor analysis has been presented well by others and is therefore omitted so that emphasis may be placed on interpretation rather than calculation.[18] In brief, the steps in a factor analysis are as follows:

1. A group of variables is analyzed for interrelationships.
2. The number of important underlying factors is determined by reviewing eigenvalues associated with each factor.
3. Factors are extracted.
4. The factor solution is rotated to maximize differences between the factors.
5. Rotated factor loadings are examined to determine a simple structure.
6. The resulting factors are interpreted.

Let's examine these steps in sequence for the 12 six-month variables. First, a correlation matrix is developed, as shown in Table 24–5. In this example, the matrix has been set up so that the theorized impairment and disability variables are close to one another. If we examine the last five columns of the matrix, which consists of the theorized disability variables, we find that they are all fairly highly correlated with the ROM and strength variables (Rows 1 through 3) and with the other disability variables (Rows 8 through 11). They are minimally correlated with the deformity variables (Rows 4 through 7). Although we can visually detect some patterns within the relationships among variables, the matrix is far too complex for simple visual analysis; hence, there is need for a mathematical tool like factor analysis.

The second step of a factor analysis is to determine the number of factors in the solution. Initially, the variables in the factor analysis problem are used to create the same number of factors. Each factor has an associated eigenvalue, which is related to the percentage of variability within the data set that can be accounted for by the factor. Some factors will account for very little variance and are therefore eliminated from the analysis. One convention for determining the number of factors in the solution is that only factors with eigenvalues of greater than 1.0 are retained. Another method is the scree method, which examines the pattern of eigenvalues

---

TABLE 24-5 **Correlation Matrix for 12-Variable Factor Analysis**

	F	E	DFC	DVV	DML	DAP	V	ADW	AAD	ASC	ARC
M6R	.56	.59	−.17	−.23	.11	−.15	.63	.68	.70	.71	.65
F		.95	−.19	.19	.04	−.05	.89	.72	.69	.75	.81
E			−.13	.24	.03	−.09	.90	.70	.65	.75	.79
DFC				.46	.45	.14	−.22	−.34	−.26	−.21	−.24
DVV					.27	−.01	.17	−.10	−.19	−.01	.02
DML						.45	−.07	−.16	−.10	−.12	.02
DAP							−.17	−.06	.02	−.17	.12
V								.80	.75	.82	.85
ADW									.83	.78	.81
AAD										.83	.81
ASC											.82

Note: M6R = 6-month range of motion; F = flexion torque; E = extension torque; DFC = deformity–flexion contracture; DVV = deformity–varus/valgus angulation; DML = deformity–mediolateral instability; DAP = deformity–anteroposterior instability; V = gait velocity; ADW = activities of daily living (ADL)–distance walked; AAD = ADL–assistive device; ASC = ADL–stair climbing; ARC = ADL–rising from chair.

graphically.[18(p635)] When a researcher is testing a theory, the number of factors he or she retains may simply be the number of theorized factors.

The factor analysis of our 12 variables shows that three factors had eigenvalues greater than 1.0; the scree method would retain either two or three factors, and our theoretical model predicted two factors. For the purpose of this example, then, two factors are selected for extraction, the third step in factor analysis. Terms that describe different extraction techniques are *principal components extraction, image factoring,* and *alpha factoring,* among others.

The fourth step in factor analysis is to rotate the factors. In essence, rotation can be thought of as resetting the zero point within the factor analysis. Doing so maximizes the appearance of differences between factors. Terms that describe different types of rotation techniques are *orthogonal, oblique, varimax,* and *quartimax,* among others. Once rotation has occurred, one speaks in terms of "factor loadings" rather than "correlation." A factor loading is essentially the correlation between each variable within a factor and the entire factor. Table 24–6 shows the rotated factor loadings determined by the factor analysis.

The fifth step in factor analysis is to determine, if possible, a simple structure for the factors. A simple structure is developed when each variable is associated with only one factor. To determine a simple structure, the researcher decides to retain in each factor only those variables that loaded above some arbitrary point, often .30. In our example, if factor loadings above .30 are retained, the flexion contracture variable remains in both factors because its loading on Factor I is −.305 and its loading on Factor II is .71. Thus, to obtain a simple structure for this analysis, we need to adopt a more restrictive criterion for variable retention. If we adopt a criterion of .35, then a simple structure is created.

The final step in factor analysis is to name and interpret the factors. This is done according to the variables that were retained in each factor and is highly subjective. Researchers often name the factors in a manner consistent with the theoretical underpinnings of the study. Factor II in

TABLE 24-6	Rotated Factor Loadings	
Variable	**Factor I**	**Factor II**
V	.94	.10
ARC	.92	.12
ASC	.91	−.03
ADW	.89	−.12
F	.89	.20
E	.88	.24
AAD	.88	−.09
M6R	.76	−.05
DML	−.07	.77
DFC	−.30	.71
DVV	−.00	.71
DAP	−.10	.44
% of variance accounted for	53.7	16.6

Abbreviations: V = gait velocity; ARC = activities of daily living (ADL)–rising from chair; ASC = ADL–stair climbing; ADW = ADL–distance walked; F = flexion torque; E = extension torque; AAD = ADL–assistive device; M6R = 6-month range of motion; DML = deformity–mediolateral instability; DFC = deformity–flexion contracture; DVV = deformity–varus/valgus angulation; and DAP = deformity–anteroposterior instability.

our solution consists of the four deformity variables and could be named "Anatomical Impairment." This name lets the reader know that Factor I consists of a subgroup of the hypothesized construct of impairment. Factor I is more difficult to name, because it consists of a combination of functional, strength, and ROM variables. A name consistent with the theoretical underpinnings would be "Physiological Impairment and Disability." Table 24–7, a modified version of Table 24–6, illustrates how a simple structure with named factors might be presented. Once the factors are named, the implications of the factors are discussed by the researcher. The following is the interpretation of this factor analysis as it might be written in a journal article:

DATA ANALYSIS

Factor analysis with principal components extraction and orthogonal varimax rotation was used to

TABLE 24-7 Rotated Factor Loadings

Variable	Factor	
	I *Physiological* *Impairment* *and Disability*	*II* *Anatomical* *Impairment*
Gait velocity	.94	
ADL–rising from chair	.92	
ADL–stair climbing	.91	
ADL–distance walked	.89	
Flexion torque	.89	
Extension torque	.88	
ADL–assistive device	.88	
Six-month range of motion	.76	
Deformity–mediolateral instability		.77
Deformity–flexion contracture		.71
Deformity–varus/ valgus angulation		.71
Deformity–anteroposterior instability		.44

ADL = activities of daily living.

test whether variables loaded as predicted on two theorized factors. A simple structure was developed by including in each factor only those variables with rotated factor loadings higher than .35.

RESULTS

Table 24–7 shows the rotated factor loadings for the two-factor solution. The first factor included all the activities of daily living (ADL) variables, as well as the gait velocity, range of motion (ROM), and torque variables. The second factor included all the deformity variables. Factor I was labeled

Physiological Impairment and Disability and accounted for 53.7% of the variance; Factor II was labeled Anatomical Impairment and accounted for 16.6% of the variance.

DISCUSSION

Our results do not fully support the hypothesized distinction between impairment and disability because some of the impairment variables loaded with the disability variables. However, the impairment variables did split among the two factors according to a physiological/anatomical distinction. The solely anatomical impairment variables (the four measures of deformity) all loaded together and were separate from the other eight variables. This indicates that the actual anatomical alignment of the knees was not related to eventual functional recovery. The variables that are more representative of physiological function than anatomical structure (flexion and extension torque and flexion ROM) loaded with the disability variables of ADL status and gait velocity. These results suggest that the constructs of impairment and disability, as defined by the World Health Organization, are not completely valid for patients who have had total knee arthroplasty.

Literature Example

Jarus and Poremba used factor analysis to determine what factors might underlie a wide range of hand evaluation items.[19] Their analysis identified four factors, which they named Pinch, Grasp, Target Accuracy, and Activities of Daily Living. The authors believed that this set of factors could be used as the basis for developing a battery of hand function tests that would be more comprehensive than existing tests, none of which include items from all four factors.

■ SUMMARY

Advanced and special relationship analysis techniques are used to analyze more than two variables simultaneously or to analyze repeated measures of the same variable. Specialized reliability correlation coefficients, in which repeated measures of the same variable are analyzed, include the Pearson product moment correlation with extensions to evaluate the slope and intercept of an associated regression line; intraclass correlation coefficients based on analysis of variance techniques; and kappa, which is used with nominal data. Multiple regression is used to predict a numerical dependent variable from many different independent variables. Logistic regression is used to predict a nominal dependent variable from many different independent variables. Factor analysis is a correlational technique that is used to determine which of many variables cluster together as a related unit separate from other, unrelated clusters.

REFERENCES

1. Delitto A, Strube MJ. Reliability in the clinical setting. *Research Section Newsletter*. 1991;24(1):2–8.
2. Müller R, Büttner P. A critical discussion of intraclass correlation coefficients. *Stat Med*. 1994;13:2465–2476.
3. Krebs DE. Intraclass correlation coefficients: use and calculation. *Phys Ther*. 1984;64:1581–1589.
4. Shrout PE, Fleiss JL. Intraclass correlations: uses in assessing rater reliability. *Psychol Bull*. 1979;86:420–428.
5. Watkins MA, Riddle DL, Lamb RL, Personius WJ. Reliability of goniometric measurements and visual estimates of knee range of motion obtained in a clinical setting. *Phys Ther*. 1991;71:90–97.
6. Diamond JE, Mueller MJ, Delitto A, Sinacore DR. Reliability of a diabetic foot evaluation. *Phys Ther*. 1989;69:797–802.
7. Cohen J. A coefficient of agreement for nominal scales. *Educ Psychol Measure*. 1960;20:37–46.
8. Cohen J. Weighted kappa: nominal scale agreement with provision for scaled disagreement or partial credit. *Psychol Bull*. 1968;70:213–220.
9. Fleiss JL. Measuring nominal scale agreement among many raters. *Psychol Bull*. 1971;76:378–382.
10. Van Dillen LR, Sahrmann SA, Norton BJ, et al. Reliability of physical examination items used for classification of patients with low back pain. *Phys Ther*. 1998;78:979–988.
11. Landis JR, Koch GG. The measurement of observer agreement for categorical data. *Biometrics*. 1977;33:159–174.
12. Dawson-Saunders B, Trapp RG. *Basic and Clinical Biostatistics*. 2nd ed. Norwalk, Conn: Appleton & Lange; 1994:213–222.
13. Andrews AW, Thomas MW, Bohannon RW. Normative values for isometric muscle force measurements obtained with hand-held dynamometers. *Phys Ther*. 1996;76:248–259.
14. Elston RC, Johnson WD. *Essentials of Biostatistics*. 2nd ed. Philadelphia, Pa: FA Davis Co; 1994:255.
15. Berg KO, Wood-Dauphinee SL, Williams JI, Maki B. Measuring balance in the elderly: validation of an instrument. *Can J Public Health*. 1992;83(suppl 2):S7–S11.
16. Shumway-Cook A, Baldwin M, Polissar NL, Gruber W. Predicting the probability of falls in community-dwelling older adults. *Phys Ther*. 1997;77:812–819.
17. Jette AM. Diagnosis and classification by physical therapists: a special communication. *Phys Ther*. 1989;69:967–969.
18. Tabachnick BG, Fidell LS. *Using Multivariate Statistics*. 2nd ed. New York, NY: Harper & Row; 1989.
19. Jarus T, Poremba R. Hand function evaluation: a factor analysis study. *Am J Occup Ther*. 1993;47:439–443.

Being a Consumer

Locating the
Literature

Types of Information
Types of Professional Literature
Focused Literature Search
  Library Holdings
  Keyword Searches
  Subject Heading Searches
  Sample Search Results
  Holdings at Other Libraries
  Single-Journal Indexes
  Multiple-Journal Databases
  Search Steps
  MEDLINE
  Cumulative Index of Nursing and Allied
    Health Literature (CINAHL)

Dissertations and Theses
Conference Proceedings
Single Article
  Science Citation Index
  Related Record Searching
Relationships Among Search
  Tools
Ongoing Literature Search
Single-Journal Contents Scanning
Multiple-Journal Contents
  Scanning
Multiple-Journal Reviews
Focused Database Scanning
Obtaining Literature Items

Becoming an educated consumer of research literature is a goal for many students and professionals. Chapters 1 to 24 of this text presented the foundations of research design and analysis that are required for knowledgeable use of the literature. This chapter and the next are devoted to two important components of becoming an informed consumer of research. Strategies for locating the literature are presented in this chapter and strategies for reviewing and critiquing that literature are offered in Chapter 26.

To make advantageous use of research, one needs to know the different types of information that are available to physical therapy clinicians and researchers and in which of two broad categories of literature that information can be found. After a brief discussion of these preliminaries, this chapter details strategies for performing a focused, short-term literature search and for maintaining an ongoing search of the literature for material related to a topic of interest. Finally, suggestions are given for obtaining copies of literature items that are not in one's local library. Throughout the chapter, different search strategies are illustrated with a sample search of the literature on the use of continuous passive motion (CPM) in patients who have undergone total knee arthroplasty (TKA). Readers should recognize that they may need to modify the strategies in this chapter in response to the rapid pace of technological change in library and information services.

TYPES OF INFORMATION

The basic goal of any literature review is to discover what is known about a certain topic. Accomplishing this goal depends on at least four types of information about the topic: theory, facts, opinions, and methods. Some references provide primarily one type of information; others contain many different types of information. The physical therapy clinician who is interested in treating patients with CPM will likely want to know (1) theories about how CPM works; (2) factual information about protocols and results from other clinics; (3) opinions of therapists and surgeons about future directions for the clinical use of CPM; and (4) methods that others have used to measure the results of CPM use. The physical therapist who is planning to conduct research in the area of CPM use after TKA needs to (1) place the topic of CPM into a conceptual, theoretical context; (2) know the facts of previous investigations of CPM; (3) understand the opinions of other researchers about important areas still in need of study; and (4) be familiar with the methods others have used to measure and analyze data in previous studies.

TYPES OF PROFESSIONAL LITERATURE

The literature is divided broadly into primary and secondary sources. *Primary sources* are those in which the authors are providing the original report of research they have conducted. Commonly encountered primary sources include journal articles describing original research, theses and dissertations, and conference abstracts and proceedings. *Secondary sources* of information are those in which the authors summarize their own work or the work of others. Book chapters and journal articles that review the literature are considered secondary sources. Secondary sources are useful because they organize the literature for the reader and provide a ready list of primary sources on the topic of interest. However, practitioners who wish to make their own judgments about the credibility of the research must read the primary literature.

FOCUSED LITERATURE SEARCH

Physical therapy practitioners may wish to conduct a focused literature search to help them plan care for individual patients, evaluate existing programs, or develop research proposals. The focused search is conducted over a short period of time to meet a specific information need. In addition to their own books and journals collected over the years, practitioners initiating such a literature search have an array of tools and strategies at their disposal. Five different categories of search tools are described in this section: library holdings, single-journal indexes, multiple-journal databases, dissertation and thesis databases, and conference papers and proceedings databases. In addition, how to use an identified article to find other citations is explained.

Practitioners who use the library should also make use of a human resource: their librarian. Librarians are educated in the art and science of retrieving information and practitioners should not hesitate to ask for their assistance as they plan and implement their literature searches.

Library Holdings

Library holdings are typically accessed through an online catalog that indexes books, conference proceedings published as books, audiovisual materials, dissertations and theses, and the titles of journals held by the library. This online catalog is accessible at the library and may be accessible from any location through an Internet connection. In addition, as is discussed later, many libraries subscribe to databases that also provide access to reference material available at other libraries.

Finding works of interest within the catalog is straightforward when users know the name of the author or the title of the work they wish to use. When specific authors or titles are not known, the user identifies works of interest by using either subject headings or keyword searches. Users need to know the distinction between subject headings and keywords so that they can take full advantage of the characteristics of each method of searching a card catalog.

KEYWORD SEARCHES. The collections of libraries with electronic catalogs can be searched by *keywords,* meaning any words that are found in the catalog's record of each volume. For example, in a recent search of an Indianapolis library, "continuous passive motion" was entered in a keyword search. The use of this keyword yielded a very valuable book authored by Robert Salter, one of the founding researchers in the area of CPM.[1] For this part of the sample search the keyword, or "free-text," method of searching led directly to a useful reference.

The problem with exclusive searching by keywords, however, is that there is limited control of synonyms. TKA procedures might be referred to as "total knee arthroplasty," "total knee replacement," and "artificial knee." In this sample search "artificial knee" as a keyword was entered and 17 references were identified. Unfortunately, only two of those references were from the 1990s. A researcher using only this keyword search would conclude—erroneously—that the library held few contemporary references about artificial knees.

An additional problem with keyword searches is that the specified words are not searched in context. This means that there are often false "hits" of references that are not relevant to the topic at hand. However, if at least one relevant reference is identified, the library user can review the complete record of that reference to find the subject headings under which it is indexed. One of the real strengths of keyword searching is that it can be an efficient route into a subject heading search.

SUBJECT HEADING SEARCHES. Library materials are organized by subject headings provided by the Library of Congress (Library of Congress Subject Headings) or the National Library of Medicine (Medical Subject Headings, or MeSH). Using subject headings for searches is known as "controlled vocabulary searching" because only specific words or phrases are recognized as subject headings. Although catalogs have cross-referencing systems to help users who search under nonstandard subject headings, valuable information is often missed by users who don't find the correct subject heading for their topic. A thesaurus of these subject headings should be available in the library, either in print or most likely online, to help the practitioner determine the terms under which the desired information is likely to be found.

In the sample search, two examples illustrate the advantages and disadvantages of subject heading searches. Using an outdated term, "artificial knee," as a subject heading yielded 8 unique references and a cross-reference to "total knee replacement." Of the 8 references under "artificial knee," only 1 was from the 1990s. Going to "total knee replacement" as suggested by the cross-reference yielded another 7 unique references, all of them from the 1990s. In this instance the cross-referencing feature of the subject headings helped identify appropriate, contemporary references.

In contrast, using the term "continuous passive motion" as a subject heading yielded no resources and no alternate terms. Looking up "continuous passive motion" in the MeSH thesaurus showed that the proper subject heading was "motion therapy, continuous passive." This subject heading yielded the Salter text identified earlier in the keyword search.[1] In this instance, the proper subject heading was neither obvious nor cross-referenced and most users would have missed the reference. Only those users who know to look up subject headings by hand—or who know to try a keyword search—would have found this reference. To avoid coming to a premature conclusion that a library does not hold the desired resources when an initial search strategy is not fruitful, users should conduct both subject heading and keyword searches, consult the thesaurus of subject headings if available, or seek assistance from a reference librarian.

SAMPLE SEARCH RESULTS. Searching the catalog of a particular library is limited in that the sources revealed are only as good as the collection of the library. However, even identification of a few key resources may lead to many others by examination of the references contained in each source. Table 25–1 shows how the identification of only two books led to 25 unique citations related to use of CPM after TKA. Of these 25 references, a good starting point for a researcher would be the seven sources that were cited within both book chapters. One obvious limitation to using library books to identify relevant primary references is that the references identified can be no more recent than the books that cite them.

HOLDINGS AT OTHER LIBRARIES. Recognizing that any one library is unlikely to hold all the desired resources, practitioners may expand their searches beyond the library walls to see what is available on a particular topic anywhere in the world. One way to do this is by searching, library-by-library, the online catalogs to which your home library has access. A more efficient way is to use a specific database, WorldCat, to simultaneously search for records of any type of material cataloged by libraries that are members of the Online Computer Library Center (OCLC). For example, searching WorldCat for English-language books on total knee replacement yielded 108 records. Each of the records includes a list of those libraries that hold the publication. With this information, the reference librarian at the home library can work with the patron to obtain an interlibrary loan of the desired item.

TABLE 25–1 **Use of Catalog of Library Holdings to Identify Literature Related to Continuous Passive Motion in Patients After Total Knee Arthroplasty**

Resource 1—Chapter within a book:
Robinson RP, Simonian PT, McCann KJ. Rehabilitation following total knee arthroplasty. In: Fu FH, Harner DC, Vince KG. *Knee Surgery*. Vol 2. Baltimore, Md: Williams & Wilkins; 1994:1409–1425.[2]

Relevant References: 9

Resource 2—Chapter within a book:
Salter RB. Clinical investigations by other clinicians. In: Salter RB. *Continuous Passive Motion (CPM): A Biological Concept for the Healing and Regeneration of Articular Cartilage, Ligaments, and Tendons: From Origination to Research to Clinical Applications*. Baltimore, Md: Williams & Wilkins; 1993:359–380.[1]

Relevant References: 23

Reference Summary:
25 unique references (7 references were cited in both chapters)
20 journal articles, 3 conference abstracts, 2 book chapters
7 published between 1990–1994, 12 between 1985–1989, 4 in 1984 or earlier

---

Single-Journal Indexes

Many professionals receive one or more journals regularly either as a benefit of belonging to a professional association or by subscribing to a journal of particular interest. One's own journals are a convenient starting point for a literature search. Most journals publish an annual subject and author index in the last issue of each volume. *Physical Therapy,* for example, publishes its annual index in each December issue and the *Journal of Orthopaedic and Sports Physical Therapy* publishes a 6-month index in every June and every December issue. Thus, readers with an interest in a particular topic can easily identify any pertinent citations from the journals in their own collection. Even if a professional decides not to retain all the journals he or she receives, this ready source of citations can be maintained by keeping at least the annual indexes from each journal. Some journals, including *Physical Therapy*, also publish cumulated indexes over several years.[3,4] Table 25–2 lists references on CPM and TKA that were identified through a review of the *Journal of Orthopaedic and Sports Physical Therapy* from 1994 through 1998.

Multiple-Journal Databases

References to articles in multiple journals, and sometimes the full text of the articles themselves, can be found by using various databases. Although most of these databases exist in hard copy as well as CD-ROM or online formats, the emphasis in this chapter is on searching the

---

TABLE 25–2 **Search Results from *Journal of Orthopaedic and Sports Physical Therapy*, 1994–1998**

Research Articles

Chiarello CM, Gundersen L, O'Halloran T. The effect of continuous passive motion duration and increment on range of motion in total knee arthroplasty patients. *J Orthop Sports Phys Ther*. 1997;25:119–127.[5]

Enloe LJ, Shields RK, Smith K, Leo K, Miller B. Total hip and knee replacement treatment programs: a report using consensus. *J Orthop Sports Phys Ther*. 1996;23:3–11.[6]

Conference Presentation Abstracts

Montgomery F, Eliasson M. Continuous passive motion compared to active physical therapy after knee arthroplasty: similar hospitalization times in a randomized study of 68 patients [abstract]. *J Orthop Sports Phys Ther*. 1996;24:48.[7]

Ververeli PA, Sutton DC, Hearn SL, Booth RE, Rothman RH. A prospective study of continuous passive motion after total knee arthroplasty: analysis of cost and benefits [abstract]. *J Orthop Sports Phys Ther*. 1994;19:57.[8]

---

databases electronically. Not long ago, most computer searches of the literature were performed by librarians from keywords supplied by patrons. Today, most computerized databases are user-friendly and designed to be used by the patrons themselves. Several common steps should be taken when searching an electronic database.[9]

SEARCH STEPS. First, the practitioner defines the information need. For the sample search the need might be defined by the following question: What is known about the effect of continuous passive motion on recovery after total knee arthroplasty? Second, the practitioner breaks the need into components. For the sample search the two main components are "continuous passive motion" and "total knee arthroplasty."

Third, the practitioner identifies synonyms for each concept. As was the case with library catalog searching, users can choose to search by subject heading or by keyword. Many databases include accurate subject headings at the bottom of each reference. This enables a person to start with a keyword search and use the information provided to refine the search by using standardized subject headings.

Fourth, the practitioner constructs logical relationships among the concepts, using the terms "AND," "OR," and "NOT." Figure 25–1 shows the relationships that are defined by the use of these terms. The use of "AND" narrows a search. In our example, searching for "continuous passive motion" AND "total knee arthroplasty" would yield only those articles containing both concepts. Another way of narrowing a search is to specify a "NOT" term. In our example, if we were not interested in TKA done for those with rheumatoid arthritis we could modify our search to look for "total knee arthroplasty" NOT "rheumatoid arthritis." This command lops off a portion of the search that is not of interest to the researcher. In contrast, the use of "OR" broadens a search to include articles that include at least one of the specified terms. If we were interested in reviewing articles documenting the use of CPM after anterior cruciate ligament reconstruc-

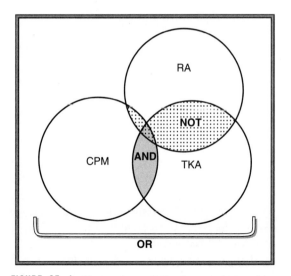

FIGURE 25–1. Illustration of Boolean relationships. Specifying "continuous passive motion (CPM) OR total knee arthroplasty (TKA)" would result in retrieval of articles in both circles, including the shaded intersection of both circles. Adding the command "NOT rheumatoid arthritis (RA)" would result in the elimination of all the stippled areas in the figure. Specifying "CPM AND TKA" would result in retrieval of articles in the shaded intersection of the two circles, including the stippled, shaded area. Specifying "CPM AND TKA NOT RA" would result in retrieval of articles in the shaded intersection, excluding the stippled, shaded region.

tion as well as after TKA, then we could specify the surgery term as "total knee arthroplasty" OR "anterior cruciate ligament reconstruction." The "AND," "OR," and "NOT" terms are known as Boolean operators, after a 19th-century logician named George Boole.[10]

Fifth, the practitioner may limit the search according to certain variables offered by the database. The most common ones are "language" and "year of publication." For example, many researchers restrict their searches to English language journals and to articles published in a certain time frame. A clinician planning a new program may scan the last 3 years of the database; a researcher who wishes to trace the history of a particular procedure may scan 20 years of a database.

For physical therapists the two major databases to consider are MEDLINE (or one of its hard copy components, *Index Medicus*) and the *Cumulative Index of Nursing and Allied Health* (CINAHL). Both are widely available in the academic libraries of institutions with physical therapy programs. The databases are supplied to libraries through various vendors or platforms, so the looks and features of the database vary from library to library, but the contents remain the same. Common vendors include OVID Technologies, OCLC FirstSearch, and SilverPlatter. Individual access to each of these databases is also available, as noted later in the chapter. Table 25–3 shows which of several journals of interest to physical therapists are indexed in each database. Readers should know that MEDLINE and CINAHL provide complete indexing of some of the journals and selective indexing of other journals. This means that even though, for example, both databases index the journal *Gerontologist*, different articles within this journal may be selected for inclusion in each of the databases. Because of the irregular overlapping of coverage within these two databases, users who wish to be as comprehensive as possible should search both databases. Even though many of the same articles are identified by both databases, each database typically identifies unique resources not identified by the other.

MEDLINE. MEDLINE is a comprehensive medically oriented online database compiled by the National Library of Medicine through its Medical Literature and Retrieval System (MEDLARS). The MEDLINE database, one of several MEDLARS databases, actually includes not only the *Index Medicus*, but also the *Index of Dental Literature*, and the *International Nursing Index*. The entries in the database are indexed according to the medical subject headings (MeSH) of the National Library of Medicine. Unfortunately, MeSH terms related to physical therapy are not always as specific as might be desired, as shown in Table 25–4. In addition to its widespread availability in academic libraries, free MEDLINE access, in formats known as PubMed and Internet Grateful Med, is available to anyone with an Internet con-

TABLE 25-3 Databases That Index Representative Journals of Interest to Physical Therapists

Journal	Database* MEDLINE	CINAHL	Journal	Database* MEDLINE	CINAHL
Acta Orthop Scand	✔	✔	J Orthop Sports Phys Ther	✔	✔
Am J Med	✔		J Phys Ther Educ		✔
Am J Occup Ther	✔	✔	J Rehabil		✔
Am J Phys Med Rehabil	✔	✔	J Rehabil Res Dev	✔	✔
Am J Physiol	✔		J Rheumatol	✔	
Am J Public Health	✔	✔	JAMA	✔	✔
Am J Surg	✔		Lancet	✔	✔
Ann Intern Med	✔	✔	Med Sci Sports Exerc	✔	✔
Arch Phys Med Rehabil	✔	✔	Muscle Nerve	✔	
Aust J Physiother		✔	N Engl J Med	✔	✔
BMJ	✔	✔	N Z J Physiother		✔
Br J Sports Med	✔	✔	Occup Ther Int		✔
Circulation	✔		Occup Ther J Res		✔
Clin Orthop	✔	✔	Orthop Clin North Am	✔	✔
Dev Med Child Neurol	✔	✔	Pediatr Phys Ther		✔
Electromyogr Clin Neurophysiol	✔		Pediatrics	✔	✔
Gerontologist	✔	✔	Percept Mot Skills	✔	
Issues Aging		✔	Phys Occup Ther Geriatr		✔
J Allied Health	✔	✔	Phys Occup Ther Pediatr		✔
J Am Geriatr Soc	✔	✔	Phys Ther	✔	✔
J Appl Physiol	✔		Phys Ther Case Rep		✔
J Biomech	✔		Phys Ther Rev		✔
J Bone Joint Surg Am	✔		Physiother Can		✔
J Burn Care Rehabil	✔	✔	Physiother Res Int	✔	✔
J Hand Surg Am	✔		Physiother Theory Pract		✔
J Hand Ther	✔	✔	Physiotherapy	✔	✔
J Head Trauma Rehabil		✔	PT—Magazine Phys Ther		✔
J Manipulative Physiol Ther	✔		S Afr J Physiother		✔
			Scand J Rehabil Med	✔	✔
			Science	✔	
J Neurosurg	✔		Spine	✔	✔

* Databases are MEDLINE and CINAHL (Cumulative Index of Nursing and Allied Health Literature). Coverage of the indicated journals is based on journal lists displayed through the respective web sites of MEDLINE (http://www.nlm.nih.gov) and CINAHL (http://www.cinahl.com). Both sites accessed March 9, 1999.

nection (http://www.nlm.nih.gov). The steps to and results of the sample search, done through MEDLINE, are shown in Table 25–5. Seven relevant articles were identified, two of which were also identified by the CINAHL search (discussed subsequently).

CUMULATIVE INDEX OF NURSING AND ALLIED HEALTH LITERATURE (CINAHL).

CINAHL was developed in 1956 to meet the needs of nonphysician health care practitioners. As illustrated in Table 25–3, many of the journals of interest to nurses and allied health professionals are not indexed in MED-

TABLE 25-4	Comparison of MeSH* and CINAHL† Terms Related to Physical Therapy

MeSH[11]	CINAHL[12]
Physical Therapy	Physical Therapy
Balneology	Baths
Ammotherapy	Drainage, Postural
Baths	Electrotherapy
Baths, Finnish	Electrical Stimulation
Mud Therapy	Functional Training
Cryotherapy	Gait Training
Cryosurgery	Home Physical Therapy
Drainage, Postural	Hydrotherapy
Electrical Stimulation Therapy	Aquatic Exercises
Electroacupuncture	Baths
Transcutaneous Electrical Nerve Stimulation	Hyperthermia, Induced
Exercise Therapy	Diathermy
Motion Therapy, Continuous Passive	Ultrasonic Therapy
Hydrotherapy	Infrared Therapy
Hyperthermia, Induced	Joint Mobilization
Ammotherapy	Massage
Diathermy	Oral Stimulation
Short-Wave Therapy	Pediatric Physical Therapy
Ultrasonic Therapy	Photochemotherapy
Manipulation, Orthopedic	PUVA Therapy
Manipulation, Spinal	Phototherapy
Massage	Prosthetic Fitting
Acupressure	Therapeutic Exercise
Myofunctional Therapy	Aerobic Exercise
Photochemotherapy	Aquatic Exercises
Hematoporphyrin Photoradiation	Breathing Exercises
PUVA therapy	Closed Kinetic Chain Exercises
Photopheresis	Conditioning, Cardiopulmonary
Phototherapy	Motion Therapy, Continuous Passive
Color Therapy	Muscle Strengthening
Heliotherapy	Isokinetic Exercises
Ultraviolet Therapy	Isometric Exercises
Rewarming	Isotonic Exercises
Thalassotherapy	Kegel Exercises
	Weight Lifting
	Neuromuscular Facilitation
	Open Kinetic Chain Exercises
	Plyometrics
	Ultraviolet Therapy

* National Library of Medicine Medical Subject Headings.

† Cumulative Index of Nursing and Allied Health Literature.

| TABLE 25-5 | Comparison of MEDLINE and CINAHL Searches |

SEARCH STRATEGY

		Number of Articles	
Steps	**Terms or Limits**	*MEDLINE*	*CINAHL*
Step 1	Continuous passive motion (CPM)	239	59
Step 2	Total knee arthroplasty (TKA)	1785	374
Step 3	CPM AND TKA	35	8
Step 4	LIMIT TO English	33	6
Step 5	LIMIT TO Publication Years 1996–1999	7	3

SEARCH RESULTS

Primary Author	**Journal, Date**	*MEDLINE*	*CINAHL*
Worland RL[13]	*J Arthroplasty*, October 1998	✔	
Yashar AA[14]	*Clin Orthop*, December 1997	✔	✔
Knight JL[15]	*Orthopedics*, November 1997	✔	
Pope RO[16]	*J Bone Joint Surg Br*, November 1997	✔	
Pham J[17]	*Am J Orthop*, February 1997	✔	
Chiarello CM[5]	*J Orthop Sports Phys Ther*, February 1997	✔	✔
Kumar PJ[18]	*Clin Orthop*, October 1996	✔	
Montgomery F[19]	*Acta Orthop Scand*, February 1996		✔

LINE. CINAHL provides a means to gain access to these journals. For example, the *Journal of Physical Therapy Education* and *Pediatric Physical Therapy* are not indexed in MEDLINE but are indexed in CINAHL. In addition to journals, CINAHL indexes books of interest to nurses and other health professionals and nursing dissertations. The CINAHL indexing terms are based on MeSH, but provide for greater specificity in the terms related to each profession represented in the index. Table 25–4 shows the MeSH and CINAHL terms used for physical therapy. CINAHL is available online by subscription to individual users. In 1999 rates ranged from as low as approximately $40 for about 20 hours of use per year to $700 for 400 hours of use (http://www.cinahl.com). Table 25–5 shows the steps to and results of the CINAHL search of the sample topic of CPM after TKA. Three relevant articles were identified, two of which were also identified by the MEDLINE search.

Dissertations and Theses

The research that students undertake as a requirement for completion of a master's or doctoral degree often is not published in the literature or is published several years after the master's thesis or doctoral dissertation has been filed with the university where the degree was completed. There are two effective ways to retrieve information on dissertations and theses. The first is to use the WorldCat database. Because dissertations and theses are generally held in the library of the institution offering the degree, and because most academic libraries participate in OCLC, this means that dissertation and thesis titles can be retrieved in a search of World-Cat. Two master's theses relevant to the sample search were identified by using the terms "continuous passive motion" and "total knee arthroplasty."[20,21] The second method is to search *Dissertation Abstracts*. Most doctoral programs and some master's degree programs require that students file a copy of the thesis or dissertation with University Microfilms International, which produces the index *Dissertation Abstracts*. Academic libraries generally maintain microfilm or computerized versions of the index. A computer search of *Dissertation Abstracts* for 1996 to 1998 identified one master's thesis related to continuous passive motion use in total knee arthroplasty[22] and several other master's theses and doctoral dissertations related to either CPM or TKA. Copies of the identified abstracts may be purchased from University Microfilms International (http://www.umi.com).

Conference Proceedings

As with dissertations and theses, research papers presented at conferences may not make it to the journal literature for several years, if at all. Access to abstracts of papers presented at conferences can often be obtained by reviewing the conference issue of journals of a particular society or association. For example, *Physical Therapy,* the American Physical Therapy Association's (APTA) journal, prints abstracts of presentations given at the Association's annual conference in a supplemental section of the May issue of the journal. At the APTA's 1998 Scientific Meeting and Exhibition, for example, the supplement shows that there was one paper presented on the topic of CPM after TKA.[23] In fact, this is a presentation of the master's thesis identified in *Dissertation Abstracts*. One sign that a comprehensive literature search is nearing completion is when redundancies among sources begin to appear.

A broader source of conference proceedings is the *Index of Scientific and Technical Proceedings* (ISTP). Published proceedings of selected conferences are indexed. The database is organized by conference sponsor, location, paper authors, geographical location of the authors, and organizational affiliation of the authors. Depending on one's interest and the information available, any of these items of information might be the starting point of a search of conference proceedings. Using the CD-ROM version of the ISTP, nine presentations related to CPM were identified in the 5-year period from 1994 through 1998. One of the presentations resulted in Yashar and associates' paper that had already been identified by the search.[14] Five of the papers were from a German conference on quality assurance in surgery, with one paper each on CPM and, respectively, ankle, knee, hip, elbow, and shoulder surgery. Although the average reader of the research on this topic would not be likely to follow up on this finding, a researcher deeply involved in evaluating the use of CPM might find it useful to make contact with the international colleagues who authored these presentations. An additional way to identify conference proceedings and conference papers is through OCLC's PapersFirst and ProceedingsFirst databases. In this example, the PapersFirst database identified a paper presentation that resulted in a publication by Ververeli and colleagues.[24] The presentation was at the February 1995 combined meeting of the Knee Society; Association for Arthritis, Hip, and Knee Surgery; and the Hip Society. The content of this presentation seems to be the same as the presentation abstract identified in the *Journal of Orthopaedic and Sports Physical Therapy* in 1994.[8] Once again, the multiple search sources are yielding redundant citations, indicating that the search is nearly complete.

Single Article

In addition to the five search tools just described, a single relevant journal article citation can be used in several different ways to identify other sources of information. It is possible to use a single article to work backward, forward, and sideways through the literature.[10(p108)] To work backward, one examines the reference list of the article and identifies relevant citations. This strategy can also be used with the reference lists of book chapters, conference proceedings, and dissertations and theses. The disadvantage of using this strategy is that it identifies only citations that are older than the source itself.

SCIENCE CITATION INDEX. Working forward through the literature from a single article, or from an influential author, can be accomplished with hard copy or electronic versions of the *Science Citation Index*. This index lists sources that have used a particular article as a reference or cited particular authors. A key citation or author is used to begin the forward search. For the sample search, we will use Salter as an author of interest since his work on CPM has been cited in many of the articles we have identified thus far in our CPM literature search. Using the computerized version of the Science Citation Index, the years from 1995 to 1998 were searched to find articles in which the work of Salter was cited. The results of this search are summarized in Table 25-6. Three relevant articles were identified through this process. Of the three, two had been identified in the MEDLINE and CINAHL searches. The third article, written by Ververeli and colleagues[24] is the published version of the conference paper identified earlier in the search.

RELATED RECORD SEARCHING. There are two ways of working sideways through the literature based on a single article. "Working sideways" means identifying additional citations that are contemporary to the original article. The first way is to call up the MEDLINE or CINAHL citation for the article and determine the subject headings under which it is indexed. Use of these terms in a new search is likely to yield related articles. The second way to work sideways takes advantage of "related-record" searching in some of the electronic databases. MEDLINE, for example, uses a complex algorithm to identify articles that are related in some way to a single article identified by the user. The algorithm includes things like shared title words, shared references, and shared subject headings. Doing a related-record search of the Chiarello[5] paper cited earlier yielded 123 related records in MEDLINE. Because they are arranged in order of relatedness, it is easy to scan down the list to determine the most relevant of the related citations.

Relationships Among Search Tools

Figure 25-2 summarizes the way in which the search tools and single-article strategies interrelate. Search tools, represented by the outer circle, are used to identify literature items. The literature items, represented as the inner circle, can then be used to identify other literature items. Practitioners conducting literature searches frequently use several strategies to identify all the literature of interest. When the citations identified by these different strategies become redundant, then the searcher can be confident that the most important references have been found.

ONGOING LITERATURE SEARCH

Regular consumers of the literature generally have developed strategies that enable them to identify articles of interest on a routine basis. Because of the enormous volume of clinical literature, practitioners must accept that they cannot remain up-to-date in all areas of their profession. Thus, the first element of an ongoing search strategy is to identify the specific topics in which one is most interested. Once these topics are selected, the basic strategies used for ongoing searches are single-journal contents scanning, multiple-journal contents scanning, multiple-journal reviews, and focused database scanning.

TABLE 25-6 Sample Use of Science Citation Index

What articles published in 1995–1998 have cited the work of SALTER–RB?
1998: 55 articles → 1 relevant to CPM after TKA (Yashar et al[14])
1997: 43 articles → 1 relevant to CPM after TKA (Pope et al[16])
1996: 51 articles → none relevant to CPM after TKA
1995: 57 articles → 1 relevant to CPM after TKA (Ververeli et al[24])

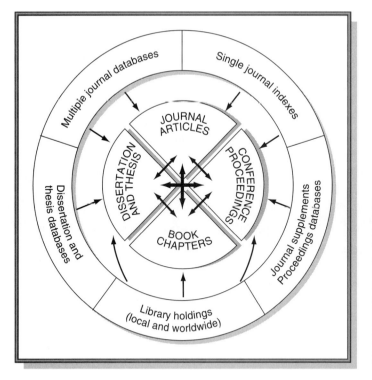

FIGURE 25–2. Relationship among search tools and types of professional literature. The search tools shown in the outer circle are used to identify relevant citations of the different literature types, as noted by the arrows. Once a citation is identified, its reference list can be used to identify other citations, as noted by the arrows between the pieces of the inner circle. For journal articles, additional tools such as citation indexes and related record searches can be used to identify other relevant sources.

Single-Journal Contents Scanning

The journals that arrive in a professional's mailbox each month can be a tremendous asset to the regular literature consumer. The most obvious resources in each journal are the articles in each issue. For a broadly ranging discipline like physical therapy, a general-interest journal such as *Physical Therapy* or *Physiotherapy Canada* may contain relatively few articles within the particular interest area of a reader. However, the regular reader of the literature should not limit his or her scanning to the articles portion of the journal's table of contents. Most journals publish book reviews and abstracts of relevant articles published in other journals. Both of these sections of the journal can point the reader to areas of interest not addressed in the present issue. In a book review it is often indicated whether the particular title being reviewed provides a thorough reference list, helpful information to the reader interested in acquiring other related citations.

Multiple-Journal Contents Scanning

Scanning the table of contents of several journals of interest is a second excellent way of keeping up with the literature outside the journals that one receives personally. Some libraries even provide a service in which the tables of contents of requested journals are sent to patrons when the journal arrives each month. This allows the consumer to scan the contents conveniently, marking for later review any articles that seem of interest. Literature consumers new to contents scanning may select a fairly large number of journals for initial scanning and reduce the number as it becomes apparent over time which journals most frequently publish articles in their area of interest.

Another way to scan new journal tables of contents is provided by a weekly publication called *Current Contents*. Different versions of this publication, such as *Current Contents: Life Sciences* or *Current Contents: Clinical Medicine*, compile and publish tables of contents from journals relevant to the version. This tool exists in hard copy and electronic formats, with institutional and individual subscription rates. *Current Contents: Clinical Medicine* contains many journals of interest to physical therapists including *Physical Therapy, Journal of Orthopaedic and Sports Physical Therapy, Archives of Physical Medicine and Rehabilitation, Journal of Bone and Joint Surgery* [American], and *Developmental Medicine and Child Neurology,* to name just a few of the approximately 1000 titles that are listed.[25]

Multiple-Journal Reviews

There are several reference products that not only inform the practitioner of new articles but also provide commentary to assist the practitioner in assessing the potential value of the articles. *Physical Therapy in Perspective* is one such product. Published six times per year, it presents detailed summaries of and brief commentaries on articles from a variety of journals of interest to physical therapists. Approximately 1000 journals are scanned and approximately 40 articles of special interest to physical therapists are abstracted in each issue. It exists in hard copy format and is available by subscription for institutions and individuals.[26]

The *ACP (American College of Physicians) Journal Club* provides a somewhat different method for gaining insight into the value of different journal articles.[27] The publication, produced in paper and electronic formats six times annually, uses stringent review methods to select articles for inclusion and provides commentary to help practitioners make "evidence-based" decisions about patient care. In contrast to the other scanning methods, the *ACP Journal Club* is the only publication that purports to evaluate the

materials in a systematic way. Although the topics included in the publication are based on the information needs of physicians, some articles of interest to physical therapists are included.

Focused Database Scanning

Regular scanning of relevant databases can be accomplished through regular visits to the library, with subscriptions to various affordable sources described in the chapter, and with use of information that is freely available through the Internet. The combination of focused database scanning, multiple-journal contents scanning, multiple-journal reviews, and single-journal contents scanning can provide the literature consumer with a solid base of literature in specific areas of interest.

■ OBTAINING LITERATURE ITEMS

If one's local library does not have a desired item, it can generally be obtained through one of six strategies: interlibrary loan, full text retrieval, document delivery systems, reprint from the author, purchase of the journal from the publisher, or use of one's network of professional colleagues. Interlibrary loan arrangements give the patron of one library access to the resources of many other libraries. The patron requests the item, and the librarian uses a computer network to determine the libraries that have the item. When a journal article is requested, the lending library usually furnishes a photocopy, often for a fee to cover photocopying and mailing.

A growing number of journals make the full text of articles available through the Internet, either directly from the journal's web site or with a link from an Internet database. For example, full text articles from *Physical Therapy* are now available through the APTA's web site (http://www.apta.org). Even easier access is provided to Internet users of MEDLINE who identify a relevant article in, for example, *BMJ (British Medical Journal)*. In the PubMed or Internet Grateful Med formats users can simply click on a hyperlink within MEDLINE that will take them to the electronic version of the article.

Most of the electronic reference services offer some form of document delivery service. Users identify the articles of interest and are able to order them from the service. The cost of these services is relatively high, and some require that the articles be delivered to a participating library rather than to the user directly.

Reprints were a common form of journal article transmission until the advent of the photocopier. The system still exists, although it is not used frequently. Authors can usually request reprints of their articles, for a fee, at the time of publication. If they order the reprints they will have a ready supply to mail out if they receive requests. Today, many authors do not buy their own reprints because they realize that interested readers will simply photocopy the item themselves or will obtain it through one of the many other ways of getting a journal article. Some authors of articles published in obscure journals are willing to mail or fax a photocopy of an article if the requesting party is able to convince them that their efforts to obtain the article through other means were unsuccessful. Students of mine who were doing a comprehensive literature review were able to obtain a particularly elusive source by faxing the author in Australia!

Back issues of journals can often be purchased from the publisher. If requests for an item through interlibrary loan have been unsuccessful, and if the author cannot be located, the most expedient way to obtain the citation may be to purchase the entire issue. This is a particularly good solution if the issue is a "special focus" issue containing many articles of interest. If a potentially important citation still eludes you, turn to your network of professional colleagues for assistance. Colleagues with an interest in the topic may have the needed article and are often willing to share their resources to foster the growth of others with that interest.

■ SUMMARY

Literature searches are undertaken to obtain information about the theory, facts, opinions, and methods related to a particular area within a discipline. Primary literature sources include journal articles, dissertations and theses, and conference proceedings. Literature search tools include catalogs of library holdings, single- and multiple-journal indexes, dissertation and thesis abstracts, and conference proceedings databases. Many of the search tools exist in either hard copy or electronic formats. Regular readers of the literature often scan the table of contents of one or more journals to identify articles of interest. Once identified, literature items can be obtained through local library holdings, interlibrary loans, full text retrieval, document delivery services, requests to authors, purchase from the publisher, or one's network of colleagues.

REFERENCES

1. Salter RB. *Continuous Passive Motion (CPM): A Biological Concept for the Healing and Regeneration of Articular Cartilage, Ligaments, and Tendons: From Origination to Research to Clinical Applications.* Baltimore, Md: Williams & Wilkins; 1993.
2. Fu FH, Harner CD, Vince KG. *Knee Surgery.* Vol 2. Baltimore, Md: Williams & Wilkins; 1994.
3. *65-Year Index to Physical Therapy.* Alexandria, Va: American Physical Therapy Association; 1987.
4. *Subject and Author Index to the Journal: A Guide to Eleven Years of Literature for the Researcher, Clinician, and Student: 1986–1996.* Alexandria, Va: American Physical Therapy Association; 1996.
5. Chiarello CM, Gundersen L, O'Halloran T. The effect of continuous passive motion duration and increment on range of motion in total knee arthroplasty patients. *J Orthop Sports Phys Ther.* 1997;25:119–127.
6. Enloe LJ, Shields RK, Smith K, Leo K, Miller B. Total hip and knee replacement treatment programs: a report using consensus. *J Orthop Sports Phys Ther.* 1996;23:3–11.
7. Montgomery F, Eliasson M. Continuous passive motion compared to active physical therapy after knee arthroplasty: similar hospitalization times in a randomized study of 68 patients [abstract]. *J Orthop Sports Phys Ther.* 1996;24:48.
8. Ververeli PA, Sutton DC, Hearn SL, Booth RE, Rothman RH. A prospective study of continuous passive motion after total knee arthroplasty: analysis of cost and benefits [abstract]. *J Orthop Sports Phys Ther.* 1994;19:57.
9. Duffel P. Constructing a search strategy. *CINAHLnews.* 1995;14(4):1–2.

10. Mann T. *The Oxford Guide to Library Research*. New York, NY: Oxford University Press; 1998.

11. *Medical Subject Headings—Tree Structures*. Bethesda, Md: National Library of Medicine; 1999:611–612.

12. *CINAHL 1998 Subject Heading List*. Glendale, Calif: Cinahl Information Systems; 1998:459.

13. Worland RL, Arredondo J, Angles F, Lopez-Jimenez F, Jessup DE. Home continuous passive motion machine versus professional physical therapy following total knee replacement. *J Arthroplasty*. 1998;13:784–787.

14. Yashar AA, Venn-Watson E, Welsh T, Colwell CW Jr, Lotke P. Continuous passive motion with accelerated flexion after total knee arthroplasty. *Clin Orthop*. 1997; 345:38–43.

15. Knight JL, Atwater RD, Grothaus L. Clinical results of the modular porous–coated anatomic (PCA) total knee arthroplasty with cement: a 5-year prospective study. *Orthopedics*. 1997;20:1025–1033.

16. Pope RO, Corcoran S, McCaul K, Howie DW. Continuous passive motion after primary total knee arthroplasty: does it offer any benefits? *J Bone Joint Surg Br*. 1997; 79:914–917.

17. Pham J, Kumar R. Heterotopic ossification after total knee arthroplasty. *Am J Orthop*. 1997;26:141–143.

18. Kumar PJ, McPherson EJ, Dorr LD, Wan Z, Baldwin K. Rehabilitation after total knee arthroplasty: a comparison of two rehabilitation techniques. *Clin Orthop*. 1996; 331:93–101.

19. Montgomery F, Eliasson M. Continuous passive motion compared to active physical therapy after knee arthroplasty: similar hospitalization times in a randomized study of 68 patients. *Acta Orthop Scand*. 1996;67:7–9.

20. Kusmer JA. *Postoperative Total Knee Arthroplasty: Initiation of Continuous Passive Motion Protocol and Achievement of Flexion* [master's thesis]. Edwardsville, Ill: Southern Illinois University at Edwardsville; 1994.

21. Prucha RJ. *Improving "Knee Society's Clinical Rating System" Knee Scores Using Continuous Passive Motion in Total Knee Arthroplasty* [master's thesis]. Atlanta, Ga: Emory University; 1994.

22. Hansen CF. *Meta-Analysis of Continuous Passive Motion Use in Total Knee Arthroplasty* [abstract]. Jackson, Miss: The University of Mississippi Medical Center; 1997. Taken from: *Master's Abstracts International*. 1998; 36(2):537.

23. Hansen C, Nick TG, Hyde J, Tsao AK, Roy W. Meta-analysis of continuous passive motion use in total knee arthroplasty [abstract]. *Phys Ther*. 1998;78:S74.

24. Ververeli PA, Sutton DC, Hearn SL, Booth RE, Hozack WJ, Rothman RR. Continuous passive motion after total knee arthroplasty: analysis of costs and benefits. *Clin Orthop*. 1995;321:208–215.

25. Institute for Scientific Information. Available at: http://www.isinet.com. Accessed March 9, 1999.

26. *Physical Therapy in Perspective*. St. Louis, Mo: CV Mosby Co. Available at: http://www.mosby.com. Accessed March 9, 1999.

27. *ACP Journal Club*. Available at: http://acponline.org. Accessed March 9, 1999.

Evaluating the Literature

Elements of a Research Article

Guidelines for Writing About Published Research

Evaluation of Single Studies

Step 1: Classify the Research and Variables

Step 2: Compare Purposes and Conclusions

Step 3: Describe Design and Control Elements

Step 4: Identify Threats to Validity

Step 5: Place the Study in the Context of Other Research

Step 6: Evaluate the Personal Utility of the Study

Evaluation of Review Articles

Step 1: Assess the Clarity of the Review Question

Step 2: Evaluate the Article Identification and Selection Strategies

Step 3: Determine How the Authors Assess Validity of the Studies

Step 4: Evaluate the Results Against the Strength of the Evidence

Step 5: Evaluate the Personal Utility of the Review

Conducting a Conceptual Review of the Literature

Step 1: Determine the Purpose of the Review

Step 2: Identify and Select Studies for Inclusion

Step 3: Identify the Designs and Constructs of the Studies

Step 4: Determine the Validity of the Individual Studies

Step 5: Make Comparisons Across Studies

Step 6: Specify Problems That Need Further Study

Critical evaluation of the literature is a necessary part of any research endeavor. If research is to make good its claim of improving patient care, researchers must study relevant clinical problems and clinicians must conduct their practices in light of relevant research results. To be effective users of the literature, practitioners must evaluate research reports before applying the results, just as they ought to evaluate new treatment methods before adopting them. There are three distinctly different levels of evaluation that are presented in this chapter. The first two levels involve an individual practitioner evaluating journal articles on an article-by-article basis. The articles that are evaluated may be (1) primary reports of single studies or (2) secondary reports that summarize or synthesize a body of literature. The third level involves an individual practitioner evaluating a body of literature—that is, doing one's own summary and synthesis rather than simply evaluating someone else's review of the literature. Before presenting guidelines for conducting each level of review, the elements of a research article and a few general rules-of-thumb for writing about published research are listed.

ELEMENTS OF A RESEARCH ARTICLE

Table 26–1 lists and describes the elements of a research article. The components encountered first are the journal article title and abstract. Following these is the body of the article, which typically consists of introduction, methods, results, discussion, conclusions, and reference sections. Several sections may contain tables, which consist of rows and columns of numbers or words; figures may also be included, which are photographs, diagrams, or graphs that illustrate important concepts or results within the study. Occasionally, an article contains an appendix of information that may be useful to readers but is too detailed for inclusion in the body of the report.

GUIDELINES FOR WRITING ABOUT PUBLISHED RESEARCH

Readers who formalize their reviews in writing or through oral presentation to others should follow three basic style guidelines:

1. Discuss the study in the past tense.
2. Clearly distinguish between your own opinions and those of the authors.
3. Qualify generalizations so they are not erroneously attributed to anyone.

Table 26–2 presents examples of inappropriate

and appropriate wording to illustrate each of the three stylistic guidelines.

EVALUATION OF SINGLE STUDIES

Single research studies should be evaluated from two major perspectives: trustworthiness and utility. *Trustworthiness* relates to whether sources of invalidity have been controlled as well as is practical, whether authors openly acknowledge the limitations of the study, and whether the conclusions drawn are defensible in light of the methods used in the study. In Chapters 7 and 20, more than 20 sources of invalidity within research studies are identified. Armed with a list of these potential problems, readers of the research literature can easily become overly critical and conclude that all studies are hopelessly flawed and offer nothing of value to the practitioner. However, as we have seen in Chapters 7 and 20, there are no perfect studies because of the reciprocal nature of many of the threats to validity. In many instances, when a researcher controls one source of invalidity, another one rears its ugly head. Thus, there is no absolute standard of trustworthiness to which every study can be held. However, because trustworthiness focuses on the design and interpretation of studies themselves, different readers can be expected to identify common areas of concern related to the trustworthiness of a study.

In contrast, the *utility* of a study relates to the usefulness of its results to a particular practitioner. Unlike the assessment of trustworthiness, the assessment of utility may vary widely among readers. The results of a well-controlled study of a narrowly defined patient population may be highly trustworthy, but of low utility to a practitioner who sees a different patient population. Conversely, a first study of a given phenomenon may be highly useful despite several methodological flaws.

When evaluating the literature, readers must balance legitimate criticisms with a realistic sense of the compromises that all researchers must

TABLE 26-1 Elements of a Research Article

Element	Characteristics
Title	Is concise, yet descriptive. Identifies major variables studied. Provides clues about whether the purpose of the research is description, relationship analysis, or difference analysis through use of phrases such as "characteristics of," "relationship between," or "effects of," respectively.
Abstract	Briefly summarizes research purpose, methods, and results. Depending on journal, is usually 150–300 words. Does not include summary of related literature or significant discussion of the limitations and implications of the research.
Introduction	Sets the stage for the presentation of the research. Usually does *not* have a heading; sometimes is subdivided into Problem, Purpose, or Literature Review sections. Whether subdivided or not, defines the broad problem that underlies the study, states the specific purposes of the study, and places the problem and purposes into the theoretical context of previous work. Often presents research hypotheses. Occasionally contains tables or figures.
Method	Describes the conduct of the study. Usually is subdivided into Subjects, Instruments, Procedures, and Data Analysis sections. Often refers to methods or procedures used by others as the basis for the present study. Often contains figures showing equipment used.
Results	Presents the results without comment on their meaning. Often is subdivided into sections corresponding to the variables studied. Is often brief because much of the information is contained in tables and figures.
Discussion	Presents the authors' interpretation of their results, along with their assessment of study limitations and directions for future research. Often refers to previous work that is related to the findings of the study. May be subdivided into Limitations, Clinical Relevance, and Future Research sections.
Conclusions	Concisely restates the important findings of the research. Presents a conclusion for each individual purpose outlined in the introduction.
References	Lists references cited in the text of the article. Occasionally is followed by a bibliography that lists relevant work that is not cited in the article.
Appendix	If included, follows the references. Typically includes survey instruments or detailed treatment protocols.

make in designing and implementing a study. Several authors have presented guidelines for evaluating the research literature.[3–7] In fact, many different scales and checklists have been developed to aid readers in evaluating the literature.[8] In addition, examples of research evaluations by experienced consumers of the literature can be found as commentaries to published reports in several journals, particularly in *Physical Therapy* beginning in the 1990s.[9] Although different evaluators of the literature structure their commentaries differently, they all assess the same basic aspects of research articles.

In this section, a six-step sequence for evaluating the literature is presented to help novice evaluators structure their critiques. The first steps emphasize classification and description of the research in order to place it in the larger context of research as a vast and varied enterprise. The middle steps emphasize identification of threats to the validity of the research. The final steps involve assessing the place the research has in both the existing literature and one's own practice. Appendix C provides a set of questions to help readers structure their critiques. Because of the great variety of research designs and analyses that appear in the published literature, readers should recognize that the questions need to be applied thoughtfully and selectively, as they are neither exhaustive nor universally applicable.

TABLE 26-2 Style Guidelines for Writing About Published Research	
Inappropriate Wording	**Appropriate Wording**
Chiarello and colleagues state that there is no difference in outcome between patients who receive short-duration CPM versus long-duration CPM.[1] (This wording implies that the authors still hold this belief.)	Chiarello and colleagues found no differences in outcome between patients who received short-duration CPM versus long-duration CPM.[1] (This wording makes it clear that the authors' statements relate to the particular study under discussion.)
Use of CPM after total knee arthroplasty decreases the need for postoperative manipulation under anesthesia. (This wording does not make it clear whether this is the conclusion of the review author or the author of the study.)	Based on their research, Ververeli and colleagues concluded that CPM after total knee arthroplasty decreased the need for postoperative manipulation under anesthesia.[2] (This wording clearly attributes the statement to the study authors.)
Patients with greater knee range of motion have better functional outcomes after surgery. (This wording implies that this relationship between range of motion and functional outcome is well established.)	Therapists and surgeons often assume that patients with greater knee range of motion have better functional outcomes after surgery. (This wording makes it clear that the relationship between range of of motion and functional outcome is an unsubstantiated assumption.)

In addition, readers need to move from merely answering the questions to interpreting the implications of the answers in the context of each study they review. For example, one of the questions in Appendix C is "Was the independent variable implemented in a laboratory-like or clinic-like setting?" In one study a tightly controlled, laboratory-like setting might be exactly what is needed to establish the effectiveness of a particular technique under ideal conditions. In another study, of a phenomenon for which effectiveness has been well established, looser, clinic-like control might be exactly what is needed to establish whether the technique can be efficacious when the vagaries of actual clinical practice apply. Thus, merely answering the question of "laboratory-like" versus "clinic-like" control of the independent variable does not tell the reader whether the control was appropriate. Rather, the reader, having determined the level of control, then needs to evaluate whether that level of control was appropriate for the study at hand.

To further assist readers embarking on a review of a study, a written critique of Gose's[10] investigation of continuous passive motion (CPM)

for patients after total knee arthroplasty (TKA) is provided as an example. The example is developed step by step as each of the six critique steps is presented. This article was selected for review because its design and its date provide many opportunities to illustrate the various control and validity issues addressed in this text. The abstract of Gose's report reads:

The purpose of this study was to evaluate the effects of adding three 1-hour sessions of continuous passive motion (CPM) each day to the entire postoperative program of patients who received a total knee replacement (TKR). A retrospective chart review was completed for 55 patients (8 with bilateral involvement, totalling 63 knees) who received a TKR between 1981 and 1984. The data analysis compared the following variables for 32 patients who received CPM and 23 patients who received no CPM: the length of hospital stay (LOS), the number of postoperative days (PODs) before discharge, the frequency of postoperative complications, and the knee range of motion at discharge. The CPM groups showed significant decreases in the frequency of complication ($p < .05$), the LOS ($p < .01$), and in the number of PODs ($p < .001$). No difference was demonstrated in the ROM of the two groups. These results support the use of postoperative applications of CPM, but not as strongly as those reported from studies that used longer periods of CPM. Further research is indicated to delineate the minimum dosage of CPM needed to obtain the maximum beneficial effects.[10(p39)]

Step 1: Classify the Research and Variables

Classification of the research and variables provides an immediate sense of where the individual piece of research belongs in the literature. The information needed to classify the research is found in the abstract, introduction, and methods sections of a journal article. If the reviewer determines that the research is experimental, then it should come as no surprise if the authors make causal statements about their results; if the reviewer determines that the research is nonexperimental, then the reader's expectations about causal statements should change. If the dependent variables of interest are range-of-motion (ROM) measures, then the reviewer should expect clean, easily understood results; if the dependent measures relate to patterns of interaction between therapists and patients, then the reviewer should expect complexity and depth. We might summarize this first evaluative step for Gose's CPM study as follows:

Gose's study of the effects of continuous passive motion (CPM) on rehabilitation after total knee arthroplasty is an example of a retrospective analysis of differences between groups. The study had one independent variable, treatment, with two levels: usual postoperative therapy and postoperative therapy supplemented with CPM. The type of treatment received by each subject was not actively manipulated, but rather was apparently determined by physician prescription.

There were five dependent variables: total length of stay in the acute care hospital, number of postoperative days in the acute care hospital,

frequency of postoperative complications, knee flexion range of motion (ROM) at discharge, and knee extension ROM at discharge. All data were gathered through retrospective chart review.

Step 2: Compare Purposes and Conclusions

Any piece of research needs to be assessed in light of the contribution it was designed to make to the profession. It is not fair to fault a study for not accomplishing a purpose that it was never designed to meet. Before reading the methods, results, and discussion sections of an article, it is often useful to compare the purposes, which may be found in the introduction, and the conclusions. This comparison serves two purposes. First, it provides an indication of whether or not the study is internally consistent. Purposes without conclusions, or conclusions without purposes, should alert the reader to look for the points at which the study strays from its original intents.

Knowing the study conclusions also provides guidance for the critique of the methods, results, and discussion. If the conclusions indicate that statistically significant relationships or differences were identified, then the reader knows to evaluate the remainder of the article with an eye to how well the researcher controlled for alternative explanations for the results and whether the statistical results are clinically important. If the conclusions do not indicate any statistically significant results, then the reader knows to evaluate the study with respect to power and the clinical importance of the results. With regard to Gose's study, we might write up this second step of our critique as follows:

The purpose of this study was clearly stated at the end of the introduction section of the paper: to compare the effects of adding three 1-hour daily sessions of CPM to a postoperative total knee arthroplasty rehabilitation program. The effects measured related to both the physical status of the patient (flexion and extension ROM and frequency of complications) and the cost-effectiveness of care (total length of stay and length of postoperative stay).

The conclusions were consistent with the purpose. There were significant differences between the CPM and non-CPM groups for three of the five dependent measures: length of stay, number of days of postoperative hospitalization, and frequency of postoperative complications. There were no significant differences between groups on the two ROM variables, knee flexion and extension.

Step 3: Describe Design and Control Elements

In the third step of the evaluation process, the reviewer completes the description of the study elements and begins to make judgments about the adequacy of the research design. The design of the study is identified so that the sequence of measurement and manipulation (if present) is clear to the reader of the review. This identification can be done in any of the three ways introduced earlier in Chapters 6 and 9:

> Making a diagram of the design
>
> Using symbols such as Campbell and Stanley's Os and Xs
>
> Using descriptive terms

The research design alone does not indicate the trustworthiness of the study. For example, a "strong" design such as a pretest-posttest control-group design may not yield trustworthy information if the independent variable is not implemented consistently for subjects in the treatment group. Thus, a critical reader of the literature needs to determine both the design of the study and the level of control the researchers

exerted over implementation of the independent variable, selection and assignment of subjects, extraneous variables related to the setting or subjects, measurement, and information. The third step in our review of Gose's CPM study can be written as follows:

As noted previously, data for this study were collected retrospectively, with group membership determined by the postoperative rehabilitation program each patient happened to have undergone. This study was therefore of a nonexperimental, ex post facto nature with nonequivalent treatment and control groups. Because all dependent variables were collected at the completion of either rehabilitation program, the study followed a posttest-only design.

The nonexperimental, retrospective nature of data collection means that many design control elements were absent. The implementation of the independent variable took place in the hospital setting and would be expected to vary accordingly. The author did not indicate the proportion of patients who received all of the intended CPM sessions. Because he later discussed how the intended dosage of CPM in this study differs from that reported in other studies, it seems important to know if the actual dosage received by the patients was equal to, greater than, or less than the intended dosage.

The selection and assignment of subjects to groups were accomplished through chart review to determine, first, whether subjects met general inclusion criteria and, second, whether they had undergone traditional or CPM-added rehabilitation. The basic inclusion criteria were having undergone a total knee arthroplasty between 1981 and 1984 at one hospital, having had ROM values recorded at admission and discharge, and having accomplished certain rehabilitation tasks by postoperative days (POD) 2 and 7. These criteria mean that patients with complications severe enough to impede the rehabilitation process were excluded from the study. Thus, the frequency of postoperative complications indicated in this study was likely less than the number of actual complications that occur after total knee arthroplasty.

Assignment of subjects to group was accomplished simply by identification of which type of rehabilitation they had undergone. The author did not indicate what factors might have led one patient to receive CPM-added rehabilitation and another patient to receive traditional rehabilitation. If, for example, certain surgeons prescribed CPM-added rehabilitation and others prescribed traditional rehabilitation, then the effects of the type of rehabilitation would be confounded by the surgeon.

If the traditional rehabilitation group had their surgery and rehabilitation in 1981 and 1982 and the CPM-added group received care in 1983 and 1984, then the effects of type of rehabilitation would be confounded with any general changes in surgical technique, knee prosthesis design, hospital staffing patterns, and the like that may have differed between the two time periods.

Because of the retrospective design, extraneous variables such as disease severity and medication received postoperatively were not controlled. In addition, there was no control over ROM measurements taken and no indication of how many different therapists recorded ROM values in the study.

Step 4: Identify Threats to Validity

Once the type of research has been defined, the purposes and conclusions reviewed, and the design and control elements outlined, the reviewer is able to examine the threats to the validity of the study. This step involves not only assessing the threats to validity but also evaluating the extent to which the authors identify the study's limitations themselves.

As described in Chapter 7, the threats to validity can be divided into construct, internal, statistical conclusion, and external validity. Our analysis of the validity of Gose's CPM study might be written as follows:

CONSTRUCT VALIDITY CONCERNS

The major construct validity concerns in Gose's study are construct underrepresentation and interaction of different treatments. The variables studied were a combination of cost-effectiveness variables related to length of stay and patient-oriented variables such as frequency of complications and knee ROM. These variables did not, however, represent a full range of outcomes for patients after total knee arthroplasty. It would have been nice if functional measures such as ambulation or stair-climbing ability had been measured. Presumably, this information would have been as available from the medical record as the ROM data were. In addition to underrepresentation of the dependent variables, the author acknowledged that the independent variable was also underrepresented: the dosage of CPM in this study was low compared with the dosage in other studies. A more complete, prospective study would assess several different dosages of CPM to determine the minimum level needed to obtain desired results.

The interaction of different treatments is always a concern with a retrospective study such as this one. We have no way of knowing, for example, whether the CPM treatments, which were administered by nursing staff, consisted of mechanical application of the unit with minimal interpersonal contact between nurse and patient or took the form of relaxed interchanges that provided an opportunity for education and discussion. If the latter was the case, then this study may have actually been assessing the effects of a combined program of CPM, education, and attention, rather than the isolated addition of CPM to the treatment regimen. The author acknowledged the possibility that differences between groups may be related to factors other than the use of CPM.

INTERNAL VALIDITY CONCERNS

The major internal validity concerns in this study are assignment, mortality, diffusion of treatment, compensatory equalization of treatments, and compensatory rivalry or resentful demoralization of subjects. Very little information was given about why a particular patient received either the CPM-added rehabilitation or the non-CPM regimen. As noted earlier, if group membership was confounded with surgeon or time frame, it would be difficult to conclude that differences between groups were related solely to the differences in their rehabilitation regimens.

Regarding the threat of mortality to internal validity, we have no way of knowing how many potential subjects in each group were not included in the study because they developed serious complications that prevented them from meeting the inclusion criteria of supervised ambulation on POD 2 and progressive ambulation by POD 7.

A third threat to internal validity comes from having patients from both groups being treated at the same time. It is plausible that members of each group were hospital roommates, and if the roommate in the CPM group extolled the virtues of this new device, perhaps the roommate in the non-CPM group compensated by moving her knee more frequently. If the therapists believed that CPM was beneficial, they could have become upset when some physicians did not prescribe it and compensated by increasing the number of ROM

repetitions they included for their patients who were not receiving CPM. Because the author did not clearly indicate whether the two regimens were in effect simultaneously or sequentially, we cannot speculate about the likelihood that these internal validity threats actually occurred.

STATISTICAL CONCLUSION VALIDITY CONCERNS

No concerns about statistical conclusion validity seem warranted. The sample sizes were reasonable (32 and 23); there was only one statistical test performed per dependent variable; the homogeneity of variance assumptions seem to have been met; the statistically significant results seem clinically important (e.g., the CPM group had an average postoperative length of stay approximately 3.5 days shorter than the non-CPM group); and the statistically insignificant results seem clinically unimportant (the difference in the mean ROM values between groups was only 1.0° for both knee flexion and extension).

EXTERNAL VALIDITY CONCERNS

The external validity of the study is strong in some areas and weak in others. The subjects seem representative of typical patients who receive total knee arthroplasties: elderly women with osteoarthritis. Therapists who work with a more predominantly rheumatoid arthritic group might find differences in patient response based on the systemic nature of rheumatoid arthritis. In addition, the retrospective nature of the study means that the treatment was implemented as it occurs in the clinical setting, with all its attendant inconsistencies. Thus, despite possible inconsistencies in application of the treatment, a clinically important reduction in length of stay was found. The study would have been strengthened by documentation of the CPM dosage delivered.

External validity is strengthened, ironically, by the relatively low dosage of CPM provided in this study. At the time the study was done, typical CPM protocols called for many hours per day—often up to 20 hours per day—of CPM. Although 3 hours of CPM per day seemed like a very low dosage at the time of the study, lower daily doses or fewer numbers of days of CPM are more common in contemporary reports. Therefore, compared with other studies of CPM administered in the early 1980s, this study has a dosage per day that more closely matches protocols in use today.

External validity is limited, however, by the dramatic changes in length of stay for almost all diagnoses and surgical procedures during the last 15 years. Although the CPM group's length of stay was significantly less in this study than the non–CPM group's, both lengths of stay (means of 16.4 and 20.0 days, respectively) were much longer than is typical today, irrespective of the nature of the rehabilitation regimen. This means that although the daily dosage of CPM may match contemporary protocols, the total dosage of CPM given across the hospital stay may be greater than typical in today's short-stay environment.

Step 5: Place the Study in the Context of Other Research

In the fifth and sixth steps of evaluation, the reviewer assesses the utility of the research. First, the reviewer determines how much new information the study adds to what is already known about a topic. Even though only a single study is being critiqued, the question of utility cannot be answered in isolation. For example, if a treatment has consistently been shown to be effective in tightly controlled settings with high internal validity, another well-controlled study may not add much to our knowledge about that treatment. In such a case what is needed is a study conducted in a realistic clinical setting,

where control is difficult. Similarly, a small one-group study of a previously unstudied area might be an important addition to the physical therapy literature, whereas the same design applied to a well-studied topic may add very little.

The best assessments of the context in which a particular study belongs are made by reviewers who have extensive knowledge of the literature on the topic. Knowledgeable reviewers can assess whether the authors of a research report have adequately reviewed and interpreted the literature they cite. Reviewers without this knowledge must rely on the authors' descriptions of the literature. Our review of the place Gose's CPM study has in the literature might be written as follows:

Despite the previously noted limitations of Gose's study, this work played an important role in the evolution of CPM from a 20-hour-per-day treatment modality to a modality that is used in varying dosages. The author indicated that previous studies of 20-hour-per-day CPM protocols found shorter lengths of stay, lower frequencies of postoperative complications, and greater early knee ROM in CPM groups compared with non–CPM groups. This study provided preliminary evidence that a low dosage of CPM can reduce the length of stay and frequency of complications in a typical group of elderly arthritic patients receiving total knee replacement. Interestingly, this question of appropriate dosage has not yet been fully answered, as indicated by a recent study comparing, in part, short-duration (3 to 5 hours per day) CPM to long-duration (10 to 12 hours per day) CPM.[1]

Step 6: Evaluate the Personal Utility of the Study

As the final step in any research critique, the reviewer determines whether the study has meaning for his or her own practice. Whereas the determination of the trustworthiness of a research article will be somewhat consistent across reviewers, the question of personal utility will be answered differently by different reviewers. Hypothetically, we might write our assessment of the personal utility of Gose's CPM study as follows:

The results of this study have some potential application for the setting in which we work. In our setting, we follow an 8- to 10-hour-a-day regimen of CPM with excellent early ROM and relatively short stays. However, for those patients who cannot sleep well with the CPM unit on, this means that they are in the CPM unit during many of their waking hours. We believe that these patients stay in bed too much and are unable to give adequate attention to the development of effective quadriceps femoris muscle power and the development of more functional skills such as walking at a relatively normal velocity and for longer distances.

Although this study provides only partial support for the effectiveness of a low dosage of CPM, its findings are consistent with other reports that have compared different dosages of CPM and found the low-dosage protocols to be as effective as the high-dosage protocols.[1,11] On the basis of the results of all of these studies, as well as our own dissatisfaction with some aspects of high dosages of CPM, we plan to implement and assess a trial of medium to low dosages of CPM in our patients who have had total knee arthroplasty.

The evaluation of personal utility is a very concrete way to conclude a review of a single research study. This ending is a reminder that the first five evaluative steps are not mere intellectual exercises, but are the means by which each reader decides whether and how to use the results of a study within his or her own practice.

EVALUATION OF REVIEW ARTICLES

Review articles provide practitioners with a time-efficient way of remaining up-to-date in areas of importance to their practice. In fact, the authors of the *Users' Guide to the Medical Literature,* a series of articles appearing in *JAMA* from 1993 to the present, recognize the importance of review articles and go so far as to recommend that "resolving a clinical problem begins with a search for a valid overview or practice guideline as the most efficient method of deciding on the best patient care."[12(p2097)] Having made this statement, though, they then indicate that clinicians need help in differentiating good reviews from poor reviews. This section of the chapter provides guidelines to help physical therapy practitioners make such judgments about review articles. Although there are mathematical ways to synthesize the results of several related studies (see Chapter 11 for a brief discussion of meta-analysis), the focus in this section is on the conceptual synthesis that is presented in many review articles. The series of points to consider has been compiled from several different resources.[7,13–15]

Step 1: Assess the Clarity of the Review Question

Readers should assess the clarity of the question being posed within the review. Well-formulated questions that can help direct practice should generally address (1) the type of exposure (to a risk factor, an intervention, or a diagnostic test); (2) the outcome of interest; (3) the type of person being studied; and (4) the comparison against which the exposure is being compared.[14] An example that illustrates these four areas is found in van der Heijden and colleagues' paper entitled "Physiotherapy for Patients with Soft Tissue Shoulder Disorders: A Systematic Review of Randomised Clinical Trials."[16] Within the body of the article the type of exposure (different forms of physiotherapy), the outcomes of interest (success rates, pain reduction, functional status, mobility, and need for drugs or surgery), the type of person being studied (those with soft tissue shoulder disorders; studies reporting on individuals postmastectomy or after fractures were excluded, as were studies reporting on shoulder pain with hemiplegia or rheumatoid arthritis), and the comparison groups (some compared various forms of physiotherapy, some compared physiotherapy with placebo treatment, and some compared physiotherapy with other interventions such as drug or injection therapies).

Step 2: Evaluate the Article Identification and Selection Strategies

The reader should determine whether the method used to identify articles was comprehensive and whether the criteria used to select articles for review were appropriate. The process of identifying articles should be as comprehensive as possible, using the strategies identified in Chapter 25 or by other authors,[14,17] and proceeding until new strategies yield only redundant studies. The search strategy should be documented clearly so that the reader has a clear sense of the time span of the review, the search terms used, and the databases that were accessed. Once a pool of articles is identified, the reviewers must cull those articles that include the information needed to answer the question posed by the review. In the study of physiotherapy for soft tissue shoulder disorders, the authors of the review reported that their search strategy yielded 47 articles that met five initial criteria: patients had shoulder pain; treatments were randomly allocated; at least one treatment included physiotherapy; outcomes included success rate, pain, mobility, or functional status; and results were published prior to January 1996. Of these 47 articles, 24 were excluded from the review because the shoulder pain was not related to soft tissue and 3 were excluded because they

represented multiple reports of the same data. Thus, 20 papers were ultimately included in the review.[16] Because the authors carefully reported their identification and selection process, readers are in a position to judge the completeness and appropriateness of the articles selected for review. Without this information, readers are left to wonder about the criteria used by the review author in selecting articles on which to report.

Step 3: Determine How the Authors Assess Validity of the Studies

The reader should determine whether and how the review authors assessed the validity of each of the studies within the review. In the study of soft tissue shoulder disorders the authors compared each trial against eight validity criteria: selection criteria, assignment procedures, similarity of groups at baseline, withdrawals from treatment, missing values, presence of additional interventions, blinded application of the intervention, and blinded assessment of the outcome.[16] Meade and Richardson indicate that readers can have a higher level of confidence in reviews in which two or more individuals have reviewed each study independently, with a process for resolving disagreements between reviewers.[7]

Step 4: Evaluate the Results Against the Strength of the Evidence

Readers should determine whether the results of the individual studies are evaluated against the strength of the evidence in those studies as well as in closely related studies. This generally means that the articles are not discussed in an article-by-article fashion (i.e., the reviews do not read as follows: Brown found x, Smith found y, Johnson found z.). Rather, the articles are discussed topic by topic, and any single article may be referred to in several different sections of the review. For example, in van der Heijden and associates' systematic review of physiotherapy for soft tissue shoulder disorders, the findings were grouped first by the type of intervention and then by the findings of those studies that were thought to have sufficiently high levels of validity.[16] For example, they first identified 6 studies that evaluated the effect of ultrasound against various alternatives and judged that 4 of the 6 studies had acceptable validity. They then summarized the findings from those 4 studies, one of which compared ultrasound to cold therapy. Later, they evaluated the effect of cold therapy against various alternatives—one of which was obviously ultrasound. Thus, the one study comparing ultrasound and cold therapy was cited at least twice—once during the general discussion of the effectiveness of ultrasound and once with the discussion of the effectiveness of cold therapy.

Step 5: Evaluate the Personal Utility of the Review

Readers should evaluate the discussion and conclusions sections of the review to determine whether this information is consistent with the findings in the review and whether it has applications to their own practice. As was the case with the evaluation of a single study, readers must place the results of the review within the context of their own practices to determine the usefulness of the information.

■ CONDUCTING A CONCEPTUAL REVIEW OF THE LITERATURE

In addition to evaluating the literature one article at a time—either the primary literature of a research report or the secondary literature of a review article—professionals may wish to conduct their own reviews of a body of literature. In a conceptual review of the literature, the reviewer evaluates several related studies to (1) synthesize their results into a summary of what is and is not

known about the topic; (2) identify areas of controversy within the literature; and (3) develop questions that need further research. Again, the focus in this section is on the conceptual synthesis that practitioners might undertake to help guide treatment or identify areas in need of further study,[18] rather than the mathematical synthesis that is developed in a meta-analysis. A six-step sequence for conducting a conceptual review is presented subsequently. Brief examples based on several studies of CPM use after total knee athroplasty are given to illustrate some of the steps.[1,2,10,11,19–21] Clearly, some of the items that were just presented as evaluative criteria for assessing the quality of a review article should be put into place when a practitioner conducts his or her own review.

Step 1: Determine the Purpose of the Review

Just as any research that involves the collection of new data should have a clearly stated purpose, so should a conceptual review of the literature. Common reasons for performing a conceptual review of the literature are

- To guide treatment decisions in one's own clinic
- To provide a basis for determining whether one's own treatment outcomes are consistent with those of others
- To determine how others measure success for particular types of patients
- To develop a research agenda in the area reviewed

Step 2: Identify and Select Studies for Inclusion

Using the techniques outlined in Chapter 25, the reader must obtain a relatively complete set of articles on the topic. Once the articles are found, the researcher then decides which are relevant to the question at hand. Which articles are selected obviously depends on the purpose for doing the review. If one is interested in how to document progress after total knee arthroplasty, then studies that involve functional assessment of patients with any type of knee pathology may be relevant; if one's interest is solely in post-TKA treatment regimens, then such articles are not relevant. If the review is to be published, the researcher needs to keep close track of search strategies and decisions about inclusion and exclusion of particular reports.[14,17]

Step 3: Identify the Designs and Constructs of the Studies

Both the nature of the studies and the nature of the variables under study must be examined carefully. What designs were used to study the topic? Was the independent variable implemented differently in different studies? What dependent measures were used consistently? Table 26–3 lists the designs and some selected variables of interest identified by examination of seven studies of CPM use after total knee arthroplasty. This review reveals, for example, that there are at least five important considerations in planning a program of CPM: when CPM is applied, how long CPM is used daily, what the starting ROM is, how much the ROM increases each day, and when CPM is discontinued. If a group of researchers were using the literature review to help them plan a new study of CPM use, they could use these five factors as the basis for planning the different levels of the CPM variable.

Step 4: Determine the Validity of the Individual Studies

After the constructs studies have been specified, it is necessary to evaluate each study individually to determine the validity of its results and conclusions. This evaluation follows the guidelines presented earlier in the chapter.

Step 5: Make Comparisons Across Studies

Once each study has been examined independently, the reviewer compares results across the studies. In our example review of seven studies of CPM after total knee arthroplasty, we see that several investigators have examined whether patients in CPM groups have less need for manipulation under anesthesia than those in non-CPM groups or those receiving less aggressive CPM protocols. Of the three authors who address this issue, Gose[10] found no difference in the rate of manipulation between patients receiving typical care and those receiving 3 hours of CPM per day; Wasilewski[19] found no difference between those receiving typical care and those receiving up to 24 hours of CPM per day; and Ververeli[2] found a difference in favor of the group receiving CPM 20 hours per day compared with the group receiving standard care. Having identified an inconsistent finding, the task of the review author is to examine this conflicting evidence carefully to determine whether there are differences among the studies that might explain the contradictory results. Similar comparisons across studies would be made for each of the factors of interest (e.g., range of motion, cost of care) within the review.

Step 6: Specify Problems That Need Further Study

By following the previous steps, we have identified the types of designs used to study CPM after total knee arthroplasty and have identified points of consensus and controversy in the literature. On the basis of this limited literature review, we might conclude that the following types of studies are needed to enhance our understanding of the phenomenon: comparison of different CPM protocols, assessment of functional outcomes after total knee arthroplasty, and further study of the relationship between CPM use and the need for manipulation under anesthesia.

| **TABLE 26-3** | **Selected Constructs in Seven Studies of Continuous Passive Motion (CPM) After Total Knee Arthroplasty** |

Constructs	Primary Author and Year of Publication[*]
Design Elements	
Timing of Data Collection	
Retrospective	Gose–1987, Wasilewski–1990
Prospective	Basso–1987, Ververeli–1995, Chiarello–1997, Pope–1997, Yashar–1997
Group Assignment	
Existing groups	Gose–1987, Basso–1987
Successive cohorts	Wasilewski–1990, Ververeli–1995
Random	Pope–1995, Yashar–1997, Chiarello–1997
Comparisons	
CPM with immobilization	Wasilewski–1990
CPM with standard care	Gose–1987, Ververeli–1995, Chiarello–1997, Pope–1997
Different CPM protocols	Basso–1987, Chiarello–1997, Pope–1997, Yashar–1997
Implementation of CPM	
Dosage	
20 or more hours per day	Basso–1987, Wasilewski–1990, Pope–1997, Yashar–1997
10 hours per day	Chiarello–1997
3–6 hours per day	Basso–1987, Gose–1987, Chiarello–1997
Decreasing duration	Ververeli–1995
Time of First Application	
Recovery room	Wasilewski–1990, Ververeli–1995, Pope–1997, Yashar–1997
2nd–3rd postoperative day	Basso–1987, Gose–1987, Chiarello–1997
Removal of CPM treatment	
3rd postoperative day	Pope–1997
At discharge or 90° of ROM	Gose–1987, Wasilewski–1990, Ververeli–1995, Chiarello–1997, Yashar–1995
Initial CPM range of motion	
0°–30° or 40°	Gose–1987, Ververeli–1995, Pope–1997
0°–60° or 70°	Wasilewski–1990, Pope–1997
70°–100°	Yashar–1997
Progression of range of motion (ROM)	
5°–10° per day	Basso–1987, Gose–1987
10° per day	Wasilewski–1990, Ververeli–1995, Chiarello–1997, Pope–1997
>10° per day	Yashar–1997
As tolerated	Chiarello–1997
Measurement of Outcomes	
Cost Measures	
Length of stay	Basso–1987, Gose–1987, Wasilewski–1990, Ververeli–1995, Yashar–1997
Cost of care	Ververeli–1995, Yashar–1997
Motion Measures	
Range of motion	Basso–1987, Gose–1987, Wasilewski–1990, Ververeli–1995, Chiarello–1997, Pope–1997, Yashar–1997
Rate of change of ROM	Chiarello–1997
Days to reach 75° flexion	Ververeli–1995
Need for manipulation under anesthesia	Gose–1987, Wasilewski–1990, Ververeli–1995

Table continued on following page

TABLE 26–3	**Selected Constructs in Seven Studies of Continuous Passive Motion (CPM) After Total Knee Arthroplasty** *Continued*
Constructs	**Primary Author and Year of Publication**[*]
Follow-Up Beyond Discharge	
Discharge only	Basso–1987, Gose–1987, Chiarello–1997
1 Year	Wasilewski–1990, Yashar–1997, Pope–1997
2 Years or more	Ververeli–1995

[*] References associated with each cited article are as follows: Chiarello,[1] Ververeli,[2] Gose,[10] Basso,[11] Wasilewski,[19] Yashar,[20] and Pope.[21]

■ SUMMARY

The major elements of a research article are the title; abstract; introduction, methods, results, discussion, conclusions, and references sections; and, sometimes, an appendix. When writing about previously published work, reviewers should use the past tense and should make clear whether statements are their own or the opinions of the authors whose study they are reviewing. Reviewers of single studies should classify the research and its variables, compare the purposes and conclusions, outline the design and control elements, determine the threats to the validity of the study, place the study in the context of previous work, and assess the study's utility for their personal practice. Evaluators of review articles should assess the clarity of the review question, evaluate the article identification and selection strategies, determine how the authors assess the validity of the studies, evaluate the results against the strength of the evidence, and evaluate the personal utility of the review. When doing a conceptual review of several related studies, the reviewer should identify the purpose of the review, conduct an appropriate literature search, identify the studies' designs and the variables examined within the studies, assess each study individually, compare results across studies for consistencies and inconsistencies, and determine what aspects of the topic require further study.

REFERENCES

1. Chiarello CM, Gundersen L, O'Halloran T. The effect of continuous passive motion duration and increment on range of motion in total knee arthroplasty patients. *J Orthop Sports Phys Ther*. 1997;25:119–127.
2. Ververeli PA, Sutton DC, Hearn SL, Booth RE Jr, Hozack WJ, Rothman RR. Continuous passive motion after total knee arthroplasty: analysis of costs and benefits. *Clin Orthop*. 1995;321:208–215.
3. Riegelman RK, Hirsch RP. *Studying a Study and Testing a Test: How to Read the Health Science Literature*. 3rd ed. Boston, Mass: Little, Brown Co; 1996.
4. Chalmers TC, Smith H Jr, Blackburn B, et al. A method for assessing the quality of a randomized control trial. *Control Clin Trials*. 1981;2:31–49.
5. Guyatt GH, Sackett DL, Cook DJ, for the Evidence-Based Medicine Working Group. Users' guides to the medical literature. II: How to use an article about therapy or prevention. A: Are the results of the study valid? *JAMA*. 1993;270:2598–2601.
6. Guyatt GH, Sackett DL, Cook DJ, for the Evidence-Based Medicine Working Group. Users' guides to the medical literature. II: How to use an article about therapy or prevention. B: What were the results and will they help me in caring for my patients? *JAMA*. 1994;271:59–63.
7. Meade MO, Richardson WS. Selecting and appraising studies for a systematic review. *Ann Intern Med*. 1997; 127:531–537.
8. Moher D, Jadad AR, Nichol G, Penman M, Tugwell P, Walsh S. Assessing the quality of randomized controlled trials: an annotated bibliography of scales and checklists. *Control Clin Trials*. 1995;16:62–73.
9. Rothstein JM. Commenting on commentaries [editor's note]. *Phys Ther*. 1991;71:431–432.
10. Gose JC. Continuous passive motion in the postoperative treatment of patients with total knee replacement: a retrospective study. *Phys Ther*. 1987;67:39–42.
11. Basso DM, Knapp L. Comparison of two continuous passive motion protocols for patients with total knee implants. *Phys Ther*. 1987;67:360–363.
12. Guyatt GH, Rennie D. Users' guides to the medical literature [editorial]. *JAMA*. 1993;270:2096-2097.

13. Oxman AD, Sackett DL, Guyatt GH. Users' guides to the medical literature: I. How to get started. *JAMA*. 1993; 270:2093–2095.

14. Counsell C. Formulating questions and locating primary studies for inclusion in systematic reviews. *Ann Intern Med*. 1997;127:380–387.

15. Shaughnessy AF, Slawson DC. Getting the most from review articles: a guide for readers and writers. *Am Fam Physician*. 1997;55:2155–2160.

16. van der Heijden GJMG, van der Windt DAWM, de Winter AF. Physiotherapy for patients with soft tissue shoulder disorders: a systematic review of randomised clinical trials. *BMJ*. 1997;315:25–30.

17. Dickersin K, Scherer R, Lefebvre C. Identifying relevant studies for systematic reviews. *BMJ*. 1994;309:1286–1291.

18. Findley TW. Research in physical medicine and rehabilitation: II. The conceptual review of the literature or how to read more articles than you ever want to see in your entire life. *Am J Phys Med Rehabil*. 1989;68:97–102.

19. Wasilewski SA, Woods LC, Torgerson WR Jr, Healy WL. Value of continuous passive motion in total knee arthroplasty. *Orthopedics*. 1990;13:291–295.

20. Yashar AA, Venn-Watson E, Welsh T, Colwell CW Jr, Lotke P. Continous passive motion with accelerated flexion after total knee arthroplasty. *Clin Orthop*. 1997; 345:38–43.

21. Pope RO, Corcoran S, McCaul K, Howie DW. Continuous passive motion after primary total knee arthroplasty: does it offer any benefits? *J Bone Joint Surg Br*. 1997; 79:914–917.

Implementing Research

Implementing a Research Project

Proposal Preparation
  General Proposal Guidelines
  Elements of the Research Proposal
    Title
    Investigators
    Problem Statement
    Purposes
    Methods
    Dissemination
    Budget
    Work Plan
    Appendices
    Approvals

Human Participants Protection
  Institutional Review Boards
  Levels of Review
  Informed Consent

Funding
  Budget
  Institution Funding
  Corporation Funding

  Foundation Funding
    Types of Foundations
    Identifying Foundations
    Applying for Foundation Funds
  Government Funding

Obtaining Participants
  Inpatient Recruitment
  Outpatient Recruitment
  Recruitment of the Lay Public

Data Collection
  Data Collection Procedures
  Safeguarding Data
  Protecting Participant Identity
  Data Recording Forms
  Pilot Study
  Scheduling Participants and
    Personnel

Data Analysis
  Data Coding
  Data Entry
  Statistical Analysis

Although the primary purpose of this text is to provide readers with the knowledge they need to become educated consumers of the research literature, some readers will want to extend that knowledge by implementing projects of their own. The final two chapters of this text, then, are designed to provide practitioners with some "nuts and bolts" guidance about implementing

research (Chapter 27) and disseminating the results of that research (Chapter 28). Readers should note, however, that published research is rarely an individual venture—most papers are written by multiple authors who provided different types of expertise to the project. Therefore, individuals beginning a research program are encouraged to identify colleagues who can provide the diverse array of skills needed to mount a successful project.

This chapter first identifies three preliminary steps that must be completed before any data are collected: (1) a research plan, or proposal, must be prepared and submitted for approval through appropriate academic or administrative channels; (2) the researchers must seek the approval of human or animal subjects protection committees, if appropriate; and (3) the researchers must secure the funds needed to implement the study. Next, the chapter presents guidelines for implementing all phases of a research project, from participant selection to data analysis. Methods of obtaining participants are discussed first, followed by the development and use of research instrumentation. Tips for managing data collection and recording are then presented, and the chapter ends with suggestions for data analysis, including guidelines for using computer statistical programs and statistical consultants.

■ PROPOSAL PREPARATION

The research proposal is a blueprint for the conduct of a research study. The proposal is also the mechanism by which the researcher sells the study idea to those individuals who are in a position to approve and fund it. Thus, the proposal must be written in a fashion that makes the purpose and methods of the study intelligible to those outside the researcher's sphere of interest. In this section of the chapter, general guidelines for proposal preparation are given, followed by specific suggestions related to each basic element of a research proposal. Detailed suggestions for proposal preparation have been provided by others.[1,2]

General Proposal Guidelines

Ideas with merit may never get to the implementation stage if the proposal does not meet the technical standards of the agency to which it is submitted, if the language is confusing, or if the appearance of the document makes it difficult to read. Thus, researchers need to prepare their proposal in the format, style, and appearance preferred by the agency to which they are submitting it. Whether one is submitting the proposal to a doctoral dissertation committee, to an institutional review board for assessment of whether the proposal contains adequate safeguards for the human participants involved in the research, or to a foundation for funding, there will be guidelines to follow for preparation of the proposal. If there is a page limit, do not exceed it. If you are required to submit one original and three copies, do not submit an original and two copies. If the proposal must be in someone's office by a certain date, do not simply mail the proposal on that date. In short, follow the directions of the group to whom the proposal will be submitted.

The proposal may need to be modified to meet different needs at different times. The format that students must use for the proposal they submit to their research advisors will likely differ from the format required for submission of the proposal to the human participants review committee, and the format required for foundation funding will probably differ from the other two formats. Word-processing programs make it relatively easy to make whatever changes in the proposal are necessary at different points in the preparation process.

The proposal must be well organized and contain clear, concise language appropriate for the individuals who will be reviewing it. A proposal submitted to one's academic advisors can be written with the assumption that the audience has basic knowledge of the area of study; a proposal submitted to a family-run philanthropic foundation must be written so that lay individuals can grasp the essential elements and importance of the proposal. The appearance of the document must both invite the reader and convey the investigator's competence. Misspellings convey the message that the proposal writer does not pay attention to details and may make the reviewer wonder whether adequate attention would be paid to the details of the research. Cramped type,

narrow margins, draft-quality print, and poor photocopying all make the document difficult to read.
Attractive documents have a good balance between text and white space, achieved through adequate margins, lots of headings for skimming,
and numbered or bulleted lists.

Elements of the Research Proposal

In many ways, the elements of a research proposal are similar to those of a research article. In
fact, a good proposal can serve as the outline for
the first draft of a research article. Table 27–1
outlines the typical sections of a proposal.

TITLE. The proposal title should be concise yet
precise, and should mention the most important

variables under study. When seeking funding for
a study, researchers may include in the title of
their study words similar to those listed as priorities by the funding agency. For example, if an
agency lists the funding of research related to
Down syndrome as one of its priorities, researchers studying children with hypotonia (including some with Down syndrome) might do
well to title their proposal "Assessment of Children with Down Syndrome and Other Hypotonic
Conditions" rather than "Assessment of Children
with Hypotonia."

INVESTIGATORS. The names, credentials, and institutional affiliations of the investigators should be
given. If cooperating institutions with whom the
researchers are not formally affiliated will be involved in the research, they should be specified

---

TABLE 27-1 **Components of a Research Proposal**

Title
  Key words
  Variables of interest
Investigators
  Names and credentials
  Affiliation
  Curricula vitae in appendix
Abstract
Problem
  Based in the work of the profession
  Backed up with literature
Purposes
  Specific objectives of the study
  Researcher hypotheses about results
Methods
  Subject selection and assignment
    Procedures
    Provisions for confidentiality
  Procedures
    Justified by literature
    Detailed enough to assess benefits and risks
    Qualifications of investigators or others to
      perform procedures
    Provisions for protection of subjects during
      testing or treatment
    Reference to informed consent form in appendix,
      if appropriate

Data analysis
  Based on best-case scenario
  May include contingency plans
References
Dissemination
  Conferences at which presentations may be given
  Journal to which results will be submitted first
  Other means by which results may be
    disseminated to the communities of interest
Budget
  Personnel, salaries, and benefits
  Supplies
  Equipment
  Mailing, printing, etc.
  Subject stipends
  Data analysis
  Presentation and publication preparation
  Presentation travel
Work plan
  All phases, from implementation to dissemination
Appendices
  Curricula vitae of investigators
  Informed consent form
  Very detailed procedures

here. A curriculum vitae, or scholar's resumé, of each investigator is often included in an appendix to the proposal.

PROBLEM STATEMENT. The problem statement in a research proposal is generated and placed in the context of related literature. A persuasive paragraph or two are needed to convince the prospective sponsors of the study's importance. The problems need to be consistent with the goals and mission of the institution at which the research will be performed and with the purposes for which an agency is making funds available.

PURPOSES. The purposes section of a proposal enumerates how the problem will be approached in the study. If there are several purposes, they should be listed in a logical sequence according to factors such as importance, underlying concepts, or timing. The format of the purposes varies depending on the type of research being proposed. For example, if the research is exploratory in nature, the purposes may take the form of questions, as in the following statement:

> The purpose of this study is to answer four questions:
> 1. To what extent do physical therapy students feel isolated from the clinical environment during their first year of study?
> 2. What difficulties do newly licensed physical therapists experience in making the transition from student to professional?
> 3. Does participation in a program in which students are matched with clinician advisors decrease feelings of isolation from the clinic?
> 4. Does participation in the clinician advisor program ease the transition from student to professional?

If the research is in a more developed area, then more formalized hypotheses may be appropriate.

METHODS. The methods section of a research proposal should include information on participant selection, procedures, and data analysis. Description of the sample must include the source of participants for the study; the sample size anticipated; the methods of assigning participants to groups, if appropriate; and the means by which the informed consent of the participants will be obtained, if appropriate. A copy of the informed consent document should be included as an appendix to the proposal (guidelines for writing informed consent statements are presented later in this chapter).

Procedures should be discussed in detail, with reference to the literature that provides justification for the choice of procedures. Any independent and dependent variables should be clearly defined. The means by which extraneous variables are controlled should be noted, and the reasons for leaving any extraneous variables uncontrolled should be given.

The data analysis procedures in the proposal are usually based on a best-case scenario, but may include contingency plans for nonnormal data or if the number of anticipated participants does not materialize. There should be a data analysis element for every research hypothesis or question. If statistical consultants have been used to develop the data analysis section of the proposal or will be available to assist with data analysis, this should be indicated here.

DISSEMINATION. Readers of the proposal will want to know how the researchers will disseminate the study findings. Conference presentation and journal article publications are the most common means of dissemination (see Chapter 28).

BUDGET. There are costs associated with any research project. If a project is self-funded by the researcher or internally funded by an organization, these costs are frequently hidden because the individuals doing the research are donating their time or the institution in which the research is being conducted simply does not actually calculate the loss of revenue from the decreased clinical productivity of the individuals involved. Externally funded projects require detailed budgets that account for both the direct and indirect costs of the research. Direct costs include equipment, supplies, computers, salaries and benefits of individuals working on the project, and the like. Indirect costs include administrative costs, overhead, and salaries and benefits of individuals peripherally involved with the study. See Funding for more detailed information on developing a budget for the research project.

WORK PLAN. The work plan details when tasks will be accomplished and who will accomplish them. All phases from planning through implementa-

tion and dissemination need to be included in the work plan. Researchers need to be realistic in estimating the amount of time needed to accomplish the project, making sure that adequate slack is included to manage unforeseen complications. Time constraints on students or considerations of the clinic may dictate that certain events happen at certain times. When this is the case, the researchers should develop the work plan by proceeding backward from a set date to ensure that all necessary preliminary tasks are accomplished. Table 27–2 shows a work plan developed for a study required for completion of

TABLE 27-2 **Work Plan for a Research Project**

Submit first draft to advisor	Nov 1, 1999
Finish revisions to first draft	Nov 30, 1999
Advisor approves proposal for degree requirements	Dec 5, 1999
Submit approved proposal to physical therapy (PT) director at hospital	Dec 8, 1999
PT director and burn clinic director review proposal and make suggestions or approve	Jan 6, 2000
Make protocol revisions if necessary	Jan 15, 2000
Submit institutional review board (IRB) materials for university approval	Jan 20, 2000
University IRB holds meeting	Jan 31, 2000
Build measuring device and test with researchers	Jan 31, 2000
Submit IRB materials for hospital approval	Feb 2, 2000
Hospital IRB holds meeting	Feb 18, 2000
Reserve video equipment for pilot and test days	Feb 20, 2000
Develop data collection forms	Feb 20, 2000
Pilot test with 1 or 2 patients	Mar 1, 2000
Revise forms and photocopy for data collection	Mar 3, 2000
Collect data at burn clinic	Mar 5, 2000
Arrange for photography for presentation and publication, to be done in April	Mar 15, 2000
Collect data at burn clinic	Apr 2, 2000
Enter data into computer program	Apr 12, 2000
Analyze data	Apr 28, 2000
Submit first draft of academic paper to advisor	June 6, 2000
Submit second draft of paper to advisor	Aug 12, 2000
Develop presentation script and submit to advisor	Sept 8, 2000
Advisor approves presentation script	Oct 4, 2000
Generate presentation slides	Oct 21, 2000
Submit abstract for presentation at conference	Nov 2, 2000
Oral presentation to faculty	Nov 11, 2000
Submit third draft of paper to advisor	Nov 27, 2000
Submit final draft of paper to advisor	Dec 1, 2000
File approved copies of paper with university	Dec 7, 2000
Revise academic paper for journal publication	Jan 31, 2001
Submit for publication	Feb 15, 2001

an academic degree in physical therapy. In this example, data collection will occur at a burn clinic held only once a month. The work plan therefore revolves around the set dates on which the clinic is held.

APPENDICES. In the appendices, the researcher provides detailed information that may be required by reviewers of the proposal but is not required for a basic understanding of what the proposal entails. Common items include the curricula vitae of the investigators, informed consent forms, and very detailed procedures such as diagrams of specific exercises and progression of repetitions for an exercise study.

APPROVALS. Once the proposal is prepared, it requires approval, sometimes from individuals at several different levels. Student proposals require the approval of research advisors and committees. Clinical research proposals require administrative approval at one or more levels in an organization. Proposals for studies using human or animal subjects require approval by human or animal subject protection committees. The procedures for obtaining academic and administrative approval vary widely from institution to institution and are not discussed further. In contrast, the procedure for obtaining approval from human participants protection committees tends to be similar at most institutions.

■ HUMAN PARTICIPANTS PROTECTION

Researchers in physical therapy must undertake many procedures to ensure the protection of the human participants they use in their studies. Researchers who use animal subjects must submit their proposals for approval from comparable animal subjects protection committees.

To protect their participants from mental and physical harm, researchers must

- Design sound studies in which dangers to participants are minimized

- Secure the informed consent of participants
- Implement the research with care and consideration for participants' safety

Review committees are the mechanisms by which the design and informed consent elements of participant safety are ensured. At many institutions, such a committee is called the *institutional review board* (IRB). Federal regulations since 1971 have specified that research conducted with government funds be subject to review by a committee concerned with the rights and welfare of participants. In addition, most scientific journals today require evidence that research with animal or human subjects has undergone a review, irrespective of the funding source of the research.

Although procedures vary from institution to institution, many IRBs base their work on federal guidelines. Consequently, most of the guidelines presented here are based on the guidelines of the federal government. These guidelines, along with thoughtful discussion of ethical issues posed within the clinical research process, have been well summarized by several authors.[3–6]

Institutional Review Boards

Federal regulations specify that an IRB be composed of at least five members with varying backgrounds representative of the type of research conducted at the university: Individuals of different sexes and races should be represented, at least one member must have a nonscientific background, and one member should be unaffiliated with the institution. This composition is designed to ensure that a closely knit group of scientists does not make the decisions about their own or their colleagues' projects.

The purpose of the IRB is to review research conducted under the auspices of the institution to ensure that the rights of human participants are protected. These rights are protected when research designs minimize risks to participants, when participant selection and assignment are equitable, when researchers have made provisions for the confidentiality of information, and when participants are provided with the information they need to make an informed decision about whether to participate in the research. The IRB accomplishes its purpose through regular meetings during which it reviews written proposals submitted in a format specified by the IRB.

Levels of Review

IRBs typically have three levels of review of research projects: exempt, expedited, and full. Research that is *exempt* from review includes

- Research that involves normal educational practices
- Survey or interview procedures that do not involve sensitive areas of behavior and in which responses are recorded in such a way that they cannot be attributed to a particular individual
- Observations of public behavior
- Study of existing data

Although federal regulations indicate that such research is exempt from review by the IRB, institutions may require researchers to submit materials (such as a proposal or questionnaires) to the IRB so that the members can determine whether the research fits the exempt category. An exempt study in physical therapy might involve retrospective chart review or opinion assessment through a mailed questionnaire.

Expedited reviews are permitted for studies that involve minimal risks to participants. Such procedures include

- Collection of hair, nails, or external secretions
- Recording of noninvasive data
- Study of small amounts of blood through venipuncture
- Study of the effects of moderate exercise in healthy volunteers

Expedited reviews sometimes may be accomplished by a single committee member. Expedited studies in physical therapy might involve measuring range of motion in a patient group or assessing strength gains following an exercise program using normal participants.

The IRB conducts a *full* review of

- Research projects that involve more risks than those identified for exempt or expedited review
- Studies of lower-risk procedures in children or others who are unable to provide meaningful consent

Examples of physical therapy studies that would require full review include assessment of the fitness level of patients with cardiovascular disease or a trial of a new exercise program in children with cerebral palsy.

Informed Consent

In the context of research, informed consent refers to an interaction between the researcher and potential participant. The researcher provides the potential participant with the information he or she needs to make an informed decision about whether to participate in the research. The potential participant then makes his or her decision and communicates it to the researcher, usually by either signing or declining to sign a written consent form.

Consent forms must be written in language that is understandable to the individuals who will be giving consent. The typical reading level of participants should be considered, as should visual acuity and native language. A copy of the consent form itself should be provided to the participant. Table 27–3 lists the elements of an informed consent statement, and Figure 27–1 presents a sample consent form document. Consent forms may not contain exculpatory language, that is, language that asks participants to waive any of their legal rights or releases the investigator or institution from liability for negli-

TABLE 27-3	Elements of a Consent Form

Statement that the study constitutes research
Explanation of study's purposes
Explanation of basis of subject selection and duration of subject involvement
Explanation of provisions for subject confidentiality
Description of procedures, with experimental procedures identified
Description of risks and discomforts
Description of potential benefits to subjects and others
Description of alternative treatments, if available
Statement of whether compensation is available for injuries
Name of person to contact if questions or injuries arise
Statement emphasizing that participation is voluntary
Statement that the subject has the right to withdraw from the study at any time
Statement of disclosure of information gained in the study that might influence subject's willingness to continue participation
Explanation of payment arrangements, if applicable
Consent statement
Date line
Subject's signature line
Investigator's signature line
Investigator's institutional affiliation and telephone number

gent acts associated with the research project. Ideally, the form is contained on a single sheet of paper, with front and back sides used as needed. If more pages are needed, they should be numbered "1 of 3," "2 of 3," and the like so that participants are assured that all the needed information has been received.

The researcher should keep the signed consent forms in a secure location. The length of time the forms are retained depends on the nature and length of the research and on the latency and duration of foreseeable complications related to the research procedures. Researchers should recognize that the signed consent form is usually the only point at which each participant's name is linked to the study. Therefore, secure storage of signed consent forms is an important part of maintaining participants' confidentiality.

There are two general situations in which consent forms may not be needed or appropriate. The first is the collection of data via a mailed survey. In this case, the elements of informed consent should be contained within the cover letter written by the researcher to the potential respondent, and return of the questionnaire by the respondent is taken as evidence of consent. The second situation is a study that is of a sensitive nature and signed consent forms would be a means by which the study participants could be identified. In this situation, informed consent may be obtained verbally.

FUNDING

Conducting research is a costly affair. The challenge for researchers is to find funding to support their research interests. Funds generally come from one of four sources: institutions, corporations, foundations, or the government. A review of the first 6 months of *Physical Therapy* in 1998 showed that approximately 40% of published research reports were apparently internally funded by the institutions at which they were conducted, none were funded by corporations, 14% were funded by foundations, 11% were funded by US government sources, and 34% were funded by sources outside the United States.

The small proportion of studies funded externally is evidence of the infancy of physical therapy research. To aid researchers who try to fund studies externally, this section of the chapter presents a typical budget for a research study and then discusses the peculiarities of the four funding sources.

Budget

Table 27–4 presents a budget for a descriptive study that would require data collection by two physical therapists and support services from

University of Anytown
1256 Holt Road
Department of Physical Therapy

Anytown, Indiana 46234
(317) 555-4300

CONSENT TO PARTICIPATE IN A RESEARCH STUDY

TITLE OF STUDY: Comparison of Integrated Electromyographic Activity and Strength Measures in the Supraspinatus Muscle in Two Positions.

You are invited to participate in a research study which measures the electrical activity and strength of the supraspinatus muscle, which is located in the back of the shoulder. You have been invited to participate based on the assumption that you have a shoulder which is free of injury or disability. Your participation would require attendance at a single measurement session lasting approximately one hour.

Prior to your participation, an investigator will take a brief medical history to determine whether you have had previous shoulder problems which would make you ineligible to participate. Weight, height, age, and sex will also be recorded. You will be assigned a subject number so that your name will not be associated with any of the findings of this study.

The research procedure consists of measurement of muscle electrical activity and strength in two positions. The electrical activity of your supraspinatus muscle will be measured by an experienced electromyographer. He will insert a 27-gauge sterile needle containing two fine-wire electrodes into your muscle. After positioning the wires, the needle will be removed and the wires will remain in place for testing in both positions. The wires will be removed on completion of data collection in both positions.

Strength will be measured with a hand-held dynamometer, which is a stationary device held by the researcher and placed at the back of your wrist. You will be asked to use your shoulder muscles to push against the device as hard as you can. This will be repeated three times in each of the two positions.

In the first position you will be seated, with your arm straight in front of you with your thumb pointing down. In the second position you will lie on your stomach with your arm out straight in front of you and with your thumb pointing up.

PAGE 1 of 2

_____ (Participant's Initials)

FIGURE 27–1. Example of a consent form.

Illustration continued on following page

one aide and one secretary. Personnel costs are determined by estimating the proportion of time each individual would be involved in the study, multiplying the salary by that proportion, and adding a reasonable percentage for benefits. Equipment costs should be estimated, including service and repair costs if appropriate. Consultants are individuals who are not employed by

CONSENT TO PARTICIPATE IN A RESEARCH STUDY (Continued)

TITLE OF STUDY: Comparison of Integrated Electromyographic Activity and Strength Measures in the Supraspinatus Muscle in Two Positions.

The risks of participation in this study include muscle fatigue or soreness from exercise, temporary discomfort from needle insertion, infection from the needle electrode, bleeding from needle insertion, and a small risk of puncture of the chest cavity which could lead to pain, difficulty breathing, and would require medical attention. To protect from infection, sterile needles and electrodes will be used and will be disposed of after each use. To protect from the risk of chest cavity puncture, the electromyographer will use needle placement designed to minimize this risk. If muscle soreness occurs, you will be instructed in procedures to minimize discomfort. No compensation is available for injuries resulting from participation in this research.

By determining the position in which the supraspinatus muscle is most effective, the results of this research may benefit patients and athletes who wish to strengthen their shoulder muscles.

If you have questions about this research or need to report an injury related to your participation in this research, contact xxxxx at (xxx) xxx-xxxx. Your participation in this research is voluntary, and your decision whether or not to participate will not affect your standing at this institution. If you elect to participate in the study, you have the right to withdraw from the study at any time without affecting your standing at the institution. You will receive a copy of this form.

CONSENT

I, _____, voluntarily consent to participate in this research study as described above. I have had a chance to ask questions of the researcher, and have had any questions answered to my satisfaction.

_____
Subject Signature

_____
Researcher Signature

_____
Date

PAGE 2 of 2

FIGURE 27–1. *Continued*

the sponsoring institution, but are engaged on a daily or hourly basis to fulfill a special need of the research project. Statistical, computer, and engineering consultants are examples. The cost of disseminating the results of the research includes the cost of manuscript preparation, the cost of creating photographs and graphs, the cost of slide presentations, and the cost of trav-

TABLE 27-4 Research Project Budget		
Item	**Explanation**	**Cost**
Personnel		
Joyce McWain, PT	10% time for 1 year	$6000
Principal Investigator	Benefits 20% of salary	
	Annual salary $50,000	
Randall Myers, PT	5% time for 6 months	$1500
Coinvestigator	Benefits 20% of salary	
	Annual salary $50,000	
Ben Riley	5% time for 6 months	$540
PT Aide	Benefits 20% of salary	
	Annual salary $18,000	
Sally Knapp	5% time for 6 months	$600
Secretary	Benefits 20% of salary	
	Annual salary $20,000	
Equipment		
Hand-held dynamometers	Two at $900 each	$1800
Consultants		
Statistician	20 hours at $100/hr	$2000
Dissemination		
Photocopying	1000 pages at $.05 per page	$50
Photography	Black and whites, $100	$500
	Slides, 40 at $10 each	
Travel	Principal investigator and	
	coinvestigator to annual	
	conference, $1500 each	$3000
Overhead	8% of $15,900	$1279
Total		$17,179

eling to conferences to present the research. The overhead costs covering the use of existing facilities is often figured as a percentage of the direct costs. This percentage is often specified by either the funding agency or the institution in which the research is conducted.

Institution Funding

As already mentioned, much of physical therapy research is funded by the institution in which it is conducted. Department managers who believe in research as an essential element of professionalism may allow staff to conduct limited amounts of research on work time. However, because research time does not produce revenue like patient care does, even the most research-oriented managers have difficulty releasing therapists from patient care to perform research. This is particularly true in the cost-cutting, high-productivity environment that is prevalent in rehabilitation settings in the late 1990s in the United States.

Corporation Funding

A corporation may fund a research project directly through its operating funds or indirectly through a grant from a foundation associated with the company. When a corporation provides research funds through direct giving, it is usually to support activities directly related to the corporation's function. For example, equipment manufacturers may be willing to provide equipment for and pay the salaries of researchers who are conducting studies that showcase their products. Some manufacturers are willing to loan equipment for the duration of a project; many students, who typically conduct research on a shoestring budget, have obtained loaner equipment simply by contacting the manufacturer or a local sales representative.

Researchers who accept funds directly from corporations need to be sure they understand who has control of the data and its dissemination. A corporation may wish to retain ownership of the data so that it has the prerogative of not releasing any data that are not favorable toward its product. Researchers who contact companies for support must decide whether they are willing to accept such terms, should the company request them.

Foundation Funding

Foundations are private entities that distribute funds according to the priorities set by their donors or their boards of trustees. There are many types of foundations; how to identify those that may be interested in your proposal and how to apply for funds from a foundation are discussed next.

TYPES OF FOUNDATIONS. Foundations that provide research grants can be broadly divided into independent, company-sponsored, and community foundations. The funds of an independent foundation usually come from a single source, such as a family, an individual, or a group of individuals. Independent foundations give grants in fields specified by the few individuals who administer the fund; giving is often limited to the local geographical region in which the fund is located. The major independent foundation that supports physical therapy research in the United States is the Foundation for Physical Therapy. In

fact, the majority of the foundation-funded studies published in *Physical Therapy* in the first half of 1998 were funded by the Foundation for Physical Therapy. This foundation is a national, independent, nonprofit corporation associated with the American Physical Therapy Association. Donors are those with interests in the physical therapy community, for example, individual physical therapists, equipment manufacturers and vendors, academic programs of physical therapy, and private physical therapy practices.

A company-sponsored foundation is an independent entity that is funded by contributions from a company. Although the foundation is independent from the corporation, it tends to give grants in fields related to the company's products or customers. Giving is often limited to the geographical region or regions in which the company is located.

Community foundations are publicly supported by funds derived from many donors. The mission of a community foundation is to meet the needs of its locale; thus the projects it funds must be directly related to the welfare of the community.

IDENTIFYING FOUNDATIONS. Large institutions supported by several grant agencies have grants administration officers who can help researchers identify appropriate funding sources. The Foundation Center, a nonprofit organization, publishes comprehensive references that can also help researchers identify foundations that fund studies in their area of interest.[7,8] These references are available in most university or public libraries. The information provided for each foundation includes the size of the fund, the amount given annually, the names of agencies to whom funds were given, and the types of projects funded (scholarships, construction of new facilities, education, or research). Several specialized indexes focus on funding projects in health or health-related areas such as aging.[9,10]

APPLYING FOR FOUNDATION FUNDS. The procedure for applying for foundation funds varies greatly from foundation to foundation. Funding decisions in independent foundations may rest with a very few individuals. Consequently, applying for funds is relatively informal. A letter of inquiry describing the research in general terms should be sent to the foundation. Ways in which the research meets the goals of the foundation should be emphasized. The reply from the foundation will indicate whether the idea is appealing to them and will ask for additional information if it is. The additional information required is likely to be fairly brief and can be assembled in a format determined by the researcher.

Corporate-sponsored foundations often have more formalized grant application procedures. However, the letter of inquiry is still the first means by which the researcher contacts the foundations. If the general area of the research is within the scope of the foundation's activities, the foundation will respond with directions for formal application for funds.

Government Funding

The federal government is a major provider of research grants in the United States. Table 27–5 provides a partial listing of the government agencies that provide funding for health sciences research. Several references provide detailed information about the grant programs of the federal government[11–13] or about strategies for applying for government grant funds.[14]

The procedure for obtaining federal grant funding is far more formal than that for obtaining foundation funding. First, the grant funds must be made available. To do this, Congress must both authorize the grant-funding program and then, in a separate legislative step, appropriate funds for the program. Administration of appropriated funds is delegated to a large grants administration bureaucracy in Washington, DC. When funds are appropriated for a grant program, notice is placed in the *Federal Register*, the daily federal government news publication. Once notice is placed in the register, application materials can be released to potential grant recipients. Applications are highly formalized, and

TABLE 27–5	**Partial Listing of Federal Government Funding Sources for Health Research***

Department of Health and Human Services
Administration for Children and Families
   Centers for Disease Control and Prevention
   National Institute for Occupational Safety and Health
   National Institutes of Health
      National Cancer Institute
      National Heart, Lung, and Blood Institute
      National Institute of Arthritis and Musculoskeletal and Skin Diseases
      National Institute of Child Health and Human Development
      National Institute of Neurological Disorders and Stroke
      National Institute on Aging
      Office of Alternative Medicine
National Science Foundation
Department of Education
   National Institute for Disability and Rehabilitation Research
Veterans Health Administration

* Compiled from the web sites of the American Physical Therapy Association (http://www.apta.org) and the US Federal Agencies Directory (http://origin.lib.lsu.edu/gov/fedgov.htm.). Both sites accessed on March 14, 1999.

grant applicants must certify that they are in compliance with a variety of federal regulations related to nondiscrimination and protection of human participants. Although the process is formalized, the individuals who direct the various grant programs are available to discuss the application process with grant writers.

The awarding of federal grants is usually accomplished by a peer review committee. Experienced researchers are assembled to review the submitted proposals and make recommendations about their disposition. Often only one or two reviewers read the entire proposal; the rest of the committee members read only the abstract of the study and hear the primary reviewers' descriptions and evaluations of the program. It is therefore imperative that the abstract of the grant proposal accurately reflect the scope of the project for which funding is sought.

Federal grant proposals will have one of three outcomes: approval with funding, approval without funding, or disapproval. A proposal is disapproved if the study does not meet the purpose of the grant or its design is not acceptable. Proposals that meet the technical requirements are approved and given a certain priority level. Only those with the highest priority level are funded.

After writing the research proposal, obtaining administrative and institutional review board approval, and securing the funds needed to implement a project, the researcher must contend with the substantial logistical details of implementing a project.[15,16] The second half of this chapter addresses a number of these concerns, including recruitment of participants, data collection, and data analysis.

▌ OBTAINING PARTICIPANTS

The time and effort required to obtain research participants are often far greater than the researcher anticipates. For example, assume that we wish to implement a study of elderly patients who have undergone total knee arthroplasty. We plan to study two groups who undergo different inpatient and outpatient postoperative rehabilitation. Measurement of certain outcomes will be taken at discharge, 3 months postoperatively, and 6 months postoperatively. If we know that 100 such surgeries are performed in a 6-month period at our facility, we may assume that there will be no difficulty obtaining two study groups of 40 participants each for our study. Table 27–6 shows, however, several ways in which the number of available participants will be far fewer than the 100 patients who undergo the surgery. If the scenario in Table 27–6 were realized, we would be faced with a situation in which fewer than 20 participants were available per group during the 6 months in which participants were to be recruited.

TABLE 27-6	Eventual Sample from a Potential 100 Patients

Reason for Participation or Nonparticipation	N	N Remaining
Total knee arthroplasties performed in 6 months	100	100
Young patient with hemophilia	3	97
Patient with perioperative complications	5	92
Patient lives more than 60 miles away or has received outpatient physical therapy at another clinic	10	82
Patient's surgeon does not wish to participate	12	70
Patient does not consent to be in study	10	60
Patient does not complete outpatient physical therapy	12	48
Patient dies before 6-month visit	2	46
Patient moves or cannot be located to schedule 6-month appointment	4	42
Patient does not come to the scheduled 6-month follow-up appointment	6	36

Researchers need to plan their participant recruitment strategy carefully to ensure an adequate number of participants. Different strategies are appropriate when recruiting inpatients, outpatients, or the general public. In all cases, recruitment of participants should take place after an institutional review board has approved both the conduct of the study and the procedures to be used for ensuring the informed consent of participants.

Inpatient Recruitment

In the inpatient setting, the admitting physician is clearly in control of the care that the patient receives while in the hospital. Thus, securing inpatients for study requires careful work with the medical staff of the institution. In fact, the best way to secure participants for study is to invite key physicians to collaborate in the entire research endeavor. In addition, the administrative chain of command within the facility will need to be followed to secure permission to implement the project.

After securing the permission of the admitting physician, the researcher contacts participants directly to secure their informed consent. As with all participant recruitment methods, patients must be approached in a manner that conveys that regardless of whether they choose to participate, their care will not be prejudiced. The physical therapist and physician should determine together the best procedure for securing patient consent: The physician may mention the study to the patients first and indicate that the therapist will visit with details; the therapist may accompany the physician on rounds so that they can jointly present the study to patients, assuring them that the different professionals are working together on the research endeavor; or the therapist may present the study first, giving patients the opportunity to discuss the study later with the physician before consenting.

Outpatient Recruitment

Outpatient recruitment is somewhat easier than inpatient recruitment because permission of the patient's physician is not always necessary. If a descriptive, correlational, or methodological study is being conducted that does not involve any procedures contraindicated by the current orders of the patient, the researcher can feel free to proceed without obtaining the individual physician's consent. As is the case with inpatients, it is wise to inform the physicians of the ongoing project, so that they will not be alarmed if patients tell them that they have participated in a research study.

After the study, it is courteous to send the physicians of participants who participated a summary of the study results, along with your assessment of how the results will allow you to serve their patients better in the future. Alternatively, collaboration with physicians may prove rewarding for both physicians and therapists while having the added benefit of providing therapists with easier access to some participants.

If the research protocol requires a departure from a physician's orders, then permission must be sought and gained from both the physician and the patient, as described in Inpatient Recruitment. Again, collaboration or communication with the physicians about the study results may make them more willing to have their patients participate in future studies.

Recruitment of patients who have completed their course of treatment requires careful consideration of the confidentiality of their medical records. Consider a case in which a university-based researcher contacts a clinic to request access to patient records to identify participants who meet certain inclusion criteria. The clinic, being interested in the project, agrees to participate in the study and provides the researcher with the names and addresses of patients with the particular diagnosis. Patients would have good reason to be concerned about breaches of confidentiality if they received a letter from an unknown researcher requesting their participation in a study based on the fact that they had had a certain surgery and were seen for treatment at a certain clinic. A procedure that protects patient privacy may involve having a clinic employee—who already has access to the clinic records—write a letter to eligible patients explaining the study and asking for their permission to release their name and address to the researcher. A form letter (and stamped return envelope) on which patients indicate their willingness to have their name released to the investigator can be included with the letter.

Recruitment of the Lay Public

When a study requires the participation of the lay public rather than patients, researchers are challenged by the need to balance their desire for convenient access to a particular group of participants with their hope that results will be generalizable beyond the particular sample studied. In the past, this balance has often been lacking: Use of physical therapy students as a convenient source of participants has limited the generalizability of many studies to young, healthy women, who make up the majority of physical therapy students.

Groups that consist of individuals with a wide range of educational, racial, and socioeconomic characteristics are desirable for many studies. If one works in a large organization, recruiting participants from employees at all levels—from upper administration to maintenance staff—often provides the sort of variety that is desired.

Researchers who require specific types of participants need to be creative in identifying existing groups from which to recruit. Examples of groups that may yield good participant pools for certain populations include churches, senior citizen or retirement centers, apartment complexes, health clubs, day care centers, and youth or adult sport leagues. For example, if one wished to study balance in the well elderly, participants might be found in church groups, senior bowling leagues, residential retirement centers, or senior citizen centers with daytime programs. The choice of which group to use would depend on the contact the researcher has with members of the groups and how seriously biased the group membership is in light of the particular research question. For instance, if a researcher's great-aunt bowls 3 days a week in a senior league, she might be able to recruit plenty of participants for a balance study. However, if the researcher believes that the senior bowlers would be biased in the direction of better balance than most of the well elderly, the bowling league may not be a good choice, no matter how easy it would be to obtain participants from the group.

Once a researcher has determined that a particular group is suitable for study, the appropriate administrative approval is needed—be it from the director of personnel, the manager of the bowling alley, the pastor of the church, or the administrator of the retirement center. When seeking such approval, the researcher needs to prepare a brief version of the study proposal, written in terms understandable to the person whose approval is sought. A blank consent form should be included along with documentation of the institutional review board approval. To gain administrative approval, the researcher will need to convince the official that the study has value; that participation in the study will not greatly disrupt the facility's routine; that participants are at minimal risk of harm and will be treated with dignity and respect; and, if appropriate, that participants may enjoy the participation and interaction with others that it affords.

Once administrative approval has been given to recruit participants from a particular facility, the researcher needs to make initial contact with potential participants. This may be done by discussing the study at a group meeting, writing letters to particular potential participants, or posting flyers in areas frequented by the members of the desired group. Whatever the format, this initial information should include the purpose of the study, the actual activities in which the participant would be participating, the time commitment required to participate, and the means by which interested parties can contact the researcher.

■ DATA COLLECTION

The three major types of data collection tools used by physical therapists are biophysiological instruments, interviews, and questionnaires. Details regarding the development and administration of interviews and questionnaires have already been presented in Chapters 13 and 16 and are not repeated here. Therefore, this section of the chapter focuses on general principles of data collection or specific data collection issues related to the use of biophysiological instruments.

Data Collection Procedures

When using existing instrumentation, the researcher must be familiar with both the manufacturer's instructions for use of the equipment and the protocols that other researchers have followed with the equipment. From this information, decisions can be made about the procedures for data collection. Although a general procedure for data collection will have been developed for the research proposal, very detailed procedural guidelines should be established and written down so that they can be implemented uniformly within the study. For example, a procedure such as height measurement seems simple and would not require detailed description in a proposal. However, before data collection is begun, the specific procedure for taking the height measurement should be developed: Will the measurement be taken with participants barefoot, stocking-footed, or in shoes? Will participants be instructed to stand comfortably or stand tall? Should the head be comfortably erect or in military axial extension? Written standardization procedures are particularly important if more than one researcher will be measuring participants.

Accuracy checks of the equipment should be conducted, if necessary. Goniometer scales can be checked against known angles, scales can be checked against known weights, and calibration of equipment can be accomplished according to manufacturer's instructions. In some instances, the researcher may wish to have an engineer or manufacturer's technician give the equipment a mechanical or electrical checkout to determine that it is operating properly before data are collected.

Safeguarding Data

When collecting data, the researcher needs to take steps to ensure quality and completeness. Although specific suggestions for data collection are provided in the following sections, all researchers must consider the overriding concern for the safety of data that have been collected. Briefcases get lost, cars get stolen, hard disks crash, dogs chew, and buildings can be destroyed by fires or floods. Given the many possible disasters that can threaten one's data, it makes sense to maintain backup copies of the information one has collected. If the data are collected and stored on computer disk, make a backup copy of the disk. If the data are collected on handwritten forms, either make copies of the completed forms or transfer the information to a data file soon after collecting it.

The two copies of the data should be stored in two different locations; it does no good to have two copies of the data if both are in the same file that was stored directly under the pipe that burst. If several researchers collaborate with one another, then different researchers should probably keep the data in different locations. If there is a single investigator, one copy can be kept at work or school and one at home.

Protecting Participant Identity

When each participant enters the trial, he or she should be assigned a number and, if appropriate, a study group according to one of the plans developed in Chapter 8. A master list specifying each participant's name, address, and phone number; study identification number; and group membership should be maintained. If data recorders and participants are blind to group membership, generally only one researcher has access to the master list. This researcher should keep the master list in a secure location where other researchers will not accidentally come across the information; a second copy should be kept separately from the original copy.

Data Recording Forms

Researchers must design forms for data collection. Today, the form may be a pen-and-paper form or one that is filled out directly on the computer. The form should contain space for each participant's identification number but not name, to ensure confidentiality of the information. The order of items on the form should be carefully considered to coincide with the order in which the information will be collected. Adequate space should be left for a readable response to the information.

In general, the information should be collected at the highest measurement level possible. For example, adult ages should be recorded as age at last birthday. Even if the researcher plans to categorize participants into age groups, such as those younger than 60 and those 60 and older, it is wise to collect the information as actual age and then code it into groups. In this way, if a later research question requires actual age, that information is available. If just the group membership (<60 or ≥60) is recorded originally, then there is no way to later determine participants' actual ages.

If data require coding (e.g., conversion of letters into numbers and collapse of actual ages into age groups) for analysis, the form should be designed to facilitate the coding process. Figure 27–2 shows a completed data collection form with space for data coding for the hypothetical total knee arthroplasty study described in Section 6 of this text (see Tables 20–1 and 20–2). The blank spaces on the right-hand side of the form are for the pieces of information that will be entered in the computer data file. Some information such as the date and the name of the therapist collecting the data may not be relevant to the final data set, but may be useful to have if there is a question about a piece of information. For two of the deformity variables, actual angular value is reduced to a category; however, there is room on the form for both the actual value and the code that corresponds to the category in which the angular value belongs.

Pilot Study

A pilot study is crucial to the smooth running of a research trial. In a pilot study, the researchers go through a dress-rehearsal of the research study, using a few volunteers similar to those who will participate in the study. The pilot study allows the researchers to take care of small glitches in the procedure and reveals the little details that need attending to: How long does it actually take to collect the data? Is the planned sequence cumbersome? Is another assistant needed for one part of the study? How much paper is used for the computer printout, and is there enough available to complete the study? Is an extension cord or extra batteries needed to power the equipment? Should office supplies be handy?

Scheduling Participants and Personnel

The pilot study allows the researcher to make educated guesses about how the data collection will proceed. Participants in the actual study should expect the researcher to provide a realistic estimate of the time it will take to complete their participation. Participants may not mind participating in a study that requires 5 hours of data collection as long as they know up-front that this is the time that will be involved. Participants will understandably be upset and may withdraw from participation if they are initially led to believe that data collection will require 1 hour and are still waiting to finish after 3 hours.

Adequate personnel need to be available for data collection. The types of tasks that need to be accomplished are greeting participants as they arrive, explaining the study and securing informed consent, phoning participants who have not arrived as expected, gathering background information and screening participants to ensure that they meet inclusion criteria, preparing participants for data collection, collecting the actual data, spotting participants for safety, and thanking participants for their assistance. In some studies, one researcher could handle all these tasks; in others, five or six researchers might be required.

TOTAL KNEE ARTHROPLASTY REHABILITATION STUDY

BACKGROUND INFORMATION

Case Number (CN)   *1*   *5*

Clinic Attended (CL)
1 =   Community Hospital
2 =   Memorial Hospital
3 =   Religious Hospital   *2*

Patient Sex (SEX)
      0 =   Male
      1 =   Female   *1*

Patient Age in years at last birthday (AGE)   *6*   *8*

Type of Prosthesis (PRO)
       1 =   Total condylar
       2 =   Posterior stabilizer
       3 =   Flat tibial plateau   *2*

Miscellaneous Information
      Surgeon   *Bennett*
      Side of Surgery   *R*
      Date of Surgery   *2-12-99*
      Diagnosis   *OA*

THREE WEEK POSTOPERATIVE DATA

Date   *3-5-99*

Three-week ROM, degrees (W3R)
Therapist   *60*   *0*   *7*   *6*

SIX WEEK POSTOPERATIVE DATA

Date   *3-25-99*

Therapist   *60*

Six-week ROM, degrees (W6R)   *0*   *7*   *0*

SIX MONTH POSTOPERATIVE DATA

Date   *8-15-99*

Six-month ROM, degrees (M6R)   *0*   *9*   *5*

Six-month Extension Torque, N•m (E)   *1*   *7*   *0*

FIGURE 27–2. Data collection form, with coding column.

Illustration continued on following page

Six-Month Flexion Torque, N•m (F)   <u>1</u> <u>0</u> <u>2</u>

Gait Velocity, cm/s (V)   <u>1</u> <u>6</u> <u>5</u>

Flexion Contracture at Six Months (DFC)

    Value   <u>8°</u>

    1 =   >15 degrees
    ②=   6 to 15 degrees
    3 =   0 to 5 degrees   <u>2</u>

Varus/Valgus Angulation in Stance (DVV)

    Value   <u>4° varus</u>

    1 =   >10 degrees valgus
    2 =   >5 degrees varus or 6 to 10 degrees valgus
    ③=   5 degrees varus to 5 degrees valgus   <u>3</u>

Mediolateral Stability (DML)
    1 =   Marked instability
    ②=   Moderate instability
    3 =   Stable   <u>2</u>

Anteroposterior Stability with Knee at 90° Flexion (DAP)
    1 =   Marked instability
    ②=   Moderate instability
    3 =   Stable   <u>2</u>

Distance Walked (ADW)
    5 =   Unlimited
    ④=   4 to 6 blocks
    3 =   2 to 3 blocks
    2 =   Indoors only
    1 =   Transfers only   <u>4</u>

Assistive Device (AAD)
    5 =   None
    4 =   Cane outside
    ③=   Cane full time
    2 -   Two canes, crutches
    1 =   Walker or unable   <u>3</u>

Stair Climbing (ASC)
    ⑤=   Reciprocal, no rail
    4 =   Reciprocal, with rail
    3 =   One at a time, with or without rail
    2 =   One at a time, with rail and assistive device
    1 =   Unable to climb stairs   <u>5</u>

Rising from Chair (ARC)
    ⑤=   No arm assistance
    4 =   Single arm assistance
    3 =   Difficult with two arm assistance
    2 =   Needs assistance of another
    1 =   Unable to rise   5

FIGURE 27–2. *Continued*

■ DATA ANALYSIS

The ease with which the data analysis is accomplished depends greatly on whether the researcher has (1) written a well-developed proposal with a sound plan for data analysis and (2) collected data carefully with an eye to the analysis stage. In discussing data analysis, this section presumes that a computer statistical package and a statistical consultant are available. For all but the smallest data sets, both are necessary. After a discussion of the roles of computers and consultants, suggestions are provided for the three steps of data analysis: data coding, data entry, and statistical analysis.

Many computer statistical packages are available for use on personal or mainframe computers. Three widely used statistical packages are Statistical Package for the Social Sciences (SPSS), Statistical Analysis System (SAS), and Biomedical Data Processing (BMDP); all three are available in mainframe or personal computer versions. In addition, many other programs are available.[17,18] The basic procedure for all of the computer statistical packages is that the variables of interest are defined, the data are coded numerically and entered into a data file, and then the analyses are run.

Statistical consultants can be used in several different ways. First, they can be consulted during the planning stages of a project to help determine whether the planned design can be analyzed in a way that will answer the research question. Second, they can help the researcher determine the sample size needed to obtain statistically significant results given certain assumptions about the size of differences between groups and the extent of variability within groups. Third, they can provide access to and are knowledgeable about statistical software. Fourth, they can check any analysis the researcher might have done on his or her own. Finally, they can review the written report of a research project to ensure that what the researcher has written about the statistical analysis is in fact what was done.

Before working with statistical consultants, the researcher must have a clear idea of the purposes of his or her research. A list of proposed variables and the values they may take is essential because statistical decisions will be based in part on the measurement characteristics of the data. Consultants may also wish to review published reports of studies similar to the one being planned so they can see the type of analysis that is the norm in the discipline or for a particular journal.

The researcher and consultant must be clear about who will do which tasks associated with the analysis. Will the consultant enter data, run the analysis, prepare summary tables, and summarize the results for the researcher? Or will the researcher enter the data, receive a stack of printouts, and contact the consultant only if there are any questions? Because the consultant will likely work for an hourly fee, the researcher should ask the consultant for an estimate of the number of hours that will be required for the level of involvement desired.

Data Coding

The first step of data analysis is to develop a coding scheme for the data. The coding scheme for our hypothetical total knee arthroplasty data was initially presented in Table 20–1. Figure 27–2 shows how the coding scheme is translated into a form that encourages simultaneous data collection and coding.

Responses that are letters or descriptors (A, B, C, and D on multiple-choice items; "strongly agree," "agree," "neutral," "disagree," and "strongly disagree" for Likert-type items) are generally converted into numbers for data analysis. Some statistical programs permit the researcher to enter the letter and convert it to a number; others require that numbers be entered.

The researcher needs to decide how to handle missing data points. One option is to simply leave them as blanks in the data set. In other instances, the researcher may want frequency counts of missing data or may wish to analyze a subgroup of individuals who did not respond to a certain question. In these cases, missing data need to be given their own code. The number 9 or 99 is often used as the code for missing data.

Some questionnaire items may permit multiple responses. For example, a multiple-choice item may ask respondents to indicate all the choices that apply to their situation. Coding of multiple responses is often best accomplished by converting the single item into several yes/no items. Assume that in our coding system a yes response is coded 1 and a no response is coded 0. The response for a respondent who checked A, C, and E out of A through F responses for a multiple-answer item would be coded as follows: A = 1, B = 0, C = 1, D = 0, E = 1, and F = 0.

Once the coding scheme is accomplished, the researcher should go through the data and convert it to codes as necessary. Although some researchers may be able to sit in front of the computer with raw data and simultaneously code and enter it, most will have a more accurate data set, and will save time in the long run, if they perform coding and entering separately. After the data have been coded initially, the codes need to be rechecked and corrected by either the original coder or another member of the research team.

Data Entry

Once the data are coded, they need to be entered into the computer for analysis. In many instances, the data file can be created through a standard spreadsheet program and then transferred into a format that can be used by the statistical software. Although the actual procedures for data entry vary from package to package, the basic structure of a data file is that the variables are represented by columns and the participants by rows, as shown initially in Table 20–2 for the hypothetical study of patients with total knee arthroplasty.

When data have already been coded before they are entered, the researcher can enter data quickly without needing to think about what the numbers actually mean. Some researchers find that data entry goes more quickly if one person reads the numbers aloud and another enters them.

After data entry, the data set needs to be edited against the data-coding sheets. Once again, this process may go more quickly if one member of the team reads the coding numbers aloud while the other checks the computer data printout. Only after the data set is edited, or "cleaned," is the researcher ready to run the statistical analyses that will answer the research questions.[19,20]

Statistical Analysis

Too often, investigators test their research hypotheses without first gaining a sense of the character of the data set. The first statistical procedure done should be running frequencies and descriptive data for each variable within the data set as a whole. In doing so, the researcher can get a sense of the distribution, means and standard deviations, and frequencies of the variables overall. If there are very extreme values for some variables, the researcher should recheck them against the original data sheets for accuracy. If the person collecting the data thought there might be an irregularity, it may be noted on the original data collection sheet. Extreme values are known as *outliers* and may sometimes be deleted from a data set with justification. A statistical consultant can help the researcher decide when it is reasonable to delete outliers.

Next, the researcher should divide the total sample into groups, if appropriate to the study purposes. For example, after the descriptive information about the total knee arthroplasty sample has been examined, frequencies, means, and standard deviations for each of the clinics under study should be run. This tells the researcher whether data are normally distributed and whether there is homogeneity of variance within the subgroups of interest. This information is essential to determining whether the assumptions for parametric testing are met. If they are not, then the researcher adopts the nonparametric contingency plan for the variables that have not met parametric assumptions.

Only after the data have been examined as noted previously can the statistical tests of interest be conducted. Many of the programs have a dizzying array of options from which to choose for a given statistical test. If uncertain about which options are appropriate, the researcher should use the services of a statistical consultant.

■ SUMMARY

A research proposal is a blueprint for a study, specifying the investigators, research problem, purposes, methods, references, methods of dissemination of results, budget, and work plan. Research proposals must be approved by facility administrators, an academic committee, an IRB, or some combination of these entities. The role of the IRB is to ensure that the investigators have put into place procedures needed to safeguard the rights of their participants. Research proposals are also used to secure funding for the study. Major sources of funding include institutions, corporations, foundations, and the government. Increasing levels of formalization of the grant application and award process are exerted as the research moves from institutional funding to government funding. Many private foundations and government agencies sponsor research that is of interest to physical therapists.

Implementation of a research project requires attention to detail at every step of the process. Recruitment of participants involves consideration of physician consent, participant consent, administrative approval, and generalizability of research findings. Researchers must attend to many details related to data collection, including specific procedures, ensuring the safety of the data, protecting the identity of participants, developing data collection forms, conducting pilot studies, and scheduling participants and personnel. Data analysis for all but the smallest data sets requires the use of a computer statistical package and a statistical consultant.

REFERENCES

1. Krathwohl DR. *How to Prepare a Research Proposal*. 3rd ed. Syracuse, NY: Syracuse University Press; 1988.
2. Brink P. *Basic Steps in Planning Nursing Research: From Question to Proposal*. 5th ed. Boston, Mass: Jones & Bartlett Publishers; 1999.
3. King NMP, Stein J, eds. *Beyond Regulations: Ethics in Human Subjects Research. Studies in Social Medicine*. Chapel Hill, NC: University of North Carolina Press; 1999.
4. Smith T. *Ethics in Medical Research: A Handbook of Good Practice*. New York, NY: Cambridge University Press; 1999.
5. Evans D, Evans M. *A Decent Proposal: Ethical Review of Clinical Research*. New York, NY: John Wiley & Sons; 1996.
6. Levine RJ. *Ethics and Regulation of Clinical Research*. 2nd ed. New Haven, Conn: Yale University Press; 1988.
7. *The Foundation Grants Index*. 26th ed. New York, NY: Foundation Center; 1998.
8. *Corporate Foundation Profiles*. 10th ed. New York, NY: Foundation Center; 1998.
9. *National Guide to Funding in Aging*. 4th ed. New York, NY: Foundation Center; 1994.
10. *National Guide to Funding in Health*. 5th ed. New York, NY: Foundation Center, 1997.
11. *Catalog of Federal Domestic Assistance*. Washington, DC: US Government Printing Office. Available at: http://www.gsa.gov. Accessed on March 14, 1999.
12. *Annual Register of Grant Support*. 31st ed. Chicago, Ill: Marquis Academic Media; 1998.
13. *Directory of Research Grants*. 23rd ed. Phoenix, Ariz: Oryx Press; 1998.
14. Reif-Lehrer L. *Grant Application Writer's Handbook*. Boston, Mass: Jones & Bartlett Publishers; 1995.
15. Selby-Harrington ML, Donat PL, Hibbard HD. Guidance for managing a research grant. *Nurs Res*. 1993;42:54–58.
16. Findley TW, Daum MC, Macedo JA. Research in physical medicine and rehabilitation: VI. Research project management. *Am J Phys Med Rehabil*. 1989;68:288–299.
17. Morgan WT. A review of eight statistics software packages for general use. *Am Stat*. 1998;52:70–82.
18. Stein PG, Matey JR, Pitts K. A review of statistical software for the Apple Macintosh. *Am Stat*. 1997;51:67–82.
19. Roberts BL, Anthony MK, Madigan EA, Chen Y. Data management: cleaning and checking. *Nurs Res*. 1997; 46:350–352.
20. Findley TW, Stineman MG. Research in physical medicine and rehabilitation: V. Data entry and early exploratory data analysis. *Am J Phys Med Rehabil*. 1989;68: 240–251.

Publishing and Presenting Research

Publication of Research	Style Issues
Types of Publications	Components of a Research Article
Peer Review Process	**Presentation of Research**
Authorship and Acknowledgment	Platform Presentations
Multiple Publication	Poster Presentations

The culmination of the research endeavor is the dissemination of the results of the research. When made public, research can fulfill its goal of adding to the base of knowledge on which clinicians draw when treating patients. This is not to say, however, that all research that is conducted should be disseminated. Some research is so flawed that valid conclusions cannot be drawn from the results. Given this caveat, once an investigator has obtained results that have something to add to the body of knowledge, he or she needs to find the appropriate way to disseminate the results. There are two main mechanisms for doing so: publication and conference presentation.

The purposes of this chapter are to describe the publication and presentation process and to present guidelines for developing effective publications and presentations. Complete guidelines for manuscript preparation, a complete manuscript, and a presentation script and slides are provided in Appendixes D through F, respectively.

■ PUBLICATION OF RESEARCH

The main vehicle for publication of research results is the journal article. This section differentiates between types of publications and journals; discusses the peer review process, authorship, and acknowledgment issues in publication; and presents a variety of language and usage issues that arise when writing about research.

Types of Publications

Professional publications usually fall into one of three categories: journals, magazines, and newsletters. Newsletters present news of interest to subscribers or members. They may occasionally highlight important research findings but do not report original research. Many state chapters of the American Physical Therapy Association (APTA) publish newsletters on a regular basis.

Magazines are publications with full-length articles about general topics of interest to professionals. Some magazine articles may refer to original research, but they do not ordinarily report original research. Articles on practice management, overviews of patient care for certain groups, and discussions of professional issues are appropriate topics for a professional magazine, exemplified by *PT—Magazine of Physical Therapy,* a professional magazine published by the APTA.

Journals have as their primary purpose the reporting of original research findings in a defined area. Although original research publication is the primary focus of a journal, this does not preclude a journal from publishing scholarly review articles, editorials, or the news of a professional association. *Physical Therapy* is the journal of the APTA, *Physiotherapy Canada* is the journal of the Canadian Physiotherapy Association, and *Physiotherapy* is the journal of the Chartered Society of Physiotherapy in the United Kingdom.

There are two types of journals: peer reviewed or non–peer reviewed. In considering a manuscript submitted for publication, editors of peer-reviewed, or *refereed,* journals contact professionals who are knowledgeable about the content area of a manuscript to determine whether the manuscript has scientific rigor and significantly adds to knowledge in the discipline. The final decision about whether a paper is published is made by an editor who is a scholar within the discipline. Publication decisions for non–peer-reviewed, or *nonrefereed,* journals may be made by individuals who are professional editors rather than scholars within the discipline. A journal's peer review status may be mentioned in its instructions to authors and can be found in directories of serials that are in the reference section of the library.[1,2]

Peer Review Process

The personnel involved in the peer review process include the journal editor, an editorial board chaired by the editor, and manuscript reviewers. All of these individuals are scholars or practitioners in the discipline. The journal editor is appointed by the managing body that publishes the journal; the editorial board is usually appointed by the editor, with the consent of the managing body that publishes the journal; the editorial board establishes qualifications for being a manuscript reviewer and accepts applications from interested professionals. For many journals, these three positions are voluntary; however, the editor of larger journals may receive a stipend or honorarium.

When a manuscript is submitted to a peer-reviewed journal for consideration for publication, a chain of events is triggered. The editor or staff reviews the manuscript to see if it meets the journal's technical requirements (length, reference style, etc.) and fits the general mission of the journal. If either of these conditions is not met, the manuscript is returned to the authors without further review. If the manuscript meets the technical and mission criteria, then it is retained for further review.

The manuscript is usually assigned for review to one editorial board member and one or more manuscript reviewers. The board and manuscript reviewers are selected on the basis of their area of expertise in the profession or their knowledge of the research methods used by the authors. The board member and reviewers critique the manuscript to determine the soundness of the research design, the importance and usefulness of the research in light of other literature and the needs of practitioners, and the clarity and readability of the manuscript.

The manuscript reviewers summarize their opinions of the manuscript to the editorial board member and indicate whether they believe it merits publication. The editorial board member synthesizes his or her opinion with the input from the various reviewers and renders an opinion about the paper to the editor.

On the basis of the information from the editorial board member and reviewers, the editor makes a decision about publication of the manuscript. A manuscript can have one of four fates:

acceptance, provisional acceptance pending revision, rejection with suggestion to rewrite, or rejection without suggestion to rewrite. Very few manuscripts are accepted for publication without revisions. Some published manuscripts were initially accepted provisionally pending revisions. This decision is made when the content and structure of the study seem sound and useful to the profession, but the article format needs to be polished. A rejection with a suggestion to rewrite usually means that the topic is important to the profession, but the article as written is too incomplete or disorganized to be able to permit judgment about the credibility of the research. A rejection without a suggestion to rewrite usually means that the topic is simply not a high priority for the journal or that the research methods are too flawed to permit valid conclusions.

As might be inferred by the process just described, peer review is time-consuming. Several months may elapse between submission and a first decision about the manuscript. Author revisions may take several more months, as will final editing of the manuscript by the journal staff. Moreover, because many journals have a backlog of articles waiting to be published, publication of an accepted paper may be delayed several more months. It is not uncommon for more than a year to elapse between submission of a manuscript and its eventual publication.

Authorship and Acknowledgment

Today, many journal articles are cowritten by multiple researchers. In addition to the authors, there are often individuals who have contributed to the study and deserve acknowledgment at the conclusion of the article. Because authorship and acknowledgment involve prestige and recognition, there are often controversies about who should be an author, in what order the authors should be presented, and who should be acknowledged.

The International Committee of Medical Journal Editors has published guidelines to help researchers make such decisions.[3] For an investigator to be listed as an author of a journal article, the committee believes that the following three requirements should be met:

- Substantial contribution to conception and design, or analysis and interpretation of data
- Drafting the article or revising it critically for important intellectual content
- Final approval of the version to be published[3(p928)]

Mere collection of the data does not meet these requirements, nor does holding an administrative post at the facility at which the research was conducted.

The order in which the authors' names are listed should reflect the relative strength of the contributions they have made to the project. This order should be discussed when tasks are being divided among the researchers in the early stages of a project. The order may change somewhat as the project progresses; before submission of the paper for publication, the authors should negotiate among themselves what the final order will be.

Authors should acknowledge individuals who have made significant contributions to the project but do not qualify to be listed as coauthors. Such contributors include those who collected or analyzed some of the data, colleagues who loaned facilities or equipment, or peers who provided critical review of early drafts of the manuscript. All acknowledged individuals should receive a copy of the manuscript and give their permission to be named.

Multiple Publication

Most journals require authors to disclose prior publication and will not accept for consideration papers that have been published in full elsewhere. In fact, most journals require that authors assign the copyright of an article to them when they submit it for publication, meaning that the authors give up the right to submit the paper elsewhere while it is being reviewed. If the first journal to which an article is submitted does not accept the manuscript for publication, the copyright reverts back to the authors, who may then submit it to another journal.

Style Issues

The research article is a specialized form of writing. Its hallmarks are precision, conciseness, and consistency. The novelist uses words to paint pictures and uses different words to convey similar meanings in different contexts. Creative use of language makes novels enjoyable—it makes research articles infuriating if several different terms are used to represent the same construct.

Each journal publishes its own instructions for authors. These instructions typically specify the types of articles accepted for review, the editorial process, the format that the manuscript should take, the reference style to use, procedures for manuscript submission, and the style manual that should be used to prepare the paper.

A style manual is a document of technical information for authors. The style manual for *Physical Therapy* is the American Medical Association's *Manual of Style;* for the *American Journal of Occupational Therapy,* it is the *Publication Manual of the American Psychological Association.*[4,5] In addition, there are good references that provide general guidelines for scientific and medical writing.[3,6,7] Style manuals specify such things as when numbers are presented as numerals (e.g., 227) and when they are written out (two hundred twenty-seven), what levels of headings and subheadings to use, how to present mathematical symbols, how to set up tables, how to cite literature in the text of an article, and what format to follow for the reference list at the end of the article. They also present useful writing style and grammar suggestions, including how to differentiate among confusing terms (e.g., *affect* and *effect*), when to use certain punctuation marks, and how to avoid exclusionary language so that sexist and racial stereotypes are not unconsciously adopted. Table 28–1 presents style problems that commonly appear in the papers of physical therapy students. This table can be used to help writers eliminate these mistakes from their papers, but it is no substitute for frequent reference to a style manual.

A set of style guidelines that should be of particular importance to physical therapists relates to references about people with disabilities. Because physical therapists frequently write about such individuals, they should pay close attention to the implications of the words they use to refer to this population. Table 28–2 presents a set of guidelines for writing about people with disabilities.[8]

Components of a Research Article

The components of a research article are as follows:

1. Title and title page
2. Abstract
3. Introduction
4. Methods
5. Results
6. Discussion
7. Conclusions
8. Acknowledgments
9. References
10. Tables
11. Figures

Appendix D provides a numbered list of guidelines for the preparation of each section; Appendix E contains a complete journal article manuscript, annotated with numbers that correspond to the items in Appendix D. Writers who expect to present a great deal of graphical data should consult more detailed texts for guidance.[9]

TABLE 28-1	Common Style Problems in Student Manuscripts	
Problem	**Example of Problem**	**Corrected Text**
Abbreviation is used without being identified at the first use.	*Rupture of the ACL is a common problem for athletes in contact sports. The ACL is a primary stabilizer of the knee.*	*Rupture of the anterior cruciate ligament (ACL) is a common. . . . The ACL is a primary stabilizer of the knee.*
Sentence begins with a numeral.	*224 responses were received.*	*Two hundred twenty-four responses were received.* or *Responses were received from 224 patients.*
Abbreviations of units of measurement are inconsistent or nonstandard. (Standard units do not have to be spelled out the first time they are used.)	*Velocity was measured in centimeters per sec, with the younger group walking at a pace of 180 cm/sec.*	*Velocity was measured in cm/s, with the younger group walking at a pace of 180 cm/s.*
Language includes jargon or informal terms understood by only a single group of professionals.	*The subjects completed 20 reps of quad sets.*	*The subjects completed 20 repetitions of a quadriceps femoris muscle setting exercise.*
Quotation marks are not used properly with punctuation. Closing quotation marks go outside periods and commas and inside semicolons and colons.	*Boswell has stated that "complacency rules when a profession does not control its own destiny".*	*Boswell has stated that "complacency rules when a profession does not control its own destiny."*
Author refers to him- or herself in the third person; the first person is now preferred, even in scientific writing.	*This author believes that Mayberry overstated the clinical applicability of his findings.*	*I believe that Mayberry overstated the clinical applicability of his findings.*
Comparative terms are used, but no comparison is made.	*Johnson found an increase in strength of the middle deltoid muscle.*	*Johnson found an increase in strength of the middle deltoid after completion of the exercise program.*
Exclusionary terms are used, or constructions to avoid them are too awkward.	*The therapist should not let his emotions cloud his judgments.* or *The therapist should not let his/her emotions cloud his/her judgment.*	*Therapists should not let their emotions cloud their judgments.* or *Emotions should not cloud the judgments of therapists.*
Male or female is used as a noun, rather than an adjective.	*We studied 50 females.*	*We studied 50 female patients.* or *We studied 50 women.*
Author unnecessarily hyphenates compound words	*The post-test scores for the noninjured leg were . . .*	*The posttest scores for the noninjured leg were . . .*

TABLE 28-2 Guidelines for Writing About People with Disabilities*

Sensational or Negative Portrayal	Straightforward, Positive Portrayal
Traumatic brain injury patient [focuses on the injury rather than the person]	*Individual with a traumatic brain injury* [focuses on the person rather than the injury; use *patient* only if the person is, in fact, undergoing medical treatment]
Physically challenged [euphemisms imply that disabilities cannot be dealt with in a straightforward manner]	*Person with a disability* [puts the person first, then the disability; acknowledges the disability directly]
Special children [attempts to glorify differences]	*Children with disabilities* [straightforward portrayal]
Wheelchair-bound [evokes a confined image contrary to the active role of many people who use wheelchairs]	*Uses a wheelchair* [describes the wheelchair as the tool that it is]
Suffers from multiple sclerosis [sensationalizes the disease]	*Has multiple sclerosis* [states the disease matter-of-factly]

* Adapted from *Guidelines for Reporting and Writing About People with Disabilities.* 5th ed. Lawrence, Kan: Research and Training Center on Independent Living, Institute for Life Span Studies, University of Kansas; 1996.

■ PRESENTATION OF RESEARCH

Presentation is the second major format by which research results are disseminated. Many professional associations hold meetings at which research presentations are made. The process of selecting a paper for presentation usually involves submission of an abstract of the study. Some associations use peer review to select abstracts for presentation; others accept any abstracts that meet the technical guidelines and can be accommodated within the conference schedule. Some associations specify that abstracts must be of studies that have not been presented previously. Because conference presentations are less permanent and less accessible than publications, multiple presentation of the same study is acceptable if each presentation is targeted to a different audience. Thus, researchers may feel comfortable presenting the results of their study at both a local and a national meeting of an association or at meetings of different types of professionals. For example, a study related to the roles of physical therapists and athletic trainers in the clinical setting might be appropriate for presentation at a conference of physical therapists and at a conference for athletic trainers.

There are two major formats for conference presentations: platform presentations and poster presentations. Publications[10,11] and videotapes[12,13] are available to guide individuals who are planning to make research presentations. Each presentation format is described and illustrated in the following sections.

Platform Presentations

A platform presentation is made by a researcher to an audience of peers attending the conference. The presentation time is usually short—anywhere from 8 to 20 minutes is common. Researchers are usually expected to show slides during the presentation. A suggested sequence for development of a research presentation is presented here. Appendix F provides a script and slides for a presentation of the manuscript presented in Appendix E.

1. COMPLETE THE MANUSCRIPT. The manuscript provides the complete picture of the study to be described in the presentation. Being able to look at a complete manuscript can help the presenter decide which elements are essential and which can be deleted for the presentation. In addition, because most research presentations follow the same sequence as a journal article, the full manuscript provides a ready-made outline for the presentation.

2. EDIT THE MANUSCRIPT TO PRESENTATION LENGTH.

Examine each paragraph to determine whether it is essential to an understanding of the presentation. A guideline for developing the script for presentation is to spend approximately

- 10% of the allotted time establishing the problem and context of the study
- 20% of the time describing the methods
- 30% of the time presenting the results
- 30% of the time discussing the results
- 10% of the time summarizing the conclusions

The introduction section of the paper can be shortened by deleting many specific references to the related literature and developing the problem conceptually. The methods section can be shortened by eliminating detail about measurement procedures and minimizing technical information about the instruments used. Remember that a presentation audience is interested in simply understanding your methods, not in replicating them in a future study.

Whereas research papers often include separate instruments and procedures sections, a presentation may flow more smoothly if the two are combined. Similarly, some repetition may be eliminated if the data analysis, results, and some parts of the discussion sections of the presentation are integrated. Conclusions should be clear and concise, reiterating the central message of the study.

Once the first edit has been done, read the text aloud, time the delivery, and note phrases that are awkward or seem too formal for your audience. Edit the script as needed for length and smooth delivery.

3. DIVIDE THE SCRIPT INTO SEGMENTS.

A general guideline for preparation of a slide presentation is to have each slide displayed for between 10 and 20 seconds. This requires that the researcher divide the script into small "sound bites" that can be illustrated with a slide. Varying the length of the segments helps maintain audience interest.

4. DESIGN THE SLIDES.

For each text segment, decide whether it is best illustrated with text, a table, a photograph, a drawing, or a graph. Most conferences are set up for horizontal projection of slides, so the presenter should design slides in a horizontal format. Some studies are best illustrated with dual projection, that is, projection of two slides side by side. Studies best suited for dual projection are those that present a great deal of visual information that needs to be reinforced by text. For example, a presentation of a study of specific exercise techniques might benefit from photographs of the exercise displayed on one side and text about the exercise on the other. Because not all conferences can accommodate dual projection, you should confirm that this equipment is available before planning an elaborate dual slide presentation.

Slides of text should generally contain no more than 10 lines of text and no more than six words per line. The style should be telegraphic, using phrases rather than complete sentences. The text in the slide should not exactly repeat the script of the presentation; audiences do not like to have slides read to them. Use of uppercase and lowercase letters is thought to be more readable than using all capital letters; simple sans serif typefaces are preferred.

Slides of tables of information should contain no more than three columns and no more than seven rows. Use of data tables as they appear in the manuscript is rarely suitable, because they contain far more information than can be absorbed in 10 to 20 seconds. Graphs are often more effective than tables in a slide presentation.

Slides of photographs should be clear enough that the audience can locate the item of interest quickly. Photographers should strive for an un-cluttered background that contrasts well with the subject. Sometimes photographs are simply not the best way to get a visual message across. For example, a line diagram of a particular piece of equipment may be able to focus attention on the relevant portion of the instrument; an illustration of an anatomical part may be more effective than a photograph.

Slides of graphs should be used to illustrate the relationships between different numbers within the data set. Pie charts show proportions well, bar graphs effectively illustrate differences in quantities between groups, and line graphs are ideal for illustrating change across time. Because the slide will be displayed for a limited time, the graph should be as simple and clear as possible. Labels should be large enough to read; words should be kept to a minimum.

5. PRODUCE THE SLIDES. Larger hospital and university settings have media services departments that can help researchers design and produce slides. Researchers who do not have access to such a resource can use commercial slide production services, which are available in any large city, or buy commercially available graphics software to design the slides and send them via modem to a production center.[14] Sometimes presenters can avoid actually making slides if the conference at which they are presenting has access to projectors that display presentation graphics directly from the computer screen.

6. PRACTICE THE COMPLETE PRESENTATION. Once the slides have been produced, the researcher needs to practice delivering the text in coordination with the slides. Often, the text needs to be reedited to help integrate the slides with the text. Figure 28–1 shows a graph and the text that highlights its important points.

The final practice is the time to decide on the format of the written materials that you will use to make the presentation. Some presenters like to use 3″ × 5″ cards on which the text for each slide and a diagram of the slide are written. Others like to use standard-sized paper on which the

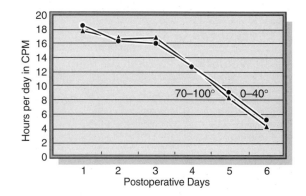

First, the two CPM groups received nearly identical hours per day in CPM, as shown by the two lines on this graph. The group starting with a CPM setting of 0–40 degrees of knee flexion is shown by the line with the circular points; the group starting at 70–100 degrees is shown by the line with the triangular points. You can observe the gradual reduction in hours of CPM per day, starting at about 18 hours per day and ending up at less than 6 hours per day by the 6th postoperative day.

FIGURE 28–1. Example of slide and text for a platform presentation. Text highlights important features of the graph shown in the slide. CPM = continuous passive motion.

text is written in paragraph form and markings are inserted to indicate when to change the slide. Still others like to use a feature of several graphics computer programs that prints out hard copies of the slides with accompanying text. Appendix F shows the text and slides for a presentation of the hypothetical paper provided in Appendix E.

Poster Presentations

Poster presentations are a common feature at conferences and are becoming increasingly accepted as a means of dissemination of scientific information. A poster session consists of a collection of large posters describing research studies. The posters are generally displayed for several hours, and presenters are required to be with their posters for a certain portion of the display time. The advantages of a poster session over a platform presentation are (1) conference attendees can view the posters when they have

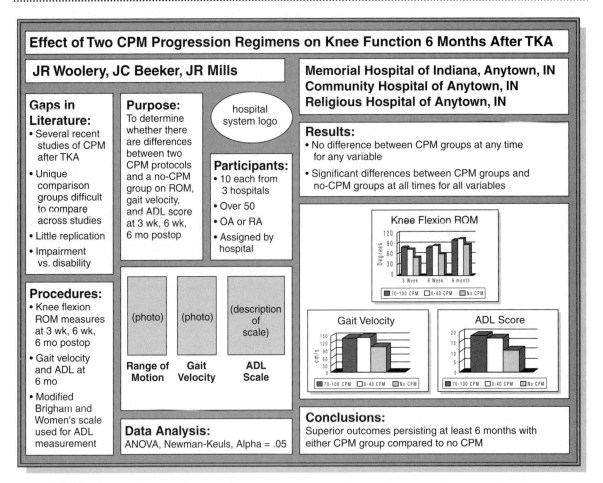

FIGURE 28–2. Schematic diagram for a poster presentation. ADL = activities of daily living; CPM = continuous passive motion; ROM = range of motion.

time and (2) the researcher has more opportunity to interact with interested colleagues.

The space available for the posters is generally about 4′ × 8′. Some presenters have professionally produced posters that they unroll from a tube and tack up onto the board. Most, however, will post a series of miniposters that are easily transported. Researchers who prepare posters should ensure that the type is readable from a distance of 2 to 3 feet and that the sequence in which the poster should be examined is clear. Figure 28–2 shows a schematic diagram of a poster.

■ SUMMARY

Research results are disseminated through either publication or presentation. Publication of research results in journals is a formal process guided by peer review. Journal articles usually follow a standard sequence: introduction, methods, results, discussion, and conclusions. Presentation of research usually occurs at conferences through a platform talk with accompanying slides or through a poster session in which the researcher can interact with conference attendees less formally than in the platform format.

Presentations usually follow the same sequence as journal articles.

REFERENCES

1. *The Serials Directory.* 13th ed. Birmingham, Ala: EBSCO Industries Inc; 1999.
2. *Ulrich's International Periodicals Directory.* 37th ed. New Providence, NJ: RR Bowker; 1999.
3. International Committee of Medical Journal Editors. Uniform requirements for manuscripts submitted to biomedical journals. *JAMA.* 1997;277:927–934.
4. American Medical Association. *Manual of Style.* 9th ed. Baltimore, Md: Williams & Wilkins; 1998.
5. *Publication Manual of the American Psychological Association.* 4th ed. Washington, DC: American Psychological Association; 1994.
6. Day RA. *How to Write and Publish a Scientific Paper.* 5th ed. Phoenix, Ariz: Oryx Press; 1998.
7. Knight KL, Ingersoll CD. Structure of a scholarly manuscript: 66 tips for what goes where. *J Athletic Training.* 1996;31:201–206.
8. *Guidelines for Reporting and Writing About People with Disabilities.* 5th ed. Lawrence, Kan: Research and Training Center on Independent Living, Institute for Life Span Studies, University of Kansas; 1996. Available at: www.lis.ukans.edu/rtcil. Accessed on March 22, 1999.
9. Cleveland WS. *The Elements of Graphing Data.* Revised ed. Murray Hill, NJ: AT&T Bell Laboratories; 1994.
10. Portney L, Craik R. Sharing your research: platform and poster presentations. *PT—Magazine of Physical Therapy.* 1998;6(4):72–81.
11. Anholt RRH. *Dazzle 'Em With Style: The Art of Oral Scientific Presentation.* New York, NY: WH Freeman Co; 1994.
12. Portney LG, Craik R. *Critiquing and Preparing a Platform Presentation* [video]. Alexandria, Va: American Physical Therapy Association; 1997.
13. Binder-McLeod S, Wolf S. *Critiquing and Preparing a Poster Presentation* [video]. Alexandria, Va: American Physical Therapy Association; 1997.
14. Seymour J. Presentation graphics: show business. *PC Magazine.* 1996;15(5):193–229.

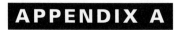

Random Numbers Table

A TABLE OF 14,000 RANDOM UNITS

Line/Col.	(1)	(2)	(3)	(4)	(5)	(6)	(7)	(8)	(9)	(10)	(11)	(12)	(13)	(14)
1	10480	15011	01536	02011	81647	91646	69179	14194	62590	36207	20969	99570	91291	90700
2	22368	46573	25595	85393	30995	89198	27982	53402	93965	34095	52666	19174	39615	99505
3	24130	48360	22527	97265	76393	64809	15179	24830	49340	32081	30680	19655	63348	58629
4	42167	93093	06243	61680	07856	16376	39440	53537	71341	57004	00849	74917	97758	16379
5	37570	39975	81837	16656	06121	91782	60468	81305	49684	60672	14110	06927	01263	54613
6	77921	06907	11008	42751	27756	53498	18602	70659	90655	15053	21916	81825	44394	42880
7	99562	72905	56420	69994	98872	31016	71194	18738	44013	48840	63213	21069	10634	12952
8	96301	91977	05463	07972	18876	20922	94595	56869	69014	60045	18425	84903	42508	32307
9	89579	14342	63661	10281	17453	18103	57740	84378	25331	12566	58678	44947	05585	56941
10	85475	36857	43342	53988	53060	59533	38867	62300	08158	17983	16439	11458	18593	64952
11	28918	69578	88231	33276	70997	79936	56865	05859	90106	31595	01547	85590	91610	78188
12	63553	40961	48235	03427	49626	69445	18663	72695	52180	20847	12234	90511	33703	90322
13	09429	93969	52636	92737	88974	33488	36320	17617	30015	08272	84115	27156	30613	74952
14	10365	61129	87529	85689	48237	52267	67689	93394	01511	26358	85104	20285	29975	89868
15	07119	97336	71048	08178	77233	13916	47564	81056	97735	85977	29372	74461	28551	90707
16	51085	12765	51821	51259	77452	16308	60756	92144	49442	53900	70960	63990	75601	40719
17	02368	21382	52404	60268	89368	19885	55322	44819	01188	65255	64835	44919	05944	55157
18	01011	54092	33362	94904	31273	04146	18594	29852	71585	85030	51132	01915	92747	64951
19	52162	53916	46369	58586	23216	14513	83149	98736	23495	64350	94738	17752	35156	35749
20	07056	97628	33787	09998	42698	06691	76988	13602	51851	46104	88916	19509	25625	58104
21	48663	91245	85828	14346	09172	30168	90229	04734	59193	22178	30421	61666	99904	32812
22	54164	58492	22421	74103	47070	25306	76468	26384	58151	06646	21524	15227	96909	44592
23	32639	32363	05597	24200	13363	38005	94342	28728	35806	06912	17012	64161	18296	22851
24	29334	27001	87637	87308	58731	00256	45834	15398	46557	41135	10367	07684	36188	18510
25	02488	33062	28834	07351	19731	92420	60952	61280	50001	67658	32586	86679	50720	94953
26	81525	72295	04839	96423	24878	82651	66566	14778	76797	14780	13300	87074	79666	95725
27	29676	20591	68086	26432	46901	20849	89768	81536	86645	12659	92259	57102	80428	25280
28	00742	57392	39064	66432	84673	40027	32832	61362	98947	96067	64760	64584	96096	98253
29	05366	04213	25669	26422	44407	44048	37937	63904	45766	66134	75470	66520	34693	90449
30	91921	26418	64117	94305	26766	25940	39972	22209	71500	64568	91402	42416	07844	69618
31	00582	04711	87917	77341	42206	35126	74087	99547	81817	42607	43808	76655	62028	76630
32	00725	69884	62797	56170	86324	88072	76222	36086	84637	93161	76038	65855	77919	88006
33	69011	65797	95876	55293	18988	27354	26575	08625	40801	59920	29841	80150	12777	48501
34	25976	57948	29888	88604	67917	48708	18912	82271	65424	69774	33611	54262	85963	03547
35	09763	83473	73577	12908	30883	18317	28290	35797	05998	41688	34952	37888	38917	88050
36	91567	42595	27958	30134	04024	86385	29880	99730	55536	84855	29080	09250	79656	73211
37	17955	56349	90999	49127	20044	59931	06115	20542	18059	02008	73708	83517	36103	42791
38	46503	18584	18845	49618	02304	51038	20655	58727	28168	15475	56942	53389	20562	87338
39	92157	89634	94824	78171	84610	82834	09922	25417	44137	48413	25555	21246	35509	20468
40	14577	62765	35605	81263	39667	47358	56873	56307	61607	49518	89656	20103	77490	18062
41	98427	07523	33362	64270	01638	92477	66969	98420	04880	45585	46565	04102	46880	45709
42	34914	63976	88720	82765	34476	17032	87589	40836	32427	70002	70663	88863	77775	69348
43	70060	28277	39475	46473	23219	53416	94970	25832	69975	94884	19661	72828	00102	66794
44	53976	54914	06990	67245	68350	82948	11398	42878	80287	88267	47363	46634	06541	97809
45	76072	29515	40980	07391	58745	25774	22987	80059	39911	96189	41151	14222	60697	59583
46	90725	52210	83974	29992	65831	38857	50490	83765	55657	14361	31720	57375	56228	41546
47	64364	67412	33339	31926	14883	24413	59744	92351	97473	89286	35931	04110	23726	51900
48	08962	00358	31662	25388	61642	34072	81249	35648	56891	69352	48373	45578	78547	81788
49	95012	68379	93526	70765	10593	04542	76463	54328	02349	17247	28865	14777	62730	92277
50	15664	10493	20492	38391	91132	21999	59516	81652	27195	48223	46751	22923	32261	85653

A TABLE OF 14,000 RANDOM UNITS

Line/Col.	(1)	(2)	(3)	(4)	(5)	(6)	(7)	(8)	(9)	(10)	(11)	(12)	(13)	(14)
51	16408	81899	04153	53381	79401	21438	83035	92350	36693	31238	59649	91754	72772	02338
52	18629	81953	05520	91962	04739	13092	97662	24822	94730	06496	35090	04822	86772	98289
53	73115	35101	47498	87637	99016	71060	88824	71013	18735	20286	23153	72924	35165	43040
54	57491	16703	23167	49323	45021	33132	12544	41035	80780	45393	44812	12515	98931	91202
55	30405	83946	23792	14422	15059	45799	22716	19792	09983	74353	68668	30429	70735	25499
56	16631	35006	85900	98275	32388	52390	16815	69298	82732	38480	73817	32523	41961	44437
57	96773	20206	42559	78985	05300	22164	24369	54224	35083	19687	11052	91491	60383	19746
58	38935	64202	14349	82674	66523	44133	00697	35552	35970	19124	63318	29686	03387	59846
59	31624	76384	17403	53363	44167	64486	64758	75366	76554	31601	12614	33072	60332	92325
60	78919	19474	23632	27889	47914	02584	37680	20801	72152	39339	34806	08930	85001	87820
61	03931	33309	57047	74211	63445	17361	62825	39908	05607	91284	68833	25570	38818	46920
62	74426	33278	43972	10119	89917	15665	52872	73823	73144	88662	88970	74492	51805	99378
63	09066	00903	20795	95452	92648	45454	09552	88815	16553	51125	79375	97596	16296	66092
64	42238	12426	87025	14267	20979	04508	64535	31355	86064	29472	47689	05974	52468	16834
65	16153	08002	26504	41744	81959	65642	74240	56302	00033	67107	77510	70625	28725	34191
66	21457	40742	29820	96783	29400	21840	15035	34537	33310	06116	95240	15957	16572	06004
67	21581	57802	02050	89728	17937	37621	47075	42080	97403	48626	68995	43805	33386	21597
68	55612	78095	83197	33732	05810	24813	86902	60397	16489	03264	88525	42786	05269	92532
69	44657	66999	99324	51281	84463	60563	79312	93454	68876	25471	93911	25650	12682	73572
70	91340	84979	46949	81973	37949	61023	43997	15263	80644	43942	89203	71795	99533	50501
71	91227	21199	31935	27022	84067	05462	35216	14486	29891	68607	41867	14951	91696	85065
72	50001	38140	66321	19924	72163	09538	12151	06878	91903	18749	34405	56087	82790	70925
73	65390	05224	72958	28609	81406	39147	25549	48542	42627	45233	57202	94617	23772	07896
74	27504	96131	83944	41575	10573	08619	64482	73923	36152	05184	94142	25299	84387	34925
75	37169	94851	39117	89632	00959	16487	65536	49071	39782	17095	02330	74301	00275	48280
76	11508	70225	51111	38351	19444	66499	71945	05422	13442	78675	84081	66938	93654	59894
77	37449	30362	06694	54690	04052	53115	62757	95348	78662	11163	81651	50245	34971	52924
78	46515	70331	85922	38329	57015	15765	97161	17869	45349	61796	66345	81073	49106	79860
79	30986	81223	42416	58353	21532	30502	32305	86482	05174	07901	54339	58861	74818	46942
80	63798	64995	46583	09765	44160	78128	83991	42865	92520	83531	80377	35909	81250	54238
81	82486	84846	99254	67632	43218	50076	21361	64816	51202	88124	41870	52689	51275	83556
82	21885	32906	92431	09060	64297	51674	64126	62570	26123	05155	59194	52799	28225	85762
83	60336	98782	07408	53458	13564	59089	26445	29789	85205	41001	12535	12133	14645	23541
84	43937	46891	24010	25560	86355	33941	25786	54990	71899	15475	95434	98227	21824	19585
85	97656	63175	89303	16275	07100	92063	21942	18611	47348	20203	18534	03862	78095	50136
86	03299	01221	05418	38982	55758	92237	26759	86367	21216	98442	08303	56613	91511	75928
87	79626	06486	03574	17668	07785	76020	79924	25651	83325	88428	85076	72811	22717	50585
88	85636	68335	47539	03129	65651	11977	02510	26113	99447	68645	34327	15152	55230	93448
89	18039	14367	61337	06177	12143	46609	32989	74014	64708	00533	35398	58408	13261	47908
90	08362	15656	60627	36478	65648	16764	53412	09013	07832	41574	17639	82163	60859	75567
91	79556	29068	04142	16268	15387	12856	66227	38358	22478	73373	88732	09443	82558	05250
92	92608	82674	27072	32534	17075	27698	98204	63863	11951	34648	88022	50148	34925	57031
93	23982	25835	40055	67006	12293	02753	14827	22235	35071	99704	37543	11601	35503	85171
94	09915	96306	05908	97901	28395	14186	00821	80703	70426	75647	76310	88717	37890	40129
95	50937	33300	26695	62247	69927	76123	50842	43834	86654	70959	79725	93872	28117	19233
96	42488	78077	69882	61657	34136	79180	97526	43092	04098	73571	80799	76536	71255	64239
97	46764	86273	63003	93017	31204	36692	40202	35275	57306	55543	53203	18098	47625	88684
98	03237	45430	55417	63282	90816	17349	88298	90183	36600	78406	06216	95787	42579	90730
99	86591	81482	52667	61583	14972	90053	89534	76036	49199	43716	97548	04379	46370	28672
100	38534	01715	94964	87288	65680	43772	39560	12918	86537	62738	19636	51132	25739	56947

Table continued on following page

A TABLE OF 14,000 RANDOM UNITS

Line/Col.	(1)	(2)	(3)	(4)	(5)	(6)	(7)	(8)	(9)	(10)	(11)	(12)	(13)	(14)
101	13284	16834	74151	92027	24670	36665	00770	22878	02179	51602	07270	76517	97275	45960
102	21224	00370	30420	03883	96648	89428	41583	17564	27395	63904	41548	49197	82277	24120
103	99052	47887	81085	64933	66279	80432	65793	83287	34142	13241	30590	97760	35848	91983
104	00199	50993	98603	38452	87890	94624	69721	57484	67501	77638	44331	11257	71131	11059
105	60578	06483	28733	37867	07936	98710	98539	27186	31237	80612	44488	97819	70401	95419
106	91240	18312	17441	01929	18163	69201	31211	54288	39296	37318	65724	90401	79017	62077
107	97458	14229	12063	59611	32249	90466	33216	19358	02591	54263	88449	01912	07436	50813
108	35249	38646	34475	72417	60514	69257	12489	51924	86871	92446	36607	11458	30440	52639
109	38980	46600	11759	11900	46743	27860	77940	39298	97838	95145	32378	68038	89351	37005
110	10750	52745	38749	87365	58959	53731	89295	59062	39404	13198	59960	70408	29812	83126
111	36247	27850	73958	20673	37800	63835	71051	84724	52492	22342	78071	17456	96104	18327
112	70994	66986	99744	72438	01174	42159	11392	20724	54322	36923	70009	23233	65438	59685
113	99638	94702	11463	18148	81386	80431	90628	52506	02016	85151	88598	47821	00265	82525
114	72055	15774	43857	99805	10419	76939	25993	03544	21560	83471	43989	90770	22965	44247
115	24038	65541	85788	55835	38835	59399	13790	35112	01324	39520	76210	22467	83275	32286
116	74976	14631	35908	28221	39470	91548	12854	30166	09073	75887	36782	00268	97121	57676
117	35553	71628	70189	26436	63407	91178	90348	55359	80392	41012	36270	77786	89578	21059
118	35676	12797	51434	82976	42010	26344	92920	92155	58807	54644	58581	95331	78629	73344
119	74815	67523	72985	23183	02446	63594	98924	20633	58842	85961	07648	70164	34994	67662
120	45246	88048	65173	50989	91060	89894	36063	32819	68559	99221	49475	50558	34698	71800
121	76509	47069	86378	41797	11910	49672	88575	97966	32466	10083	54728	81972	58975	30761
122	19689	90332	04315	21358	97248	11188	39062	63312	52496	07349	79178	33692	57352	72862
123	42751	35318	97513	61537	54955	08159	00337	80778	27507	95478	21252	12746	37554	97775
124	11946	22681	45045	13964	57517	59419	58045	44067	58716	58840	45557	96345	33271	53464
125	96518	48688	20996	11090	48396	57177	83867	86464	14342	21545	46717	72364	86954	55580
126	35726	58643	76869	84622	39098	36083	72505	92265	23107	60278	05822	46760	44294	07672
127	39737	42750	48968	70536	84864	64952	38404	94317	65402	13589	01055	79044	19308	83623
128	97025	66492	56177	04049	80312	48028	26408	43591	75528	65341	49044	95495	81256	53214
129	62814	08075	09788	56350	76787	51591	54509	49295	85830	59860	30883	89660	96142	18354
130	25578	22950	15227	83291	41737	79599	96191	71845	86899	70694	24290	01551	80092	82118
131	68763	69576	88991	49662	46704	63362	56625	00481	73323	91427	15264	06969	57048	54149
132	17900	00813	64361	60725	88974	61005	99709	30666	26451	11528	44323	34778	60342	60388
133	71944	60227	63551	71109	05624	43836	58254	26160	32116	63403	35404	57146	10909	07346
134	54684	93691	85132	64399	29182	44324	14491	55226	78793	34107	30374	48429	51376	09559
135	25946	27623	11258	65204	52832	50880	22273	05554	99521	73791	85744	29276	70326	60251
136	01353	39318	44961	44972	91766	90262	56073	06606	51826	18893	83448	31915	97764	75091
137	99083	88191	27602	90113	57174	35571	99884	13951	71057	53961	61448	74909	07322	80960
138	52021	45406	37945	78314	24097	86978	22644	87779	23753	99926	63898	54886	18051	96314
139	78755	47744	43776	83098	03225	14281	83637	55984	13300	52319	58781	14905	46502	04472
140	25282	69106	59180	16257	22810	43609	12224	25643	89884	31149	85423	32581	34374	70173
141	11959	94202	02743	86847	79725	51811	12998	76844	05320	54236	53891	70226	38632	84776
142	11644	13792	98190	01424	30078	28197	55583	05197	47714	68440	22016	79204	06862	94451
143	06307	97912	68110	59812	95448	43244	31262	88880	13040	16458	43813	89416	42482	33939
144	76285	75714	89585	99296	52640	46518	55486	90754	88932	19937	57119	23251	55619	23679
145	55322	07589	39600	60866	63007	20007	66819	84164	61131	81429	60676	42807	78286	29015
146	78017	90928	90220	92503	83375	26986	74000	30885	88567	29169	72816	53357	15428	86932
147	44768	43342	20696	26331	43140	69744	82928	24988	94237	46138	77426	39030	55596	12655
148	25100	19336	14605	86603	51680	97678	24261	02464	86563	74812	60069	71674	15478	47642
149	83612	46623	62876	85197	07824	91392	58317	37726	84628	42221	10268	20692	15699	29167
150	41347	81666	82961	60413	71020	83658	02415	33322	66036	98712	46795	16308	28413	05417

A TABLE OF 14,000 RANDOM UNITS

Line/Col.	(1)	(2)	(3)	(4)	(5)	(6)	(7)	(8)	(9)	(10)	(11)	(12)	(13)	(14)
151	38128	51178	75096	13609	16110	73533	42564	59870	29399	67834	91055	89917	51096	89011
152	60950	00455	73254	96067	50717	13878	03216	78274	65863	37011	91283	33914	91303	49326
153	90524	17320	29832	96118	75792	25326	22940	24904	80523	38928	91374	55597	97567	38914
154	49897	18278	67160	39408	97056	43517	84426	59650	20247	19293	02019	14790	02852	05819
155	18494	99209	81060	19488	65596	59787	47939	91225	98768	43688	00438	05548	09443	82897
156	65373	72984	30171	37741	70203	94094	87261	30056	58124	70133	18936	02138	59372	09075
157	40653	12843	04213	70925	95360	55774	76439	61768	52817	81151	52188	31940	54273	49032
158	51638	22238	56344	44587	83231	50317	74541	07719	25472	41602	77318	15145	57515	07633
159	69742	99303	62578	83575	30337	07488	51941	84316	42067	49692	28616	29101	03013	73449
160	58012	74072	67488	74580	47992	69482	58624	17106	47538	13452	22620	24260	40155	74716
161	18348	19855	42887	08279	43206	47077	42637	45606	00011	20662	14642	49984	94509	56380
162	59614	09193	58064	29086	44385	45740	70752	05663	49081	26960	57454	99264	24142	74648
163	75688	28630	39210	52897	62748	72658	98059	67202	72789	01869	13496	14663	87645	89713
164	13941	77802	69101	70061	35460	34576	15412	81304	58757	35498	94830	75521	00603	97701
165	96656	86420	96475	86458	54463	96419	55417	41375	76886	19008	66877	35934	59801	00497
166	03363	82042	15942	14549	38324	87094	19069	67590	11087	68570	22591	65232	85915	91499
167	70366	08390	69155	25496	13240	57407	91407	49160	07379	34444	94567	66035	38918	65708
168	47870	36605	12927	16043	53257	93796	52721	73120	48025	76074	95605	67422	41646	14557
169	79504	77606	22761	30518	28373	73898	30550	76684	77366	32276	04690	61667	64798	66276
170	46967	74841	50923	15339	37755	98995	40162	89561	69199	42257	11647	47603	48779	97907
171	14558	50769	35444	59030	87516	48193	02945	00922	48189	04724	21263	20892	92955	90251
172	12440	25057	01132	38611	28135	68089	10954	10097	54243	06460	50856	65435	79377	53890
173	32293	29938	68653	10497	98919	46587	77701	99119	93165	67788	17638	23097	21468	36992
174	10640	21875	72462	77981	56550	55999	87310	69643	45124	00349	25748	00844	96831	30651
175	47615	23169	39571	56972	20628	21788	51736	33133	72696	32605	41569	76148	91544	21121
176	16948	11128	71624	72754	49084	96303	27830	45817	67867	18062	87453	17226	72904	71474
177	21258	61092	66634	70335	92448	17354	83432	49608	66520	06442	59664	20420	39201	69549
178	15072	48853	15178	30730	47481	48490	41436	25015	49932	20474	53821	51015	79841	32405
179	99154	57412	09858	65671	70655	71479	63520	31357	56968	06729	34465	70685	04184	25250
180	08759	61089	23706	32994	35426	36666	63988	98844	37533	08269	27021	45886	22835	78451
181	67323	57839	61114	62192	47547	58023	64630	34886	98777	75442	95592	06141	45096	73117
182	09255	13986	84834	20764	72206	89393	34548	93438	88730	61805	78955	18952	46436	58740
183	36304	74712	00374	10107	85061	69228	81969	92216	03568	39630	81869	52824	50937	27954
184	15884	67429	86612	47367	10242	44880	12060	44309	46629	55105	66793	93173	00480	13311
185	18745	32031	35303	08134	33925	03044	59929	95418	04917	57596	24878	61733	92834	64454
186	72934	40086	88292	65728	38300	42323	64068	98373	48971	09049	59943	36538	05976	82118
187	17626	02944	20910	57662	80181	38579	24580	90529	52303	50436	29401	57824	86039	81062
188	27117	61399	50967	41399	81636	16663	15634	79717	94696	59240	25543	97989	63306	90946
189	93995	18678	90012	63645	85701	85269	62263	68331	00389	72571	15210	20769	44686	96176
190	67392	89421	09623	80725	62620	84162	87368	29560	00519	84545	08004	24526	41252	14521
191	04910	12261	37566	80016	21245	69377	50420	85658	55263	68667	78770	04533	14513	18099
192	81453	20283	79929	59839	23875	13245	46808	74124	74703	35769	95588	21014	37078	39170
193	19480	75790	48539	23703	15537	48885	02861	86587	74539	65227	90799	58789	96257	02708
194	21456	13162	74608	81011	55512	07481	93551	72189	76261	91206	89941	15132	37738	59284
195	89406	20912	46189	76376	25538	87212	20748	12831	57166	35026	16817	79121	18929	40628
196	09866	07414	55977	16419	01101	69343	13305	94302	80703	57910	36933	57771	42546	03003
197	86541	24681	23421	13521	28000	94917	07423	57523	97234	63951	42876	46829	09781	58160
198	10414	96941	06205	72222	57167	83902	07460	69507	10600	08858	07685	44472	64220	27040
199	49942	06683	41479	58982	56288	42853	92196	20632	62045	78812	35895	51851	83534	10689
200	23995	68882	42291	23374	24299	27024	67460	94783	40937	16961	26053	78749	46704	21983

From Beyer WH, ed. *Standard Mathematical Tables.* Boca Raton Fla: CRC Press; 1984:555–558.

Table: Areas in One Tail of the Standard Normal Curve

This table shows the shaded area

z	.00	.01	.02	.03	.04	.05	.06	.07	.08	.09
0.0	.500	.496	.492	.488	.484	.480	.476	.472	.468	.464
0.1	.460	.456	.452	.448	.444	.440	.436	.433	.429	.425
0.2	.421	.417	.413	.409	.405	.401	.397	.394	.390	.386
0.3	.382	.378	.374	.371	.367	.363	.359	.356	.352	.348
0.4	.345	.341	.337	.334	.330	.326	.323	.319	.316	.312
0.5	.309	.305	.302	.298	.295	.291	.288	.284	.281	.278
0.6	.274	.271	.268	.264	.261	.258	.255	.251	.248	.245
0.7	.242	.239	.236	.233	.230	.227	.224	.221	.218	.215
0.8	.212	.209	.206	.203	.200	.198	.195	.192	.189	.187
0.9	.184	.181	.179	.176	.174	.171	.169	.166	.164	.161
1.0	.159	.156	.154	.152	.149	.147	.145	.142	.140	.138
1.1	.136	.133	.131	.129	.127	.125	.123	.121	.119	.117
1.2	.115	.113	.111	.109	.107	.106	.104	.102	.100	.099
1.3	.097	.095	.093	.092	.090	.089	.087	.085	.084	.082
1.4	.081	.079	.078	.076	.075	.074	.072	.071	.069	.068
1.5	.067	.066	.064	.063	.062	.061	.059	.058	.057	.056
1.6	.055	.054	.053	.052	.051	.049	.048	.048	.046	.046
1.7	.045	.044	.043	.042	.041	.040	.039	.038	.038	.037
1.8	.036	.035	.034	.034	.033	.032	.031	.031	.030	.029
1.9	.029	.028	.027	.027	.026	.026	.025	.024	.024	.023
2.0	.023	.022	.022	.021	.021	.020	.020	.019	.019	.018
2.1	.018	.017	.017	.017	.016	.016	.015	.015	.015	.014
2.2	.014	.014	.013	.013	.013	.012	.012	.012	.011	.011
2.3	.011	.010	.010	.010	.010	.009	.009	.009	.009	.008
2.4	.008	.008	.008	.008	.007	.007	.007	.007	.007	.006
2.5	.006	.006	.006	.006	.006	.005	.005	.005	.005	.005
2.6	.005	.005	.004	.004	.004	.004	.004	.004	.004	.004
2.7	.003	.003	.003	.003	.003	.003	.003	.003	.003	.003
2.8	.003	.002	.002	.002	.002	.002	.002	.002	.002	.002
2.9	.002	.002	.002	.002	.002	.002	.002	.001	.001	.001
3.0	.001									

Adapted from Croxton [25]. Permission sought: Colton T. *Statistics in Medicine*. Boston, Mass: Little, Brown & Co; 1974 and Croxton FE. *Elementary Statistics with Applications in Medicine*. New York, NY: Prentice-Hall; 1953.

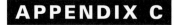

Questions for Evaluating a Research Article

STEP ONE
Classification of Research and Variables

○ Was data collection prospective or retrospective? (Chapter 6)

○ Was the purpose of the research description, relationship analysis, difference analysis, or some combination? (Chapter 6)

○ Was the study experimental or nonexperimental? (Chapter 6)

○ Was the study conducted according to the assumptions and methods of the quantitative, qualitative, or single-system paradigms? (Chapter 5)

○ What were the independent variables? (Chapter 6)

○ What were the dependent variables? (Chapter 6)

STEP TWO
Analysis of Purposes and Conclusions

○ Is there a conclusion for every purpose?

○ Is there a purpose for every conclusion?

○ Are there significant results that should be evaluated for possible alternative explanations and clinical importance? (Chapter 20)

○ Are there nonsignificant results that should be evaluated for power and clinical importance? (Chapter 20)

STEP THREE
Analysis of Design and Control Elements

○ What was the design of the study? (Chapters 9 through 11)

○ Was the independent variable implemented in a laboratory-like or clinic-like setting? (Chapter 6)

○ Was selection of subjects done randomly, by cluster, by convenience, or purposively? (Chapter 8)

○ Were subjects assigned to groups through individual random assignment, block assignment, systematic assignment, matched assignment, or consecutive assignment? (Chapter 8)

○ Were extraneous experimental-setting variables under tight laboratory-like control or loose, clinic-like control? (Chapter 6)

○ Were extraneous subject variables under laboratory-like or clinic-like control? (Chapter 6)

○ What was the level of control over measurement techniques? (Chapters 6, 17, and 18)

○ Was information controlled through incomplete information, subject blinding, or researcher blinding? (Chapter 6)

STEP FOUR
Validity Questions

   ○ Construct Validity (Chapter 7)

Were the variables in the study defined and implemented in meaningful ways?

Construct Underrepresentation

Were variables well developed and defined?

Were there enough levels of the independent variable? Was treatment administered as an all-or-none phenomenon or in varying levels?

Do the dependent variables provide information in all areas important to the phenomenon under study?

Was the independent variable administered at a lower intensity or in a different manner than would be typical in a clinical setting?

Experimenter Expectancies

Were the experimenter's expectations transparently obvious to subjects?

Were there differences between the construct as labeled and the construct as implemented, based on the influence of the experimenter?

Interaction of Different Treatments

What uncontrolled treatments might have interacted with the independent variable?

Interaction of Testing and Treatment

Could any of the measurements used in the study have contributed to a treatment effect?

○ Internal Validity (Chapter 7)

Was the independent variable the probable cause of differences in the dependent variables?

History and Interaction of History and Assignment

What events other than implementation of the independent variable occurred dur-

ing the study that might have plausibly caused changes in the dependent variable?

If any historical events took place, did the events have an equal impact on treatment and control groups?

Maturation and Interaction of Maturation and Assignment

Could changes in the dependent variable have been the result of the passage of time, rather than the implementation of the independent variable?

If a control group was present, were the same maturational influences at work for them as for the treatment group?

Testing

Is familiarity with testing procedures a likely explanation for differences in the dependent variable?

Were tests conducted with equal frequency for treatment and control groups so that any testing effects were consistent for all groups within the study?

Instrumentation and Interaction of Instrumentation and Assignment

Were instruments calibrated appropriately?

Were measurements taken under controlled environmental conditions such as temperature or humidity?

If the instrument was a human observer, what measures were taken to ensure consistency of observations?

Were instruments expected to be equally sensitive across the values expected for both the treatment and control groups?

Statistical Regression to the Mean

Were subjects selected for the study based on an extreme score on a single administration of a test?

Can improvements or declines in performance be attributed to statistical regression rather than true change?

Assignment

Were subjects assigned to groups randomly?

If not assigned randomly, what factors other than the one of interest might have influenced their assignment?

Mortality

What proportions of subjects were lost from the treatment and control groups?

Were the proportions of subjects lost equal for the treatment and control groups?

What are possible explanations for differential loss of subjects from the groups?

Diffusion or Imitation of Treatments

Were treatment and control subjects able to share information about their respective routines?

Was either the treatment or control regimen likely to have been perceived as more desirable by subjects in the other group?

Compensatory Equalization of Treatments

Were researchers aware of which subjects were in which group?

Were those implementing the treatments likely to have paid extra attention to control group subjects because of the presumed inferiority of care they received?

Compensatory Rivalry or Resentful Demoralization

Did subjects know whether they were in the treatment or control group?

Were control-group subjects likely to have either tried harder or withdrawn their efforts because they knew they were in the control group and perceived it to be a less desirable alternative than being in the treatment group?

○ Statistical Conclusion Validity (Chapter 20)

Were statistical tools used appropriately?

Low Power

Are statistically insignificant results related to small sample size, high within-group variability, or small between-groups differences?

Do statistically insignificant differences seem clinically important?

Lack of Clinical Importance

Are statistically significant results clinically important?

Error Rate Problems

If multiple statistical tests were performed, did the researcher set a conservative alpha level to compensate for alpha level inflation?

Are identified significant differences isolated and difficult to explain, or is there a pattern of significant differences that suggests true differences rather than Type I errors?

Violated Assumptions

Were tests used appropriately for independent and dependent samples?

Were normal-distribution and homogeneity of variance assumptions satisfied?

○ External Validity (Chapter 7)

To whom and under what conditions can the research results be generalized?

Selection

Were volunteers used for study? In what ways do these volunteers differ from clinical populations?

Are results from normal subjects generalized to patient populations?

Do the authors limit their conclusions to subjects similar to those studied?

Setting

To what extent did the experimental setting differ from the setting to which the researchers wish to generalize the results?

Were control elements implemented fastidiously, as in a laboratory, or pragmatically, as in a clinic?

Time

How much time elapsed between the collection of the data in the study and the present time?

Do differences in overall clinical management of patients make the studied procedures less appropriate today than when the study was implemented?

STEP FIVE
Place Study into Literature Context

○ Do results confirm or contradict the findings of others?

○ Does this study correct some of the deficiencies identified in other studies?

○ Does the study examine constructs or variables unstudied by others?

○ How do the sample size and composition compare with those of other studies?

○ How does the validity of this study compare with that of related studies?

STEP SIX
Personal Utility Questions

○ Are your setting and the research setting similar enough to warrant application of the results of the research to your clinical practice?

○ Does the study cause you to question some of the assumptions under which you have managed patients?

○ Do the methods of this study suggest ways in which you can improve on the design of a study you are planning?

Guidelines for Preparing a Journal Article Manuscript

1. General Guidelines

   1.1 Double-space everything, including block quotes, tables, and references.

   1.2 Margins should be a minimum 1 inch; some journals will request more generous margins.

   1.3 Don't right-justify the text or hyphenate words at the ends of lines. These adjustments may make an attractive document but hinder the editing process.

   1.4 Generally plan for 15 pages of text, plus title page, abstract page, tables, references, and figures. Consult journal instructions to authors for more specific length guidelines.

   1.5 Manuscript pagination is as follows: Title page is page 1, but is not labeled; abstract page is page 2; text begins on page 3. Tables follow the references. Each table begins on a new page, and table pages are numbered consecutively with the manuscript. The final numbered manuscript page is the one on which the figure legends are written; it starts on a separate page following the tables.

   1.6 Determine formats for headings and subheadings and use them consistently. One common scheme:

METHODS   (First-level side heading in uppercase letters, set off from text with extra spacing above and below the heading)

Subjects   (Second-level side heading, upper- and lowercase letters, set off from text with extra spacing above and below the heading)

Facility A.   (Third-level side heading, indented with period following heading; leave extra space above heading, and run in text after heading)

2. Title and Title Page

   2.1 Be concise, yet specific. Include important variables under study. "Knee Function after Total Knee Arthroplasty" is too concise if the study is really one of "Effect of Two Continuous Passive Motion Regimens on Knee Function Six Months After Total Knee Arthroplasty."

   2.2 Titles may be descriptive (such as "Effect of Continuous Passive Motion on Knee Range of Motion After Total Knee Arthroplasty") or assertive (such as "Continuous Passive Motion Does Not Improve Knee Range of Motion After Total Knee Arthroplasty"). Some journal editors prefer the latter, which summarizes results in the title; others prefer to let readers draw their own conclusions.

   2.3 Consider using terms that are indexed in the databases interested readers are likely to search; for example, use "total knee arthroplasty" rather than "total knee replacement" because "arthroplasty" is indexed and "replacement" is not.

2.4 Refer to journal requirements for author and affiliation format because these vary widely among journals.

3. Abstract

3.1 Generally limit the abstract to less than 250 words.

3.2 Summarize the study's purpose, procedures, results, and major conclusions, using a structured abstract with headings if required.

3.3 Use major indexing terms because users of computer databases often search abstracts as well as titles.

3.4 Do not cite references or provide p values because these are meaningful only in the context of the study.

4. Introduction

4.1 No heading is used for the introduction; just begin the first paragraph.

4.2 In a paper of 15 pages, the introduction section is typically 2 to 3 pages.

4.3 Cite only the most relevant citations about the topic area. A journal article does not contain an exhaustive review of the literature, but rather it places the problem into the context of the literature.

4.3.1 American Medical Association (AMA)-style citations in the text use superscript numerals in sequential order.

4.3.2 If superscripts are unavailable, then the number should be enclosed in parentheses.

4.3.3 If the text refers to an author's name, the numeral follows the name directly. If the author's name is not mentioned and the entire sentence is related to the citation, the numeral goes at the end of the sentence. If the citation refers to only part of the sentence, the numeral is placed at the conclusion of that part.

4.3.4 When using a numbered reference style like the AMA, writers often cite references with the author name in parentheses in early drafts of the paper. This prevents repeated renumbering of references as the paper is edited. For the final draft, the names and parentheses are removed and the correct numbers inserted.

4.3.5 The other most frequently encountered reference style is the name-date style, in which the author's name and the date of publication are placed in parentheses within the text. Journals that follow the *Publication Manual of the American Psychological Association* use the name-date citation format.

4.4 Suggested first paragraph: Broadly state the problem, with documentation as needed.

4.5 Suggested second through fourth paragraphs, as needed: Summarize what is known about the problem, that is, what others have found out about the problem in their own research.

4.6 Suggested last paragraph: Identify the gap in the literature that needs to be filled, and then state the purpose of your research. State research hypotheses if appropriate. Identify major variables, using the names that you will use throughout the rest of the paper. If you have several purposes, place them in order of importance or in the order that they will be discussed in the rest of the paper.

5. Methods

5.1 The methods section is usually subdivided into "Subjects," "Instruments," "Procedures," and "Data Analysis."

5.2 In a paper of 15 pages, the methods section is typically 3 to 5 pages long.

5.3 Cite literature needed to justify the methods you used, or cite others' procedures if they are too lengthy to be repeated in your article.

5.4 The subjects subsection should describe inclusion and exclusion criteria, sampling and assignment methods, and source of the subjects.

5.5 The instruments subsection should describe each instrument used in data collection.

    5.5.1 Present instruments in the order that you will eventually present your results. For example, if you have taken range of motion, strength, and functional measures and plan to discuss them in that order, describe the goniometers first, the dynamometers second, and the functional scale last.

    5.5.2 If you developed the instrument, provide details about the instrument development process.

    5.5.3 If you performed reliability or validity testing with the instruments but this was not the primary purpose of the research, present reliability or validity information here. If the research is methodological, then reliability or validity information belongs in the results section.

5.6 The procedures subsection should describe what you did in enough detail that others can replicate the study. Refer to other authors if necessary to justify your procedures.

    5.6.1 If the measurement order is irrelevant, then present the procedures in the same order as you described the instruments. If the measurement order is critical, describe it.

    5.6.2 Consider combining the instrument subsection with the procedures subsection if the equipment used is nontechnical and familiar to most professionals to whom the article would be of interest.

5.7 The data analysis subsection should include data reduction procedures and statistical testing for each variable.

    5.7.1 If possible, present information about the data analysis in the order of variables presented earlier in the paper.

    5.7.2 State the statistical package used and alpha level if appropriate.

    5.7.3 If necessary, justify or clarify your use of statistical procedures with references.

6. Results

6.1 Sometimes the results section is subdivided by variables or class of variables.

6.2 Text is often short, with much of the information presented in tables and figures. Tables and figures should substitute for information in the text, not repeat it. Tables and figures are numbered separately in order of their appearance in the text (see Sections 11 and 12).

6.3 Present variables in previously established order.

6.4 Don't discuss the implications of the results here; just present the appropriate descriptive and statistical information.

6.5 In a paper of 15 pages, the results section is typically only 1 to 2 pages long, supplemented by figures and tables.

7. Discussion

7.1 The discussion is the heart of the paper, the place for interpretation of the results.

7.2 In a paper of 15 pages, the discussion is typically 3 to 4 pages long.

7.3 Additional references are often cited to place the results into a broader context.

7.4 Suggested first section: Restate the major results in terms of your original hypotheses.

7.5 Suggested second section: Examine the expected results, showing reinforcement of the theory that led you to a hypothesis that was supported.

7.6 Suggested third section: Examine the unexpected results, providing theoretical explanation through examination of related literature.

7.7 Suggested fourth section: Discuss the limitations of the study.

7.8 Suggested fifth section: Discuss the clinical implications of the findings.

7.9 Suggested sixth section: Discuss directions for future research.

8. Conclusions

8.1 Not all articles have a conclusions section. If the conclusions are not a separate section, they are addressed in the discussion.

8.2 In a paper of 15 pages, the conclusions are typically less than a page long. The conclusions are stated concisely, in the order in which the questions were posed in the purpose section of the study.

9. Acknowledgments

9.1 Each person acknowledged should have given permission to be acknowledged.

9.2 Be specific about the contribution of each person: "critical review," "manuscript preparation," or "data collection."

9.3 Place acknowledgments on a separate page so that they can be removed from the manuscript to maintain authors' anonymity when the paper is sent out for review.

10. References

10.1 Begin references on a separate page.

10.2 Remember to double-space references.

10.3 List only references cited in the study.

10.4 The *Manual of Style* of the AMA numbers references in the reference list in the order they are cited in text. If you are submitting to a journal that follows another style, consult their style manual and order the references appropriately.

10.5 Place references into proper format. Pay attention to punctuation, capitalization, and abbreviation of journal article title. AMA formats for the different elements of a journal article citation are as follows:

10.5.1 *Authors*: Smith DL, Riley JW, Anderson MD.
There is no internal punctuation within each name; names are separated by commas; a period follows the final name.

10.5.2 *Journal article title*: Effects of prolonged sitting on attention span: a study of physical therapy students.
Only the first word is capitalized unless there is a proper name within the title; the first word after a colon starts with a lowercase letter; a period follows the title.

10.5.3 *Journal name: Phys Ther.* Use the *Index Medicus* abbreviation for the journal name. The journal abbreviation or name is italicized (or underlined if an italicized font is not available), and a period follows. For a list of journals and journal abbreviations used frequently by physical therapists, see Table 25–3.

10.5.4 *Year, volume, issue and pages*: 1987;67:3002-3007. The year comes first, followed by a semicolon; the volume number comes next, followed by a colon; an issue number is required only if each issue begins with page 1 (if the issue number is necessary, it is enclosed in parentheses); the page numbers are last, followed by a period. Inclusive page numbers are listed and the full page number is repeated on each side of the hyphen.

10.6 Consult the appropriate style manual for detailed directions on specific formats for different types of references (e.g., book, chapter in a book, dissertation).

11. Tables

11.1 Tables consist of rows and columns of numbers or text.

11.2 Vertical lines are not used in tables; use horizontal lines only.

11.3 Tables should not repeat information in the text. If a table can be summarized in a sentence or two, then it should probably not be a table.

11.4 Number tables (Table 1, Table 2, Table 3 . . .) according to their order in the paper. Refer to each table in the text, highlighting the most important information. If there is only one table, it is not numbered.

11.5 Table titles should describe the specific information contained within the table; for example, "Data" is too general a title; "Mean Knee Function Variables by Clinic" is more specific.

11.6 Each table begins on a separate page placed after the references. Tables may be continued onto additional pages.

12. Figures

12.1 Figures are illustrative materials such as graphs, diagrams, or photographs.

12.2 Figures should not repeat information in text or tables. They should be used only when visual information is more effective than tabular or text information.

12.3 Figures are numbered (Figure 1, Figure 2, Figure 3 . . .) in order of their appearance in the paper. If there is only one figure, it is not numbered.

12.4 Figure legends are listed on a separate sheet following the tables. The legend should make the figure meaningful on its own by explaining any abbreviations and describing concisely the important points being illustrated.

12.5 The figure itself is not labeled or numbered on its face. Figures are identified on the back using lightly penciled writing or a gummed label; be careful not to damage the figure by labeling it. When submitting a manuscript, encase the figures in cardboard to protect them.

12.6 Identification of figures in theses or dissertations will deviate from this format. Because they are used in the format prepared by the author, rather than being typeset in a journal, figure numbers and legends must accompany the figures themselves.

REFERENCES

American Medical Association. *Manual of Style.* 9th ed. Baltimore, Md: Williams & Wilkins; 1998.

Day RA. *How to Write and Publish a Scientific Paper* 5th ed. Phoenix, Ariz: Oryx Press; 1998.

International Committee of Medical Journal Editors. Uniform requirements for manuscripts submitted to biomedical journals. *JAMA.* 1997;277:927–934.

Publication Manual of the American Psychological Association. 4th ed. Washington, DC: American Psychological Association; 1994.

Sample Manuscript for Hypothetical Study

The following manuscript on continuous passive motion use after total knee arthroplasty is based, with a few changes in the demographic variables, on the hypothetical data set presented in Chapter 20 in Tables 20–1 and 20–2. The literature cited in the manuscript is from the conceptual review of the literature presented in Chapter 26. However, an exhaustive review of the literature related to continuous passive motion and total knee arthroplasty was not developed for use in this example. Although the individual studies are cited appropri-

ately, readers should realize that the hypothetical problem statement may not accurately reflect the overall state of research in this area.

The ninth edition of the American Medical Association's *Manual of Style* was used to guide the preparation of the sample manuscript. Writers should consult the particular journal's instructions for authors to determine whether another style manual should be followed. The circled numbers in the manuscript correspond to guidelines listed in Appendix D.

Effect of Two Continuous Passive Motion Progression
Regimens on Knee Function Six Months After Total Knee
Arthroplasty   ←(2.1)

Jan R. Woolery

Jodi C. Beeker

Jonathon V. Mills

JR Woolery, PT, PhD, is Research Therapist, Department of
Physical Therapy, Memorial Hospital of Indiana, 555 Main Street,
Anytown, IN 46234 (USA). Address all correspondence to Dr.
Woolery.

JC Beeker, PT, MS, is Senior Physical Therapist, Department of
Rehabilitation Services, Community Hospital of Anytown, Anytown,
IN.

JV Mills, PT, MS, is Staff Therapist, Physical Therapy
Department, Religious Hospital of Anytown, Anytown, IN.

The results of this study were presented in a platform
presentation at the Conference, Association, City, State, Date.

This study was approved by the institutional review boards of
Memorial Hospital of Indiana, Community Hospital of Anytown, and
Religious Hospital of Anytown.

ABSTRACT

(3.2)

Context: The optimal progression of motion in continuous passive motion (CPM) devices used after total knee arthroplasty (TKA) is not well established, despite their use for over 15 years. **Objective:** To compare the effects of two different CPM regimens to no CPM on knee motion, strength, and function up to 6 months after TKA. One CPM regimen began with range of motion (ROM) set at 70° to 100° of knee flexion and progressed toward full extension. The other regimen began with ROM set at 0° to 40° of knee flexion and progressed toward full flexion. **Design:** Nonrandomized controlled trial with up to 6-month follow-up. **Setting:** Three community hospitals in the midwestern region of the United States. **Patients:** Ten consecutive patients over the age of 50 years and undergoing unilateral TKA at each of three different hospitals. **Interventions:** Patients were assigned by hospital to receive 70° to 100° of CPM, 0° to 40° of CPM, or no CPM. CPM treatment began in the recovery room and continued for 6 days. **Outcome Measures:** Knee flexion ROM at 3 and 6 weeks postoperatively and knee flexion ROM, gait velocity, and activities of daily living (ADL) score at 6 months postoperatively. **Results:** Significant differences among groups were identified for all dependent variables. The CPM groups scored significantly higher on all variables than did the no-CPM group. There were no significant differences between the CPM groups for any of the dependent variables.

Conclusions: CPM initiated at 70° to 100° ROM resulted in similar outcomes after TKA as CPM initiated at 0° to 40° ROM. Both CPM groups experienced better outcomes than the no-CPM group and these differences persisted for 6 months after surgery.

3

(4.1)→   Total knee arthroplasty is a common surgical procedure used to reduce pain and enhance function for individuals with knee impairment secondary to osteoarthritis or rheumatoid arthritis. Continuous passive motion (CPM) is used routinely to encourage early motion of the knee joint after total knee arthroplasty (TKA). Despite its widespread clinical use, the optimal CPM regimen to maximize short-term and long-term function of patients after TKA has not been identified.

The first limitation of the literature about CPM after TKA is that the comparison groups in each study have been unique, with little direct replication of results across studies. Several different studies have compared CPM to standard care.[1-4] In addition, two of these studies also   ←(4.3.1) compared more than one CPM regimen.[3,4] Two other studies compared different CPM regimens without comparing to a group that did not receive CPM.[5,6]

The four studies comparing CPM to standard care found at least weak short-term evidence in favor of CPM. Gose,[1] in a study published in 1987, found shorter lengths of stay for patients receiving 3 hours of CPM per day compared to those receiving no CPM. In 1995 Ververeli and colleagues[2] reported that patients initially treated with CPM for 20 hours per

4

day, with continued CPM during daytime hours until discharge, had significantly more knee flexion at discharge and required fewer manipulations under anesthesia than those receiving no CPM. In a 1997 report, Chiarello and associates[3] reported that there was an increased rate of change of knee flexion for those patients receiving from 4 to 8 hours of CPM per day compared with those not receiving CPM. Also in 1997, Pope and colleagues[4] reported significantly better 1-week postoperative ROM for patients receiving CPM 20 hours per day for 2 days compared with those not receiving CPM.

The four studies comparing different CPM regimens have found few short-term differences among groups and no long-term differences. Basso and Knapp,[5] in a 1987 study, ←(4.3.3) found no discharge differences in knee excursion or length of stay between groups who received 20 or 5 hours of CPM per day. Chiarello and colleagues[3] also failed to identify discharge differences in ROM between groups receiving 4 versus 8 hours of CPM per day. Pope and colleagues[4] compared a group receiving CPM beginning at 0° to 40° of knee flexion to one receiving CPM beginning at 0° to 70° of knee flexion. Each group's ROM was advanced 10° per day for each of 2 days of CPM treatment. The only difference found between CPM groups was that the 0° to 70° CPM group had significantly more postoperative blood loss than the 0° to 40° CPM group. Finally, in 1997, Yashar and associates[6] reported on their comparison of a group receiving typical CPM beginning at 0° to 30° of flexion with a group receiving accelerated flexion in CPM beginning at 70° to 100° of flexion. The accelerated flexion group had significantly more flexion ROM on the third postoperative day and at discharge, but these differences disappeared by 4 weeks after surgery. Despite these consistent findings of no differences between varying CPM protocols, none of the particular comparisons have been replicated.

The second limitation of the literature is that few authors have studied outcomes other than ROM and length of hospital stay. Disability level outcomes such as gait velocity or ADL have not been measured.

(4.6)   To fill these gaps in the literature, we designed a study that would replicate the least studied variation in CPM protocol (direction of progression of ROM in the CPM unit) and extend it by comparing the CPM variants to a group that does not undergo CPM. In addition, we measured both short-term knee flexion ROM as well as long-term functional outcomes after different CPM regimens.

6

Specifically, the purpose of this study was to determine whether there were differences between two CPM protocols (initial ROM of 0° to 40° vs. initial ROM of 70° to 100°) and no CPM on knee flexion ROM at 3 and 6 weeks postoperatively and on knee flexion ROM, gait velocity, and ADL score at 6 months postoperatively. We hypothesized that there would be no differences between the 0° to 40° and 70° to 100° groups at any time; that there would be differences between the no-CPM group and both CPM groups at 3 and 6 weeks postoperatively, and that there would be no differences among the groups at 6 months postoperatively.

METHODS

Subjects

Subjects were patients who were at least 50 years old, had a diagnosis of either osteoarthritis or rheumatoid arthritis, and underwent TKA in 1999 at one of three hospitals in Anytown, Indiana: Community Hospital, Memorial Hospital, and Religious Hospital. Before beginning this study, the characteristics of patients undergoing TKA and the postoperative rehabilitation regimens of patients after TKA were compared across the three participating hospitals. All used similar regimens, which included preoperative instructions from a physical therapist; CPM application of 0° to 40° of knee flexion within 24 hours after surgery and maintenance of CPM approximately 20 hours daily; twice-daily physical therapy beginning within 36 hours of surgery; and weight-bearing, progression of ROM, and strengthening exercises as tolerated by the patient. The comparison showed nearly identical patient characteristics on the variables of age, sex, diagnosis, and type of prosthesis implanted. Because of the similarity of both patient characteristics and rehabilitation regimens at the three hospitals, we decided to assign the CPM protocol randomly to hospitals rather than individually to patients. Patients at Community Hospital received 70° to 100° of CPM, patients at Religious Hospital received 0° to 40° of CPM, and patients at Memorial Hospital received no CPM. For the two CPM groups the units were applied in the recovery room and used for 20 hours per day the first postoperative day. On subsequent days the ROM was advanced 10° (toward more flexion for the 0° to 40° group and toward extension for the 70° to 100° group) per day and the time in the unit was reduced by about 2 hours per day. The first 10 patients in 1999 who met the inclusion criteria were selected for study at each hospital. Table 1 shows that the background ←(11.4) characteristics of the subjects are nearly identical across facilities.

INSTRUMENTS ←(5.5.1)

   CPM Units. ACME CPM (ACME Orthopedics, 123 Canyon Road, Roadrunner, AZ, 44304) units were used to deliver the CPM treatment at all three facilities.

   Goniometers. ROM measurements were taken with the 12-inch, full-circle, plastic universal goniometers available at each facility.

ADL Scale. We modified the Brigham and Women's Knee Rating Scale[7] to assess ADL (Table 2). The values for each of the four subscales (distance walked, assistive device, stair climbing, and rising from a chair) were added for each person to give a single ADL score that could range from a low of 4 to a high of 20.

Procedure

Patients underwent the appropriate postoperative rehabilitation protocol described above. For patients in the CPM groups the ROM was increased up to 10° per day. Each day the time spent in CPM was recorded for each patient, as were the ROM settings for the unit. Knee flexion ROM measurements were taken with patients supine according to the procedures described by Norkin and White,[8] with values recorded to the nearest degree. The 3-week and 6-week ←(5.3) measures were taken by the treating therapists at each hospital when patients came for their routine outpatient physical therapy visits. The 6-month measures were all taken in the physical therapy department at Community Hospital. One investigator (JRW) measured 6-month ROM for all subjects. Velocity was measured by having the subject walk at a comfortable pace across a 20-m measured distance. Each

subject was timed with a stopwatch during the center 10 m
of the walk. This time was converted to cm/s for analysis.
One investigator (JCB) took all the velocity measures. The
modified Brigham and Women's Knee Rating Scale was
administered to each subject by the third investigator
(JVM). Use of an assistive device, rising from a chair, and
stair climbing were actually observed and rated; distance
walked was a self-reported measure. All subjects completed
the functional scale first, the ROM measures second, and the
gait velocity measure last.

Data Analysis

An analysis of variance (ANOVA) was used to test for
differences between groups for each of the following
dependent variables: 3-week ROM, 6-week ROM, and 6-month
ROM; gait velocity; and ADL score. The Newman-Keuls
procedure was used for post hoc analysis. Alpha was set at
.05 for each analysis. SPSS for Windows Release 8.0.0 was
used for the data analysis.[*]

---

[*]SPSS Inc, 444 N. Michigan Avenue, Chicago, Ill, 60611.

11

RESULTS ←(6.2)

Figure 1 shows that the average time spent in CPM per day was similar for the two CPM groups. Figure 2 shows the progression of ROM for each group by plotting the adjustable ROM across days. Table 3 shows the group means for each of the dependent variables, accompanied by the F and p values for the ANOVA. There were significant differences between groups for all variables. Post hoc analysis showed that for all variables the CPM groups were not statistically different from one another, but that both were significantly different from the no-CPM group.

DISCUSSION

Of our three hypotheses, two were supported: (1) that there ←(7.4) would be no differences between the CPM groups at any time and (2) that there would be 3- and 6-week differences between the no-CPM group and both the CPM groups. Most reports comparing CPM to no CPM have found weak evidence of the effectiveness of CPM in improving short-term postoperative ROM. Our study is consistent with this evidence and strengthens the case for using CPM to improve short-term postoperative ROM after TKA.

12

Our finding of no differences between the CPM groups is consistent with the work of Yashar and colleagues,[6] who also found no difference in ROM outcome between groups with initial 0° to 40° or 70° to 100° ROM settings. Further, the addition of gait velocity and ADL measures in our study provides evidence that both impairment and disability level outcomes are similar regardless of the direction in which ROM is progressed with CPM.

Our final hypothesis--that differences between the no-CPM group and the CPM groups would not be present at 6 months-- was not supported. This is in contrast to the findings of Ververeli and associates[2] who found no differences between CPM and non-CPM groups at 2 years postoperatively. Although we had initially believed that patient status would stabilize by 6 months postoperatively, we plan to continue the study to determine if the differences in all variables disappear 1 or 2 years postoperatively.

The functional importance of our gait and ADL findings is apparent if one looks at the mean values for the different groups. Gait velocities of the CPM groups (144.0 and 145.6 cm/s) were well above that needed to cross a typical city street (approximately 80 cm/s).[9] The no-CPM

← (7.3)

group had an average gait velocity of only 107.6 cm/s; this is sufficient to cross many streets, but certainly well below the averages of the other two groups.

The ADL scores of the CPM groups were approximately 18 and 17 of 20, respectively. This indicates minor impairment on two of the components or moderate impairment on one of the components. In contrast, the average ADL score for the no-CPM group was 11, indicating moderate to severe impairment in one or more of the ADL components.

In interpreting these results, several limitations or alternative explanations must be considered. First, because the treatments were assigned by hospital and not by patient, there may have been systematic differences between care at the hospitals that could explain the difference in results. Second, because the investigators were not blinded to the group membership of the subjects, their expectations may have influenced subject performance. Third, there may be differences among groups that are important but were not measured. For example, if a greater proportion of patients in the no-CPM group live with family members who assist them in ADL, perhaps they have less incentive to achieve higher levels of function than individuals who live alone.

14

Despite these limitations, the results have clinical implications for facilities using CPM for patients after TKA. Our results seem to indicate that patients who receive CPM--regardless of whether the CPM works from extension into flexion or from flexion into extension--do better on important outcome measures until at least 6 months after surgery compared with patients who do not receive CPM. Further research must be done to see if these results can be replicated, to see whether differences between CPM and no-CPM groups persist longer than 6 months, and to determine whether there are other important differences among CPM groups (e.g., blood loss or analgesic use) that would suggest an optimal direction for increasing motion after surgery.

CONCLUSIONS ←8.2

Patients who underwent TKA and received CPM in either of two progressions (starting at 70° to 100° of flexion or starting at 0° to 40° of flexion) had significantly better knee flexion ROM at 3 weeks and 6 weeks and significantly better knee flexion ROM, gait velocity, and ADL scores at 6 months postoperatively than did those who did not receive CPM.

15

ACKNOWLEDGMENTS

We would like to thank Ben Counter, PhD, for assistance with   ←(9.2)
the statistical analysis of the study, and Ellen Redline,
PT, PhD, for her critical review of an earlier draft of the
manuscript.

REFERENCES ←(10.1)

1. Gose JC. Continuous passive motion in the postoperative treatment of patients with total knee replacement: a retrospective study. *Phys Ther.* 1987;67:39-42.

2. Ververeli PA, Sutton DC, Hearn SL, Booth RE Jr, Hozack WJ, Rothman RR. Continuous passive motion after total knee arthroplasty: analysis of costs and benefits. *Clin Orthop.* 1995;321:208-215.

3. Chiarello CM, Gundersen L, O'Halloran T. The effect of continuous passive motion duration and increment on range of motion in total knee arthroplasty patients. *J Orthop Sports Phys Ther.* 1997;25:119-127.

4. Pope RO, Corcoran S, McCaul K, Howie DW. Continuous passive motion after primary total knee arthroplasty: does it offer any benefits? *J Bone Joint Surg Br.* 1997;79:914-917.

5. Basso DM, Knapp L. Comparison of two continuous passive motion protocols for patients with total knee implants. *Phys Ther.* 1987;67:360-363.

6. Yashar AA, Venn-Watson E, Welsh T, Colwell CW Jr, Lotke P. Continuous passive motion with accelerated flexion after total knee arthroplasty. *Clin Orthop.* 1997;345:38-43.

17

7. Ewald FC, Jacobs MA, Miegel RE, Waller PS, Poss R, Sledge CB. Kinematic total knee replacement. *J Bone Joint Surg Am*. 1984;66:1032–1040.

8. Norkin CC, White DJ. *Measurement of Joint Motion: A Guide to Goniometry*. 2nd ed. Philadelphia, Pa: FA Davis Co; 1995:142–143.

9. Lerner-Frankiel MB, Vargas S, Brown M, Krusell L, Schoneberger W. Functional community ambulation: what are your criteria? *Clin Manage Phys Ther*. 1986;6(2):12–15.

18

(11.6)→ Table 1. Patient Characteristics

Variable	Hospital and Regimen		
	Community 70°–100° CPM	Religious 0°–40° CPM	Memorial No CPM
Mean age in years	73.2	71.7	72.5
Sex			
Women (%)	50	40	60
Men (%)	50	60	40
Diagnosis			
Osteoarthritis	70	80	70
Rheumatoid arthritis	30	20	30

19

Table 2. Modified Brigham and Women's Knee Rating Scale[7]

Variable	Scoring Criteria
Distance walked	5 = Unlimited
	4 = 4 to 6 blocks
	3 = 2 to 3 blocks
	2 = Indoors only
	1 = Transfers only
Assistive device	5 = None
	4 = Cane outside
	3 = Cane full time
	2 = Two canes or crutches
	1 = Walker or unable
Stair climbing	5 = Reciprocal, no rail
	4 = Reciprocal, rail
	3 = One at a time, with or without rail
	2 = One at a time, with rail and assistive device
	1 = Unable

20

Table 2 (continued). Modified Brigham and Women's Knee
Rating Scale[7]

Rising from a chair	
	5 = No arm assistance
	4 = Single arm assistance
	3 = Difficult with two arm assistance
	2 = Needs assistance of another
	1 = Unable

21

Table 3. Outcomes of 70°–100° CPM, 0°–40° CPM, and No-CPM Groups

| | Group | | | ANOVA Results | |
Variable	70°–100° CPM	0°–40° CPM	No CPM	*F*	*p*
Mean 3-week range of motion (ROM) (°)	77.6	72.6	49.1	7.21	.0031
Mean 6-week ROM (°)	78.9	82.8	58.6	8.53	.0031
Mean 6-month ROM (°)	100.0	103.3	85.8	15.63	.0000
Mean gait velocity (cm/s)	144.0	145.6	107.6	8.25	.0016
Mean activities of daily living (ADL) score	18.3	17.0	11.0	16.24	.0000

22

FIGURE LEGENDS ←(12.4)

FIGURE 1. Mean daily time in continuous passive motion (CPM) for patients in each CPM group.

FIGURE 2. Average daily adjustable range of motion for patients in each continuous passive motion (CPM) group. The line for the group that initiated movement at 70° to 100° of flexion shows the progression toward full extension. The line for the group that initiated movement at 0° to 40° of flexion shows the progression toward full flexion. The constant end of the range of motion (100° of flexion for the 70° to 100° CPM group and 0° of flexion for the 0° to 40° CPM group) is not shown for either group.

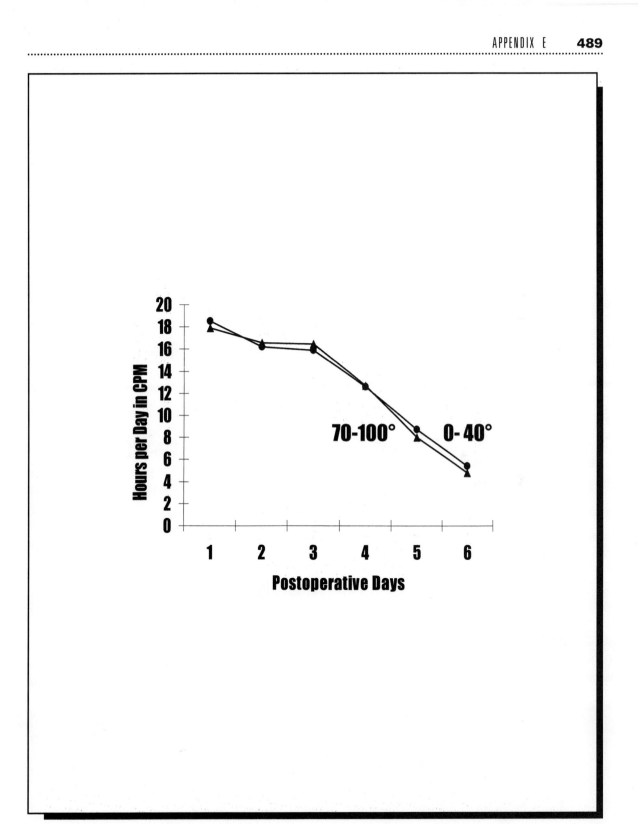

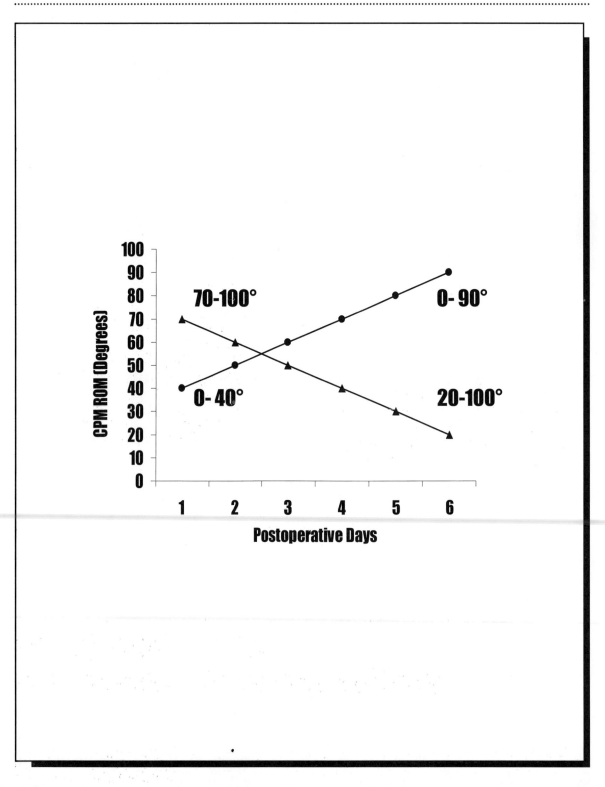

Sample Platform Presentation Script with Slides

1. Good afternoon. I'm pleased to be here in Denver to present the results of our study of the effect of two continuous passive motion progression regimens on knee function 6 months after total knee arthroplasty.

Effect of Two CPM Progression Regimens on Knee Function 6 Months After TKA

Jan R. Woolery, PT, PhD
Memorial Hospital of Indiana, Anytown, IN
Jodi C. Beeker, PT, MS
Community Hospital of Anytown, IN
Jonathon V. Mills, PT, MS
Religious Hospital of Anytown, IN

2. We were prompted to do this study because we had trouble defending our choice of CPM protocols after total knee arthroplasty.

- **Problem**
- Method
- Results
- Discussion
- Conclusions

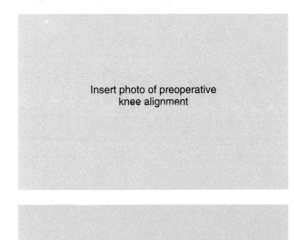

Insert photo of preoperative knee alignment

Insert photo of CPM in use

CPM Comparisons

• CPM to No CPM
- ⇩ LOS
  (Gose, 1987)
- ⇩ Manipulations
  (Ververeli, 1995)
- ⇧ Rate of Δ in flexion
  (Chiarello, 1997)
- ⇧ 1-week ROM
  (Pope, 1997)

• CPM Variations
- No Δ in ROM or LOS
  (Basso, 1987)
- No Δ in ROM
  (Chiarello, 1997)
- No Δ except blood loss
  (Pope, 1997)
- No Δ in 4-week ROM
  (Yashar, 1997)

Outcomes in CPM Literature

• Impairment and Cost Outcomes
- Reported often
- Range of motion
- Length of stay

• Disability Outcomes
- Reported rarely
- Gait velocity
- Activities of daily living

3. As you know, total knee arthroplasty is a common surgical procedure used to reduce pain and enhance function for individuals with knee impairment and disability secondary to osteoarthritis or rheumatoid arthritis.

4. CPM is used routinely in our facilities to encourage early motion of the knee joint after total knee arthroplasty. Despite its widespread clinical use, the optimal CPM regimen for maximizing the short-term and long-term function of patients after total knee arthroplasty has not been established.

5. Although there are a fair number of studies on CPM use after total knee arthroplasty, the comparisons across groups have generally been unique, with little direct replication. Four studies comparing CPM to no CPM have all found at least weak short-term evidence in favor of CPM, as shown in the left column. Four studies comparing different CPM protocols have all found few, if any, differences between the protocols, as shown in the column on the right.

6. Another aspect of the CPM literature is that authors have often reported on impairment and cost outcomes such as range of motion and length of hospital stay. Disability level outcomes such as gait velocity or activities of daily living have rarely been reported.

7. To fill these gaps in the literature, we designed a study that would replicate comparisons among CPM protocols and extend them by comparing the CPM variations to a group that did not receive CPM. In addition, we studied disability level outcomes after total knee arthroplasty.

CPM Research Needs

- Replicate and extend comparisons of CPM

- Study disability level outcomes

8. Specifically, the purpose of this study was to determine whether there were differences between two CPM protocols and a no-CPM group. The two CPM groups differed in their initial ROM, with one group starting at 0° to 40° and the other group at 70° to 100°. The dependent measures were knee flexion range of motion at 3 and 6 weeks postoperatively, and ROM, gait velocity, and ADL score 6 months postoperatively.

Purpose

- Determine whether there are differences between two CPM protocols and a no-CPM group

- Initial ROM of 0-40° versus 70-100° of knee flexion

- Flexion ROM, gait velocity, ADL score

- 3 weeks, 6 weeks, 6 months postoperatively

9. We hypothesized that there would be no differences between the CPM groups at any time; that there would be differences between the CPM and no-CPM groups at 3 and 6 weeks postoperatively, and that there would be no differences among the groups at 6 months postoperatively.

Hypotheses

- No differences between CPM groups at any time

- Differences between CPM and no-CPM groups at 3 weeks and 6 weeks

- No difference between CPM and no-CPM groups at 6 months

10. The study was a nonequivalent control group design with . . .

- Problem
- **Method**
- Results
- Discussion
- Conclusions

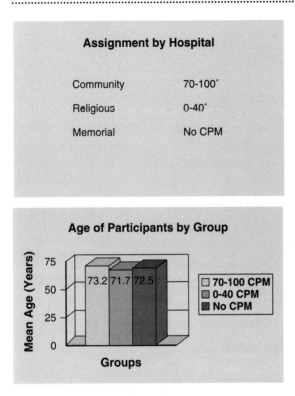

Assignment by Hospital

Community	70-100°
Religious	0-40°
Memorial	No CPM

Age of Participants by Group

Mean Age (Years)

73.2 71.7 72.5

☐ 70-100 CPM
☐ 0-40 CPM
■ No CPM

Groups

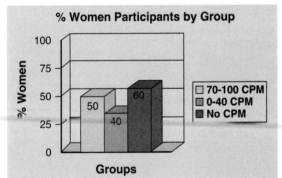

% Women Participants by Group

% Women

100

75

50 60

50

40

25

☐ 70-100 CPM
☐ 0-40 CPM
■ No CPM

0

Groups

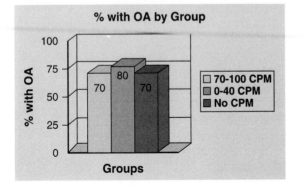

% with OA by Group

% with OA

100

75 80

70 70

50

25

☐ 70-100 CPM
☐ 0-40 CPM
■ No CPM

0

Groups

11. . . . assignment to group based on the hospital at which the surgery was done. Patients were at least 50 years old, had a diagnosis of osteoarthritis or rheumatoid arthritis, and underwent unilateral total knee arthroplasty in 1999 at any one of three hospitals in Anytown, Indiana. The first 10 patients who met all inclusion criteria were selected for study.

12. The average age of participants in the three groups was very similar, as shown in the graph.

13. In addition, the proportion of men and women was fairly evenly distributed across the groups as shown.

14. Finally, the distribution of osteoarthritis and rheumatoid arthritis among the groups was fairly similar, as shown by the graph.

15. We took knee flexion measures as shown in the slide. We used a 12-inch, full-circle goniometer according to the procedures outlined by Norkin and White.

Insert photo of therapist
using goniometer

16. Gait velocity measures were taken 6 months after surgery as shown, by timing the participant with a stopwatch during the middle 10 meters of a 20-meter walkway. The data were converted to centimeters per second.

Insert photo of
gait velocity measure

17. The Modified Brigham and Women's Knee Function Scale was administered 6 months after surgery by observing assistive device use, stair climbing, and rising from a chair. The distance each participant was able to walk was a self-reported measure. The four activity scores are summed to create a single ADL score with the highest level of function scored as 20.

Modified Brigham and Women's Scale

- **Distance walked**
  -Unlimited = 5, transfers only = 1
- **Assistive device**
  -None = 5, walker = 1
- **Stair climbing**
  -Reciprocal no rail = 5, unable = 1
- **Rising from chair**
  -No arm assistance = 5, unable = 1

18. We used an analysis of variance to test for differences between groups for each of the dependent variables. The Newman-Keuls procedure was used for post hoc analysis. Alpha was set at .05 for each analysis.

Data Analysis

- ANOVA
- Newman-Keuls post-hoc tests
- Alpha = .05

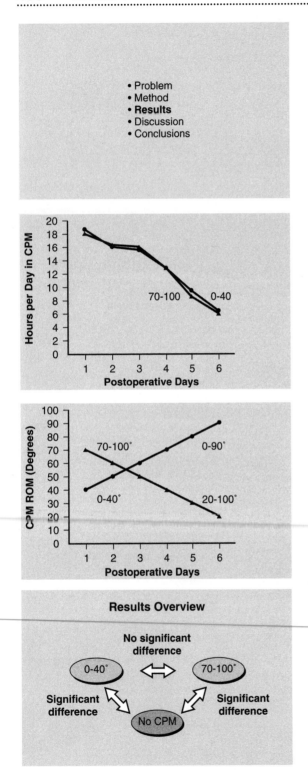

- Problem
- Method
- **Results**
- Discussion
- Conclusions

19. Our results showed several things.

20. First, the two CPM groups received nearly identical hours per day in CPM, as shown by the two lines on this graph. The group starting with a CPM setting of 0° to 40° of knee flexion is shown by the line with the circular points; the group starting at 70° to 100° is shown by the line with the triangular points. You can observe the gradual reduction in hours of CPM per day, starting at about 18 hours per day and ending up at less than 6 hours per day by the 6th postoperative day.

21. This graph shows the range of motion progression of each CPM group. The 0° to 40° group started motion at 0° to 40° and ended up at 0° to 90° of flexion by the 6th postoperative day. The 70° to 100° group started motion at 70° to 100° and moved toward extension each day, ending up at 20° to 100° of motion.

22. The overview of the results of our statistical analysis shows that there were no differences between the two CPM groups, represented by the light ovals, for any of the dependent variables. In addition, both CPM groups had statistically superior results on all variables when compared to the no-CPM group, represented by the darker oval. The specific findings are shown for each dependent variable on the next series of slides.

23. Mean knee flexion ROM at 3 weeks, 6 weeks, and 6 months after surgery can be seen to increase across time for all groups. The CPM groups both achieved better than 90° of flexion by 6 months but the group that did not receive CPM had slightly less than 90° of flexion by then.

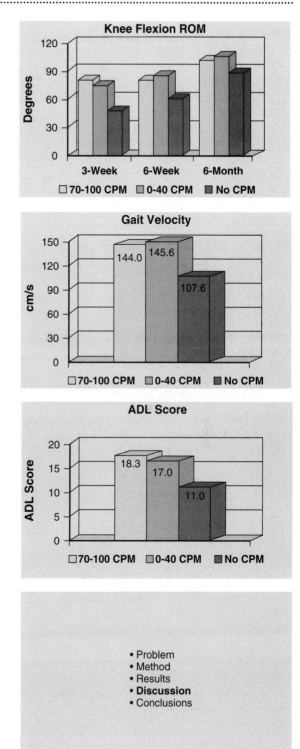

Knee Flexion ROM

Degrees
120
90
60
30
0

3-Week   6-Week   6-Month
☐ 70-100 CPM   ☐ 0-40 CPM   ■ No CPM

24. Mean gait velocity for both CPM groups was close to 150 centimeters per second; for the non-CPM group it was less than 110 centimeters per second.

Gait Velocity

cm/s
150
120
90
60
30
0

144.0   145.6   107.6

☐ 70-100 CPM   ☐ 0-40 CPM   ■ No CPM

25. The mean ADL scores for the two CPM groups were 18 and 17 out of 20; the mean score for the non-CPM group was 11.

ADL Score

ADL Score
20
15
10
5
0

18.3   17.0   11.0

☐ 70-100 CPM   ☐ 0-40 CPM   ■ No CPM

26. Discussion of the results will address the level of support for our hypotheses, the limitations of the study, the functional importance of the differences between groups, and directions for further study.

• Problem
• Method
• Results
• **Discussion**
• Conclusions

Partial Support of Hypotheses

- **Supported**
  - No differences between CPM groups
  - Differences between CPM and no-CPM groups at 3 weeks and 6 weeks

- **Not supported**
  - No difference between CPM and no-CPM groups at 6 months

Functional Implications

- **Gait velocity**
  - Fast enough to cross city street
  - No-CPM group 40 cm/s slower than CPM groups

- **ADL score**
  - CPM groups → minimal to moderate limitation
  - No-CPM group → moderate to severe limitation

Limitations

- Nonrandom assignment to groups

- Investigators aware of group membership

Future Research

- Can results be replicated?

- Do differences between CPM and no-CPM groups persist longer than 6 months?

- Other important variables to measure (blood loss, analgesic use)?

27. We found support for 2 of our 3 hypotheses. The two hypotheses that were supported were that there would be no differences between CPM groups and that there would be differences between the CPM and no-CPM groups at 3 weeks and 6 weeks after surgery. The hypothesis that was not supported was that the differences between the CPM and no-CPM groups would disappear by 6 months after surgery. Instead, we found that the differences between groups persisted at 6 months after surgery.

28. For gait velocity, the difference between the CPM and no-CPM groups seems important. Although all groups could walk fast enough to cross a city street, the no-CPM group was 40 cm/sec or 7/10 of a mile per hour slower than the CPM groups. The difference in ADL scores also appears to be important, with participants in the CPM groups demonstrating minimal to moderate limitations in 1 of the 4 tasks and the participants from the no-CPM group demonstrating moderate to severe limitations in 1 to 2 tasks.

29. There are two main limitations of our research design. First, because the treatments were assigned by hospital and not by patient, there may have been systematic differences between care at the hospitals that could explain the differences in results. Second, because the investigators collecting the data were aware of group membership of the participants, our expectations may have influenced their performance.

30. Future research in the area should focus on replicating these results, studying whether differences between the CPM and no-CPM groups persist longer than 6 months, and determining whether other important variables—such as postoperative blood loss or analgesic use—should be investigated.

31. In conclusion, we found that . . .

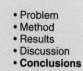

- Problem
- Method
- Results
- Discussion
- **Conclusions**

32. One, there was no difference in outcome after total knee arthroplasty with CPM initiated at 0° to 40° or at 70° to 100°. Two, there were superior outcomes after total knee arthroplasty for both CPM groups compared to no-CPM. Three, these differences persisted for 6 months after surgery.

Conclusions

- No difference in outcome after TKA with CPM progression from 0-40° or 70-100°

- Superior outcomes after TKA for CPM groups compared to no-CPM groups

- Differences persisted for 6 months

33. I'd be happy to take any questions at this time.

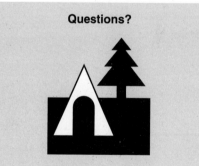

Questions?

Glossary

A-B designs. A family of single-system designs in which baseline (A) and intervention (B) phases are alternated. Common forms are A-B, A-B-A, B-A-B, A-B-A-B.

Absolute reliability. The extent to which a score varies on repeated measurements; it is quantified by the standard error of measurement.

Ad hoc theory. Descriptive theory in which a nonexhaustive list of characteristics is used to describe a phenomenon.

Adjusted rates. Rates that enable valid comparisons across populations with different proportions of various subgroups; calculated by adjusting the rates for one population based on the composition of the population to which it is being compared; contrast with *crude rates*.

Alpha level. The probability of concluding that the null hypothesis is false, when in fact it is true. The alpha level is set by the researcher before data analysis; contrast this with *probability level*, which is generated by the data analysis.

Alternating-treatment design. A single-system design including the use of different treatments, each administered independently of the other.

Analysis of covariance (ANCOVA). A form of analysis of variance in which the effect of an intervening variable is mathematically removed from the analysis.

Analysis of variance (ANOVA). A family of statistical tests used to analyze differences between two or more groups; based on partitioning the sum of squares into that attributable to between-group differences and that attributable to within-group differences.

Archival data. Records or documents of the activities of individuals, institutions, or governments found in sources such as medical records, voter registration rosters, newspapers and magazines, and meeting minutes.

Artifacts. Physical evidence, particularly within a qualitative research design, which contributes to the understanding of the research question.

Assignment threat. An internal validity threat that is realized when subjects are assigned to groups in ways that do not ensure their equivalence.

Attribute variable. A variable created not by manipulation, but through division of subjects into groups based on an existing attribute such as sex or age; also called *classification variable*.

Autonomy. The moral principle that individuals should be permitted to be self-determining.

Beneficence. The moral principle that people should act to promote the welfare of others.

Beta-weight. Used to interpret multiple-regression equations by standardizing the slopes associated with each independent variable within the equation.

Between-subjects design. An experimental design in which all of the independent variables are between-subjects factors.

Between-subjects factor. An independent variable whose different levels are administered to different groups of subjects.

Bimodal distribution. A frequency distribution in which there are two modes, or most frequently occurring scores.

Block. A grouping of subjects based on a classification or attribute variable, such as age, sex, or diagnosis.

Bonferroni adjustment. Divides the total alpha level for an experiment by the number of statistical tests conducted to control for alpha level inflation.

Case-control design. An epidemiological research design in which groups of patients with and without a desired effect are compared to determine whether they have different proportions of presumed causes; contrast with *cohort design,* which proceeds from cause to effect.

Case report. Systematic, nonexperimental description of clinical practice; contrast with *case study* and *single-system design.*

Case study. Method of structuring a qualitative research project by detailed analysis of a well-defined unit or case; contrast with *case report* and *single-system design.*

Categorical theory. Descriptive theory in which the characteristics that describe a phenomenon are exhaustive.

Causal-comparative research. Nonexperimental research in which assignment to groups is based on preexisting characteristics, or attributes, of subjects; also called *ex post facto research.*

Celeration line. Method of analyzing single-system research by determining a trend line in one phase, extrapolating the trend into the next phase, and determining whether the data in the second phase differ significantly from the extrapolated trend line.

Chi-square distribution. A distribution of squared z scores; it forms the basis for chi-square tests of differences between groups when the dependent variable is in the form of a frequency or percentage.

Classification variable. A variable created not by manipulation, but through division of subjects into groups based on an existing attribute such as sex or age; also called *attribute variable.*

Closed-format item. Questionnaire items that require a specific type of response, such as a "yes or no" question; contrast with *open-format item.*

Coefficient of determination. The square of the correlation coefficient; indicates the percentage of variance shared by the variables.

Cohort. In general, any group. More specifically, groups that follow one another in time, as in subsequent school-year classes.

Cohort design. An epidemiological research design that works forward from cause to effect; contrast with *case-control design,* which works from effect to cause.

Compensatory equalization of treatments. A threat to internal validity that is realized when a researcher who has preconceived notions about which treatment is more desirable showers attention on subjects receiving the treatment perceived to be less desirable.

Compensatory rivalry. This threat to internal validity is realized when members of one group react competitively to the perception that they are receiving a less desirable treatment than the other groups.

Concept. A phenomenon expressed in words; sometimes used as a more concrete term than *construct.*

Conceptual framework. Theory that specifies relationships between variables but does not have a deductive component; used interchangeably with *model.*

Concurrent validity. The extent to which a developing measure is comparable to a measurement standard.

Confidence interval. A range of scores around a statistic; represents a specified probability that the true value is within the range.

Construct. A property that is invented for a specific purpose; sometimes used as a more abstract term than *concept*.

Construct underrepresentation. A threat to construct validity that is realized when the independent or dependent variables are poorly developed.

Construct validity. Threats to construct validity are realized when the independent or dependent variables within a study are not well developed or are incorrectly labeled.

Content analysis. A process by which the text of archival records is reduced to quantifiable information.

Continuous variable. A variable that theoretically can be measured to finer and finer degrees.

Contrast. Comparison of two means; specifically, multiple-comparison tests conducted as part of complex analysis of variance tests.

Correlation coefficient. Mathematical expression of the degree of relationship between two or more variables; several different forms exist.

Criterion-referenced measure. A measurement framework in which each individual's performance is evaluated with respect to some absolute level of achievement.

Criterion validity. The extent to which one measure is systematically related to other measures or outcomes; subdivided into concurrent and predictive validity.

Cross-sectional study. Study documenting the status of a group at a particular point in time.

Crude rates. Rates calculated using the entire population at risk; contrast with *specific* and *adjusted rates*.

Deductive reasoning. Reasoning that proceeds from the general to the specific.

Degrees of freedom. The number of items that are free to vary. For example, the degrees of freedom for the mean is $n - 1$, meaning that if a certain mean score is desired, $n - 1$ of the values are free to fluctuate as long as one can control the final value.

Delphi technique. A survey design in which several rounds of a questionnaire are administered, each round building on information collected in previous rounds.

Dependent variable. The measured variable; used to determine the effects of the independent variable.

Descriptive theory. The least restrictive form of theory, simply describing the phenomenon of interest.

Deviation score. Calculated by subtracting the mean of a data set from each raw score.

Dichotomous variable. A variable that can take only two values, such as male/female or present/absent.

Diffusion of treatments. This threat to internal validity is realized when subjects in treatment and control groups share information about their respective treatments.

Discrete variable. A variable that can assume only distinct values. An example is a ligamentous laxity scale, which can assume values of hypomobile, normal, and hypermobile.

Effect size. Method of quantifying differences by expressing them in standard deviation units by calculating the ratio of the difference between the means to the pooled standard deviation of the groups being compared; standardizes the magnitude of change across many different variables.

Effectiveness. Usefulness of a particular treatment to the individuals receiving it under typical clinical conditions, usually determined by nonexperimental methods in outcomes research; contrast with *efficacy*.

Efficacy. Biological effect of treatment delivered under carefully controlled conditions, usually determined by randomized controlled trial; contrast with *effectiveness*.

Epidemiology. The study of disease, injury, and health in a population. Epidemiological research documents the incidence of a disease or injury, determines causes for the disease or injury, and develops mechanisms to control the disease or injury.

Ethnographic research. Research whose purpose is to develop an in-depth picture of the culture of a particular group or unit.

Ex post facto research. Nonexperimental analysis of differences in which the independent variable is not manipulated. An example is research that examines differences between men and women on various dependent variables. Also called *causal-comparative research*.

Experimental research. Research in which at least one independent variable is subjected to controlled manipulation by the researcher.

Experimenter expectancy. A threat to construct validity that is realized when the subjects are able to guess the ways in which the experimenter wishes them to respond.

Explanatory theory. Theory that examines the *why* and *how* questions that undergird a problem.

External criticism. Concerns about the authenticity of archival records.

External validity. Concerns the issue of to whom, in what settings, and at what times the results of research can be generalized.

Facets. The factors of interest within a generalizability study; examples of facets might be raters, days, and times of measurement.

Factor analysis. A multivariate correlational technique used to reduce a large number of variables into a smaller number of factors by clustering related variables.

Factorial design. A design in which there are at least two independent variables, and all levels of each independent variable are crossed with all other independent variables.

F distribution. A distribution of squared *t* statistics; the basis of analysis of variance.

Fisher's exact test. A modified chi-square statistic that is sometimes used if the dependent variable consists of only two categories.

Frequency distribution. A tally of the number of times each individual score is represented in a data set; can be presented visually as a histogram or a stem-and-leaf plot.

Friedman's ANOVA. The nonparametric version of the repeated measures analysis of variance.

Generalizability theory. An extension of classical measurement theory that quantifies the extent of variability on repeated measures that can be attributed to different facets of interest.

Grounded theory. A qualitative research approach that starts from an atheoretical perspective and develops theory that is grounded in the information gathered.

Health-related quality of life (HRQL). Quality of life concept that includes elements related to physical, psychosocial, and social functioning; measured by generic tools such as the Short Form-36, Sickness Impact Profile, and Functional Status Questionnaire.

Heuristic. Discovering or revealing relationships that may lead to further development of a particular line of research.

Historical research. Research in which past events are documented because they are of inherent interest or because they provide a perspective that can guide decision making in the present.

History. This threat to internal validity is realized when events unrelated to the treatment of interest occur during the course of the study and cause changes in the dependent variable.

Homoscedasticity. One of the assumptions that should be met before calculating a correlation coefficient. Homoscedasticity means that for each value of one variable, the other variable has equal variability.

Hypothesis. A conjectural statement of the relationship between variables. Sometimes used interchangeably with *proposition*.

Idiographic. Pertaining to a particular case in a particular time and context; the opposite of *nomothetic*.

Incidence. The rate of new cases of a condition that develop during a specified period of time; the formula is *new cases during a time period/population at risk during a time period*.

Independent *t* test. A parametric test of differences between two independent samples.

Independent variable. The presumed cause of a measured effect. In experimental research, at least one independent variable is manipulated by the researcher.

Informed consent. A process by which health care practitioners or investigators provide potential subjects with the information they need to make informed decisions about treatment or participation within a study. Four components are required for autonomy in making such decisions: disclosure, comprehension, voluntariness, and competence.

Instrumentation. This threat to internal validity is realized when changes in measuring tools themselves are responsible for observed changes in the dependent variable.

Interaction. A research question in which the effect of one variable is assessed to determine whether it is consistent across the different levels of a second independent variable.

Interaction of different treatments. A threat to construct validity that may be realized when treatments other than the one of interest are administered to subjects.

Internal criticism. Concerns about the neutrality of the interpretation of information found in archival records.

Internal validity. Concerns whether the independent variable is the probable cause of changes in the dependent variable.

Interrater reliability. The consistency among different judges' ratings of the same object or response. In its purest form, interrater reliability is determined by having the judges perform the ratings of one group of subjects at the same point in time.

Interval scale. Has the real-number system properties of order and distance, but lacks a meaningful origin.

Intraclass correlation coefficient (ICC). A family of correlation coefficients that allows comparison of two or more repeated measures; used to analyze measurement reliability.

Intrarater reliability. The consistency with which one rater assigns scores to a single set of responses on two or more occasions.

Kappa. A reliability coefficient designed for use with nominal data; corrects agreement percentages to account for chance agreements.

Kruskal-Wallis test. The nonparametric version of the one-way analysis of variance.

Level. A value of the independent variable; for example, a design in which the independent variable consists of a treatment group and a control group is said to have two levels of the independent variable.

Likert-type items. Used to assess the strength of response to a declarative statement. The most typical set of responses is "strongly agree," "agree," "undecided," "disagree," and "strongly disagree."

Logistic regression. Regression technique used to predict dichotomous outcomes from numerical independent variables.

Mann-Whitney test. The nonparametric version of the independent t test.

Maturation. This threat to internal validity is realized when changes within a subject due to the passage of time occur during the course of a study and cause changes in the dependent variable.

McNemar test. A statistical test that analyzes frequency or percentage data collected on repeated occasions.

Mean. The sum of observations divided by the number of observations.

Median. The middle score of a ranked distribution.

Member checking. Method of verification in qualitative research by which informants review results generated by the researcher to correct technical errors or challenge the researcher's interpretation of their situation.

Meta-analysis. A means by which research results across several different studies are synthesized in a quantitative way.

Mixed design. A design in which some of the independent variables are between-subjects factors and some of the independent variables are within-subject factors; also called a *split-plot design*.

Mode. The most frequently occurring score within a distribution; if there are two modes, the distribution is called *bimodal*.

Model. A theory that specifies relationships between variables but does not have a deductive component; used interchangeably with *conceptual framework*.

Mortality. This threat to internal validity is realized when subjects are lost from the different study groups at different rates or for different reasons.

Multiple baseline design. A single-system design in which several subjects are studied after baselines of varying lengths.

Multiple regression. Extension of simple correlation and regression techniques to use multiple independent variables to predict a numerical dependent variable.

Multivariate analyses. Statistical tools designed for simultaneous analysis of multiple dependent variables.

Naturalistic. One term for qualitative research; refers specifically to the philosophy that qualitative researchers should study subjects in their natural setting.

Negative predictive value. The percentage of individuals identified by a test as negative who actually do not have the diagnosis.

Nested design. A design in which there are at least two independent variables, but not all levels of the independent variables are crossed.

Newman-Keuls test. A multiple-comparison procedure.

Nominal scale. Has none of the properties of a real-number system; provides classification without placing any value on the categories within the classification.

Nomothetic. Relating to general or universal principles; opposite of *idiographic*.

Nondirectional. A t-test hypothesis in which the researcher is open to the possibility that one mean is either greater than or less than the other mean.

Nonexperimental research. Research in which there is no manipulation of an independent variable.

Nonmaleficence. The moral principle of doing no harm.

Nonparametric tests. Statistical tests that do not rest on assumptions related to the distribution of the populations from which the samples are drawn.

Nonprobability sample. A form of sampling that does not use randomization.

Normal curve. A symmetric, bell-shaped frequency distribution that can be defined in terms of the mean and standard deviation of a set of data.

Norm-referenced measure. A measure that judges individual performance in relation to group norms.

Null hypothesis. The statistical hypothesis that there is no difference between groups; contrast with *research hypothesis.*

Number. A numeral that has been assigned quantitative meaning.

Numeral. A symbol that does not necessarily have quantitative meaning; it is a form of naming.

Odds ratio. Method of estimating relative risk by calculating the ratio of the odds that each of two groups will possess a certain characteristic.

Omnibus test. An overall test of a hypothesis within an analysis of variance; if the omnibus test identifies a significant difference between groups, then multiple-comparison procedures are needed to determine the location of the differences.

Open-format item. An interview or survey item allowing respondents freedom to structure their responses as desired; contrast with *closed-format item.*

Operational definition. A specific description of the way in which a construct is presented or measured within a study.

Ordinal scale. Has only one of the properties of a real number system: order. Ordinal scales do not ensure that there are equal intervals between categories or ranks.

Outcomes research. Analysis of clinical practice as it actually occurs for the purpose of determining effectiveness of clinical methods.

Paired-*t* test. A statistical test that determines the difference between two paired measures.

Paradigm. A belief system researchers use to organize their discipline.

Parameter. A characteristic of a population; estimated by sample statistics.

Parametric tests. Statistical tests that rest on assumptions related to the distribution of the populations from which the samples are drawn.

Pathokinesiology. The application of anatomy and physiology to the study of abnormal human movement.

Pearson correlation coefficient. Analysis of the relationship between two variables; ranges in value from $+1.0$ to -1.0; calculated by determining the average of the crossproducts of the z scores of both variables.

Phenomenology. A qualitative research approach whose purpose is to describe some aspect of life as it is lived by the participants.

Positive predictive value. The percentage of individuals identified by the test as positive who actually have the diagnosis.

Positivism. A research tradition that rests on the objective measurement of reality; the traditional method of science.

Post hoc comparisons. Tests that are used to make pair-wise comparisons of means after an omnibus test has identified significant differences between more than two means.

Postpositivist. The qualitative research tradition, resting on the assumption of multiple constructed realities.

Power. The ability of a statistical test to detect a difference when it exists.

Predictive theory. A theory that is used to make predictions based on the relationships between variables.

Predictive validity. The ability of a measurement made at one point in time to predict future status.

Prevalence. The proportion of a population who exhibit a certain condition at a given point in time; the formula is *existing cases/population examined at a given point in time*.

Primary sources. Scholarly works that constitute the first documentation of the results of a study; the traditional primary source in the health sciences is the journal article, which reports the findings of original research.

Probability (*p*) level. The probability of obtaining a certain test statistic if the null hypothesis is true; the probability level is generated by the data analysis itself. Contrast with *alpha level,* which is set by the researcher.

Proportion. A fraction in which the numerator is a subset of the denominator; the formula is *a/a + b*.

Proposition. A statement of the relationship between concepts. Sometimes used interchangeably with *hypothesis*.

Prospective research. A research approach in which the researcher completes data collection after the research question is developed. Also used by epidemiologists as a synonym for *cohort design*.

Purposive sampling. A sampling technique, commonly used in qualitative research, involving selection of individuals for diversity of views rather than for representativeness.

Q-sort. A survey research technique in which respondents generate a forced-choice ranking of many alternatives.

Qualitative research. A research paradigm based, in part, on assumptions of multiple constructed realities, interdependence of investigator and participant, and time- and context-dependency of information.

Quasiexperimental research. A form of experimental research characterized by nonrandom assignment of subjects to groups or repeated treatments to the same group.

Questionnaire. A written self-report instrument used in survey research.

Randomized block design. A design in which the levels of at least one independent variable are randomly assigned and the levels of at least one independent variable are determined by blocks.

Randomized clinical trial. The name often given to clinical research in which subjects are randomly assigned to treatment and control groups.

Rate. A proportion expressed over a particular unit of time, often multiplied by a constant to obtain whole number values.

Ratio. Expresses the relationship between two numbers by dividing the numerator by the denominator; the simple formula is *a/b*.

Ratio scale. Exhibits all three components of a real-number system: order, distance, and origin. All the arithmetic functions of addition, subtraction, multiplication, and division can be applied to ratio scales.

Receiver-operator curve (ROC). Method of graphing test data to determine cutoff points that balance *sensitivity* and *specificity*.

Relative reliability. Exists when individual measurements within a group maintain their position within the group on repeated measurement; quantified by correlation coefficients.

Relative risk. Comparison of the probability that different groups with different characteristics will be affected by disease or injury in some way.

Reliability. The extent to which measurements are repeatable.

Repeated measures analysis of variance. One of a family of analysis of variance techniques; used to determine differences between two or more dependent samples.

Research hypothesis. A statement that makes predictions about the expected outcome of the study; contrast with *null hypothesis.*

Resentful demoralization. This threat to internal validity is realized when members of one group react negatively to the perception that they are receiving a less desirable treatment than the other groups.

Residual. The amount of variability left unexplained after a data analysis; part of some analysis of variance and linear regression procedures.

Retrospective research. A research approach in which data are collected before the research question is developed. Also used by epidemiologists as a synonym for *case-control design.*

Reversed treatment design. A design in which the subjects or groups receive treatments that are expected to cause changes in opposite directions. This is in contrast to typical control-group designs, in which the control group is not expected to change.

Risk ratio. Method of calculating relative risk by creating a ratio of the incidence rate for one subgroup and the incidence rate for another subgroup; contrast with *odds ratio.*

Robust. Describes statistical procedures that tolerate violation of their assumptions without distortion of the probability of making a Type I error.

Sampling distribution. A distribution of sample means formed by drawing repeated samples from the same population. Ordinarily, the sample distribution is a theoretical distribution with a standard deviation estimated by dividing a single sample standard deviation by the square root of the number within the sample.

Scheffé test. A multiple-comparison procedure.

Secondary sources. Scholarly works, such as book chapters or literature reviews, that are interpretations of original sources such as journal article reports of original research.

Selection. This threat to external validity is realized when the selection process is biased because it yields subjects who are in some manner different from the population to whom researchers hope to generalize their results.

Self-report measures. These measures are the foundation of survey research; it is assumed that meaningful information can be obtained by asking the parties of interest what they know, what they believe, and how they behave.

Semantic differential items. A type of closed-format item that uses adjective pairs, such as "invigorating–dull" to represent different ends of a continuum.

Semistructured interview. An interview technique based on predeveloped questions, but with latitude for the interviewer to clarify questions as needed for the interviewee, thereby obtaining more information for the study.

Sensitivity. The percentage of individuals with a particular diagnosis who are correctly identified as positive by a test.

Setting. This threat to external validity is realized when peculiarities of the setting in which the research was conducted make it difficult to generalize results to other settings.

Single-system design. Experimental research designs in which the unit of interest is a single person or setting, studied over time under baseline and treatment conditions.

Skewed. A distribution that is not symmetric, that is, one with a long tail at its upper or lower end.

Slope. A characteristic of a line; the ratio of the change in Y that accompanies a change of one unit of X.

Snowball sampling. A nonprobability sampling technique employing a few key informants to identify others who have had similar experiences.

Specificity. The percentage of individuals without a particular diagnosis who are correctly identified as negative by a test.

Specific rates. Rates calculated for specific subgroups of the population; contrast with *crude rates.*

Split-plot design. A design in which some of the independent variables are between-subjects factors and some are within-subject factors; also called a *mixed design.*

Standard deviation. The square root of the variance; expressed in the units of the original measure.

Standard error of measurement. A measure of absolute reliability; represents the standard deviation of measurement errors.

Standard error of the estimate. The standard deviation of the difference between individual data points and the regression line through them.

Standard error of the mean. The standard deviation of the sampling distribution.

Standard normal distribution. A normal distribution with a mean of 0.0 and a standard deviation of 1.0.

Statistic. A characteristic of a sample; used to estimate population parameters.

Statistical conclusion validity. Concerns whether statistical tools have been used and their results interpreted properly within a study.

Statistical regression to the mean. This threat to internal validity may be realized when subjects are selected on the basis of extreme scores on a single administration of a test.

Structured interview. Oral administration of a written questionnaire without deviation from the wording of the questionnaire.

Survey. A research method based on self-reported information from participants rather than on observations or measurements taken by researchers.

Survival analysis. Mathematical tool used to analyze the changing proportion of individuals exhibiting a certain characteristic (often survival) over time after a naturally occurring event or a treatment or research manipulation.

t **distribution.** A flattened standard normal curve; the basis for *t* tests, which are used to assess the differences between two groups or between paired data.

Testing. This threat to internal validity is realized when repeated testing itself is likely to result in changes in the dependent variable.

Test-retest reliability. The ability of a measurement to be repeated from one test occasion to another.

Theory. A body of interrelated principles that present a systematic view of phenomena; a theory is testable and tentative.

Time. This threat to external validity is realized when the results of a study are applicable to limited time frames.

Transform. Mathematical manipulation of data, usually to make it fit a normal distribution.

Trend. Related to data analysis of single-system research designs; describes whether the direction of change during a study phase is upward or downward.

Triangulation. A method of establishing reliability in qualitative research; consists of comparing responses across several different sources.

Tukey test. A multiple-comparison procedure.

Two standard deviation band analysis. A method of analyzing single-system data by calculating a two standard deviation band around the baseline data and observing the pattern of intervention data that fall within and outside the band.

Unstructured interview. An interview technique wherein the order and way in which the topics are covered are left to the interviewer as he or she interacts with participants.

Utility. The moral principle that we should act to bring about the greatest benefit and the least harm.

Validity. The meaningfulness of test scores as they are used for specific purposes.

Variance. Conceptually, the average of the squared deviations about the mean. The *population variance* is found by dividing the sum of the squared deviations by the number within the sample; the *sample variance* is found by dividing the sum of the squared deviations by n − 1.

Wilcoxon rank sum test. The nonparametric version of the independent *t* test; synonymous with *Mann-Whitney test.*

Wilcoxon signed rank test. The nonparametric version of the paired-*t* test.

Withdrawal design. A family of single-system designs characterized by implementation and withdrawal of treatment over the course of the study; known generically as A-B-A designs.

Within-subject design. A design in which all of the factors are within-subject factors.

Within-subject factor. An independent variable whose different levels are administered to the same group of subjects. The comparison of interest is within the subject group.

Yates' correction. A correction factor sometimes used with chi-square tests in which the expected frequency in several cells is very small.

z score. A deviation score divided by the standard deviation; indicates how many standard deviations the raw score is above or below the mean.

Index

Note: The letter "t" following a page number represents tables; the letter "b" following a page number represents boxed material; and *italic* page numbers indicate illustrations.

A

A-B designs, 127–128
A-B-A designs, 128–129
Absolute reliability, 234–235
Accelerometer, 254
Acceptance region, 296
Accessible population, 96
ACP Journal Club, 391
Action-knowledge conflict, 43
Activities of daily living, basic 252, 253
   instrumental 252, 253
Actuarial analysis, 341
Ad hoc theories, 16
Adjusted rates, 176–177, *177*
Agency for Health Care Policy Research
   (AHCPR) report, 8
Alpha level, 292–293, 298–299
Alternating-treatment designs, 129–131,
   131
Alternative hypothesis, 46
American Physical Therapy Association
   (APTA), 12
Analysis of covariance (ANCOVA), *334,*
   334–336, *335,* 335t
Analysis of differences, 144, 300
   across several dependent variables,
      332–333, 333t
   advanced ANOVA techniques for,
      326–336, 326t, *327,* 327t, 328t,
      329, 330t, *331,* 333t, *334, 335,*
      335t
   assumptions for, 302–304
   between more than one independent
      variable, 326–332, 326t, *327,*
      327t, 328t, *329,* 330t, *331*
   between two dependent samples,
      316–320, 317t, 319t, 320t
   between two independent groups,
      305–310, 306t, 308t
   between two or more dependent
      samples, 320–323, 321t, 322t
   between two or more independent
      groups, 310–320, 310t, 311t,
      315t, 317t, 319t, 320t

Analysis of differences *(Continued)*
   distributions for, *301,* 301–302
   effect of removing intervening variable
      on, *334,* 334–336, *335,* 335t
   hypothesis testing with confidence
      intervals for, 341–344
   power analysis and effect size for,
      344–345
   prospective, 145–146
   retrospective, 144–145
   single-system design analysis for,
      336, 336–340, *337, 338, 340*
   steps in, 304, 305t
   using survival analysis, 340–341
Analysis of relationships, 142–143,
   347–348
   prospective, 143–144
   retrospective, 143
   using correlation, 348–356, 348t, *349,*
      350t, *351, 352, 353, 355*
   using factor analysis, 372–375, 373t,
      374t, 375t
   using linear regression, 356–358, *357*
   using logistic regression, 370–372, *371*
   using multiple regression, 367–370,
      369
   using reliability analysis, 360–367,
      361t, *362, 363,* 364t, 365t, 366t
Analysis of variance (ANOVA),
      advanced techniques for, 326–336,
      326t, *327,* 327t, 328t, *329,* 330t,
      331, 333t, *334, 335,* 335t
   Friedman's, 323
   multivariate, 332–333, 333t
   one-way, 310–313, 311t
   repeated measures, 321–322, 322t,
      364–365
   two-way, between subjects, 326–329,
      326t, *327,* 327t, 328t, *329*
   mixed design, 329–332, 330t, *331*
ANCOVA (analysis of covariance), *334,*
   334–336, *335,* 335t
ANOVA. See *Analysis of variance
   (ANOVA).*

Anthropometric characteristics, 249–251,
   250t, *251*
APTA (American Physical Therapy
   Association), 12
Archives, 138
Arousal (alertness) measurement,
   251–252
Artifacts, 163–164
Ashworth Scale of Spasticity, 260
Assignment to groups, 105
   and internal validity, 85
   consecutive, 108
   defined, 95
   matched, 107t, 108
   maturation, history, or
      instrumentation in, 86–87
   methods of, 108–109
   random, block, 106t, 107–108, 122
      individual, 105–106, 105t, 106t
   significance of, 95–96
   systematic, 107t, 108
Attribute variable, 70
Authorship, 438
Autonomic functions, 267
Autonomy, principle of, 31

B

Back issues, 392
BADL (basic activities of daily living),
   252, 253
Balance, measurement of, 256–257
Barthel Index, 253
Basement effect, 87
Basic activities of daily living (BADL),
   252, 253
Belmont definition, 28–29
Bench research, 149
Benchmarking, 198
Beneficence, principle of, 30
Berg Balance Scale, 256
Between-groups differences, 293, 297
Between-groups independent
   variable, 64

Between-subjects design, 116, 122–123, *123*
  in mixed-design two-way ANOVA, 329–332, 330t, *331*
  in repeated measures ANOVA, 321
  in two-way ANOVA, 326–329, 326t, *327,* 327t, 328t, *329*
Between subjects factor, 329–330
Bimodal distribution, 284
Black box, 56
Blinding, 75
Block grouping, 70
  by random assignment, 106t, 107–108, 122
Blood flow, 266
Blood pressure, 265–266
Body composition, 251
Bonferroni adjustment, 292–293
Boolean operators, 383–384, *384*
Budget, proposed, 420–423, 423t
b-weight, 367, 368

C

Calibration, 83
Canonical correlation, 350t, 351
Cardiovascular functions, 265–266
Case-control studies, 145, 184–185, 185–187
Case mix adjustments, 198–199
Case report(s), 140
  case study *versus,* 148
  contributions of, *149,* 149–150, *150*
  defined, 148–149
  format of, 152–153
  purposes of, 150–152
  single-system paradigm *versus,* 58, 126–127
Case study(ies), 140
  case report *versus,* 148
  defined, 148–149
  qualitative designs as, 155–157
  single-system paradigm *versus,* 58, 126–127
Case-to-case generalizability, 126, 132
Categorical theories, 16
Causal-comparative research, 144
Causal conclusions, 71
Cause and effect, with qualitative paradigm, 55
  with quantitative paradigm, 52
Ceiling effect, 87
Celeration line analysis, 337, *337*
  level, trend, and slope analysis with, *338,* 338–339
Central tendency, 283–284, 284t
Chi-square distribution, 301, *301,* 302
Chi-square test, of association, 309–310, 314–316, 315t
  of goodness of fit, 315
CI. See *Confidence interval (CI).*
CINAHL (Cumulative Index of Nursing and Allied Health Literature), 384–387, 386t, 387t

Classical measurement theory, 231–232
Classification variable, 70
Clever Hans, 51
  experimenter expectancies and, 89–90
Clinical case report. See *Case report(s); Case study(ies).*
Clinical pathways, 152
Clinical Test of Sensory Interaction and Balance, 256
Closed-format survey items, 206–207
Cluster sampling, 101–103, *102*
Coding systems, 165, 166b
Coefficient of determination, 354
  confidence intervals around, 354–355
Cognition, 251–252
Cohort studies, 117–118, 184–185, 187
Compensatory equalization, of treatment, 88
Compensatory rivalry, 88
Competence, in informed consent, 32
Comprehension, in informed consent, 31
Computer statistical packages, 433
Concept, 16–17
Conceptual dependent variable, 67
Conceptual framework, 17
Conceptual model, 17
Concurrent cohort study, 187
Concurrent validity, 237, 246
Confidence interval (CI), around correlation coefficient, 354–355
  around mean, 342
  of sampling distribution, 290–291
  testing hypotheses with, 341–344
    foundations for, 342–343
    interpretation and examples for, 343–344
Confidentiality, 36
Confounding variable, 72
Consecutive assignment, 108
Consecutive sampling, 104
Consistency, internal, 232
Constant, 63, 367
Construct, 16–17
  underrepresentation of, 89
Construct validity, 77, 88–89, 235–236, 244–245
  threat(s) to, evaluation of, 400–401
    experimenter expectancies as, 89–90
    testing–treatment interactions as, 91
    treatment interactions as, 90
    underrepresentation as, 89
Content analysis, 138
Content validity, 236, 245–246
Contingency table, 315, 315t
Continuous variable, 225
Contrast, 312
  planned, 313
Control, and internal validity, 78
  independent variable implementation as, 71–72
  of extraneous setting variables, 72

Control *(Continued)*
  of extraneous subject variables, 72–74, *74*
  of information received by subject and researcher, 74–76
  of maturation effects, 80–82, *81–82*
  of measurement variation, 74
  of subject selection and assignment, 72
  with qualitative paradigm, 57–58
  with quantitative paradigm, 54
  with single-system paradigm, 59
Controlled vocabulary searching, 381
Corporation funding, 423–424
Correlation, canonical, 350t, 351
  defined, 142
  multiple, 350t, 351
  partial, 350t, 351
Correlation coefficient(s), 228–230, 230t, 234, 235
  alternative, 350–351, 350t
  analysis of relationships using, 348–356, 348t, *349,* 350t, *351, 352, 353, 355*
  assumptions of, *351,* 351–353, *352, 353*
  calculation of Pearson Product Moment correlation and, 348–349, 348t
  coefficient of determination to evaluate, 354
  confidence intervals around, 354–355
  interpretation of, 353–356, *355*
  intraclass, 350, 350t, 364–365, 364t, 365t
  literature examples of, 356
  statistical significance of, 354
  strength of, 354
Correlation matrix, 349, *349,* 350t, 373, *373*
Correlational research, 142
Counterbalancing, 73
Cover letter, for mailed questionnaire, 212, *213, 214*
Cox log-rank test, 341
Cox regression model, 341
Criterion-referenced measure, 231
Criterion validity, 236, 246
Cross-sectional studies, 138, 184, 185
Crossproduct, 349
Crude rates, 176, *176*
Cumulative Index of Nursing and Allied Health Literature (CINAHL), 384–387, 386t, 387t
Current Contents, 391

D

Data analysis, 433–435
  in qualitative designs, 164–168, 166b, *168*

Data coding, 433–434
  verification of, by multiple
    researchers, 167
Data collection, artifact examination for,
    163–164
  control of measurements for, 74
  for prospective descriptive research,
    141–142
  interview for, 161–162
  observation for, 162–163
  pilot study for, 430
  procedures for, 429
  recording forms for, 429–430,
    431–432
  safeguarding methods of, 429
  scheduling participants and
    personnel for, 430
  surveys for, 207–208
  timing of, 68–69
Data entry, 434
Data management, 165
Data set(s), central tendency of,
    283–284, 284t
  dependence of, 303–304
  frequency distribution of, 278–283,
    279t, 280t, 281t, 282t, 283t
  hypothetical, 278, 279t, 280t
  independence of, 303–304
  measurement levels of, 303
  normal distribution of, *287,* 287–289,
    288, 289t
  sampling distribution of, 289–291,
    289t
  significant difference in, 291–296, *294*
  statistical errors with, 295–297
  transformation of, 302
  variability of, 284–287, 286t
Database(s), data missing from, 199
  in outcomes research, 196–198
  in-house development of, 197–198
  of insurance claims, 197
  survival analysis in, 199
Declaration of Helsinki, 32
Deductive reasoning, 17–18, *18*
Degrees of freedom, 285–286, 301
Delphi technique, 215
Demoralization, resentful, and internal
    validity, 88
Department of Health and Human
    Services, research-governing
    regulations of, 32
Dependent variable(s), comparisons
    across, 199–200
  component of, independent variable
    as, 70–71
  conceptual, 67
  defined, 63
  operational, 67
  types of, 63–67
Descriptive research, 138
  prospective, 140–142
  retrospective, 138–140
Descriptive theory, 16

Developmental research, 141
Deviation score, 226, 285
Diagnostic tests, *180,* 180–184, *181,*
    182, 183
Dichotomous variable, 225
Diffusion of treatment, and internal
    validity, 87–88
Digitizing, cinematographic, 254
Disclosure, in informed consent, 31
Discrete variable, 225
Dissertation Abstracts, 387–388
Dissertations, 387–388
Distance of numbers, 222
Distribution(s), chi-square, 301, *301,*
    302
  chi-square test of association,
    309–310
  chi-square test of goodness of fit, 315
  F, 301, *301,* 302
  normal, *287,* 287–289, *288*
    percentages of, *287,* 287–289, *288*
    random selection from population
      of, 302
    standard, 287
  sampling, 289–291, 289t
  t, 301, *301,* 302
Document delivery service, 392
Documents, written, 164
Double-blind study, 75
Dummy coding, 367
Dynamometry, hand, 259
  hand-held, 258, *258*
  isokinetic, 259–260

E
Economic risks, 36
Effect size, 199–200, *201,* 345
Effectiveness, defined, 190–191
Efficacy, defined, 190
Eigenvalue, 373–374
Electrical activity, of muscle, 260, *260*
Electrogoniometer, 263
Electromyography (EMG), 254–255, 260,
    260, 261
Empiricism, 51
Epidemiological research, 140
  nonexperimental, *184,* 184–187
Epidemiology, 170–187, 171b
  defined, 140, 170
Error(s), sampling, 322
  statistical, *295,* 295–297, *296*
  systematic, 234
Error rate problems, 298–299
Ethics, concerns about, as barrier to
    research, 11
  explicit attention to, 35
  informed consent and, 31–32, 75
  moral principles of action and, 29–31
  of case-control studies, 186
  of research problem, 47
    and control of interaction between
      treatments, 90

Ethics *(Continued)*
  practice–research boundaries and,
    28–29
  research codes of, 32–35, 33b
  research problems related to,
    qualitative designs with, 163
  single-system designs and, 132
  research risks related to, 35–36
Ethnographic design, 157–158
Evaluation research, 140
Ex post facto research, 144–145
Exclusion characteristics, 97
Experimental design(s), multiple factor,
    118–123, *119, 120, 121, 122, 123*
  single-factor, 115–118
  true, *versus* quasiexperimental,
    69–70
  with surveys, 205
Experimental research, 69–71. See also
    Research.
  controlled manipulation with, 71
  design of. See *Research design(s).*
  group. See *Quantitative paradigm(s).*
  internal validity in, 78
  purposes of, 67–68
Experimenter expectancy, 89–90
Explanatory theory(ies), 18, *18*
External validity, 77–78, 91
  group designs for, 126
  selection and, 91–92
  setting and, 92–93
  threats to, 401–402
  time and, 93
Extraneous variables, 72–74

F
Facet(s), 231–232
Factor, 63
Factor analysis, in relationships,
    372–375, 373t, 374t, 375t
  literature examples of, 375
  steps in, 373–375, 373t, 374t, 375t
Factorial design, 119
  versus nested designs, *119,* 119–122,
    120, 121, 122
Familiarization, equipment, 83
Fastidious design, 72–73
F distribution, 301, *301,* 302
FEV (forced expiratory volume),
    measurement of, 267
Field studies, 149
FIM (Functional Independence
    Measure), 253
Financial resources, 10, 12, 47
Fisher's exact test, 315
Fitness, measurement of, 266, *266*
Floor effect, 87
Focus on Therapeutic Outcomes
    (FOTO) database, 194
Force platform, 255
Forced expiratory volume (FEV),
    measurement of, 267

FOTO (Focus on Therapeutic Outcomes) database, 194
Foundation funding, 424–425
Framework(s), conceptual, 17
  for research problem, *44*, 44–45, *45*
  for outcomes research, 191–193, *192*
    issues and refinements of, 192–193
  functional, for physical therapy, 20–22, *21*
  measurement of, 230–231
Frequency distribution, 225, 225t, *226*, 278–283, 281t, 282t, 283t
  histogram, 281, *283*
  stem-and-leaf plot, 283, 283t
  with percentages, 278–281, 281t, 282t
  grouped, 281, 282t
Friedman's analysis, of variance, 323
FSQ (Functional Status Questionnaire), 195
F statistic, with one-way ANOVA, 310–313
  with repeated measures ANOVA, 321–322
Functional Independence Measure (FIM), 253
Functional Reach test, 256
Functional Status Questionnaire (FSQ), 195
Funding, 420–426
  budget for, 420–423, 423t
  corporate, 423–424
  foundation, 424–425
  government, 425–426, 425t
  institutional, 423
  lack of, 10

G

Gait, biomechanical analysis of, 254–255, *255*
GCS (Glasgow Coma Scale), 252
Generalizability theory, 53, 231–232
Generalizing, randomness, 126
  in single-system designs, 132
  sample-to-population, 126
Get-up and Go test, 257
Girth, 250, *251*
Givens, 43
Glasgow Coma Scale (GCS), 252
Gold standard, 143, 180
Goniometer, electro-, 263
  gravity-referenced, 263, *263*
  universal, 262–263
Government funding, 425–426, 425t
Grand mean, 310–311
Grand theory, 19–22, *20*, *21*
Grateful Med, Internet, 384
Grounded theory design, 159

H

Hand dynamometers, 259
Hand-held dynamometers, 258, *258*
Health-related quality of life (HRQL), 194–195

Heart rate, measurement of, 265
Height, 250
Heuristic research, 142
Hislop's model, of pathokinesiology, 20–21, *21*
Histogram, 281, *283*
Historical cohort study, 187
Historical research, 140
Homoscedasticity, *351*, 351–352
Howevers, 43
HRQL (health-related quality of life), 194–195
Human instruments, 83
Human participant. See *Subject(s)*.
Hypothesis, 17
  case reports to develop, 151
  directional, 307
  nondirectional, 307
  null, 291–292
  research, defined, 46
  testing of, confidence intervals for, 341–344

I

IADL (instrumental activities of daily living), 252, 253
ICCs (intraclass correlation coefficients), 350, 350t, 364, 364t, 365t
Idiographic research, 55, 154
If–then statements, 17–18, *18*
Incidence, 174–175
  versus prevalence, 175
Inclinometer, 263, *263*
Inclusion characteristics, 97
Independent *t* test, 306–308, 306t
Independent variable(s), as component of dependent variable, 70–71
  between-group, 64
  defined, 63
  implementation of, 71–72
  in single-system paradigm, 127
  interaction between, 326
  levels and types of, 63–67, 63t, *64*, *66*
  nonmanipulated, categories of 70–71
  within-group, 65
Index Medicus, 384
Inferential statistics, 291
Informants, 160. See also *Subject(s)*.
Informed consent, 31–32, 32–33, 33b, 75, 419–420, 420t, *421–422*
Inpatient recruitment, 426–427
Institution funding, 423
Institutional review board (IRB), 34–35, 418–419
Instrument, accuracy of, 246
  familiarization with, 83
  reliability of, 232–233
Instrumental activities of daily living (IADL), 252, 253
Instrumentation effects, and internal validity, 83
  assignment and, 86–87
Insurance claims databases, 197

Integrity in Physical Therapy Research, 32
Integument, measurement of, 257
Interaction between treatments, 90
Interaction designs, 131
Interlibrary loan, 391
Internal consistency, 232
Internal validity, defined, 78
  threat(s) to, assignment to groups as, 85, 96
    compensatory equalization of treatments as, 88
    compensatory rivalry as, 85
    diffusion or imitation of treatments as, 87–88
    evaluation of, 401
    history as, 78–80, *79*
    instrumentation as, 83
    interactions between, 86–87
    maturation as, 80–82, *81–82*
    mortality as, 85–86
    resentful demoralization as, 88
    sampling methods as, 95–96
    single-system designs as, 132
    statistical regression to mean as, 83–85, *84*
    testing as, 82–83
International Classification of Impairments, Disabilities, and Handicaps, 191, *192*
  issues with and refinements to, 192–193
Interrater reliability, 233
Interval scales, 224
Interview(s), closed-format items in, 206–207
  implementation of, 216–217
  in qualitative paradigm, 161–162
  personal, data collected from, 207–208, 208t
  prospect motivation for, 216
  prospective descriptive research and, 141–142
  prospective subjects for, 215–216
  survey research by, 215–217
  telephone, data collected from, 207–208, 208t
  location for, 216–217
Intraclass correlation coefficients (ICCs), 350, 350t, 364, 364t, 365t
Intrarater reliability, 233
Intrasubject reliability, 232
IRB (institutional review board), 34–35, 418–419

J

Joint motions, extrinsic, 262–264, *263*, *264*
  intrinsic, 264
  linear, 263
Joint position, 264–265

Journal article(s), citation of, 388–389, 389t
  components of, 439
  elements of, 395, 396t
  evaluation of single study of, 395–403
  evaluation questions for, 455–458
  preparation guidelines for, 459–463
  review, evaluation of, 403–405
    guidelines for writing, 395, 397t
Journal literature searching, item retrieval in, 391–392
  multiple-journal reviews for, 391
  scanning in, focused database, 391
    multiple-journal, 390–391
    single-journal, 390
  using multiple-journal databases, 383–387, *384,* 385t, 386t, 387t
  using single-journal indexes, 382–383
Journal types, 437

K

Kaplan-Meier analysis, 341
Kappa coefficient, 350–351, 350t, 365–367, 366t
Kendall's tau, 350, 350t
Keyword searches, 381
Kinematics, 254
Kinetics, 254–255
Knowledge-knowledge conflict, 43
Knowledge void, 43–44
Kruskal-Wallis test, 314

L

Latin square technique, 74, *74*
Lay public recruitment, 427–428
Level, with celeration line analysis, *338,* 338–339
Library holdings, catalogue of, 380–382, 382t
  using interlibrary loan, 382
Likelihood ratios, 180
Likert-type survey items, 207
Linear regression, 356–358, *357*
Literature, correlation coefficient examples in, 356
  factor analysis examples in, 375
  logistic regression examples in, 371–372
  manuscript sample in, 465–478
  multiple regression examples in, 370
  obtaining, 391–392
  preparation guidelines in, 459–463
  types of information in, 380
Literature review, conceptual, 405–407, 407t–408t
  evaluation questions for, 455–458
  of review articles, 403–405
  of single studies, 395–403
Literature search, catalogue of library holdings for, 380–382, 382t
  focused, 380–389, 382t, 383t, *384,* 385t, 386t, 387t, 389t
  on-going, 389–391

Literature search *(Continued)*
  relationships among tools for, 389, *390*
  using dissertation and theses databases, 387–388
  using multiple-journal databases, 383–387, *384, 385,* 386t, 387t
  using related record searching, 389
  using single article citation, 380–381, 389t
  using single-journal indexes, 382–383, 383t
Locomotion, biomechanical analysis of, 254–255, *255*
Logical positivism, 50
Logistic regression, 370–372, *371*
Longitudinal study design, 138
Lysholm Knee Rating Scale, 195

M

Macroethnography, 157
Magazines, 436–437
Main effects, 120
Manipulation, as research design component, *67,* 69–71
  controlled, interpretation based on, *71*
  in qualitative paradigm, 57–58
  in quantitative paradigm, 53–54
  in single-system paradigm, 59
  of independent variables, *69–71*
  retrospective, *70*
Mann-Whitney rank sum test, 308–309, 308t
MANOVA (multivariate analysis of variance), 332–333, 333t
Mantel log-rank test, 341
Manuscript, components of, 439
  sample, 465–478
Matched assignment, 107t, 108
Maturation effects, and internal validity, 80–82, *81–82*
  assignment and, 86–87
McGill Pain Questionnaire, 262
McNemar Test, 318–319, 320t
Mean, 226, 283
  grand, 310–311
Mean designs, 243–244
Measurement(s), analysis of relationships as, 142–143
  biophysiological, 232
  control of techniques for, 74
  criterion-referenced, 231
  definitions of, 222
  levels of, in parametric testing, 303
  linear, of joint movements, 263–264
  norm-referenced, 230–231
  observational, 232–233
  of anthropometric characteristics, 249–251
  of arousal, mentation, and cognition, 251–252

Measurement(s) *(Continued)*
  of autonomic functions, 267
  of balance, 256–257
  of basic activities of daily living, 252, 253
  of cardiovascular functions, 265–266
  of community and work integration, 252–254
  of condition-specific functions, 253–254
  of gait, locomotion, and balance, 254–257, *255*
  of home management functionality, 252–254
  of independent variable treated as dependent variable, 70–71
  of instrumental activities of daily living, 252, 253
  of integumentary integrity, 257
  of joint integrity and mobility, 262–265
  of muscle performance, 257–261
  of neuromotor development, 261
  of nonmanipulated variable, 70
  of pain, 261–262
  of pulmonary functions, 266–267
  of self-care functionality, 252–254
  of sensory integration, 261
  of sensory integrity, 265
  of task-specific functions, 253
  of ventilation, respiration, circulation, aerobic capacity, and endurance, 265–267
  reliability of, 231–235
  repeated, 73
    problems with, 126
  scales of, 222–225, *223*
    determination of, 224–225
  self-report, 232
  standard error of, 230, 235, 362
  standardization levels for, 240–242
  validity of, 143, 235–237, 244–246
  variability in, sources of, 240, 240t
  with qualitative paradigm, 53
  with quantitative paradigm, 53
  with single-system paradigm, 59
Measurement frameworks, 230–231
Measurement theory, 53, 225–230, 225t, *226,* 227t, *228, 229,* 230t
  classical, 231–232
  generalizability, 53, 231–232
Measurement tools, 248–267
  for outcomes research, 193–196
    condition-specific, 195
    design issues, 196–200, *200, 201*
    health-related quality of life, 194–195
    quality of life, 194
    satisfaction, 195–196
Median, 284, 284t
Medical Literature and Retrieval System (MEDLARS), 384

Medical Outcomes Study (MOS), 194
Medical records, 196–197
MEDLARS (Medical Literature and Retrieval System), 384
MEDLINE, 384–385, 385t, 387t
Member checking, 167
Mentation, 251–252
MeSH (National Library of Medicine Medical Subject Headings), 356, 381, 384
Meta-analysis, 145
Method, paradigm *versus*, 50
Methodological research, 141, 239–246
Microethnography, 157
Middle-range theory(ies), 22, 22–25, 23, 24, 25t
Mini-Mental State Examination (MMSE), 252
Mixed experimental designs, 122–123, 123
MMSE (Mini-Mental State Examination), 252
Mode, 284, 284t
Model, conceptual, 17
    of pathokinesiology, Hislop's, 20–21, 21
Mortality, and internal validity, 85–86
MOS (Medical Outcomes Study), 194
Movement science, 8
Multiple constructed realities, 54–55, 55b, 154
Multiple correlation, 350t, 351
Multiple-factor experimental research, 118–119
    between-subjects, 116, 122–123, 123
    completely randomized *versus* randomized-block, 122
    factorial *versus* nested, 119, 119–122, 120, 121, 122
    mixed design, 122–123, 123
    questions leading to, 119
    within-subjects, 118, 122–123, 123
Multiple publication, 438–439
Multiple regression, equation interpretation in, 368–370, 369
    for analysis of relationships, 367–370, 369
    literature examples of, 370
    variable entry in, 367–368
Multiple-baseline designs, 129, 130
Multiple-choice survey items, 207
Multivariate analysis of variance (MANOVA), 332–333, 333t
Multivariate statistics, 200
Muscle(s), cable tensiometers to evaluate, 258–259
    dynamometer testing of, hand, 259
    hand-held, 258, 258
    isokinetic, 259–260
    electrical activity of, 260, 261
    electrical stimulation to strengthen, middle range theory and, 22, 22–23, 23

Muscle(s) (*Continued*)
    force generating capacity of, 257–260, 258, 259
        electromyographic signal and, 260
    manual testing of, 257–258
    measures of performance of, 257–260, 258, 259
    microscopic composition of, 261
    strain gauges to evaluate, 258–259
    weights to evaluate, 258
Muscle tone, measurement of, 260–261

N

Nagi formulation, 192–193
National Commission for Protection of Human Subjects of Biomedical and Behavioral Research, Belmont report of, 28–29
National Library of Medicine Medical Subject Headings (MeSH), 356, 381, 384
Naturalistic paradigm, 54
Negative predictive value, 183, 183–184
Nested design, 121
    versus factorial design, 119, 119–122, 120, 121, 122
Neuromotor development, 261
Newsletters, 436
Nominal scales, 222
Nomothetic research, 52
Nonconcurrent cohort study, 187
Nondirectional hypothesis, 307
Nonequivalent control-group design, 117–118
Nonexperimental research, 69–71, 137–138, 138, 139t
    analysis of differences as, 144–146
    analysis of relationships as, 142–144
    descriptive, 138–142
    internal validity in, 78
    to determine effectiveness, 191
    with surveys, 205
Nonmaleficence, principle of, 29–30, 34
Nonmethodological studies, reliability in, 244
Nonparametric tests, 302–304
Nonprobability sampling, 97, 103
    convenience, 103–104, 104
    purposive, 104–105
    snowball, 104, 160
Nonproportional stratified sampling, 100, 101t
Nonrefereed journals, 437
Norm-referenced measure, 230–231
Normal curve, 227–228, 228, 229, 287, 287, 288
    areas in one tail of, 453t
Normal distribution(s). See *Distribution(s), normal.*
Normative research, 143–144
Null hypothesis, 46, 291–292

Number, 222
Numeral, 222
Nuremberg Code, 32

O

Objective observer, 163
Observation, in qualitative design, 162–163
    measurement reliability with, 232–233
    prospective descriptive research and, 141
Observer-as-participant models, 163
OCLC (Online Computer Library Center), 382
Odds, *versus* proportions, 179–180
Odds ratio, 179–180
Omnibus F test, 312
Online Computer Library Center (OCLC), 382
Open-format survey items, 206
Operational definition, 236
Operational dependent variable, 67
Opportunistic research, 162–163
Optimization designs, 243–244
Order of numbers, 222
Ordinal scales, 222–224, 223
Origin of numbers, 222
Oswestry Low Back Pain Disability Index, 195
Outcomes research, 144
    analysis issues in, 198–200
    case mix adjustments in, 198–199
    comparisons across scales in, 199–200, 201
    design issues in, 196–200, 200, 201
    frameworks for, 191–193, 192
    measurement tools for, 193–196
    missing data in, 199
    multivariate statistics in, 200
    overview of, 189–190
    purpose of, 190–191
    survival analysis in, 199, 200
    using databases for, 196–198
Outliers, 434
Outpatient recruitment, 427
Oximeter, noninvasive, 267
Oxygen saturation, measurement of, 267

P

Pain, measurement of, 261–262
Paired-*t* test, 317–318
Paradigm(s), competing, 50
    method *versus*, 50
    qualitative, 49–50, 54–58, 55b
    quantitative, 49–50, 50–54, 51t, 52t
    relationships among, 59–60
    single-system, 49–50, 58–59
    terminology for, 50, 50t
Parameter, 287
Parametric tests, 302–304. See also specific tests, e.g., *Analysis of variance (ANOVA).*

Participant-as-observer models, 162–163
Participant–observers, 157
Paternalism, 31
Pathokinesiology, 8
  Hislop's conceptual model of, 20–21, *21*
Patient. See *Subject(s)*.
Pearson Product Moment Correlation, 348–349, 348t
  with extensions, 361–364, 361t, *362, 363*
Peer review process, 437–438
Peer-reviewed journals, 437
Pendulum test, 261
Performance Oriented Mobility Assessment, 256–257
Phenomenologic design, 158
Phi coefficient, 350, 350t
Physical Performance Test (PPT), 253
Physical risks, 35–36
Physical therapist, patient interaction with, ethics of, 28–29
  in research environment, 57
Pilot study, 430
Placebo, 75
Platform presentations, 441–443, *443*
  sample, 479–487
Point-biserial correlation, 350, 350t
Policy research, 140
Policy–action conflict, 43
Population(s), 96–97, 96t
  defined, 96
  normally distributed, 302
  variance of, 285
Positive predictive value, *183,* 183–184
Positivism, 50
Poster presentations, 443–444, *444*
Posttest-only control-group design, 83, 116–117
Posturography, 256
Power, statistical. See *Statistical power.*
PPT (Physical Performance Test), 253
Practice, theory, and research, *25,* 25–26
  case report contributions to, *149,* 149–150, *150*
Practice guidelines, 152
Pragmatic design, 72–73
Predictive theory, 17
Predictive validity, 237, 246
Predictive value, 182–184, *183*
Presentation of research, 441–444, *443, 444*
Pretest-posttest control-group design, 116
Prevalence, 173–174
  versus incidence, 175
Primary sources, 380
Probability determinants, 293–295
Probability sampling, 97
  cluster, 101–103, *102*
  simple random, 97–98, 99t

Probability sampling *(Continued)*
  stratified, 100, 101t
  systematic, 98–100, 100t
p value(s), determinants of, 341–342
Problem-solving, case reports in, 151
Profession, characteristics of, 7, 7t
Proportional hazards model, 341
Proportional stratified sampling, 100, 101t
Proportions, 172, 172t
  versus odds, 178–179
Proposal, data analysis for, 433–435
  data collection for, 426t, 428–432, *431–432*
  elements of, 415–418, 415t, 417t
  funding for, 420–426
  general guidelines for, 414–415
  human participant protection in, 418–420, 420t, *421–422*
  obtaining participants for, 426–428
  preparation of, 414–418, 415t, 417t
Proposition, 17
Prospective study design, analysis of differences using, 145–146
  analysis of relationships using, 143–144
  case reports as, 148–149
  defined, 68, 184–185
  descriptive, 140–142
  single-system paradigm and, 127
Proxy consent, 32
Psychological risks, 36
Publication(s), 11
  acknowledgments in, 438
  authorship of, 438
  components of, 439
  integrity of, 35
  multiple, 438–439
  peer review process for, 437–438
  style issues with, 439, 440t, 441t
  titles of, variable identification from, 63
  types of, 436–437
PubMed, 384
Pulmonary functions, measurement of, 266–267
Purposive sampling, 104–105

Q
Q-sort survey items, 207
Qualitative paradigm, 49–50, 51t, 52t, 54–58, 55b
  assumptions of, 51t, 54–56, 55b, 154–155
  data analysis with, 164–168, 166b, *168*
  data collection with, 161–164
  data meaning generation in, 165–167
  methods used with, 159–168
  other paradigms and, 59–60
  sampling methods with, 160–161
Quality of life, health-related, 194–195

Quantitative, defined, 50
Quantitative paradigm(s), 49–50, 50–54, 51t, 52t
  assumptions of, 51–52, 51t
  designs for, 155–159, 156t
  methodological issues with, 52–54, 52t
  other paradigms and, 59–60
  problems with, 125–126
Quasiexperimental research, *versus* true experimental research, 69–70
Quebec Task Force on Spinal Disorders report, 4–5, *5*
Questionnaire(s), closed-format items in, 206–207
  drafting of, 209–210, *211*
  expert review of, 210
  final revision of, 212
  first revision of, 210
  mailed, 208
    development of, 209–212
    implementation details in, 208–215
    motivating prospects to respond to, 212
    researcher-developed *versus* existing, 209
    sampling frame for, 209
    survey data collected by, 207–208, 208t
  open-format items in, 206
  pilot test for, 211–212
  prospective descriptive research and, 142

R
Random assignment to groups, 69, 73–74, 78, 122
  by block, 106t, 107–108
    completely randomized *versus,* 122
  consecutive, 108
  control of assignment threats with, 85, 87
  deciding on method of, 108–109
  individual, 105–106, 106t
  matched, 107t, 108
  systematic, 107t, 108
  testing effect minimization with, 82–83
Random numbers table, 448t–451t
  use of, 98
Random sampling, from a normally distributed population, 302
  simple, 97–98, 99t
Random start with rotation, 73–74
Randomization. See *Random assignment to groups.*
Randomized clinical trial. See *Randomized controlled trial (RTC).*
Randomized controlled trial (RTC), defined, 69, 116
  N of 1, 131
  to determine efficacy, 190

Randomized design, *versus* randomized-block designs, 122
Range, 285
Range of motion, joint integrity and mobility and, 262–265
Range-of-motion measurements, 260–261
Ranking, 223
Rates, 172–173, 172t
  adjusted, *176,* 176–177, 177t
  crude, 176, *176*
  specific, 176, *176*
Ratio scales, 224
Ratios, 172, 172t
Real-number system, 222
Receiver-operator curves, 181–182, *182*
Records, 164
  medical, 196–197
Refereed journals, 437
Regression. See *Statistical regression to mean;* specific regression topic, e.g., *Logistic regression.*
Rejection region, 296
Relative reliability, 234
Relative risk, 177–180, *178, 179*
Reliability, absolute, 234–235, 360, 361
  analysis of, 360–367, 361t, *362, 363,* 364t, 365t, 366t
  components of, 232–233
    standardization levels for, 240–242
    variability due to, 240, 240t
  defined, 231
  highly standardized approach to, 241–242
  in nonmethodological studies, 244
  instrument, 232–233
  interrater, 233
  intrarater, 233
  intrasubject, 233
  nonstandardized approach to, 241
  optimization designs for, 243–244
  parallel-form, 232
  partially standardized approach to, 242
  quantification of, 233–235
  range of scores to determine, 243
  relative, 234, 360, 361
    Pearson product moment correlation to measure, 361–364, 361t, *362, 363*
  subject selection and, 242–243
  test-retest, 232
  theories of, 231–232
Repeated measures design, 73, 118
Repeated treatment design, 73, 118
  and maturation effects, 82
Reprints, 392
Research. See also *Experimental research.*
  as body of knowledge, 7–8, 7t
  as challenge to status quo, 4–6, *5*
  as creative endeavor, 6

Research *(Continued)*
  as systematic endeavor, 7
  barrier(s) to, 9–11, *10*
  Belmont definition of, 28–29
  contributions to, acknowledgment of, 438
  definitions of, 4–7
  ethics of, 27
    codes for, 32–35, 33b
    informed consent and, 31–32
    moral principles of action in, 29–31
    practice–research boundaries and, 28–29
  financial support of, 12
  history of, 11–13
  idiographic, 55
  nomothetic, 52
  practice, theory, and, *25,* 25–26
  purposes of, 67–68
    data collection timing and, 68–69
  reasons for, 7–9
  risks of, 35–36
  theory and. See *Theory(ies).*
  to establish physical therapy efficacy, 8
  to improve patient care, 8–9
Research article. See *Journal article(s).*
Research design(s), control of, 71–76, *74*
  dimensions of, *67,* 67–71
  experimental. See *Experimental research.*
  for qualitative paradigms, 155–159, 156t
  group, multiple-factor, 118–123, *119, 120, 121, 122, 123*
    problems with, 125–126
    single-factor, 115–118
  nonexperimental. See *Nonexperimental research.*
  power analysis during, 344–345
  prospective, 68, 184–185
  reliability, 239–244, 240t
  retrospective, 68
  single system, 127–131, *130, 131*
    analysis of, *336,* 336–340, *337, 338, 340*
    characteristics of, 126–127
    limitations of, 132
  validity of, 244–246
  variable identification in, 63–67, 63t, *64, 66*
Research hypothesis. See *Hypothesis.*
Research problem. See also *Research question; Research topic.*
  development of, 41–46, *42, 44*
  ethicalness of, 47
  evaluation of, 46–48
  feasibility of, 46–47
  identification and selection of, 43–44
  interest of, 47
  novelty of, 47

Research problem *(Continued)*
  relevance of, 47–48
  theoretical framework for, *44,* 44–45, *45*
  versus research question, 42
Research proposal. See *Proposal.*
Research question. See also *Research problem; Research topic.*
  identification and selection of, 46
  versus research problem, 42
Research topic, 44. See also *Research problem; Research question.*
  identification and selection of, 42–43
Research validity, 77–78, 235
Researcher, as human instrument, 83
  blinding of, 75
  expectancies of, construct validity and, 89–90
  observational role of, 162–163
  questionnaire development by, 209–212
Resentful demoralization, and internal validity, 88
Residual, 321, 357
Restrictiveness of theories, 15–19, 16t, *18*
Retrospective study design, analysis of differences with, 144–145
  analysis of relationships with, 143
  case reports as, 148
  defined, 68, 185
  descriptive, 138–140
  manipulation and, 70
Review article(s), evaluation of, 403–405
  guidelines for writing, 395, 397t
Risk(s), ethical handling of, 35–36
Risk ratio, 178–179
Rivalry, compensatory, and internal validity, 88
Robust statistical tests, 302
Romberg test, 256
Rotation, random start with, 73–74
Roy Adaptation Model, 20, *20*
RTC (randomized controlled trial), 69, 116
  N of 1, 131
  to determine efficacy, 190

S

Sample(s), defined, 96
  dependent, 303–304
  independent, 303–304
  of convenience, 103–104, *104*
  size of, determining, 109–110, 109t, *110*
    statistical power and, 297, 345
    statistical probabilities and, 294, *294*
Sample variance, 285
Sample-to-population generalizability, 126, 132

Sampling, defined, 95, 96
for qualitative research, 160–161
nonprobability, 97, 103–105, *104,* 160
probability, 97–103, 99t, 100t, 101t, *102*
significance of, 95–96
with replacement, 98
without replacement, 97
Sampling distribution, 289–291, 289t
confidence intervals of, 290–291
Sampling error, 97
Sampling frame, 97
for mailed questionnaires, 209
Scales, of measurement, 222–225, *223*
Science Citation Index, 389, 389t
Scree method, 373–374
Screening tests, *180,* 180–184, *181, 182, 183*
Secondary analysis, 139
Secondary sources, 380
SEE (standard error of estimate), 357–358, *358*
Segmental length, 250
Selection, and external validity, 91–92
in qualitative paradigm, 56
in quantitative paradigm, 53
in single-system paradigm, 59
Self-reported information, 232
SEM (standard error of mean), 289–291, 289t, 342
Semantic differential survey items, 207
Semistructured interview, 161
Sensitivity, 180–181, *181*
likelihood ratios calculated from, 182
receiver-operator curves for, 181–182, *182*
Sensory integration, 261
Sensory integrity, 265
Sensory Organization Test, 256
Setting, and external validity, 92–93
extraneous variables in, 72
Short Form-12 (SF-12), 194
Short Form-36 (SF-36), 194
Sickness Impact Profile (SIP), 194–195
Significant difference, 291–295
Single-blind study, 75
Single-factor experimental designs, 115–116
nonequivalent control-group design for, 117–118
posttest-only control-group design for, 116–117
pretest-posttest control-group design for, 116
repeated measures for, 118
repeated treatment designs for, 118
single-group pretest-posttest design for, 117
time series design for, 118
Single-group studies, 80
pretest-posttest design for, 117
Single-subject research, 58

Single-system designs, 126–127
A-B, 127–128
A-B-A, 128–129
alternating treatment, 129–131, *131*
analysis of, *336,* 336–340, *337, 338, 340*
group designs *versus,* 125–126
interaction, 131
limitations of, 132
multiple-baseline, 129, *130*
two standard deviation band analysis, 339–340, *340*
withdrawal, 128–129
Single-system paradigm, 49–50, 58–59, 126–127
assumptions of, 58
methodological issues with, 59
other paradigms and, 59–60
SIP (Sickness Impact Profile), 194–195
Skewed plot, 306
Slides, 442–443, *443*
Slope, with celeration line analysis, *338,* 338–339
Snowball sampling, 104, 160
Social risks, 36
Solomon four-group design, 91
Spasticity, measurement of, 260–261
Spearman's rho, 350, 350t
Specific rates, 176, *176*
Specificity, 180–181, *181*
Spirometer, 267
Split-plot design, 122–123, *123*
SSB (between-group sum of squares), 311t, 312
SST (total sum of squares), 311, 311t
SSW (within-group sum of squares), 311t, 312
Standard deviation, 227, 286–287
band analysis, two, 339–340, *340*
Standard error of measurement, 230, 235
extended Pearson reliability analysis with, 362
Standard error of estimate (SEE), 357–358, *358*
Standard error of mean (SEM), 289–291, 289t, 342
Standard normal distribution(s), 287
Standardization designs, 243
Statistical analysis, multivariate results and, 200
single-system designs and, 132
Statistical conclusion validity, threats to, 297–299
evaluation of, 401
Statistical power, 297
analysis of, 344–345
low, and statistical conclusion validity, 298
of group designs, 125–126
Statistical regression to mean, and internal validity, 83–85, *84*
extended Pearson reliability analysis with, 362, *362, 363*

Statistics, defined, 287
inferential, 291
Stem-and-leaf plot, 283, 283t
Strain gauges, 258–259
Stratified sampling, 100–101, 101t
Structured interview, 161
Style guidelines, 439, 440t, 441t
Subject(s), blinding of, 75
codes of ethics for, 32–35, 33b
extraneous variables related to, 72–74, *74*
incomplete information given to, 74–75
informants as, 160
informed consent and, 31–32
interviewed, access to, 215–216
moral principles of action and, 29–30
obtaining, 426–428, 426t
practice–research boundaries with, 28–29
protection of, 418–420, 420t, *421–422,* 429
risks involving, 35–36
satisfaction of, 195–196
selection and assignment of, 72
in reliability studies, 242–243
qualitative, 56–57
Subject heading searches, 381–382
Sum of squares, between-group, 311t, 312
total, 311, 311t
within-group, 311t, 312
Survey instruments, cover letters for, 212, *213, 214*
researcher-developed *versus* existing, 209
Survey research, 204
data collection methods in, 207–208, 208t
defined, 204, 205
information types in, 206
item types in, 206–207
scope of, 204–206
self-report measurement for, 232
using interviews, 215–217
using mailed questionnaires, 208–215
Survival analysis, 199, 340–341
Survival curves, 340–341
Systematic assignment, 107t, 108
Systematic sampling, 98–100, 100t

T

Target population, 96
t distribution, 301, *301, 302*
Tensiometer, cable, 258–259
Tentativeness, of theories, 18–19
Test development, 372
Testability, of theories, 19
theory of, use of case reports to carry out, 152
Testing effects, and construct validity, 91
and internal validity, 82–83

Test–retest reliability, 232
Theory(ies), ad hoc, 16
  categorical, 16
  definitions of, 15–19, 16t, *18*
  descriptive, 16
  explanatory, 18, *18*
  factor analysis in, 372
  grand, 19–22, *20, 21*
  grounded, 159
  middle-range, *22,* 22–25, *23, 24,* 25t
  of measurement, 225–230, 225t, *226,* 227t, *228, 229,* 230t
  predictive, 17
  qualitative studies and, 58
  quantitative method selection and, 52–53
  research, practice, and, *25,* 25–26
    contributions of case reports to, *149,* 149–150, *150*
  research question development and, 42, 46
  scope of, 19–25, *20, 21, 22, 23, 24,* 25t
  testing of, 372
  with qualitative method selection, 56
  with single-system paradigm, 59
Therefores, 43
Theses, 387–388
Time, and external validity, 93
  as barrier to research, 10–11
Time series design, 118
Trend, with celeration line analysis, *338,* 338–339
Triangulation, 167, 233
Trustworthiness, 395
t test, independent, 306–308, 306t
  paired-, 317–318
    extended Pearson reliability analysis with, 361–362
Tuskegee Syphilis Study, 33b
Twister cables, 36
Two standard deviation band analysis, 339–340, *340*
Type I error, *295,* 295–297, *296*
Type II error, *295,* 295–297, *296,* 345

U

University Microfilms International, 388
Unstructured interview, 161–162
Utility, 395
  of study, evaluation of, 402–403, 405
  principle of, 30

V

Validity, analysis of relationships for, 77–78, 143
  concurrent, 237, 246
  construct, 77, 88–89, 235–236, 244–245
    threats to, 89–91
      evaluation of, 400–401
  content, 236, 245–246
  criterion, 236–237, 246
  cumulative relationships and, 93
  external, threats to, 77–78, 91–93, 126
    evaluation of, 401–402
  internal, 78
    threats to, 78–86, *79, 81–82, 84*
      evaluation of, 401
  measurement of, 235–237
  predictive, 237, 246
  reciprocal relationships and, 93–94
  research, 77–78, 235
  sampling and assignment for, 95–96
  statistical conclusion, 297–299
    threats to, 78, 297–299
      evaluation of, 401
  threats to, 400–402
Variability, 284–287, 286t
  between-group, 310
  coefficient of determination for, 354
  sources of, 240, 240t
  standardization levels for, 240–242
  within-group, 293–294, *294,* 297, 310
Variable(s), 62
  analysis of relationships among, 142–144
  confounding, 72
  continuous, 225
  defined, 63
  dependent. See *Dependent variable(s).*
  dichotomous, 225
  discrete, *225*
  extraneous, *72–74, 74*
  homoscedasticity of, *351,* 351–352
  identification of, 63–67, 63t, *64, 66*
  independent. See *Independent variable(s).*
  linear relationship of, 351, *351*
  manipulation of, 69–71
  nonlinear relationship of, 351, *351*
  variability of, 352–353, *353*
  variance shared by, 348t, 354

Variance, 226–227, 227t, 285–286
  Friedman's analysis of, 323
  homogeneity of, 303
  population, 285
  sample, 285
VAS (visual analogue scale), 262
Videotaping, 254
Vignette, 207
Visual analogue scale (VAS), 262
Volume, 251
Voluntariness, in informed consent, 31–32

W

Weight, 250
Weights, to test muscle performance, 258
Wilcoxon rank sum test, 308–309, 308t, 341
Wilcoxon signed rank test, 318, 319t
Withdrawal designs, 128–129
Within-group independent variable, 65
Within-group variability, 293–294, *294,* 297
Within-subject designs, 118, 122–123, *123*
  in mixed-design two-way ANOVA, 329–332, 330t, *331*
  in repeated measures ANOVA, 321
Within-subject factor, 330
Work plan, 417–418, 417t
World Health Organization, Declaration of Helsinki by, 32
  International Classification of Impairments, Disabilities, and Handicaps by, 191, *192*
  issues with and refinements to, 192 193
WorldCat database, 302, 307
Wound measurement, 257

Y

Yates' correction, 315

Z

z score, 227, 286t, 287